McArdle Library APH

B10188

D1341958

This book is due for return on or before the last date shown below.

CANCELLED

2 AUG 2014 CANCELLED

- 6 MAR 2015 CANCELLED

CANCELLED

2 3 OCT 2020

Don Gresswell Ltd., London, N21   Cat. No. 1208   DG 02242/71

Evidence-Based Management of Low Back Pain

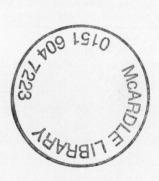

Editors

Simon Dagenais, DC, PhD
Division of Orthopaedic Surgery and Department of
Epidemiology and Community Medicine
University of Ottawa
Ottawa, Ontario, Canada
Department of Social and Preventive Medicine
University at Buffalo
Buffalo, New York, USA

Scott Haldeman, DC, MD, PhD
Department of Neurology
University of California, Irvine
Irvine, California, USA
Department of Epidemiology
University of California, Los Angeles
Los Angeles, California, USA
Southern California University of Health Sciences
Whittier, California, USA

ELSEVIER
MOSBY

3251 Riverport Lane
St. Louis Missouri 63043

EVIDENCE-BASED MANAGEMENT OF LOW BACK PAIN   ISBN: 978-0-323-07293-9
© 2012 by Mosby, Inc., an affiliate of Elsevier Inc.

All rights reserved. No part of this publication may be reproduced or transmitted in any form or by any means, electronic or mechanical, including photocopy, recording, or any information storage and retrieval system, without permission in writing from the publisher. Details on how to seek permission, further information about the Publisher's permissions policies and our arrangements with organizations such as the Copyright Clearance Center and the Copyright Licensing Agency, can be found at our website: www.elsevier.com/permissions.

This book and the individual contributions contained in it are protected under copyright by the Publisher (other than as may be noted herein).

Notices

Knowledge and best practice in this field are constantly changing. As new research and experience broaden our understanding, changes in research methods, professional practices, or medical treatment may become necessary.

Practitioners and researchers must always rely on their own experience and knowledge in evaluating and using any information, methods, compounds, or experiments described herein. In using such information or methods they should be mindful of their own safety and the safety of others, including parties for whom they have a professional responsibility.

With respect to any drug or pharmaceutical products identified, readers are advised to check the most current information provided (i) on procedures featured or (ii) by the manufacturer of each product to be administered, to verify the recommended dose or formula, the method and duration of administration, and contraindications. It is the responsibility of practitioners, relying on their own experience and knowledge of their patients, to make diagnoses, to determine dosages and the best treatment for each individual patient, and to take all appropriate safety precautions.

To the fullest extent of the law, neither the Publisher nor the authors, contributors, or editors, assume any liability for any injury and/or damage to persons or property as a matter of products liability, negligence or otherwise, or from any use or operation of any methods, products, instructions, or ideas contained in the material herein.

ISBN: 978-0-323-07293-9

Vice President and Publisher: Linda Duncan
Senior Editor: Kellie White
Senior Developmental Editor: Jennifer Watrous
Publishing Services Manager: Julie Eddy
Project Manager: Marquita Parker
Design Direction: Margaret Reid

Printed in the United States of America

Last digit is the print number: 9 8 7 6 5 4 3 2 1

Working together to grow
libraries in developing countries

www.elsevier.com | www.bookaid.org | www.sabre.org

ELSEVIER   BOOK AID International   Sabre Foundation

Contributors

Editorial Assistant:
Erin K. Galloway, B. Eth.

Venu Akuthota, MD
Associate Professor and Vice Chair
Director, Spine Center and Pain Fellowship
Department of Physical Medicine and Rehabilitation
University of Colorado, Denver
Aurora, Colorado

Carlo Ammendolia, DC, PhD
Assistant Professor, University of Toronto
Clinician-Researcher, Mount Sinai Hospital
Associate Scientist, Institute for Work and Health
Toronto, Ontario
Canada

Paul A. Anderson, MD
Professor, Department of Orthopedic Surgery and
   Rehabilitation
University of Wisconsin
Madison, Wisconsin

Ray M. Baker, MD
Director, Swedish Spine Program
Clinical Professor of Anesthesiology (Affiliate)
University of Washington, Department of Anesthesiology
Seattle, Washington

**Nikolai Bogduk, BSc (Med), MB, BS, PhD, MD, DSc,
   FAFRM, FFPM (ANZCA), MMed, Dip Anat**
Conjoint Professor of Pain Medicine
University of Newcastle; Newcastle Bone and Joint
   Institute; Royal Newcastle Centre
Newcastle, New South Wales
Australia

Joanne Borg-Stein, MD
Assistant Professor of Physical Medicine and Rehabilitation
Harvard Medical School
Director, Sports Medicine Fellowship
Spaulding Rehabilitation Hospital
Medical Director, Newton Wellesley Hospital Spine Center
Medical Director, Spaulding-Wellesley Rehabilitation
   Center
Team Physician, Wellesley College
Boston, Massachusetts

Jeffrey S. Brault, DO
Assistant Professor, Physical Medicine and Rehabilitation
Mayo Clinic College of Medicine
Rochester, Minnesota

Gert Bronfort, DC, PhD
Professor and Vice President of Research
Northwestern Health Sciences University
Bloomington, Minnesota

Lucie Brosseau, PhD
Professor, School of Rehabilitation Sciences
Faculty of Health Sciences
University of Ottawa
Ottawa, Ontario
Canada

Jens Ivar Brox, PhD, MD
Consultant
Oslo University Hospital, Rikshospitalet
Oslo, Norway

Victor H. Chang, MD
Assistant Professor, Department of Physical Medicine and
   Rehabilitation
University of Colorado, Denver
Aurora, Colorado

Simon Dagenais, DC, PhD
Division of Orthopaedic Surgery and Department of
   Epidemiology and Community Medicine
University of Ottawa
Ottawa, Ontario
Canada
Department of Social and Preventive Medicine
University at Buffalo
Buffalo, New York

Richard Derby, MD
Medical Director
Spinal Diagnostics and Treatment Center
Daly City, California

Michael J. DePalma, MD
Medical Director
Virginia Commonwealth University Spine Center Program
Director, Interventional Spine Care Fellowship
Associate Professor
Department of Physical Medicine and Rehabilitation
Virginia Commonwealth University/Medical College of
   Virginia Hospitals
Richmond, Virginia

Angus Shane Don, FRACS, MBChB, BHB
Spinal Surgeon
Auckland City Hospital
Auckland, New Zealand

Ronald Donelson, MD, MS
President
SelfCare First, LLC
Hanover, New Hampshire

Trish Dryden, RMT, MEd
Associate Vice President, Research & Corporate Planning
Centennial College
Toronto, Ontario
Canada

Hege R. Eriksen, PhD
Professor
Department of Health Promotion and Development
University of Bergen; Uni Health
Bergen, Norway

Roni Evans, BA, DC, MS
Dean of Research and Director, Wolfe-Harris Center for
    Clinical Studies
Northwestern Health Sciences University
Bloomington, Minnesota

Andrea D. Furlan, MD, PhD
Associate Scientist
Institute for Work & Health
Assistant Professor
Department of Medicine
University of Toronto
Toronto, Ontario
Canada

Joel J. Gagnier, ND, MSc, PhD
Assistant Professor
Department of Orthopaedic Surgery
University of Michigan
Ann Arbor, Michigan

Robert J. Gatchel, PhD, ABPP
Professor and Chairman, Nancy P. & John G. Penson
    Endowed Professor of Clinical Health Psychology
Department of Psychology, College of Science
The University of Texas at Arlington
Arlington, Texas

Ralph E. Gay, MD, DC
Assistant Professor of Physical Medicine and Rehabilitation
Mayo Clinic College of Medicine
Rochester, Minnesota

Peter G. Gonzalez, MD
Assistant Professor; Director, EVMS Sports Medicine
Department of Physical Medicine and Rehabilitation
Eastern Virginia Medical School
Norfolk, Virginia

Margreth Grotle, PhD
Research Leader/Senior Researcher
Oslo University Hospital, FORMI and Diakonhjemmet
    Hospital, National Resource Center for Rehabilitation in
    Rheumatology
Oslo, Norway

Mitchell Haas, DC, MA
Associate Vice President of Research
University of Western States
Portland, Oregon

Scott Haldeman, DC, MD, PhD
Department of Neurology
University of California, Irvine
Irvine, California
Department of Epidemiology
University of California, Los Angeles
Los Angeles, California
Southern California University of Health Sciences
Whittier, California

Hamilton Hall, MD, FRCSC
Professor, Department of Surgery
University of Toronto
Toronto, Ontario
Canada

Marta Imamura, MD, PhD
Division of Physical Medicine and Rehabilitation
Department of Orthopedics and Traumatology
University of Sao Paulo School of Medicine
Sao Paulo, Brazil

Aage Indahl, Professor II, MD, PhD
Department of Research and Development
Clinic Physical Medicine and Rehabilitation
Vestfold Hospital Trust
Stavern, Norway
Department of Health Promotion and Development
University of Bergen; Uni Health
Bergen, Norway

Emma L. Irvin, BA
Director, Research Operations
Institute for Work & Health
Toronto, Ontario
Canada

Gregory Kawchuk, BSc, DC, MSc, PhD
Canada Research Chair in Spinal Function and Associate
    Professor
University of Alberta
Edmonton, Alberta
Canada

Chang-Hyung Lee, MD, PhD
Physical Medicine and Rehabilitation Specialist
Sports Medicine Subspecialist
Assistant Professor, Department of Physical Medicine and
    Rehabilitation
Pusan National University School of Medicine
Yangsan, Gyeongnam
South Korea

Jeong-Eun Lee, PT
Graduate School Student
Graduate School of Medicine, Korea University
Seoul, South Korea
Research Analyst
Spinal Diagnostics and Treatment Center
Daly City, California

Gerard A. Malanga, MD
Director, Pain Management Overlook Hospital
Summit, New Jersey
Clinical Professor, Physical Medicine and Rehabilitation
University of Medicine and Dentistry of New Jersey, New
    Jersey Medical School
Newark, New Jersey

Stephen May, MA, FCSP, Dip MDT, MSc, PhD
Senior Lecturer in Physiotherapy
Sheffield Hallam University
Sheffield, United Kingdom

John Mayer, DC, PhD
Lincoln Endowed Research Chair
College of Medicine
School of Physical Therapy and Rehabilitation Sciences
University of South Florida
Tampa, Florida

Tom G. Mayer, MD
Clinical Professor of Orthopedic Surgery
University of Texas Southwestern Medical Center
Medical Director, Productive Rehabilitation Institute of
    Dallas for Ergonomics
Dallas, Texas

Daniel Mazanec, MD
Associate Director, Center for Spine Health
Neurological Institute
Cleveland Clinic
Associate Professor of Medicine
Cleveland Clinic Lerner College of Medicine
Cleveland, Onio

Irina L. Melnik, MD
Diplomate of ABDM&R
Spinal Diagnostics and Treatment Center
Daly City, California

Vert Mooney, MD (deceased)
Formerly:
Medical Director, US Spine and Sport Foundation
Clinical Professor, Department of Orthopaedic Surgery
University of California, San Diego
San Diego, California

Stephane Poitras, PT, PhD
Assistant Professor, School of Rehabilitation Sciences
Faculty of Health Sciences
University of Ottawa
Ottawa, Ontario
Canada

Ben B. Pradhan, MD, MSE
Spine Surgeon, Director of Research
Risser Orthopedic Group
Pasadena, California

Sebastian Rodriguez-Elizalde, MD, FRCS(C)
Adult Hip and Knee Reconstruction Fellow
The Hospital for Special Surgery
New York, New York

Darren M. Roffey, PhD
Clinical Research Coordinator
Clinical Epidemiology Program, Ottawa Hospital Research
    Institute; University of Ottawa Spine Unit, Division of
    Orthopedic Surgery, The Ottawa Hospital
Ottawa, Ontario
Canada

Kathryn H. Rollings, PhD Candidate
The University of Texas at Arlington
Arlington, Texas

Jerome Schofferman, MD
SpineCare Medical Group
Daly City and San Francisco, California

Curtis W. Slipman, MD
Miami Beach, Florida

Kjersti Storheim, PT, PhD
Oslo University Hospital Ullevål, NAR, Department of
    Orthopedics and FORMI
Oslo, Norway

Andrea C. Tricco, PhD
Researcher, Li Ka Shing Knowledge Institute
St. Michael's Hospital
Toronto, Ontario
Canada

Torill Helene Tveito, PhD
Postdoctoral Research Fellow
Harvard School of Public Health
Boston, Massachusetts
University of Bergen, Uni Health
Bergen, Norway

Maurits van Tulder, PhD
Professor of Health Technology Assessment
Department of Health Sciences, Faculty of Earth and Life
    Sciences, VU University Amsterdam
Amsterdam, the Netherlands

Eugene K. Wai, MD, MSc, CIP, FRCSC
Assistant Professor and Chief Attending Spine Surgeon
Division of Orthopedic Surgery, University of Ottawa, The
    Ottawa Hospital
Clinical Investigator
Clinical Epidemiology Program, Ottawa Hospital Research
    Institute
Ottawa, Ontario
Canada

Erin T. Wolff, MD
Assistant Professor of Rehabilitation Medicine
University of Miami Miller School of Medicine
Miami, Florida

Foreword

Spine care has enjoyed a most dramatic evolution in the decades from 1980 to the present. Many would expect me to extol the technologic advances of imaging, internal fixation, and other surgical technologies that have unquestionably changed the face of spine care. In fact, the changes in interventional or physiatric spine care have been as (or more) dramatic and pervasive. The integration of both approaches and respective innovations into the profession and professional societies delivering spine care may in fact be the most significant evolutionary development. The fact that a neurosurgical spine surgeon is introducing a text focussing primarily on the evidence for alternatives to surgical care is witness to this.

Scott Haldeman and Simon Dagenais, recognizing a gap in the literature documenting the evidence for the host of approaches to low back pain care, proposed a supplement to *The Spine Journal*, the official journal of the North American Spine Society, the largest multidisciplinary spine care society in the world. This supplement would be a compilation of the evidence, and the actions supported by the evidence, for the host of spine care interventions currently in use. This evidence and supported recommendations would be presented in an algorithmic or standardized format allowing the reader to compare and contrast different treatments for different conditions in a cohesive format. The result of this effort was so striking and compelling that as Editor in Chief, I chose to publish this as a distinct issue of *The Spine Journal*, ensuring that this compilation would not be relegated to supplement status, but incorporated in the medical literature as a quality review of spine care evidence. This issue was well received and referenced. This success compelled Drs. Dagenais and Haldeman to expand the scope of their initial effort, and the result is this truly remarkable reference text, *Evidence-Based Management of Low Back Pain*.

This is a remarkable contribution for a host of reasons. The editors and authors bridge the fields of chiropractic and allopathic spine care. Contributors represent an international compendium of spine care experts. The approach is novel and highly educational and is a "must read" for all spine care practitioners, no matter what the lineage, tradition, or current area of expertise. This is a bold claim that I will support with the following considerations.

A perusal of the table of contents reveals the breadth of the scope of this effort. The entire spectrum of spine care from conventional to complementary or alternative therapies are included. Each modality is addressed in a similar format with a thorough description or review of that specific modality, followed by a standardized presentation of the evidence of efficacy, safety, cost effectiveness, and an overall assessment. A brief educational opportunity in the form of a quiz is included in each chapter as well. The entire experience provides a valuable reference for the practitioner in a specific field, and meaningful insight into the modalities of spine care

that might be unfamiliar. The editors and authors are to be congratulated for this truly remarkable work.

The challenges or concerns generated from a work such as this must be acknowledged as well. This highly detailed reference will likely be out of date even at the moment of publication with newly published evidence potentially impacting the conclusions offered. Harnessing current information technology to create a living contemporary edition of this work would be a laudable aspiration. The title of this work, *Evidence-Based Management of Low Back Pain*, conjures up much of the ambiguity that plagues our current nomenclature and undermines our efforts to clearly define the most appropriate treatment for a specific condition. Although the editors and authors of each section have made laudable effort to clarify the conditions, treatments, and outcomes, our nomenclature and definition of specific conditions continues to be a challenge. This reality contributes to the worrisome overall conclusions of this work that there is little evidence to support the value of the myriad of therapies that are currently applied in the management of nonspecific low back pain. These conclusions could be misused or misappropriated by health care systems to reject or limit access to reasonable care and must not be construed as an absolute guideline.

As we move into the era of value determination in all of health care, this work will serve as a pillar upon which to build our knowledge base. The model for value analysis must include a clear definition of the specific spinal condition, an understanding of the therapeutic modality, the available evidence for efficacy and safety, and the gaps that must be filled, the direct and indirect costs or resource utilization, and the durability of benefit. This work by Haldeman and Dagenais lays down a pattern upon which value analysis should begin and be developed. For this contribution, they are to be congratulated.

For the spine care provider thirsty for enlightenment or a more thorough understanding of the myriad of therapeutic options currently employed in the treatment of low back pain, this work will undoubtedly quench that thirst, but as with any masterful culinary experience, will leave one longing for more.

Charles L. Branch Jr., MD

Eben Alexander Jr. Professor and Chair
Department of Neurosurgery
Wake Forest University Health Sciences
Winston Salem, North Carolina

Former Editor in Chief
The Spine Journal—Official Journal of the
North American Spine Society
Past President
North American Spine Society

vii

Preface

BACKGROUND

The concept for this textbook was initially proposed in 2006 by the North American Spine Society (NASS), one of the largest associations of health professionals involved in caring for patients with spine conditions. NASS has more than 5000 members in Canada, the United States, Mexico, and around the world. Its members include primary care physicians, medical specialists, spine surgeons, chiropractors, physical therapists, nurses, physician assistants, researchers, policy makers, among many others. Although they come from varied backgrounds, members of NASS all share a common interest of wanting to improve spinal health.

NASS's scientific publication, *The Spine Journal*, was created in 2001 to provide its members and others in the scientific and health care communities with a medium to share important scientific discoveries, disseminate study results, and discuss important concepts and opinions related to the management of spinal conditions. Although most of its members are spine surgeons, NASS recognizes the importance of a multidisciplinary approach to spine care. *The Spine Journal* has always attempted to include a variety of articles related to all aspects of caring for patients with both common and rare spine conditions that may be of interest to its readers.

Low back pain (LBP) is one of the most common reasons for consulting with primary care, specialty care, and allied health professionals involved in the management of spinal conditions. The number of treatment approaches available for the management of LBP has grown rapidly in recent decades following advances in surgical techniques, discoveries of new medications, and focused interventions developed in response to a greater understanding of the etiology of LBP. This constant growth in the number of available treatments has made it challenging for those involved in the management of LBP to select among these myriad options.

There is also a growing reluctance among spine surgeons to offer surgical treatments to patients with LBP who do not have clear indications that are expected to benefit from decompression, fusion, or other surgical approaches. This evolution has largely occurred due to lackluster outcomes from high-quality randomized controlled trials comparing the long-term results of both surgical and nonsurgical interventions for LBP. As those involved in spine care have become increasingly familiar with evidence-based medicine, the view toward surgery has shifted and it is no longer widely accepted as *the* gold standard treatment for common LBP. This shift makes it even more important for surgeons to become familiar with nonsurgical approaches to LBP.

To help its many surgeon members understand the many nonsurgical treatments now available for LBP, NASS proposed that a special issue of *The Spine Journal* be dedicated to the management of LBP without surgery. A decision was made to concentrate on chronic LBP because patients with longstanding symptoms are often viewed as the most clinically challenging and are apt to try numerous treatments. The number of nonsurgical interventions initially proposed for this special issue was quite small but grew rapidly as word spread about this project and NASS members volunteered to write review articles about specific treatments that had not yet been considered. The special issue eventually included review articles on 24 types of nonsurgical interventions, as well as a brief overview of surgical approaches for LBP to identify the instances in which surgery was beneficial or even necessary.

The list of interventions reviewed in that special issue should not be viewed as exhaustive, nor should the inclusion or exclusion of a particular intervention be perceived as a reflection of its clinical or scientific merit. The primary goal of the special issue was to openly discuss both the advantages and the disadvantages of various treatments currently being offered to patients with LBP, and not merely to restrict the conversation to those interventions which had been pre-screened or approved by NASS, *The Spine Journal*, or the editors of the special issue. The result was an eclectic mix of interventions that included education, exercise, manual therapies, injections, medications, complementary and alternative medicine, minimally invasive interventions, as well as a brief discussion of various surgical approaches.

The format of the review articles in the special focus issue was discussed at length by those involved in its planning to determine the critical aspects necessary to evaluate and compare various interventions for LBP. It was determined that each review article should contain four sections: (1) description, (2) theory, (3) efficacy, and (4) harms. The first section should begin by explaining and defining any relevant terminology, summarize historical milestones, describe the intervention, estimate its costs, and outline third-party reimbursement policies. The second section should then describe the intervention's proposed mechanism of action, and list its indications, contraindications, and required diagnostic testing. The third section should then review the evidence evaluating its efficacy, focusing on high-quality evidence from clinical practice guidelines, systematic reviews, and randomized controlled trials, resorting to observational studies only if nothing else was available. The fourth section should then discuss harms, including both minor, self-limiting side effects and rare but serious adverse events.

Authors invited to contribute to that special issue included both expert clinicians who were personally experienced with administering these interventions, as well as academic researchers experienced in applying evidence-based medicine (EBM) to evaluate such interventions scientifically.

Although it was the intention that the special issue be centered on scientific evidence, authors were given considerable leeway to provide information they felt was most clinically important within each of the required sections. The review articles contained in the special issue were therefore a blend of narrative and systematic reviews. The term *evidence-informed* was chosen over the more traditional *evidence-based* following spirited discussions in which clinicians and academics debated both the intent and the application of EBM.

Although some felt that strictly "evidence-based" reviews were synonymous with methodologically rigorous systematic reviews of high-quality randomized controlled trials with clear-cut results, others were willing to accept a broader definition of evidence that also included expert opinion when necessary. Some clinicians shared their discouragement after having read the conclusions of previous "evidence-based" reviews, which often stated that insufficient high-quality evidence was available to support making a decision either for or against an intervention. It was suggested that those reviews, although scientifically rigorous, were rarely helpful to clinicians who were nevertheless required to make such decisions on a daily basis, and would gladly accept expert clinical opinion while waiting for more robust evidence. Conversely, some academics were opposed to simple narrative review articles that did not adhere to commonly accepted EBM methodology because their conclusions could simply not be considered meaningful. The term "evidence-informed" was therefore offered and adopted as an alternative to those opposed to interpretations of the term "evidence-based" that were felt to be either too loose or too rigid.

The special issue on "Evidence-informed management of low back pain without surgery" was published as the January/February 2008 issue of *The Spine Journal* and was the largest ever at 278 pages. The initial response to that special issue from a variety of sources both within NASS and from those outside the spine community was very encouraging. In addition to being distributed to thousands of NASS members, as well as individual and institutional subscribers to *The Spine Journal*, hundreds of additional copies were purchased as reprints by health care professionals, students, and other decision makers involved in the management of LBP.

The editors and authors involved in the special issue were then invited to present findings at a number of professional society meetings related to spine care, including the American Back Society, Florida Chiropractic Association, NASS, American Academy of Physical Medicine and Rehabilitation, Association of Chiropractic Colleges-Research Agenda Conference, and American Physical Therapy Association. Shorter versions of these presentations were also offered to medical, chiropractic, and physical therapy students eager to learn about the numerous interventions available to patients with LBP. Feedback from those presentations was also quite positive and continued to generate interest in this project.

Based largely on this feedback, Elsevier, the publisher of *The Spine Journal*, conceived the notion of a textbook based on that special issue. The goals initially identified for this textbook were to build upon the interest that had been demonstrated in the topic of multidisciplinary management of LBP using a variety of interventions while improving the content and presentation of this information for both students and clinicians. After many of the authors who had originally contributed review articles to the special issue agreed to also participate in this endeavor, the decision was made to proceed with this textbook. The numerous changes that were made by the editors and authors of this textbook to the articles that originally appeared in that special issue are described below.

CHANGES MADE TO TEXTBOOK BASED ON SPECIAL ISSUE

Upon carefully reviewing the special issue on which this textbook is based numerous times in order to extract materials used in presentations given to both practitioners and students, it became apparent that the review articles were somewhat heterogeneous in their content and/or style. Some of the required information in each of the four sections was occasionally given only a cursory consideration, which made it difficult to compare and contrast different articles. It was often unclear, for example, whether differences noted in the nature, quality, and quantity of evidence reviewed were truly reflective of the scientific literature or simply related to the amount of effort spent by authors in trying to search and obtain this information.

In order to facilitate comparisons between interventions, it was first necessary to ensure that a minimum amount of information was provided in each of the required sections and subsections without regard to the quality of the underlying evidence supporting that information. For better or worse, it was reasoned that some information was better than none, so every effort was made to avoid leaving a section or subsection completely blank. It was then necessary to standardize the style and content in each required section and subsection by reducing, expanding, or modifying the information originally provided.

To retain the original goal of centering a discussion of advantages and disadvantages of various interventions on the best available scientific evidence, it was then important to standardize the methods used to search for, present, and summarize evidence related to efficacy, safety, and costs. This required consistently reviewing and summarizing evidence from high-quality sources such as evidence-based clinical practice guidelines (CPGs), systematic reviews (SRs), randomized controlled trials (RCTs), and health economic evaluations related to the interventions discussed in this textbook. For CPGs and SRs, brief findings were summarized in both table and text format to emphasize important conclusions about specific interventions. For RCTs, basic elements of study design were summarized in both table and text format so that readers could appreciate the types of research questions that these studies could have addressed. Important outcomes from RCTs were also summarized, emphasizing both within and between study groups for the last available follow-up in each study. Although this information cannot replace the details provided in the many CPGs, SRs, and RCTs that have been published on various interventions for

LBP, they provide a succinct summary for readers who may not otherwise be familiar with these studies.

An effort was made to expand the information provided on safety, which had often been overlooked in the special issue because details about harms were often not provided in the SRs and RCTs focused on efficacy. A new section was also created within each chapter to discuss information related to costs, including not only fees and current procedural terminology codes, but also some insight into third-party reimbursement policies. Health economic evaluations such as cost effectiveness and cost utility analyses were also summarized when available. Although EBM has often focused on comparative effectiveness, other aspects such as relative safety and costs are increasingly important when efficacy alone is unable to establish clear superiority among the many interventions being offered for LBP.

Multiple choice questions and answers were created to help readers, whether students or clinicians, gauge their learning efforts. Information provided in each of the five sections (description, theory, efficacy, safety, and costs) within each chapter was also summarized at the end of each chapter to reinforce the important messages within each section.

A more detailed description of how the textbook was developed is provided in Chapters 1–4 to help guide readers.

Simon Dagenais
Scott Haldeman

Acknowledgments

This textbook evolved from a project proposed by the North American Spine Society (NASS) for its scientific publication, *The Spine Journal* (TSJ). Their vision and commitment to create a credible and comprehensive source of information for its members on a variety of treatment approaches to low back pain should be acknowledged as the genesis of this effort. In particular, the encouragement provided by Dr. Charles Branch was much appreciated. He gave us the highest compliment possible after having been handed the completed draft of the special issue, which was many hundreds of pages long: Charlie admitted to having read it cover to cover.

The feedback provided by readers of the special issue should also be acknowledged, as it provided the impetus to continue this project. This feedback came through emails, blog posts, and conversations at various professional, educational, and scientific meetings in the past few years. Clinicians genuinely seemed to appreciate the effort that had been put into finding, evaluating, and summarizing the best available evidence supporting various common treatment approaches to low back pain.

This encouragement is a testament to the excellent work of the contributing authors, a group that includes some of the most qualified and experienced spine care clinicians and scientists in the world. Although they were all busy with clinical practice, research, teaching, and other writing commitments, they graciously agreed to share their expertise and knowledge with readers. I also wish to thank them for allowing us to edit their material to enhance consistency throughout the textbook, and apologize in advance for any errors that may have resulted from this process.

Robin Campbell, the managing editor of TSJ, should be acknowledged for his role in putting us in touch with his colleagues at Elsevier, including Kellie White and Jennifer Watrous. Their guidance was instrumental in helping us transform the special issue from a series of independent review articles in a scientific, peer-reviewed journal into didactic articles written with a common style and format that now form a textbook. Although this process seemed rather simple at first, it required a great deal of effort to reappraise each article and identify where it could be expanded, shortened, or enhanced in a consistent manner to facilitate comparison of its contents across interventions. This work was largely performed by a team of researchers with expertise in clinical epidemiology and systematic review, including Dr. Andrea Tricco, Carmen Ng, and Erin Galloway. Without their attention to detail and commitment, this project simply could not have been completed. Linda Smith is a medical billing expert who was instrumental in providing and verifying the information presented in this textbook related to fees, procedure codes, and reimbursement.

Support for this project was initially provided by CAM Research Institute, a nonprofit research organization whose goal is to investigate various forms of complementary and alternative medical (CAM) therapies for low back pain. Funding for this organization has been generously provided by the philanthropists Michael Marcus and Janet Zand, who are committed to evaluating promising but unconventional therapies that may otherwise be overlooked by the scientific and medical communities.

Additional support was later provided by Palladian Health, a company founded by Dr. Kevin Cichocki to manage specialty benefits on behalf of health plans and insurers. I've been fortunate to collaborate with Kevin and help develop a program aimed at improving the care of low back pain by promoting informed decision making based on the scientific evidence reviewed in this textbook. Implementing this Coordinated Spine Care program in a commercial environment could provide an opportunity to measure the impact of providing high quality, scientifically based information to both clinicians and patients at the point of care.

Dr. Louis Sportelli and the NCMIC Foundation have also provided support that allowed me to pursue training in health economics and gain an additional perspective into the challenges faced by third-party payers and other stakeholders when evaluating interventions for low back pain. I am much indebted to my mentor, Dr. Scott Haldeman, who has provided me with tireless counsel since we began working together and countless chances for me to expand my professional development as a spine clinician and researcher. I hope that Scott's emphasis on patient-centered, clinical and scientific excellence in the area of spine care can be advanced with this textbook.

Last but not least, the support provided by my wife throughout this project cannot be overstated. She has been a constant source of encouragement throughout the inevitable ups and downs that occur when the requirements of a project of this magnitude clash with those of everyday life. Thank you all.

Simon Dagenais
Hamburg, New York
March, 2010

About the Editors

Simon Dagenais, DC, PhD

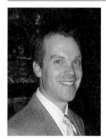

Dr. Simon Dagenais is currently the Chief Scientific Officer at Palladian Health, a health management company in West Seneca, New York. Simon also holds an academic appointment as Assistant Professor in Orthopaedic Surgery and Epidemiology and Community Medicine at the University of Ottawa, as well as Research Assistant Professor in the Department of Preventive and Social Medicine at the University at Buffalo. Simon is an active member of the North American Spine Society, Associate Editor for *The Spine Journal*, and a peer reviewer for several scientific journals related to spine care. Simon previously advised physicians and surgeons at The Ottawa Hospital on clinical research methodology. He previously cofounded CAM Research Institute in Irvine, California, a nonprofit organization devoted to conducting research into promising complementary therapies for spinal pain. Simon obtained a PhD in Environmental Health, Science, and Policy, specializing in Epidemiology and Public Health, at the University of California, Irvine, and a Doctor of Chiropractic from Southern California University of Health Sciences. He is currently completing a Master's degree in Health Economics, Policy, and Management, at the London School of Economics and Political Science. Simon has published articles in peer-reviewed scientific journals, contributed to textbook chapters, previously edited a textbook on chiropractic care, and has given presentations on evidence based care of spinal pain to students and clinicians from a variety of disciplines. His main research interest is to use the best available scientific evidence to help patients and clinicians make informed decisions about the management of spinal, musculoskeletal, and pain disorders.

Scott Haldeman, DC, MD, PhD, FRCP(C), FCCS(C), FAAN

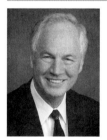

Dr. Scott Haldeman holds the positions of Adjunct Professor, Department of Epidemiology, School of Public Health, University of California, Los Angeles; Clinical Professor, Department of Neurology, University of California, Irvine; and Adjunct Professor, Department of Research, Southern California University of Health Sciences. He is past President of the North American Spine Society, the American Back Society, the North American Academy of Manipulative Therapy, and the Orange County Neurological Society. He is currently chairman of the Research Council of the World Federation of Chiropractic. He serves as President of World Spine Care, a nonprofit organization with the goal of helping people in underserved regions of the world who suffer from spinal disorders. He sits on the editorial boards of eight journals. He has published more than 190 articles or book chapters, more than 70 scientific abstracts, and has authored or edited eight books. He is certified by the American Board of Neurology and Psychiatry, is a Fellow of the Royal College of Physicians of Canada, and is a Fellow of the American Academy of Neurology. He is a Diplomate of the American Board of Electrodiagnostic Medicine, the American Board of Electroencephalography and Neurophysiology, and the American Board of Clinical Physiology. He served on the US department of Health AHCPR Clinical Guidelines Committee on *Acute Low Back Problems in Adults* as well as four other Clinical Guidelines Committees. He presided over *The Bone and Joint Decade 2000 to 2010 Task Force on Neck Pain and Its Associated Disorders*. He was awarded an honorary Doctor of Humanities degree from the Southern California University of Health Sciences and an honorary Doctor of Science degree from the Western States Chiropractic College. He received the David Selby Award from the North American Spine Society. A resident of Santa Ana, California, he maintains an active clinical practice.

Contents

SIMON DAGENAIS
SCOTT HALDEMAN

CHAPTER 1

Evidence-Based Management of Low Back Pain

A number of books have been published related to various aspects of low back pain (LBP). There are textbooks on the anatomic and physiological mechanisms that have been proposed to explain the etiology of LBP. There are textbooks that discuss the methods and diagnostic tests that have been developed to identify the many suspected causes of LBP. There are several textbooks that describe a unique or specific method of assessing and managing the approach to LBP using a particular technique or system. There are textbooks describing one or more of the many treatment methods available to relieve symptoms of LBP. There are also books aimed at the general public to help them understand why they have LBP and what they should do to find relief from their symptoms. On the surface, it would appear that so much has already been published on the topic of LBP that nothing new could be offered.

However, most of the information that has been published to date on LBP has generally focused on only one or a few of the many interventions available in an isolated context, making it difficult to develop a comprehensive and widely accepted approach to this challenging clinical problem. Narrow perspectives about LBP ignore the reality that the list of available treatment approaches is very long and continues to grow. This reality has reached the point where there is demand for a logical and scientific approach to be developed to deal with the problem that is LBP. This is especially true given the current climate within the wider health care debate on comparative effectiveness, cost effectiveness, and how to reasonably distribute limited health care resources.

It is important that all stakeholders be aware of the confusion, frustration, costs, and disability related to LBP and recognize that its deep societal impact will only worsen if we fail to develop strategies to improve its management. In this introduction, we present the challenges that have been associated with LBP in an attempt to paint a picture of the current burden on society and a few of the reasons for our failure to develop a cohesive approach to the problem. We also outline the solutions that have been proposed to address these challenges, including a brief overview of how evidence is currently being interpreted. We then explain our attempt to provide readers with information that, on one hand, covers the broad scope of treatments available to clinicians and their patients and, on the other hand, provides a means to compare the scientific basis, rationale, and indications for approaching this universal problem. In the summary chapter, we offer our opinion as to what constitutes an evidence-based approach to managing LBP.

CHALLENGES ASSOCIATED WITH LOW BACK PAIN

There are many challenges involved in the management of common LBP that have made it difficult for all stakeholders, including patients, clinicians, third-party payers, and policy makers, to deal with this universal problem. These challenges relate to its epidemiology, etiology, clinical characteristics, prognosis, temporality, risk factors, diagnostic testing, subgroups, diagnostic classifications, health care professionals, direct health care costs, and indirect non–health care costs. Each is briefly discussed below.

Epidemiology

The magnitude of LBP as a health concern can be illustrated by reviewing its epidemiologic characteristics and perhaps most importantly its prevalence. Studies of adults from the general population in a number of developed countries have reported that the prevalence of LBP is quite high, and increases according to the time span considered. The point prevalence of bothersome LBP has been estimated at 25%, whereas the 1-year prevalence has been estimated at 50% and

1

the lifetime prevalence has been estimated at 85%.[1-3] These statistics mainly hold true regardless of age, sex, or country and vary only slightly between occupations. The odds of someone never experiencing LBP in their life are therefore stacked 6:1 against them. There is some evidence to suggest that everyone will at some point in their life experience LBP and that surveys suggesting otherwise are including people who are young and have not yet experienced LBP or have experienced LBP in the past and have simply forgotten this fact.[4] The sheer number of people with LBP must always be considered when examining how this condition should be optimally managed, because solutions should ideally be available to the masses rather than the few.

Clinical Characteristics

Many episodes of common LBP are trivial, often beginning with minor aches and pains in the lower spine that can occur without reason or shortly after an unusually heavy bout of physical activity, or without any obvious reason at all, and resolving within a few days without receiving any particular intervention.[5,6] Other instances of LBP, however, can be much more severe, frightening, and debilitating. Symptoms may include muscle spasms seemingly precipitated by any movement, as well as searing, burning pain that radiates into the thigh, leg, or foot, or even numbness, tingling, and weakness throughout the lower extremities. The sudden appearance of one or more of these symptoms can be frightening and can severely impact a person's ability to carry out activities of daily living, whereas their gradual worsening can impact one's general mood and outlook on life.

Prognosis

It is common wisdom that a substantial majority of those who suddenly develop LBP will quickly improve on their own regardless of the care received. This belief is founded on studies conducted a few decades ago in which those who recently developed LBP were followed prospectively and asked about the severity of their symptoms after various time intervals.[7] In these studies, patients often reported that their symptoms had improved markedly within several weeks.[7] By carrying forward this observed reduction in severity, it was natural for researchers to conclude that symptoms should disappear entirely within, at most, a few months.

However, this assumption has been questioned by other epidemiologists who found it difficult to reconcile this theoretically favorable prognosis with the substantial number of patients who still reported symptoms many years after their original episode of LBP. When researchers reexamined those original studies, another hypothesis emerged for their results. Although symptoms often do recede within a few months, the follow-up periods were often too short to capture the longer-term recurrences and exacerbations of symptoms that were common with LBP. By truncating the length of follow-up, these studies failed to observe the true pattern of waxing and waning symptoms. Currently, LBP can be considered a recurrent disorder that can occur at any time in a person's life and fluctuates between a status of no pain or mild pain, and pain that reaches a point where it interferes with activities of normal living or becomes debilitating.

Temporality

The current consensus on the prognosis of LBP has become more nuanced. The prognosis for LBP is generally favorable for those with recent symptoms, but somewhat grim for those with longstanding symptoms. It became important to adopt a universal terminology to define the temporality of LBP to appreciate this distinction. People whose symptoms lasted less than 6 weeks since onset were generally categorized as having "acute LBP," progressing to "subacute LBP" if symptoms lasted 6 to 12 weeks, and "chronic LBP (CLBP)" if symptoms persisted beyond 12 weeks.[8] Further gradations have been suggested for those with longstanding symptoms that disappeared for a time and reappeared, which can be considered "recurrent" or "episodic" LBP.[9]

Although acknowledging that the duration of symptoms affects the prognosis of LBP was important, the demarcation of patients into those with acute, subacute, or chronic LBP has never been as clear as many had wished. Both the severity and duration of symptoms vary from episode to episode, and episodes often become intertwined, with no clear beginning and end. This makes it difficult to define patients using such simple temporal labels. The perception that acute LBP goes away rapidly without returning has been proven false, but so has the seemingly gloomy prognosis attributed to someone who has crossed the 3-month threshold and been labeled as "chronic," a term often perceived as incurable rather than longstanding by patients. Another phenomenon that has been noted is that as the length of follow-up in clinical studies increased, the results of all treatments studied generally grew less impressive as outcomes gradually regressed to the mean.

Etiology

One of the greatest mysteries surrounding common LBP is its etiology. Epidemiologic, anatomic, biomechanical, and pathologic studies into the etiology of common LBP have yet to create a clear link between precise risk factors or a specific tissue injury and particular symptoms. In fact, such studies have identified abundant theories and hypotheses about the origins of LBP, few of which have withstood scientific scrutiny over time.[8,10] Exploration of a condition's etiology often begins by identifying risk factors thought to contribute to its onset in the hope that it will provide information about the precise nature of any pathognomonic injuries. The number of studies conducted in recent decades that have attempted to evaluate potential risk factors for common LBP is impressive, but their findings are often difficult to interpret because they are diverse, nonspecific, and frequently disputed among clinicians and researchers.[11,12]

Risk Factors

Sociodemographic factors such as age, gender, education, and marital status have all been identified as risk factors for developing or prolonging episodes of common LBP.[9,13] Similarly, occupational factors such as work satisfaction, autonomy, supervisor empathy, monotonous or repetitive tasks, and prolonged exposure to heavy physical activities including lifting, carrying, and manual handling, have also been identified as risk factors for common LBP.[2,14-16] General health factors including tobacco use, body weight, physical activity levels, and the presence of systemic, physical, or psychological comorbidities have also been implicated in LBP.[6,9,17] Socioeconomic factors including income level, involvement in worker's compensation, personal injury, or other litigation, and availability of supplemental disability insurance are also thought to impact the severity or duration of common LBP.[9,16] Genetic factors have also been identified that may increase the risk for development of lumbar degenerative disc disease, which may lead to LBP.[18]

Diagnostic Testing

Even though few of the suspected risk factors for LBP are able to elucidate a clear mechanism of injury and identify a specific anatomic structure that can be targeted with an intervention, diagnostic tests are often ordered to find tissue pathology. These tests include plain film x-ray studies, magnetic resonance imaging (MRI), and computed tomography (CT). Although diagnostic imaging occasionally identifies serious pathology that may be responsible for symptoms of LBP and requires urgent and targeted intervention, this is the exception rather than the rule. Too often, diagnostic imaging reports list findings that should be considered normal signs of aging (e.g., disc degeneration) or normal anatomic variants (e.g., minor positional misalignments or disc bulging).[2,19,20] Further clouding the interpretation of diagnostic imaging reports is that findings may not correlate with the clinical presentation, making their significance dubious at best (e.g., left-sided disc protrusion at L4 with symptoms of right-sided thigh numbness). In fact, there are a number of studies that have shown that adults who are not reporting LBP having significant abnormalities on x-ray studies, CT scans, and MRI.[21-26] The results of diagnostic testing for common LBP must therefore be interpreted with caution.

Subgroups

Currently, LBP is viewed as a symptom rather than a medical diagnosis because it can be caused by a variety of conditions, including some that may originate outside the lumbar spine. For example, one of the first symptoms of kidney stones may be LBP, but applying a diagnosis of LBP to such a patient and prescribing analgesics would be ignoring the underlying illness. Conversely, a prolonged search for a specific diagnosis for a patient in otherwise good health who reports moderate LBP will likely prove fruitless because nociceptive input can be triggered by dozens of anatomic structures and result in similar symptoms. Clinicians faced with a patient who reports LBP must therefore balance these two extremes. First, clinicians must be vigilant to avoid missing rare but potentially serious pathology that may manifest itself as LBP.

Second, they must refrain from ordering unnecessary diagnostic tests that will not change their recommended management approach and could confound what is an otherwise simple clinical scenario.

Diagnostic Classifications

Numerous diagnostic classifications have been proposed for LBP in an attempt to simplify the dozens of potentially underlying pathologies that may account for a group of related symptoms. One of the simplest has been extrapolated from an increasingly popular method of defining neck pain. Under this terminology, patients presenting with LBP can be divided into four categories or diagnostic groups, each of which requires a different management approach. Group 1 is common, nonspecific, and nondebilitating LBP that does not impact activities of daily living. Group 2 includes people with LBP that has become disabling and is interfering with activities of daily living; people in this group commonly seek care. Group 3 includes people who have demonstrable neurologic deficits, including motor, sensory, or reflex changes that are suggestive of an anatomic lesion compressing a neurologic structure. Group 4 includes people with serious and often progressive spinal pathology, which can be differentiated into two subgroups. The first is likely to require surgery (e.g., spinal tumor, spinal abscess, spinal fracture, cauda equina syndrome). The second is likely to respond to medical intervention, although surgery may become necessary if the problem is not resolved by medical intervention (e.g., infection, osteoporosis, ankylosing spondylitis, rheumatoid arthritis).

Several terms are often used to describe LBP that falls into groups 1 and 2, including *nonspecific LBP* (i.e., no specific cause has been identified for these symptoms), *mechanical LBP* (i.e., symptoms appear to be exacerbated when a mechanical load is applied to the lumbar spine), *common LBP*, *musculoskeletal LBP*, or *simple LBP*. These terms are often used interchangeably and generally indicate that a working diagnosis of common LBP has been established after reasonable efforts have been made by a clinician to rule out a specific cause of LBP. It has been estimated that less than 1% of LBP is associated with potentially serious spinal pathology requiring surgery, 1% with specific spinal pathology requiring medical intervention, and 5% to 10% with substantial neurologic involvement.[27,28]

Given our current understanding, it does not appear to be possible to establish a specific diagnosis for more than 90% of patients with LBP.[19,27,28] The vast majority of patients can simply be said to have common LBP that may or may not be impacting their activities of daily living. This notion of common LBP can be difficult for both patients and clinicians to accept, in that it seems to contradict the basic sequence of events used in many other areas of modern medicine: elicit a history, develop a differential diagnosis, examine the patient, refine the differential diagnosis, order diagnostic tests, further refine the differential diagnosis, apply an intervention targeted at the diagnosis, and implement a cure. This can make it difficult for some patients and clinicians trained in the classical method of treating disease to accept the uncertainty of a diagnosis of nonspecific LBP and address the problem according to the current scientific evidence.

Health Care Professionals

Further compounding the clinical challenge presented by common LBP is the number of health care professionals involved in its diagnosis and management, each of whom may approach a patient with LBP according to their particular training and experience with this condition. Unlike many other medical conditions that are clearly identified with a particular health care discipline (e.g., cancer and oncology, tooth disease and dentistry), a variety of clinicians must contend with common LBP, whether by choice or by chance. Care for common LBP is also sought in many different settings across the health care spectrum, including primary, secondary, and even tertiary medical care, as well as allied health, and complementary and alternative medicine practitioners. Health care professionals who are routinely consulted for LBP are listed in Box 1-1.

In the absence of clear scientific evidence about the etiology and ideal management of LBP, many health care disciplines have developed their own views on how to deal with this condition. Naturally, these views are shaped by the extent

---

BOX 1-1	Health Care Professionals Involved in Managing LBP

Acupuncturists
Anesthesiologists
Behavioral medicine specialists
Chiropractors
Family practice physicians
General practice physicians
Homeopaths
Internal medicine physicians
Interventional radiologists
Massage therapists
Naprapaths
Naturopaths
Neurologic spine surgeons
Neurologists
Nurses
Nurse practitioners
Nutritionists
Occupational medicine physicians
Orthopedic spine surgeons
Osteopathic physicians
Pain management physicians
Pharmacists
Physical medicine and rehabilitation physicians
Physical therapists
Physician assistants
Psychiatrists
Psychologists
Radiologists
Rheumatologists
Sports medicine physicians
Traditional Chinese medicine practitioners

---

and nature of their academic and clinical experience, as well as their scope of practice, state licensing laws, third-party reimbursement policies, and patient demand for specific services. In aggregate, these factors have resulted in health care professionals from different disciplines using treatment strategies as divergent as acupuncture, traction therapy, anticonvulsant medications, cognitive behavioral therapy, facet neurotomy, arthrodesis, and spinal manipulation under anesthesia, to name only a few interventions. For particularly severe or recalcitrant cases of LBP, multiple interventions may be used simultaneously (e.g., opioid analgesics with epidural steroid injections and massage).

Direct Health Care Costs

Given the high number of patients who report common LBP and seek care from a variety of health care professionals who then order multiple diagnostic tests before recommending a panoply of interventions, it should come as no surprise that the direct health care costs associated with LBP are substantial. In the United States, yearly direct health care costs associated with back and neck problems—most commonly LBP—were estimated to have doubled over 7 years, from $52.1 billion in 1997 to $102 billion in 2004, before settling to $85.9 billion in 2005.[29] This increase in health care costs cannot solely be attributed to the number of people afflicted with LBP because the prevalence on which those estimates are based was 13.7% in 1997 and 15.2% in 2005, an annualized increase of only 1.5%, whereas costs rose at an annual rate of 7.5%. Similarly, high direct health care costs have been reported for LBP in other developed countries, including the United Kingdom, the Netherlands, Sweden, Australia, Belgium, and Japan.[30] LBP often ranks among the 10 most expensive medical conditions, with costs similar to those associated with cancer, cardiovascular disease, or diabetes.[30]

The problem is that disability associated with LBP appears to be increasing even though more money is being spent to relieve its symptoms. As noted by Martin and colleagues,[29] there was a substantial increase in the expenditure for all categories of treatment for LBP. At the same time, the estimates of self-reported physical limitations of those with LBP increased from 20.7% in 1997 to 24.7% in 2005. This study also noted that there was a marked increase in the overall health care expenditure in patients who experienced LBP compared with those who were not experiencing LBP. In 2005, the mean age- and sex-adjusted medical expenditure among respondents with spinal problems was $6096, compared with $3516 among respondents without spinal problems. Not all of this increase can be attributed to treatment directed at their spinal problems, but it may be a marker for increased overall health seeking behavior among those with LBP.

Indirect Non–Health Care Costs

Although direct health care costs related to diagnostic tests, outpatient visits, inpatient visits, professional services, medication, physical therapy, surgery, and other services for LBP are substantial, they often pale in comparison with indirect non–health care costs associated with lost productivity. From a societal perspective, such indirect non–health care costs associated with a particular medical condition are just as important as the more familiar direct health care costs in that they have an impact not only on the individual affected, but also on their employer, family, and society at large.[31] This is particularly true for common LBP, which often afflicts adults between the ages of 30 and 50 during their most economically productive years. The economic value of any reduction in workplace, household, or personal productivity that occurs as a result of LBP can be estimated using various methods to arrive at indirect non–health care costs.

When direct health care costs are combined with indirect non–health care costs, the total cost of illness of a particular disease can be estimated and its societal impact more fully understood. Relatively few studies have estimated the cost of illness associated with LBP, and none are currently available in the United States. Estimates from cost of illness studies in other countries have reported that direct health care costs may only represent 15% of total costs.[30] If similar results were to occur in the United States, the total cost of illness associated with LBP could exceed $500 billion per year.

The simplest costs associated with lost productivity are those due to absenteeism, in which an injured worker is unable to perform his or her job duties due to LBP. Because the economic value of a person's productivity can be difficult to estimate, wages are often used as a more readily available substitute. Absenteeism may be temporary or permanent depending on the type of injury, circumstances under which it occurred, resulting physical disability, and private or public insurance provisions for such injuries.

Human Capital Approach to Lost Productivity Costs

Health economists often disagree about the more appropriate of two commonly used methods to estimate lost productivity due to absenteeism (i.e., human capital approach and friction period approach). The human capital approach assumes that employees are similar to other capital assets with an expected duration of productivity (e.g., machinery). The lost productivity of a worker who is unable to resume employment following an injury is therefore assumed to be the value of future earnings until his or her expected retirement at age 65 years. This method results in much higher estimates of lost productivity for younger workers with a higher earning potential.

Friction Period Approach to Lost Productivity Costs

The friction period approach assumes instead that injured workers who are unable to return to work due to LBP will eventually be replaced, thereby negating much of the economic value of lost productivity associated with a long-term absence. This method is only concerned with the economic value of productivity lost during the period in which a new employee is recruited and trained until his or her output can match that of the injured worker being replaced, which is termed the *friction period*. This method results in higher estimates of lost productivity for more specialized, educated, and experienced workers for whom it may take more time to find suitable replacements. Studies in which the economic value of lost productivity due to absenteeism resulting from LBP has been estimated using both the human capital approach and the friction period approach have reported a wide disparity between these two methods. In one instance, the estimate was 97% lower when using the friction period approach.[30]

CURRENT APPROACHES TO MANAGEMENT OF LOW BACK PAIN

The many challenges outlined above are confronted by clinicians attempting to provide the highest quality health care possible, by patients seeking safe, effective, and affordable relief from their symptoms, by employers wishing to minimize the economic impact of injured workers by returning them to full productivity promptly, and by third-party payers faced with rising direct health care costs who desire the most cost effective approaches. Although these challenges are numerous and considerable, solutions are available to help surmount them, including acknowledging the bio-psychosocial model of LBP, adopting a multidisciplinary approach, fostering shared and informed decision making, and applying the principles of evidence-based medicine (EBM) to evaluate and compare the efficacy, safety, and cost effectiveness of available interventions.

Bio-Psychosocial Model

The failure to reliably identify a clear anatomic structure and pathophysiology that could account for the observed symptoms and be cured by an intervention targeted at that anatomic structure has led to great frustration among those involved in the management of common LBP. Findings from various studies that socioeconomic factors often predict prognosis better than clinical characteristics led to theories that common LBP was merely a social or psychological issue.[32] Because opposing viewpoints can rarely be simultaneously correct, the truth often lies somewhere in the middle. The bio-psychosocial model to common LBP was proposed in the 1990s in an attempt to reconcile these theories.[33] This model postulates that the initial trigger for common LBP is likely an injury to one or more anatomic structures in the lumbosacral spine (e.g., intervertebral disc, muscles, ligaments, articulations, nerves) that may occur following exposure to one of several suspected risk factors (e.g., acute or repeated mechanical loading).

However, once that injury occurs, an individual's response to persistent common LBP will be dictated not only by the injury itself, but also by a host of psychosocial factors, most notably prior experiences with LBP, beliefs about LBP, general and psychological health, job satisfaction, economic status, education, involvement in litigation, and social well-being at home. It is therefore conceivable under this model that the original anatomic injury can heal while the subsequent symptoms and disability persist. Interventions aimed solely at anatomic structures are therefore likely to fail, and a more holistic approach must be taken.

Multidisciplinary Approach

Reviewing the list of health care disciplines involved in the management of common LBP and contemplating the varied nature of the interventions currently offered could easily lead someone who is poorly informed to conclude that many of these approaches should simply be eliminated prima facie. Upon further inquiry, however, it will likely be noted that each of the many treatments offered for common LBP has strong and vocal adherents—both clinicians and patients—who will readily attest to having observed marked clinical improvements following their use. Rather than dismissing some interventions altogether and denigrating approaches with which clinicians of a particular health care discipline may be unfamiliar, it may be constructive to learn enough about each one to appreciate its ideal role (if any) in the management of common LBP. Because no single intervention can claim to have perfect effectiveness, and no two patients are exactly alike, a coordinated multidisciplinary approach based on solid scientific evidence has been proposed as an appropriate method of tackling this vexing clinical challenge. There is concern, however, that this approach may result in increased cost and frustration if multiple treatments are attempted simultaneously or sequentially without success.

Shared and Informed Decision Making

One of the important roles played by clinicians involved in the management of common LBP is that of an informed agent who provides the information required by the patient to help decision making. The first step in this process is to conduct a thorough assessment of the patient's symptoms in order to be reasonably confident that the problem at hand (e.g., common LBP) has been identified, and to convey this information to the patient, who may have imagined terrible scenarios that could account for his or her symptoms. The second step is to propose a course of action that may be taken by the particular health care professional that the patient has chosen to consult with, outlining information related to efficacy, safety, and costs that are necessary to fully evaluate a proposed intervention. The third step is to engage in an informed discussion of available alternatives to those originally proposed by the clinician, which, for common LBP, may require a lengthy conversation of the relative advantages and disadvantages of scores of interventions. The final step is for the patient and clinician to openly review this information and make a decision based on patient preference and the experience of the clinician.

Evidence-Based Medicine

The process by which clinicians become knowledgeable about the many interventions available for LBP can be daunting. But it is this process that determines the information that will be given to patients and drive treatment decisions. Ideally, the most current and best available scientific evidence should guide this process. The framework in which scientific evidence is evaluated, summarized, and reconciled with clinical training and experience to make an informed decision is known as *EBM*. The concept of EBM is not particularly new, having been first introduced in the 1970s and grown rapidly in prominence in the 1990s.[34]

At its best, EBM offers decision makers a framework for evaluating multiple competing interventions to determine which one is supported by high-quality evidence and should therefore be selected or, alternatively, which one has been convincingly shown to be ineffective or dangerous and should be abandoned. Few would dispute the principles of EBM, which have long guided medical decision making. However, debates frequently occur among clinicians and clinical epidemiologists about the practice, implementation, and consequences of EBM, which continues to evolve as new research methods are developed and novel challenges emerge.[35-37] These debates often occur following instances in which EBM is unable to clearly categorize an intervention as effective and therefore recommended, or ineffective and therefore not recommended. The challenges in EBM often concern the middle ground, in which insufficient evidence is available to make that decision.

Applying Evidence-Based Medicine to Low Back Pain

In some areas of medicine, the application of EBM has resulted in marked improvement in important clinical outcomes (e.g., myocardial infarction survival) whereas with common LBP, no such victory can be claimed. Attempts to apply EBM too rigorously for conditions in which uncertainty about clinical outcomes abounds and insufficient high-quality evidence is the norm can make this process seem like a mirage. This phenomenon has been acknowledged by many trained in EBM, and can occasionally result from well intentioned but poorly executed attempts to develop strict rules to an approach based on relative rather than absolute merits.

Uncertainty and Evidence-Based Medicine

When dealing with common LBP, whose etiology remains unknown, clinicians must simply accept that decisions will be made even in the absence of the highest possible type, quantity, and quality of evidence that some mistakenly believe is required by EBM. When first proposed, EBM was intended to be a flexible, practical approach that could be adapted to different scenarios as required, rather than a rigid, obdurate rejection of all treatments that fail to meet sometimes impossibly high standards that can lead one to nihilism. At its core, EBM is based on the principles of clinical epidemiology, which evaluates the relative strengths and weaknesses of available scientific studies before making a clinical decision that is informed by that process.[38] EBM is therefore conducted in three broad steps: (1) identifying available studies, (2) evaluating their methodologic quality, and (3) summarizing evidence.

Identifying Available Studies

In order for the decisions made when using EBM to be valid, they should be based on the best available scientific evidence. This requires conducting a thorough review of the literature to uncover the best available evidence. Unfortunately, the methods used to search the literature can introduce bias in the evidence uncovered. This can perhaps be illustrated at its extreme by imagining clinicians who form their opinion of an intervention based solely on the results of a randomized controlled trial (RCT) published in the latest issue of the only medical journal they read each month. Unless that RCT reports on a completely novel technique that has never previously been discussed in the literature, it is unlikely to encompass all available evidence.

When clinicians are aware of the possibility that a poorly developed literature search can result in bias, numerous incremental steps can be taken to improve its quality. For example, clinicians can search major medical databases such as MEDLINE or PubMed, which contain information about millions of articles published in thousands of journals over several decades. Other medical databases are also available that may include different journals, such as EMBASE, CINAHL, and The Cochrane Library, among many others. It should be acknowledged here that the efforts devoted to searching the health literature often have rapidly diminishing returns. Although important studies are occasionally reported in obscure medical journals that are not indexed in any of the main medical databases, these situations are fairly rare. For most clinicians, a simple but educated search of the literature using several keywords in PubMed should be sufficient to provide most of the essential information. Such searches will often uncover systematic reviews (SRs) that have previously been conducted on that topic using much more thorough and exhaustive literature searching methods than those accessible and practical for clinicians to reproduce themselves.

Categorizing Studies by Design

Once available studies have been identified, it can be helpful to categorize them according to their study design, which commonly includes clinical practice guidelines (CPGs), SRs, RCTs, non-RCTs, prospective observational studies (OBSs), retrospective OBSs, case reports, and expert opinion.

Clinical Practice Guidelines

CPGs are often broad recommendations made for clinicians facing specific scenarios, and are usually conducted by a multidisciplinary panel of expert clinicians, scientists, decision makers, and patients who interpret the best available scientific evidence at that time.[38,39] CPGs are often sponsored by professional medical societies or government entities, and usually begin by conducting an SR of the literature.

Systematic Reviews

SRs are studies that search, evaluate, summarize, and synthesize the results of available studies related to one or more important but specific research questions.[38,39] The methods used in SRs are becoming increasingly standardized, and the validity of their conclusions is dependent on the way they were conducted. Organizations such as the Cochrane Collaboration conduct and disseminate high-quality SRs on a variety of topics. SRs differ from traditional narrative reviews by clearly stating their objectives, specific search methods and results, study eligibility criteria, screening methods, methodologic quality evaluation criteria, and methods to summarize results. Meta-analyses are SRs in which the results of multiple studies are combined statistically to increase the ability to detect clinically meaningful differences.

Randomized Controlled Trials

RCTs are clinical studies in which willing participants with a particular medical condition who meet stated eligibility criteria are assigned, by chance, to an intervention and their results are compared with those of participants assigned, by chance, to another intervention designated as a control group.[34] Although the control group for RCTs evaluating medications is often a placebo, the control group may also be another medication, a medical or surgical procedure, an educational, exercise, or manual therapy intervention, or any other intervention against which the first is compared to answer the stated research question. RCTs are very important in EBM because the process of assigning participants to an intervention by chance minimizes the possibility of biased results common to OBSs.[38]

Nonrandomized Controlled Trials

Non-RCTs are clinical studies in which willing participants with a particular medical condition who meet stated eligibility criteria are assigned to an intervention and their results are compared with those of participants assigned to another intervention designated as a control group. The control group may be a placebo, a medication, a medical or surgical procedure, an educational, exercise, or manual therapy intervention, or any other intervention against which the first is compared to answer the stated research question. Because participants are not assigned at random, their assignment to a particular intervention or control group may be based on factors that are also related to their expected success and personal preference. This nonrandomized method of assigning patients to groups may increase the possibility of observing biased results.[39] There is also a substantial risk that the results will be confounded by factors that caused the patient to choose a treatment approach and the groups being compared may differ substantially in multiple characteristics that invalidate any conclusions.[34,38,39]

Prospective Observational Studies

Prospective OBSs are clinical studies in which willing participants with a particular medical condition who meet other stated eligibility criteria receive an intervention and their results are measured over time. Because they often lack a control group, it is difficult to attribute the results observed in these studies solely to the intervention, in that other factors may also be important (e.g., natural history of the disease). These studies may, however, be useful in determining prognostic factors that influence outcome and the incidence of harms that result from a treatment approach.[39,40]

Retrospective Observational Studies

Retrospective OBSs are clinical studies in which the results of patients with a particular medical condition who received an intervention are aggregated based on information available from their medical records. Because they often lack a control group, did not collect sufficient outcomes data, are unaware of other interventions participants may have received, and have fairly heterogeneous populations, it is difficult to attribute the results observed in these studies solely to the intervention because other factors may also be important (e.g., natural history of the disease).[41] The results of these studies are rarely accepted as valid information because they do not usually have a prospective information gathering process or properly considered research question, and patients are either not informed of the study or cannot be located for follow-up.

Case Reports/Series

Case reports and case series are clinical studies in which clinicians describe in some detail the clinical characteristics of one (case report) or several (case series) particularly interesting patients whose management they were involved in. Opinions and theories are then offered about the results observed, which may be helpful to discover new or unusual manifestations of clinical conditions, or provide an initial report of novel interventions. These case reports may also be of some value in documenting rare negative outcomes or harms that result following a treatment approach.[38]

Expert Opinion

Expert opinion can take many forms in the published literature, but is typically characterized by an abundance of opinions, theories, conjectures, and personal philosophies and a dearth of specific, objective, or measurable data to offer independent support for those statements. Expert opinion can nevertheless be important to opine on controversial areas, in which no other data are available or forthcoming, or to stimulate thought and encourage specific research projects.

Pyramid of Evidence

Once a clinician has conducted a literature search and categorized studies according to their design, their respective merits must then be evaluated. If multiple homogeneous RCTs are identified, their results may be combined and compared fairly easily. Similarly, results from multiple homogeneous OBSs may also be combined. However, there is no universally accepted quantitative method for combining results from studies with different designs. This has often led to results from studies other than RCTs being dismissed entirely from literature reviews. While this is occasionally appropriate, EBM generally encourages clinicians to consider all available evidence, not only that from RCTs.[42] This does not mean that results from OBSs will be given the same weight as those from RCTs, but they should nevertheless be considered. In some instances, results from a well conducted OBS study may be more clinically important to the decision being made

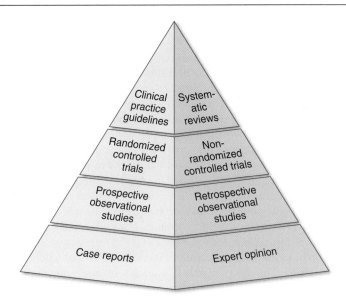

Figure 1-1 Pyramid of evidence-based medicine.

than those from a poorly conducted RCT that is only tangentially relevant.

This process is qualitative and it can be quite challenging for a clinician to reconcile positive results reported in a prospective OBS with poor results reported in an RCT. To facilitate this process, it can be helpful to refer to the pyramid of evidence. This concept is based on the premise that specific study designs are more likely to report uncertain results that may later be contradicted by more rigorously performed studies. Each study design has its strengths and weaknesses, and may be the most appropriate or relevant at a particular time. However, when viewed globally, some study designs are more prone to bias and confounding. This concept is illustrated as a pyramid, in which more robust study designs are placed at the top and are built on the results of the more numerous and less robust studies below[43]; this concept is illustrated in Figure 1-1.

Evaluating Methodologic Quality

The hierarchy of evidence is an important concept to help illustrate the relative merits of different study designs, but ignores the methodologic quality of studies. Not all CPGs, SRs, RCTs, and OBSs are created equally, and notable differences do exist in the methodologic rigor with which they were designed, conducted, and reported. Because the methodologic quality of a study is related to the probability that its results are biased, it is important for clinicians to understand and acknowledge the criteria used to evaluate the methodologic quality for common study designs, including CPGs, SRs, RCTs, and OBSs.

Clinical Practice Guidelines

The methodologic quality of CPGs can be evaluated using a tool proposed by the Appraisal of Guidelines Research & Evaluation (AGREE) group, which contains 23 items in six dimensions, as well as an overall assessment of whether the CPG is useful.[44] Each item can be answered on a scale from

1 (strongly agree) to 4 (strongly disagree), although no total score should be calculated when using this tool.[44] No thresholds are available to determine whether a CPG is of higher or lower methodologic quality. The criteria suggested by this tool to evaluate CPGs are summarized in Box 1-2. Numerous other criteria are also available to help evaluate the methodology and reporting quality of CPGs.

Systematic Reviews

The methodologic quality of SRs can be evaluated using a tool proposed by the Cochrane Collaboration, which contains 10 questions that should be considered. Answers are not scored, and no thresholds are available to determine whether an SR is of higher or lower methodologic quality. The criteria suggested by this tool to evaluate SRs are summarized in Box 1-3. Numerous other criteria are also available to help evaluate the methodology and reporting quality of SRs.

Randomized Controlled Trials

The methodologic quality of RCTs can be evaluated using a tool proposed by the Cochrane Back Review Group (CBRG), which is the Cochrane Collaboration group tasked with the development of SRs related to back and neck pain and other spinal disorders. This tool contains 11 questions, which can be answered "yes", "no", or "unsure."[45] Studies in which at least six of the questions can be answered "yes", and in which no serious flaws are identified, can be considered of higher methodologic quality, whereas others are of lower methodologic quality.[45] The criteria suggested by this tool to evaluate RCTs are summarized in Box 1-4. Numerous other criteria are also available to help evaluate the methodology and reporting quality of RCTs.

Observational Studies

The methodologic quality of RCTs can be evaluated using the Newcastle-Ottawa Scale (NOS), which contains eight questions across three dimensions with two to four multiple choice answers.[46] Answers are not scored, and no thresholds are available to determine whether an OBS is of higher or lower methodologic quality.[46] The criteria suggested by the NOS tool to evaluate OBSs are summarized in Box 1-5. Numerous other criteria are also available to help evaluate the methodology and reporting quality of OBSs.

Summarizing Evidence

After having identified available studies through a literature search, categorized them according to their study design, considered their relative propensity for reporting biased results according to the pyramid of evidence, and evaluated their methodologic quality using various criteria, clinicians are then left with the task of summarizing this evidence. Several systems have been proposed for doing this in the context of EBM. They usually involve determining which of several categories (or levels) of evidence is most appropriate for a particular conclusion based on the type, quantity, and quality of available studies. Levels of evidence are often assigned both alphabetic (e.g., level A/I, B/II, C/III, D/IV) and descriptive nomenclature (e.g., strong, moderate, limited,

---

BOX 1-2	Criteria for Evaluating Clinical Practice Guidelines

Scope and Purpose
1. Overall objectives of the guideline are specifically described.
2. Clinical questions covered by the guideline are specifically described.
3. Patients to whom the guideline is meant to apply are specifically described.

Stakeholder Involvement
4. Guideline development group includes individuals from all the relevant professional groups.
5. Patients' views and preferences have been sought.
6. Target users of the guideline are clearly defined.
7. Guideline has been piloted among target users.

Rigor of Development
8. Systematic methods were used to search for evidence.
9. Criteria for selecting the evidence are clearly described.
10. Methods used for formulating the recommendations are clearly described.
11. Health benefits, side effects, and risks have been considered in formulating the recommendations.
12. There is an explicit link between the recommendations and the supporting evidence.
13. Guideline has been externally reviewed by experts before its publication.
14. A procedure for updating the guideline is provided.

Clarity and Presentation
15. Recommendations are specific and unambiguous.
16. Different options for management of the condition are clearly presented.
17. Key recommendations are easily identifiable.
18. Guideline is supported with tools for application.

Applicability
19. Potential organizational barriers in applying the recommendations have been discussed.
20. Potential cost implications of applying the recommendations have been considered.
21. Guideline presents key review criteria for monitoring or audit purposes.

Editorial Independence
22. Guideline is editorially independent from the funding body.
23. Conflicts of interest of guideline development members have been recorded.

Overall Score
24. Would you recommend these guidelines for use in practice?

Development and validation of an international appraisal instrument for assessing the quality of clinical practice guidelines: the AGREE project. Qual Saf Health Care 2003;12:18-23.

BOX 1-3	Criteria for Evaluating Systematic Reviews

1. Did the review address a clearly focused question?
2. Did the authors look for the appropriate sort of papers?
3. Do you think the important, relevant studies were included?
4. Did the authors do enough to assess the quality of included studies?
5. If the results of the review have been combined, was it reasonable to do so?
6. What is the overall result of the review?
7. How precise are the results?
8. Can the results be applied to the local population?
9. Were all the important outcomes considered?
10. Are the benefits worth the harms and costs?

From Del Mar CB, Glasziou PP. Antibiotics for sore throat (Cochrane review) in The Cochrane Library Issue 3, 1999 Oxford: Update Software. http://ssrc.tums.ac.ir/SystematicReview/Glasgow.asp.

BOX 1-4	Criteria for Evaluating Randomized Controlled Trials

1. Was the method of randomization adequate?
2. Was the treatment allocation concealed?
3. Was the patient blinded to the intervention?
4. Was the care provider blinded to the intervention?
5. Was the outcome assessor blinded to the intervention?
6. Was the dropout rate described and acceptable?
7. Were all randomized participants analyzed in the group to which they were allocated?
8. Are reports of the study free of suggestion of selective outcome reporting?
9. Were the groups similar at baseline regarding the most important prognostic indicators?
10. Were co-interventions avoided or similar?
11. Was the compliance acceptable in all groups?
12. Was the timing of the outcome assessment similar in all groups?

Furlan AD, Pennick V, Bombardier C, van TM. 2009 Updated method guidelines for systematic reviews in the Cochrane Back Review Group. Spine (Phila Pa 1976) 2009;34:1929-1941.

BOX 1-5	Criteria for Evaluating Observational Studies

Selection
1. Representativeness of the exposed cohort
2. Selection of the nonexposed cohort
3. Ascertainment of exposure
4. Demonstration that outcome of interest was not present at start of study

Comparability
5. Comparability of cohorts on the basis of the design or analysis

Outcome
6. Assessment of outcome
7. Was follow-up long enough for outcomes to occur
8. Adequacy of follow up of cohorts

Wells G, Shea B, O'Connel D, et al. Newcastle-Ottawa scale (NOS) for assessing the quality of non randomised studies in meta-analysis. http://www.ohri.ca/programs/clinical_epidemiology/oxford.htm.

TABLE 1-1	Levels of Evidence	
Level	Evidence	Supporting Evidence
A	Strong	Generally consistent findings provided by systematic review of multiple high-quality RCTs
B	Moderate	Generally consistent findings provided by systematic review of: i. at least four low-quality RCTs ii. at least two high-quality RCTs
C	Limited	One RCT (either of low or high quality) Inconsistent findings from systematic review of at least four RCTs
D	None	No RCTs

RCT, randomized controlled trial.
Data from American College of Occupational and Environmental Medicine. Low back disorders. In: Occupational medicine practice guidelines: evaluation and management of common health problems and functional recovery in workers, edited by L.S. Glass, Elk Grove Village, (IL): American College of Occupational and Environmental Medicine (ACOEM), 2006.

none). The number of levels of evidence used in these systems varies from three to eight, although the criteria required to meet the highest and lowest levels are often similar; one such classification system is summarized in Table 1-1.

THE GOAL OF THIS TEXTBOOK

As noted in this introduction, there remain considerable challenges that face the development of a cohesive approach to LBP that is likely to reduce its burden to both individuals and to society. It is our opinion that none of the current books on the topic provide the information on the different treatment approaches that are available to patients and clinicians in a manner that allows for adequate comparison of the different management options. The goal of this book is to reduce the confusion amongst clinicians and patients and to allow stakeholders to place the different approaches to the management of LBP in some context. The intention is that readers of this book will be able to compare the rationale for each treatment, the cost and reimbursement, the evidence supporting each treatment approach, and the indications, contraindications, and potential harms posed by each treatment. This book provides the information necessary for clinicians, patients, and policy makers to make informed decisions when considering the different treatment approaches to LBP.

The current scenario in which clinicians involved in the management of common LBP work in silos and make recommendations based mostly on their personal experience cannot continue. Because no single health care discipline has all of the answers when it comes to managing LBP, clinicians must learn to work together to offer multidisciplinary and coordinated care centered on the patient. This first requires that clinicians learn about the multitude of available treatment options using a common metric and language. In this book, we asked our authors to apply the principles of EBM and present the relative merits of different study designs, assess their methodologic quality, and summarize their results into levels of evidence-based support, thereby allowing the clinician to determine the confidence that can be placed in the underlying studies.

The clinicians and stakeholders who use this text will be informed about each of the different treatment options available to patients with LBP and will be aware of the best available scientific evidence on each of these approaches. Only then can clinicians appreciate where their professional experience and opinion are most necessary to fill in the gaps. With this knowledge, clinicians can then educate their patients about the relative advantages and disadvantages of the approach they are recommending and compare that approach with available options to achieve truly informed consent. This book assembles the information that is necessary to begin this process. A description of the information contained in each section is provided in the next chapter. In the summary chapter, we review the available evidence and provide the reader with a review of how the information from the chapters in this text is currently being interpreted.

REFERENCES

1. Walker BF. The prevalence of low back pain: a systematic review of the literature from 1966 to 1998. J Spinal Disord 2000;13:205-217.
2. Airaksinen O, Brox JI, Cedraschi C, et al. European guidelines for the management of chronic nonspecific low back pain. Eur Spine J 2006;15(Suppl 2):192-300.
3. Nielens H, van Zundert J, Mairiaux P, et al. Chronic low back pain, Vol. 48C. Brussels: KCE Reports; 2006.
4. Burton AK, Clarke RD, McClune TD, et al. The natural history of low back pain in adolescents. Spine 1996;21:2323-2328.
5. Gozna E. For the Workplace Health Safety and Compensation Commission of New Brunswick. Guidelines for the diagnosis and treatment of low back pain. New Brunswick, Canada: WHSCC of New Brunswick; 2001.
6. Bogduk N. Evidence-based clinical guidelines for the management of acute low back pain. Submitted to the Medical Health and Research Council of Australia, November 1999.
7. Coste J, Delecoeuillerie G, Cohen de LA, et al. Clinical course and prognostic factors in acute low back pain: an inception cohort study in primary care practice. BMJ 1994;308:577-580.
8. van Tulder M, Becker A, Bekkering T, et al. European guidelines for the management of acute nonspecific low back pain in primary care. Eur Spine J 2006;15(Suppl 2):169-191.
9. University of Michigan Health System. Acute low back pain. Ann Arbor, MI: University of Michigan Health System; 2003.
10. Deyo RA, Cherkin D, Conrad D, et al. Cost, controversy, crisis: low back pain and the health of the public. Annu Rev Public Health 1991;12:141-156.
11. Loeser JD, Volinn E. Epidemiology of low back pain. Neurosurg Clin N Am 1991;2:713-718.
12. Leboeuf-Yde C, Lauritsen JM, Lauritzen T. Why has the search for causes of low back pain largely been nonconclusive? Spine 1997;22:877-881.
13. Skovron ML. Epidemiology of low back pain. Baillieres Clin Rheumatol 1992;6:559-573.
14. McIntosh G, Hall H. Low back pain (chronic). Clin Evid (Online) 2008;pii:1116.
15. McIntosh G, Hall H. Low back pain (acute). Clin Evid (Online) 2008;pii:1102.
16. UK Clinical Standards Advisory Group. Clinical guidelines for the management of acute low back pain. London: Royal College of General Practitioners; 2001.
17. Deyo RA, Bass JE. Lifestyle and low-back pain. The influence of smoking and obesity. Spine 1989;14:501-506.
18. Zhang Y, Sun Z, Liu J, Guo X. Advances in susceptibility genetics of intervertebral degenerative disc disease. Int J Biol Sci, 2008;4:283-290.
19. Australian Acute Musculoskeletal Pain guidelines Group. Evidence-based management of acute musculoskeletal pain. Brisbane, Australia: Australian Academic Press Pty Ltd; 2003.
20. Danish Institute for Health Technology Assessment. Low-back pain: frequency, management, and prevention from an HTA perspective. Copenhagen, Denmark: National Board of Health; 1999.
21. Jensen MC, Brant-Zawadzki MN, Obuchowski N, et al. Magnetic resonance imaging of the lumbar spine in people without back pain. N Engl J Med 1994;331:69-73.
22. Boden SD, Davis DO, Dina TS, et al. Abnormal magnetic-resonance scans of the lumbar spine in asymptomatic subjects. A prospective investigation. J Bone Joint Surg Am 1990;72:403-408.
23. Boos N, Semmer N, Elfering A, et al. Natural history of individuals with asymptomatic disc abnormalities in magnetic resonance imaging: predictors of low back pain-related medical consultation and work incapacity. Spine 2000;25:1484-1492.
24. Borenstein DG, O'Mara JW Jr, Boden SD, et al. The value of magnetic resonance imaging of the lumbar spine to predict low-back pain in asymptomatic subjects: a seven-year follow-up study. J Bone Joint Surg Am 2001;83-A:1306-1311.
25. Weishaupt D, Zanetti M, Hodler J, et al. MR imaging of the lumbar spine: prevalence of intervertebral disk extrusion and sequestration, nerve root compression, end plate abnormalities, and osteoarthritis of the facet joints in asymptomatic volunteers. Radiology 1998;209:661-666.
26. Wiesel SW, Tsourmas N, Feffer HL, et al. A study of computer-assisted tomography. I. The incidence of positive CAT scans in an asymptomatic group of patients. Spine 1984;9:549-551.
27. Borkan J, Reis S, Werner S, et al. [Guidelines for treating low back pain in primary care. The Israeli Low Back Pain Guideline Group]. Harefuah 1996;130:145-151.
28. The Norwegian Back Pain Network, The Communication Unit. Acute low back pain: interdisciplinary clinical guidelines. Oslo, Norway: The Norwegian Back Pain Network; 2002.
29. Martin BI, Deyo RA, Mirza SK, et al. Expenditures and health status among adults with back and neck problems. JAMA 2008;299:656-664.
30. Dagenais S, Caro J, Haldeman S. A systematic review of low back pain cost of illness studies in the United States and internationally. Spine J 2008;8:8-20.

31. Koopmanschap MA, Rutten FF. Indirect costs in economic studies: confronting the confusion. Pharmacoeconomics 1993;4:446-454.

32. Andersson GB. Epidemiological features of chronic low-back pain. Lancet 1999;354:581-585.

33. Waddell G. Biopsychosocial analysis of low back pain. Bailliere's Clin Rheumatol 1992;6:523-557.

34. Manchikanti L, Heavner JE, Racz GB, et al. Methods for evidence synthesis in interventional pain management. Pain Physician 2003;6:89-111.

35. Straus SE, McAlister FA. Evidence-based medicine: a commentary on common criticisms. CMAJ 2000;163:837-841.

36. Feinstein AR, Horwitz RI. Problems in the "evidence" of "evidence-based medicine." Am J Med 1997;103:529-535.

37. Guyatt G, Cook D, Haynes B. Evidence based medicine has come a long way. BMJ 2004;329:990-991.

38. Manchikanti L, Abdi S, Lucas LF. Evidence synthesis and development of guidelines in interventional pain management. Pain Physician 2005;8:73-86.

39. Chou R. Evidence-based medicine and the challenge of low back pain: where are we now? Pain Pract 2005;5:153-178.

40. Hoppe DJ, Schemitsch EH, Morshed S, et al. Hierarchy of evidence: where observational studies fit in and why we need them. J Bone Joint Surg Am 2009;91(Suppl 3):2-9.

41. Hess DR. Retrospective studies and chart reviews. Respir Care 2004;49:1171-1174.

42. Sackett DL, Rosenberg WM, Gray JA, et al. Evidence based medicine: what it is and what it isn't. BMJ 1996; 312:71-72.

43. Bernstein J. Evidence-based medicine. J Am Acad Orthop Surg 2004;12:80-88.

44. Development and validation of an international appraisal instrument for assessing the quality of clinical practice guidelines: the AGREE project. Qual Saf Health Care 2003; 12:18-23.

45. van Tulder M, Furlan A, Bombardier C, et al. Updated method guidelines for systematic reviews in the Cochrane Collaboration Back Review Group. Spine 2003;28:1290-1299.

46. Wells G, Shea B, O'Connel D, et al. Newcastle-Ottawa scale (NOS) for assessing the quality of non randomised studies in meta-analysis. http://www.ohri.ca/programs/clinical_epidemiology/oxford.htm.

SIMON DAGENAIS
SCOTT HALDEMAN

CHAPTER 2

Guide to Using This Textbook

BOOK SECTIONS

This book is organized into 11 sections, including one section for introductory chapters and ten sections pertaining to broad categories of interventions for low back pain (LBP). Those ten categories include educational therapies, exercise therapies, medications, physical modalities, manual therapies, complementary and alternative medicine, behavioral therapies, injection therapies, minimally invasive therapies, and surgical therapies. These categories are not meant to be mutually exclusive, and it is recognized that the division between certain categories may be quite blurry. An attempt was also made to present these categories in the order in which a typical patient with common LBP may navigate through the maze of available therapies, from least to most invasive. This presentation is imperfect and does not apply to all (or even most) patients with common LBP, some of whom may need to proceed immediately to surgical therapies while others may only resort to medications. This ordering is simply offered as a method of organizing the contents of this book and should not be interpreted as ascribing any particular worth to the interventions discussed in each chapter.

CHAPTER FORMAT

The main goal of this book is to educate clinicians from a wide variety of health care disciplines about the relative merits of the many interventions currently offered for the management of LBP based on the best available supporting scientific evidence and expert opinion. To achieve this goal and facilitate comparing the information available for different treatments, each intervention uses a common chapter format. This format reflects the information that was thought to be most important for clinicians to understand and evaluate the many different interventions with which they may not be familiar. Each chapter contains five main sections: (1) description, (2) theory, (3) efficacy, (4) safety, and (5) costs. In addition, each chapter contains a summary section. A description of the information presented in each of these sections is provided below.

Section 1—Description

This section is intended to provide basic information about the interventions discussed so that a clinician who is not familiar with that particular approach may understand basic terminology, any relevant subtypes found within that intervention, a brief description of its history, an estimate of the frequency with which those with common LBP may use it, the type of health care practitioner who offers this intervention, in which settings and locations it is available, a description of how it is performed, and the regulatory status of any medication or medical device relevant to that intervention. Additional information on each segment in this section follows.

Terminology and Subtypes

Practitioners often use medical or technical jargon that can be misunderstood even by highly trained health providers from slightly different disciplines. This can create a barrier to effective communication and lead to misunderstandings about the concepts being discussed. This segment is intended to list and define any special terminology that may be important to understanding the interventions reviewed, including commonly used synonyms. This segment should also make readers aware of any subtypes that may be relevant to understanding how a particular intervention fits within the broader context of other similar approaches.

History and Frequency of Use

Some of the interventions used for LBP can trace their origins back to approaches used thousands of years ago (e.g., spinal manipulation), whereas others are based on relatively recent discoveries or inventions (e.g., X-STOP).[1] Interventions that were once in favor may be discarded, only to be rediscovered decades later (e.g., manipulation under anesthesia).[2] Understanding the genesis and evolution of interventions can be helpful to evaluating their role in the management of LBP. This segment is intended to briefly describe the origins and important milestones of an intervention. This segment is also intended to provide some estimate about the frequency of use for a particular intervention to give some idea of how commonly it is employed by those with LBP, often based on health care utilization surveys, if available.

Practitioner, Setting, and Availability

Numerous clinicians are involved in the management of LBP, few of whom know much about the specific interventions offered by those outside their specialty. Although some clinicians are primarily associated with one type of therapy (e.g., surgeons and surgery), others may in fact be trained to offer a multitude of therapies but do not routinely practice all of them (e.g., physiatrists and medication, injections, and minimally invasive interventions). Some interventions are widely offered by a variety of clinicians (e.g., spinal manipulation and chiropractors, physical therapists, and osteopaths), whereas others are fairly atypical with few qualified practitioners (e.g., prolotherapy). This segment is intended to describe the type of clinician most commonly associated with a particular intervention, as well as the clinical setting in which it is administered, and provide some estimate of its availability across the United States.

Procedure

Some of the interventions used for LBP have nomenclature that is fairly descriptive and provides a general idea about what is actually involved (e.g., artificial disc replacement), whereas others have names that may seem somewhat misleading when details are sought about the procedure (e.g., minimally invasive interventions). Others may have names that do not provide any information about the nature of the treatment (e.g., X-STOP). Clinicians may therefore be acquainted with the names of many interventions, but may not be familiar with their precise nature. This segment is intended to provide a broad description of how the intervention is actually performed, although it is not intended to be a teaching manual for those interested in learning new techniques.

Regulatory Status

Many of the interventions used for LBP are techniques or procedures practiced by licensed health care professionals (e.g., massage therapy given by massage therapists) that are not subject to specific regulatory approval by federal authorities, such as the US Food and Drug Administration (FDA). In the United States, only medications and medical devices used to address specific health conditions are subject to regulation and approval by the FDA.[3] The regulatory approval process for medications in the United States is fairly rigorous. Manufacturers must first submit an investigational new drug application to the FDA summarizing the results of preclinical studies demonstrating safety and efficacy in different species of animals.[4] They can then obtain permission to conduct progressively larger clinical studies in healthy humans or participants with the targeted disease using different medication doses and lengths of follow-up (e.g., phase 1, 2, and 3).[4] Final approval is then sought from the FDA to market a medication for the defined indication studied in the clinical trials through a new drug application.[4]

The regulatory approval process for medical devices depends on the three classes recognized by the FDA (e.g., class I, II, and III).[5] Class I medical devices generally pose a very low risk of harms when used correctly (e.g., bandages, thermometers).[5] Class II medical devices are more complex and require greater training and prudence in their usage (e.g.,

x-ray machine, surgical sutures).[5] Class III medical devices include implants (e.g., joint replacement) and equipment used to monitor life-preserving function (e.g., pacemaker).[5] The supporting information required by the FDA increases substantially for each class. Medical devices may also be approved based on their similarity to previously approved medical devices, although greater latitude is used in the interpretation of this tenet for medical devices than medications.

Use of a medication for conditions other than its FDA approved indication is termed "off-label" and is generally left to the prescribing physician's discretion.[6] However, off-label use cannot be promoted by its manufacturer and supporting information must be provided to the FDA to formally expand the approved indication for a medication that is already on the market. Because manufacturers often pursue the indication most likely to be approved based on the supporting evidence provided, it can be revealing to discover that a medication often used for one purpose (e.g., sciatica) was in fact approved for another (e.g., postherpetic neuralgia).

Section 2—Theory

This section is intended to provide basic information about the scientific and clinical theories related to the interventions discussed, for clinicians who may not be familiar with that particular approach, including its proposed mechanism of action, indication, and any diagnostic testing required. Additional information on each segment in this section is provided below.

Mechanism of Action

Interventions are often developed in response to the specific etiology of a medical condition (e.g., antipyretic medication for acute fever). Understanding the disease process can therefore provide some insight into its appropriate management by matching the intervention to the observed pathophysiology. However, this process can be quite challenging for a condition such as common LBP whose etiology is so poorly understood. Numerous anatomic structures have been implicated in the development of LBP (e.g., intervertebral discs, vertebrae, nerve roots) with corresponding interventions aimed at their eradication (e.g., discectomy, laminectomy, rhizotomy). Similarly, many disease constructs have been proposed to explain the presence of LBP (e.g., poor motor control or strength, hypomobility, emotional distress), also with analogous interventions (e.g., exercise therapy, spinal manipulation, cognitive behavioral therapy). This segment is intended to discuss the proposed mechanism of action for various interventions, if known, and to discuss any basic science studies supporting that mechanism.

Indication

Although this book is focused on the management of LBP, not every treatment discussed is appropriate for each patient with LBP. It is reasonable to assume that interventions intended to alleviate instability (e.g., arthrodesis) should be targeting a different group of patients with LBP than those that aim to improve hypomobility (e.g., spinal manipulation under anesthesia). Expert clinicians who routinely manage LBP often develop specific indications for the interventions they offer. This segment is intended to highlight some of the specific indications (if any) for the interventions discussed beyond simply having LBP.

Assessment

Despite the difficulty faced by clinicians who attempt to pursue a specific anatomic source for common LBP, many interventions do in fact require some form of diagnostic testing before being implemented. It is assumed that all interventions discussed in this book require a clinician to first rule out the possibility that symptoms may be related to potentially serious spinal or other pathology. Rather than repeating the steps involved in the basic assessment of LBP for each intervention, that process is described in detail in one of the introductory chapters. This segment is intended to describe any specific diagnostic testing required before initiating a particular intervention once a basic assessment has been conducted to rule out serious or specific pathologies related to LBP.

Section 3—Efficacy

This section is often the longest in a chapter and may be the one on which more attention is focused by clinicians evaluating various interventions. A distinction is often made by clinical researchers between efficacy, which is how well an intervention works in a controlled research setting such as a clinical trial, and effectiveness, which is how well an intervention works in the real world after the clinical trials are completed and it is more widely adopted by practicing clinicians. Not surprisingly, the effectiveness of interventions for common LBP is often less impressive than their preliminary efficacy as their use grows beyond simply the ideal patient.

Such differences are also noted in the efficacy reported by various study designs. Large improvements noted in prospective observational studies (OBSs) may diminish in randomized controlled trials (RCTs), or positive results noted in some RCTs may be offset by negative results in other RCTs

when systematic reviews (SRs) are conducted. It is therefore important for clinicians to reconcile the evidence available from a variety of study designs. To facilitate this process, the evidence in this section is presented by study design according to the hierarchy suggested by the pyramid of evidence discussed in Chapter 1. Attempts were also made to standardize the sources of information summarized in this section, as described here.

Clinical Practice Guidelines

An SR was recently conducted to identify clinical practice guidelines (CPGs) related to the diagnosis and management of LBP, that had been sponsored by national organizations and for which English language reports had been published in the past decade; 10 such CPGs were found (Table 2-1).[7] This segment of the section on efficacy is intended to provide a succinct summary of the conclusions from these CPGs on the interventions reviewed. Not all CPGs reviewed each of the interventions in this book, and not all interventions were in fact evaluated in any of these CPGs; some chapters also discussed conclusions from CPGs other than those listed in Table 2-1.

Systematic Reviews

The Cochrane Back Review Group (CBRG) is one of 50 review groups focused on specific topics, which together form the Cochrane Collaboration.[8] As of February 2010, the CBRG has conducted 45 SRs on a variety of topics related to spinal disorders, including 31 related to interventions for LBP. In addition, the two CPGs related to LBP that were sponsored by the American Pain Society (APS) and the American College of Physicians (ACP) were each accompanied by two SRs that evaluated and summarized the best available scientific evidence for many interventions.[9-14] This segment of the section on efficacy is intended to briefly summarize the conclusions from these specific SRs, which are summarized in Table 2-2. Not all interventions were discussed in this group of SRs; some chapters also discussed conclusions from SRs other than those listed in Table 2-2 where the authors deemed this appropriate.

TABLE 2-1	Recent National Clinical Practice Guidelines	
Country	**Year**	**Title**
Australia	2003	Evidence-based management of acute musculoskeletal pain
Belgium	2006	Chronic low back pain. Good clinical practice
Europe	2006	European guidelines for the management of acute nonspecific low back pain in primary care
Europe	2005	European guidelines for the management of chronic nonspecific low back pain in primary care
Italy	2006	Diagnostic therapeutic flow charts for low back pain patients: the Italian clinical guidelines
New Zealand	2004	Acute low back pain guide
Norway	2002	Acute low back pain: interdisciplinary clinical guidelines
United Kingdom	2009	Low back pain: early management of persistent nonspecific low back pain
United States	2009	Interventional therapies, surgery, and interdisciplinary rehabilitation for low back pain: an evidence-based clinical practice guideline from the American Pain Society
United States	2007	Diagnosis and treatment of low back pain: a joint clinical practice guideline from the American College of Physicians and the American Pain Society

TABLE 2-2	Recent Systematic Reviews	
Organization	Year	Topic
APS	2009	Interventional therapies, surgery, and interdisciplinary rehabilitation for low back pain
APS	2009	Surgery for low back pain
APS/ACP	2007	Medications for acute and chronic low back pain
APS/ACP	2007	Nonpharmacologic therapies for acute and chronic low back pain
CBRG	2000	NSAIDs for low back pain
CBRG	2003	Back schools for non-specific low back pain
CBRG	2003	Muscle relaxants for nonspecific low back pain
CBRG	2003	Work conditioning, work hardening, and functional restoration for workers with back and neck pain
CBRG	2003	Radiofrequency denervation for neck and back pain. A systematic review of randomized controlled trials
CBRG	2004	Spinal manipulative therapy for low back pain
CBRG	2005	Exercise therapy for treatment of non-specific low back pain
CBRG	2005	Acupuncture and dry needling for low back pain
CBRG	2005	Behavioral treatment for chronic low back pain
CBRG	2005	Surgery for degenerative lumbar spondylosis
CBRG	2006	Opioids for chronic low back pain
CBRG	2006	Herbal medicine for low back pain
CBRG	2007	Traction for low back pain with or without sciatica
CBRG	2007	Prolotherapy injections for chronic low back pain
CBRG	2008	Individual patient education for low back pan
CBRG	2008	Antidepressants for nonspecific low back pain
CBRG	2008	Massage for low back pain
CBRG	2008	TENS versus placebo for chronic low back pain
CBRG	2008	Injection therapy for subacute and chronic low back pain

ACP, American College of Physicians; APS, American Pain Society; CBRG, Cochrane Back Review Group; NSAIDs, nonsteroidal anti-inflammatory drugs; TENS, transcutaneous electrical nerve stimulation.

Randomized Controlled Trials

RCTs are often viewed as the gold standard clinical evidence to determine the true relative efficacy of an intervention.[15] There are several advantages to RCTs when compared with OBSs, chiefly their ability to reduce bias and confounding that may be associated with factors that could otherwise influence both group assignment and prognosis.[15] However, it can be quite challenging to design and conduct high-quality RCTs for common LBP which does not have clear diagnostic criteria that are easily transferable from one study to another, and for which outcomes are largely self-reported and therefore subjective. This is only magnified by the difficulties associated with devising methods for blinding and selecting appropriate control groups for interventions that are much more complex than tablets or capsules. These caveats are mentioned to provide context to clinicians interpreting reports of RCTs. This segment of the section on efficacy is intended to summarize RCTs that were included in the SRs summarized in the previous segment (e.g. SRs from CBRG and ACP/APS). The conclusion of RCT methodological quality as reported in the CBRG reviews (e.g. higher or lower quality) was also indicated in this segment when such evaluations were available from previous SRs. Some chapters also discussed other RCTs not previously reviewed in SRs from the CBRG or ACP/APS; methodological quality was not formally evaluated for those RCTs.

Observational Studies

OBSs are often the starting point for evaluating the efficacy of interventions that are deemed promising by clinicians or researchers.[16] It can often be difficult to interpret their results, because these studies are rarely designed to answer the same research questions as RCTs.[16,17] Issues of bias and confounding are common, and it is unclear whether the results reported by participants are truly attributable to the interventions studied.[15] The methodologic quality of OBSs may also vary as it is less established and standardized than for RCTs. Nevertheless, OBSs offer an initial estimate of efficacy to identify interventions that may later be evaluated through RCTs. This segment of the section on efficacy is intended to summarize certain OBSs in instances in which there were no RCTs available, or when specific OBSs discussed were nevertheless thought to be important by the authors.

Section 4—Safety

Many clinicians involved in the management of LBP focus their attention on the efficacy of various interventions. This is understandable since most patients are seeking care in the hope of alleviating their symptoms, and the probability of this happening is related to an intervention's efficacy. In doing so, clinicians may overlook the importance of one of the basic tenets of medicine, *primum non nocere*, which requires a careful evaluation of an intervention's safety.[18] This discussion encapsulates both contraindications, which are important to improve safety, and adverse events (AEs), which describe previously reported safety concerns.

Contraindications

Contraindications are patient characteristics that may suggest that a patient is at an increased risk of experiencing poor outcomes with a given intervention that may be best avoided when those factors are present.[19] Contraindications may be related to age, gender, obesity, smoking status, general health, systemic, psychiatric, or genetic comorbidities, medication use, personal preferences, or a variety of other factors. Contraindications may also be relative (suggesting that the intervention carries some risk but may still be appropriate in that patient) or absolute (suggesting that the risk presented by the intervention exceeds its expected benefit and should not be performed). Contraindications may be important when considering various treatment options, some of which may be eliminated from contention if they are not appropriate for a given patient.

Adverse Events

The term *adverse event* is used instead of terms such as *side effects* or *complications,* which can be difficult to distinguish and may carry certain unintended connotations (e.g., side effects are "normal"; complications are the doctor's fault).[20] An AE is simply any unfavorable medical occurrence observed in a clinical research participant, including any abnormal sign, symptom, or disease.[21] Detecting an AE does not mean that it was caused by a particular study intervention, only that it was observed and reported. The goal is to remove blame from the reporting process to ensure that all AEs, even those that are later dismissed as not related to an intervention, are nevertheless reported and examined. Although AEs are typically identified in clinical trials, they may also be reported by clinicians through postmarket surveillance systems such as MedWatch, operated by the FDA, or directly to medication or medical device manufacturers.[22] AEs are classified as "serious" if they result in hospitalization, permanent disability, birth defects, or death.[21] The term *harms* can also be used to describe AEs. If no AEs have been reported for a particular intervention, potential AEs based on the nature of the procedure are discussed instead.

Section 5—Costs

In addition to efficacy and safety, costs are also an important but often overlooked consideration when contemplating various treatment options for LBP. Costs are borne not only by third-party payers such as private insurers and the government, but also by health care providers, patients, and their families, friends, and employers. The societal costs associated with common LBP are substantial, making it one of the most expensive medical conditions in the United States. This section discusses general charges associated with an intervention, as well as gives some indication of third-party reimbursement policies. Because costs must always be evaluated

in conjunction with outcomes, evidence related to cost effectiveness is also reviewed where available.

Charges and Reimbursement

Fees charged by different health care providers for the same interventions, and even by the same providers for different patients or third-party payers, can vary substantially according to a variety of factors. Fees can also be quite different than the actual amount paid. It is therefore very difficult to specify the exact charges that apply to an intervention for common LBP with any degree of certainty. This problem is exacerbated by the reluctance that health care providers and third-party payers often have in making specific fees, charges, and amounts reimbursed publicly available. This segment is intended to provide an estimate of the charges associated with different interventions for clinicians to compare their relative costs. To facilitate this comparison, the Medicare Fee Schedule (MFS) was chosen to serve as a baseline for providers to develop an associated charge for the services described.

The MFS is publicly available and has been developed using the Resource Based Relative Value Scale (RBRVS), created at Harvard University in 1988, which assigns procedures a relative value unit (RVU) based on three factors: physician work, practice expense, and malpractice expense.[23] MFSs may vary from area to area, in that the RBRVS payment methodology also applies a geographical adjustment factor (GAF) to each locality. Values from the 2010 MFS are provided for both California (Los Angeles) and New York (New York City); the GAFs for those areas are among the highest in the country, affect a large population, and may approximate fee schedules for private health insurers.[24] The 2010 participating physician, non-facility fees are displayed in each chapter.

A conversion factor (CF) is calculated annually by the Centers for Medicare and Medicaid Services (CMS) and applied to the RVU and GAF, which determines the reimbursement amounts listed in the referenced data. Although some third-party payers continue to base their reimbursements on the outdated "usual, customary, and reasonable" payment methodology, the majority have developed reimbursement tables based on the RBRVS used by Medicare. The CF applied by other third-party payers is typically a negotiated rate and should result in reimbursements that are generally much higher than the Medicare rates referenced.

Cost Effectiveness

The charges associated with an intervention are important when evaluating its costs, but do not give any idea of its value. The outcomes that can be obtained with an intervention are also essential because they are the reason for seeking treatment. Studies in which both the costs and the outcomes associated with an intervention are evaluated and compared relative to other interventions are known as *cost effectiveness analyses* (CEAs).[25] The results of CEAs are typically reported as the costs associated with obtaining a particular health outcome of interest (e.g., dollars per life saved). Outcomes used in CEAs can vary, which makes it difficult to compare their results.

TABLE 2-3	Cost Effectiveness Analyses Related to Low Back Pain	
Reference	**Title**	**Year**
29	The functional restoration approach to the treatment of chronic pain in patients with soft tissue and back injuries	1994
30	The treatment of acute low back pain—bed rest, exercises, or ordinary activity?	1995
31	Health economic assessment of behavioural rehabilitation in chronic low back pain: a randomised clinical trial	1998
32	Efficiency and costs of medical exercise therapy, conventional physiotherapy, and self-exercise in patient with chronic low back pain. A pragmatic, randomized, single-blinded, controlled trial with 1-year follow-up	1998
33	A comparison of physical therapy, chiropractic manipulation, and provision of an educational booklet for the treatment of patients with low back pain	1998
34	Randomised controlled trial of exercise for low back pain: clinical outcomes, costs, and preferences	1999
35	Cost-minimisation analysis of three conservative treatment programmes in 180 patients sick-listed for acute low-back pain	2000
36	Randomized trial comparing traditional Chinese medical acupuncture, therapeutic massage, and self-care education for chronic low back pain	2001
37	Cost-benefit and cost-effectiveness analysis of a disability prevention model for back pain management: a six year follow up study	2002
38	Relative cost-effectiveness of extensive and light multidisciplinary treatment programs versus treatment as usual for patients with chronic low back pain on long-term sick leave: a randomized controlled study	2002
39	Does early intervention with a light mobilization program reduce long-term sick leave for low back pain: a 3-year follow-up study	2003
40	A randomized trial of combined manipulation, stabilizing exercises, and physician consultation compared to physician consultation alone for chronic low back pain	2003
41	Treatment- and cost-effectiveness of early intervention for acute low-back pain patients: a one-year prospective study	2003
42	United Kingdom back pain exercise and manipulation (UK BEAM) randomised trial: cost effectiveness of physical treatments for back pain in primary care	2004
43	Mini-interventions for subacute low back pain: two-year follow-up and modifiers of effectiveness	2004
44	Botulinum toxin A versus bupivacaine trigger point injections for the treatment of myofascial pain syndrome: a randomised double blind crossover study	2005
45	Cost-utility analysis of physiotherapy treatment compared with physiotherapy advice in low back pain	2006
46	Effectiveness and cost-effectiveness of adding a cognitive behavioral treatment to the rehabilitation of chronic low back pain	2006
47	A randomised controlled trial of acupuncture care for persistent low back pain: cost effectiveness analysis	2006
48	Active exercise, education, and cognitive behavioral therapy for persistent disabling low back pain: a randomized controlled trial	2007
49	Low back pain in general practice: cost-effectiveness of a minimal psychosocial intervention versus usual care	2007
50	Effectiveness and cost-effectiveness of three types of physiotherapy used to reduce chronic low back pain disability: a pragmatic randomized trial with economic evaluation	2007
51	A brief pain management program compared with physical therapy for low back pain: results from an economic analysis alongside a randomized controlled trial	2007
52	Economic evaluation of an intensive group training protocol compared with usual care physiotherapy in patients with chronic low back pain	2008
53	Cost-effectiveness of naturopathic care for chronic low back pain	2008

Studies in which the health outcome of interest is measured as health-related quality of life are known as *cost utility analyses* (CUAs).[26] *Utility* is an economic term used to describe the value or preference that someone expresses for a given outcome.[25] When applied to health, utility may be expressed from 0 (no health) to 1 (perfect health).[26] It can be estimated from generic health-related quality of life questionnaires such as the short form 36 (SF-36), EQ-5D, or Health Utilities Index (HUI), among others.[26] Because utility is intended to reflect overall health, it may not be as precise as disease-specific questionnaires for common LBP such as the Roland Morris Disability Questionnaire (RMDQ) or Oswestry Disability Index (ODI).

Utility can also be applied to a specific time period to yield a commonly used metric in CUAs known as *quality-adjusted life-years* (QALYs).[25] This metric is helpful when evaluating CUAs in which interventions may impact not only the quantity of life (e.g., death), but also its quality (e.g., utility). Results of CUAs are often reported as the costs associated with achieving one QALY (e.g., dollars/QALY). When comparing the cost effectiveness of two interventions, one is said to dominate the other if both its costs are lower and its outcomes are superior. However, if one intervention has higher costs but also better outcomes than another, results are reported in terms of incremental costs and outcomes (e.g., dollars/QALY).[25] This can be interpreted as the additional costs associated with obtaining superior outcomes with a more expensive intervention.

Two SRs have recently been conducted on interventions for the management of LBP.[27,28] Together, these two SRs evaluated a total of 25 CEAs and CUAs, which are presented in Table 2-3.[29-53] This segment summarizes their findings for the interventions reviewed in this textbook. Results are summarized for clinical outcomes, direct costs (e.g., health care costs), indirect costs (e.g., lost productivity costs), total costs (direct and indirect costs), and cost effectiveness metrics (e.g., dollars/QALY) or conclusions (e.g., one intervention dominated the other).

SUMMARY

This book is intended to help clinicians learn more about various interventions available for the management of common LBP, starting with basic information related to their description. Proposed mechanisms of action of interventions are also discussed to understand why they are used. During this process, the relative merits of different interventions can be assessed and compared. Where possible, these comparisons should be based on the best available scientific evidence, which has been summarized from CPGs, SRs, RCTs, and OBSs. Aspects that may be particularly important in determining the relative advantages and disadvantages of different interventions include efficacy, safety, and costs. Armed with this information, health care professionals involved in the management of common LBP may not only make better clinical decisions, but also convey their rationale for making these decisions with their patients in an effort to share the decision making process and improve the informed consent process.

REFERENCES

1. Wiese G, Callender A. History of spinal manipulation. In: Haldeman S, Dagenais S, Budgell B, et al, editors. Principles and practice of chiropractic. 3rd ed. New York: McGraw-Hill; 2005.
2. Kohlbeck FJ, Haldeman S. Medication-assisted spinal manipulation. Spine J 2002;2:288-302.
3. US Food and Drug Administration. About FDA. http://www.fda.gov/AboutFDA/CentersOffices/default.htm.
4. Rutherford EM. The FDA and "privatization"—the drug approval process. Food Drug Law J 1995;50 Spec:203-225.
5. Maisel WH. Medical device regulation: an introduction for the practicing physician. Ann Intern Med 2004;140:296-302.
6. Stafford RS. Regulating off-label drug use—rethinking the role of the FDA. N Engl J Med 2008;358:1427-1429.
7. Dagenais S, Tricco AC, Haldeman S. Synthesis of recommendations for the assessment and management of low back pain from recent clinical practice guidelines. Spine J 2010;10:514-529.
8. Cochrane Back Review Group. Cochrane Back Review Group. http://www.cochrane.iwh.on.ca.
9. Chou R, Qaseem A, Snow V, et al. Diagnosis and treatment of low back pain: a joint clinical practice guideline from the American College of Physicians and the American Pain Society. Ann Intern Med 2007;147:478-491.
10. Chou R, Loeser JD, Owens DK, et al. Interventional therapies, surgery, and interdisciplinary rehabilitation for low back pain: an evidence-based clinical practice guideline from the American Pain Society. Spine 2009;34:1066-1077.
11. Chou R, Huffman LH. Medications for acute and chronic low back pain: a review of the evidence for an American Pain Society/American College of Physicians clinical practice guideline. Ann Intern Med 2007;147:505-514.
12. Chou R, Huffman LH. Nonpharmacologic therapies for acute and chronic low back pain: a review of the evidence for an American Pain Society/American College of Physicians clinical practice guideline. Ann Intern Med 2007;147:492-504.
13. Chou R, Baisden J, Carragee EJ, et al. Surgery for low back pain: a review of the evidence for an American Pain Society Clinical Practice Guideline. Spine 2009;34:1094-1109.
14. Chou R, Atlas SJ, Stanos SP, et al. Nonsurgical interventional therapies for low back pain: a review of the evidence for an American Pain Society clinical practice guideline. Spine 2009;34:1078-1093.
15. Chou R. Evidence-based medicine and the challenge of low back pain: where are we now? Pain Pract 2005;5:153-178.
16. Benson K, Hartz AJ. A comparison of observational studies and randomized, controlled trials. N Engl J Med 2000;342:1878-1886.
17. Silverman SL. From randomized controlled trials to observational studies. Am J Med 2009;122:114-120.
18. Smith CM. Origin and uses of *primum non nocere*—above all, do no harm! J Clin Pharmacol 2005;45:371-377.
19. Dugdale DC. MedlinePlus: Contraindications. http://www.nlm.nih.gov/medlineplus/ency/article/002314.htm.
20. World Alliance for Patient Safety. WHO draft guidelines in adverse event reporting and learning systems. Geneva, Switzerland: World Health Organization; 2005.
21. Office for Human Research Protections (OHRP), Department of Health and Human Services (HHS). Guidance on reviewing and reporting unanticipated problems involving risks to subjects or others and adverse events. Washington, DC: US Department of Health and Human Services; 2007.
22. US Department of Health and Human Services. MedWatch. http://www.fda.gov/safety/MedWatch/default.htm, 2010.
23. Centers for Medicare and Medicaid Services. Physician fee schedule. http://www.cms.hhs.gov/PhysicianFeeSched.
24. TrailBlazer Health. Medicare fee schedule. http://www.trailblazerhealth.com/Tools/Fee%20Schedule/MedicareFeeSchedule.aspx, 2009.
25. Detsky AS, Naglie IG. A clinician's guide to cost-effectiveness analysis. Ann Intern Med 1990;113:147-154.
26. Tosteson AN. Preference-based health outcome measures in low back pain. Spine 2000;25:3161-3166.

27. van der Roer N, Goossens MEJB, Evers SMAA, et al. What is the most cost-effective treatment for patients with low back pain? A systematic review. Best Pract Res Clin Rheumatol 2005;19:671-684.

28. Dagenais S, Roffey DM, Wai EK, et al. Can cost utility evaluations inform decision making about interventions for low back pain? Spine J 2009;9:944-957.

29. Mitchell RI, Carmen GM. The functional restoration approach to the treatment of chronic pain in patients with soft tissue and back injuries. Spine 1994;19:633-642.

30. Malmivaara A, Hakkinen U, Aro T, et al. The treatment of acute low back pain—bed rest, exercises, or ordinary activity? N Engl J Med 1995;332:351-355.

31. Goossens ME, Rutten-Van Molken MP, Kole-Snijders AM, et al. Health economic assessment of behavioural rehabilitation in chronic low back pain: a randomised clinical trial. Health Econ 1998;7:39-51.

32. Torstensen TA, Ljunggren AE, Meen HD, et al. Efficiency and costs of medical exercise therapy, conventional physiotherapy, and self-exercise in patients with chronic low back pain. A pragmatic, randomized, single-blinded, controlled trial with 1-year follow-up. Spine 1998;23:2616-2624.

33. Cherkin DC, Deyo RA, Battie M, et al. A comparison of physical therapy, chiropractic manipulation, and provision of an educational booklet for the treatment of patients with low back pain. N Engl J Med 1998;339:1021-1029.

34. Moffett JK, Torgerson D, Bell-Syer S, et al. Randomised controlled trial of exercise for low back pain: clinical outcomes, costs, and preferences. BMJ 1999;319:279-283.

35. Seferlis T, Lindholm L, Nemeth G. Cost-minimisation analysis of three conservative treatment programmes in 180 patients sick-listed for acute low-back pain. Scand J Prim Health Care 2000;18:53-57.

36. Cherkin DC, Eisenberg D, Sherman KJ, et al. Randomized trial comparing traditional Chinese medical acupuncture, therapeutic massage, and self-care education for chronic low back pain. Arch Intern Med 2001;161:1081-1088.

37. Loisel P, Lemaire J, Poitras S, et al. Cost-benefit and cost-effectiveness analysis of a disability prevention model for back pain management: a six year follow up study. Occupat Environ Med 2002;59:807-815.

38. Skouen JS, Grasdal AL, Haldorsen EM, et al. Relative cost-effectiveness of extensive and light multidisciplinary treatment programs versus treatment as usual for patients with chronic low back pain on long-term sick leave: randomized controlled study. Spine 2002;27:901-909.

39. Molde Hagen E, Grasdal A, Eriksen HR. Does early intervention with a light mobilization program reduce long-term sick leave for low back pain: a 3-year follow-up study. Spine 2003;28:2309-2315.

40. Niemisto L, Lahtinen-Suopanki T, Rissanen P, et al. A randomized trial of combined manipulation, stabilizing exercises, and physician consultation compared to physician consultation alone for chronic low back pain. Spine 2003;28:2185-2191.

41. Gatchel RJ, Polatin PB, Noe C, et al. Treatment- and cost-effectiveness of early intervention for acute low-back pain patients: a one-year prospective study. J Occup Rehabil 2003;13:1-9.

42. UK Beam Trial Team. United Kingdom back pain exercise and manipulation (UK BEAM) randomised trial: cost effectiveness of physical treatments for back pain in primary care. BMJ 2004;329:1381.

43. Karjalainen K, Malmivaara A, Mutanen P, et al. Mini-intervention for subacute low back pain: two-year follow-up and modifiers of effectiveness. Spine 2004;29:1069-1076.

44. Graboski CL, Gray DS, Burnham RS. Botulinum toxin A versus bupivacaine trigger point injections for the treatment of myofascial pain syndrome: a randomised double blind crossover study. Pain 2005;118:170-175.

45. Rivero-Arias O, Gray A, Frost H, Lamb SE, et al. Cost-utility analysis of physiotherapy treatment compared with physiotherapy advice in low back pain. Spine 2006;31:1381-1397.

46. Schweikert B, Jacobi E, Seitz R, et al. Effectiveness and cost-effectiveness of adding a cognitive behavioral treatment to the rehabilitation of chronic low back pain. J Rheumatol 2006;33:2519-2526.

47. Ratcliffe J, Thomas KJ, MacPherson H, et al. A randomised controlled trial of acupuncture care for persistent low back pain: cost effectiveness analysis. BMJ 2006;333:626.

48. Johnson RE, Jones GT, Wiles NJ, et al. Active exercise, education, and cognitive behavioral therapy for persistent disabling low back pain: a randomized controlled trial. Spine 2007;32:1578-1585.

49. Jellema P, van der Roer N, van der Windt DAWM, et al. Low back pain in general practice: cost-effectiveness of a minimal psychosocial intervention versus usual care. Eur Spine J 2007;16:1812-1821.

50. Critchley DJ, Ratcliffe J, Noonan S, et al. Effectiveness and cost-effectiveness of three types of physiotherapy used to reduce chronic low back pain disability: a pragmatic randomized trial with economic evaluation. Spine 2007;321474-321481.

51. Whitehurst DGT, Lewis M, Yao GL, et al. A brief pain management program compared with physical therapy for low back pain: results from an economic analysis alongside a randomized clinical trial. Arthritis Rheum 2007;57:466-473.

52. van der Roer N, van Tulder M, van Mechelen W, et al. Economic evaluation of an intensive group training protocol compared with usual care physiotherapy in patients with chronic low back pain. Spine 2008;33:445-451.

53. Herman PM, Szczurko O, Cooley K, et al. Cost-effectiveness of naturopathic care for chronic low back pain. Altern Ther Health Med 2008;14:32-39.

SIMON DAGENAIS
ANDREA C. TRICCO
SCOTT HALDEMAN

CHAPTER 3

Assessment of Low Back Pain

Common low back pain (LBP) is a frequent complaint for which numerous health care providers are routinely consulted.[1] While the management of common LBP can quickly become complicated, it is important to remember the basic goals of patients who seek care. First, patients wish to be reassured that despite any excruciating pain they may be feeling, their health is not in imminent danger. Patients may have waited weeks, months, or even years before consulting a clinician. It is quite possible that the severity or debilitating nature of their symptoms may have led them to imagine horrible scenarios about their cause. Although this is very rarely the case with common LBP, clinicians nevertheless need to conduct a thorough assessment to eliminate this remote possibility and demonstrate to the patient that their concerns are being heard and addressed.[2,3]

Second, patients wish to learn something about the general nature of their condition, including possibly a differential or working diagnosis. There are many diagnostic modalities available to clinicians that portend to facilitate this process, but an overreliance on such testing overlooks one of the fundamental principles of common LBP: its unclear and nonspecific origins.[1,4] There is mounting evidence of overuse of diagnostic testing for LBP, especially magnetic resonance imaging (MRI).[5] Wide regional disparities have also been noted in the use of MRI for common LBP in the United States. Not only are there substantial costs associated with MRI for LBP but there are also clinical consequences to their overuse.[6,7]

Studies have reported that patients with common LBP who are made aware of MRI findings, none of which were significant or revealed any serious spinal pathology, did not improve as rapidly as those who were not aware of the mostly minor anatomic variants noted on those reports.[8] Even though clinicians may dismiss such inconsequential MRI findings, patients may not be so cavalier. Simply knowing that they have "abnormalities" in their lumbar spine that can be pointed to on an MRI scan may cloud their potential for quick recovery. A correlation has also been established between the rate of diagnostic testing such as MRI for common LBP and the rate of subsequent medical or surgical procedures aimed at correcting their findings, including epidural steroid injections and lumbar decompression or fusion.[8] Whereas some of these procedures are in fact warranted when patients have serious spinal pathology or other accepted indications, in many instances they are not strictly necessary and may incur negative ramifications such as costs and harms.[9-12]

RECENT CLINICAL PRACTICE GUIDELINES

To balance the necessity of conducting a thorough clinical assessment of common LBP with the obligation that clinicians have to minimize the harm resulting from unnecessary diagnostic testing, it may be helpful to receive guidance from clinical practice guidelines (CPGs). Numerous evidence-based CPGs have been conducted to identify, evaluate, summarize, and synthesize the results of hundreds or even thousands of studies related to the assessment of common LBP. Such CPGs were developed specifically to help practicing clinicians make practical decisions about their patients, and are therefore considered important tools to the practice of evidence-based medicine.[13-16] Although recommendations from CPGs are not intended to replace expert clinical judgment, they can enhance decision making by providing guidance for uncertain scenarios. Clinicians may also feel more confident about their clinical judgment when it is based on recommendations from well-conducted CPGs.

The findings from 10 CPGs sponsored by national organizations throughout the world and published in English during the past decade were compared and summarized to provide clinicians with an overview of the best available evidence to guide their assessment of patients with common LBP. An equal number of the CPGs summarized evidence related to acute LBP (i.e., less than 12 weeks) and chronic LBP (CLBP) (i.e., more than 12 weeks), using definitions recommended by the Cochrane Back Review Group (CBRG).[17] It was unclear why two of the CPGs reviewed defined CLBP as lasting more than only 4 to 6 weeks.[6,18] Such temporal classifications are somewhat arbitrary, but they do facilitate comparison of recommendations when used consistently.[18] It was also unclear why some CPGs excluded LBP with neurologic involvement from their scope when this presentation is found in a substantial proportion of patients with LBP.[7] The results of these 10 CPGs are presented according to the stated goals of the assessment, rather than by diagnostic modality.

GOALS OF ASSESSMENT FOR LOW BACK PAIN

There was general agreement among the 10 recent CPGs reviewed that there are 5 main goals when conducting an assessment of LBP and that these goals can be considered

21

TABLE 3-1	Goals of the Assessment for Patients with Low Back Pain										
Country	Australia	Belgium	Europe (Acute)	Europe (Chronic)	Italy	New Zealand	Norway	United Kingdom	United States (1°)	United States (2°)	Count
Reference	4	19	10	11	20	7	13	18	6	21	
Goals of Assessment											
Assess risk factors for chronicity	X		X	X	X				X		5
Assess severity of symptoms and function	X	X	X		X	X			X		6
Rule out neurologic involvement	X	X	X	X	X	X	X	X	X		9
Rule out potentially serious pathology	X	X	X	X	X	X	X	X	X		9
Rule out specific causes	X			X	X			X	X		5

1°, primary care; 2°, secondary care.

TABLE 3-2	Elements of the Patient History Related to Low Back Pain										
Country	Australia	Belgium	Europe (Acute)	Europe (Chronic)	Italy	New Zealand	Norway	United Kingdom	United States (1°)	United States (2°)	Count
Reference	4	19	10	11	20	7	13	18	6	21	
Patient History											
Pain characteristics	X	X	X		X	X			X		6
Red flags	X	X	X		X	X	X		X		7
Review of systems	X		X						X		3
Risk factors for chronicity	X	X			X	X			X		5

1°, primary care; 2°, secondary care.

sequentially, in that the findings from each goal can be pertinent to achieving the next goal. These five goals include (1) ruling out potentially serious spinal pathology,[4,6,7,10,11,13,18-21] (2) ruling out specific causes of LBP,[4,6,11,18,20] (3) ruling out substantial neurologic involvement,[4,6,7,10,11,13,18-20] (4) evaluating the severity of symptoms and functional limitations,[4,7,10,11,19,20] and (5) identifying risk factors for chronicity.[4,6,10,11,22] Findings from the 10 recent CPGs that were pertinent to each of these goals are discussed below and summarized in Tables 3-1 and 3-2.

Ruling Out Potentially Serious Spinal Pathology

All CPGs discussed the possibility that symptoms of LBP—in very rare cases—could be due to potentially serious spinal pathology. It was generally suggested that clinicians screen such conditions by identifying items indicating the presence of potentially serious spinal pathology known as *red flags* which are signs, symptoms, or patient characteristics that may indicate the need for additional screening to eliminate the possibility of underlying medical conditions. The number of red flags for LBP specified in each CPG ranged from 7 to 17, with a mean of 11. Overall, 22 red flags were identified, the most common being age older than 50 years (n = 9), history of cancer (n = 9), and steroid use (n = 9); the least common were gait abnormality (n = 2) and weakness in limbs (n = 1). Of the 22 red flags, 8

were potentially associated with spinal cancer, 6 with cauda equina syndrome, 5 with spinal fracture, and 5 with spinal infection; one red flag (age older than 50 years) was associated with both cancer and fracture. One red flag (age younger than 20 years) was not reported as being associated with any specific serious spinal pathology. Findings from the 10 recent CPGs that were pertinent to serious pathology are summarized in Table 3-3.

Red flags suggesting spinal cancer included a history of cancer, unexplained weight loss, nonresponsiveness to care, night pain, pain at multiple sites, pain at rest, age older than 50 years, and urinary retention; x-ray studies and blood tests or MRI was suggested in those patients. Red flags suggesting cauda equina syndrome included fecal incontinence, gait abnormality, saddle numbness, urinary retention, weakness in limbs, and widespread neurologic symptoms; surgical evaluation or MRI was generally recommended in those patients. Red flags suggesting spinal fracture included age older than 50 years, osteoporosis, steroid use, structural deformity, and trauma; x-ray studies and blood tests or MRI/computed tomography (CT) was recommended in those patients. Red flags suggesting spinal infection included fever, immune suppression, intravenous drug use, systemic unwellness, and trauma (one CPG[4] reported this); blood tests and x-ray studies or MRI was recommended in those patients. Findings from the 10 recent CPGs that were pertinent to red flags and serious spinal pathology are summarized in Table 3-4.

TABLE 3-3 | **Serious Pathology and Specific Causes of Low Back Pain**

Country	Australia	Belgium	Europe (Acute)	Europe (Chronic)	Italy	New Zealand	Norway	United Kingdom	United States (1°)	United States (2°)	Count
Reference	4	19	10	11	20	7	13	18	6	21	
Red Flags Definition											
Nonmusculoskeletal origins		X									1
Potentially serious disorder	X		X	X		X	X		X		6
Require additional investigation	X	X	X	X	X				X		6
Require urgent evaluation	X					X	X		X		4
Specific cause of LBP		X							X		2
Specific Causes of LBP											
Aortic aneurysm	X				X				X		3
Inflammatory disorder	X		X	X	X		X	X	X		7

1°, primary care; 2°, secondary care; LBP, low back pain.

TABLE 3-4 | **Categories of Red Flags and Recommended Follow-up Examinations***

Red Flag	Potentially Serious Spinal Pathology				Diagnostic Testing Suggested					References
	Cancer	Infection	Fracture	Cauda Equina Syndrome	X-rays	Blood Tests	MRI	CT	Surgical Evaluation	
Age <20 yr					X					10, 11, 13, 19
Age >50 yr	X		X		X	X				4, 6, 7, 10, 11, 13, 18-20
Fecal incontinence				X			X		X	6, 7, 10, 13, 18, 20
Fever		X			X	X	X			4, 6, 7, 10, 11, 13, 18-20
Gait abnormality				X			X		X	7, 10, 13, 18, 20
History of cancer	X				X	X	X			4, 6, 7, 10, 11, 13, 18-20
Immune suppression		X			X	X	X			4, 6, 10, 11, 13, 18-20
Intravenous drug use		X			X	X	X			4, 6, 7, 10, 11, 13, 18-20
Night pain	X				X	X	X			4, 6, 7, 10, 11, 13, 18-20
Nonresponsive to care	X				X	X	X			4, 6, 10, 11, 13, 18-20
Osteoporosis			X		X	X	X			4, 6, 13, 18, 20
Pain at multiple sites	X				X	X	X			4, 10, 11, 13, 18-20
Pain at rest	X				X	X	X			4, 7, 10, 11, 13, 18-20
Saddle numbness				X			X		X	6, 7, 10, 13, 18, 20
Steroid use			X		X	X	X	X		4, 6, 7, 10, 11, 13, 18-20
Structural deformity			X		X					11, 13, 19
Systemic unwellness		X			X	X	X			10, 11, 13, 18-20
Trauma		X	X		X	X	X	X		4, 7, 10, 13, 18, 20
Unexplained weight loss	X				X	X	X			4, 6, 7, 10, 11, 13, 18-20
Urinary retention	X			X			X		X	4, 6, 7, 10, 13, 18, 20
Weakness in limbs				X			X		X	7, 10, 13, 18, 20
Widespread neurologic symptoms				X			X		X	4, 6, 7, 10, 11, 13, 18-20

*References are cited if they recommended any of the diagnostic tests for any of the suspected underlying serious pathology, not all references suggested all forms of diagnostic testing.

CT, computed tomography; MRI, magnetic resonance imaging.

Ruling Out Specific Causes of LBP

CPGs also discussed the need to rule out rare but specific causes of LBP other than serious spinal pathology, most commonly related to systemic inflammatory disorders (n = 7). The most common systemic inflammatory disorder discussed was ankylosing spondylitis. Characteristics reported for ankylosing spondylitis included a gradual onset of symptoms, night pain, morning stiffness, symptoms that improve with exercise, alternating buttock pain, and a family history of spondyloarthritis; x-ray study of the spine and pelvis along with blood tests were recommended in those patients.[6,20] Characteristics reported for aortic aneurysm included age older than 60 years, atherosclerosis, pulsating abdominal mass, night pain, pain at rest, and radiating leg pain; referral to a surgeon was recommended in those patients.[20] Other specific causes of LBP reported in CPGs were enteropathic, reactive, or psoriatic spondyloarthritis, as well as endocarditis, nephrolithiasis, or pancreatitis; little information was provided on the characteristics of these conditions and their respective follow-up assessment procedures.[6,20]

Ruling Out Substantial Neurologic Involvement

In the CPGs reviewed, LBP with substantial neurologic involvement was generally defined as LBP with moderate, severe, or progressive (collectively termed substantial) signs or symptoms of neurologic dysfunction in the lower extremities secondary to neural impingement from common causes such as spinal stenosis or intervertebral foramen stenosis; mild radiculopathy, referred pain, and cauda equina syndrome were generally excluded from this category. The CPGs generally recommended ruling out substantial neurologic involvement such as severe lower extremity pain, sensory or motor deficits, or abnormal deep tendon reflexes (DTRs), which may stem from irritation or compression of spinal nerve roots (Figure 3-1). Although minor neurologic signs or symptoms are frequently noted with common LBP, these rarely require specific interventions. Only when such signs or symptoms are progressive, severe, or markedly interfere with a patient's activities of daily living should clinicians consider interventions aimed at addressing them. Neurologic signs and symptoms may be indicative of spinal nerve root compression, central canal stenosis, foraminal encroachment, inflammation, neuropathic pain, or other neurologic conditions. The main tools suggested by CPGs to rule out substantial neurologic involvement were the patient history and neurologic examination. Findings from the 10 recent CPGs that were pertinent to physical examination are summarized in Table 3-5. Assessment of standing lumbosacral range of motion is illustrated in Figures 3-2 through 3-5.

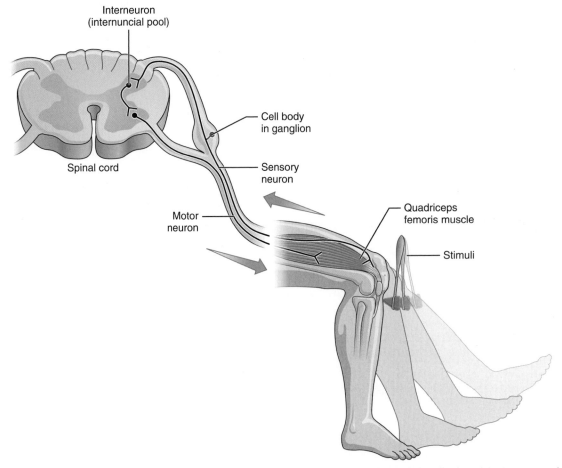

Figure 3-1 Spinal nerve roots and lower extremity deep tendon reflexes. (Modified from Patton KT, Thibodeau GA: Anatomy and Physiology, ed. 7. St. Louis, 2010, Elsevier.)

TABLE 3-5	Elements of the Patient Examination Related to Low Back Pain									
Country	Australia	Belgium	Europe (Acute)	Europe (Chronic)	Italy	New Zealand	Norway	United Kingdom	United States (1°)	United States (2°)	Count
Reference	4	19	10	11	20	7	13	18	6	21	
Examination											
Deep tendon reflexes							x		x		2
Dermatomes	x				x		x		x		4
Manual: palpation	x				x		x				3
Manual: provocative	x			x			x				3
Myotomes	x				x		x		x		4
Straight leg raise			x		x		x		x		4
Visual: inspection	x						x				2
Visual: range of motion							x				1

1°, primary care; 2°, secondary care.

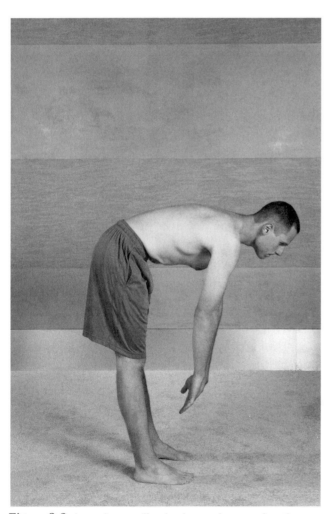

Figure 3-2 Assessing standing lumbosacral range of motion: flexion.

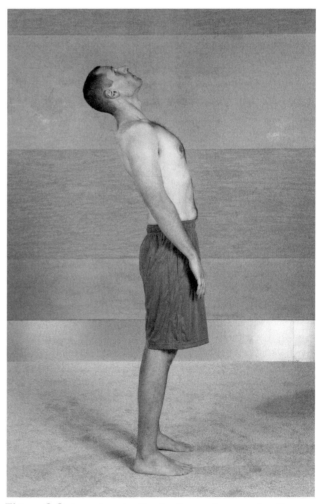

Figure 3-3 Assessing standing lumbosacral range of motion: extension.

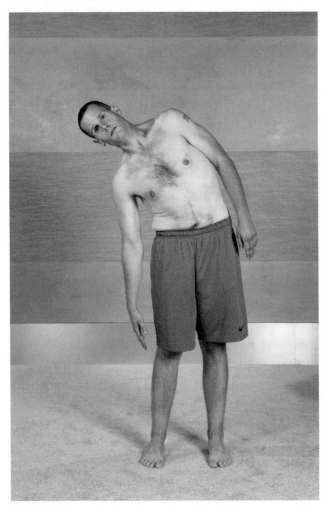

Figure 3-4 Assessing standing lumbosacral range of motion: lateral bending.

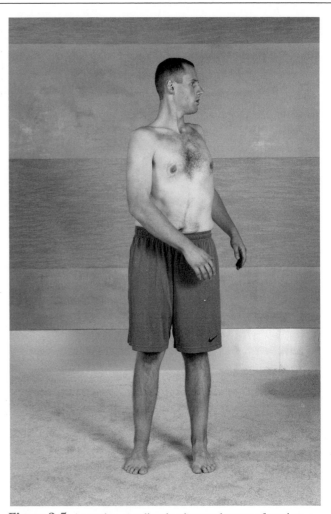

Figure 3-5 Assessing standing lumbosacral range of motion: rotation.

It was often recommended that the patient history include detailed inquiry into specific characteristics of symptoms in the lower extremities, including their exact location, description, duration, and any noted aggravating or ameliorating factors.[4,6,7,10,19,20] A neurologic examination of the lower extremities should be performed, focusing on the myotomes, dermatomes, and DTRs of L4, L5, and S1, as illustrated in Figures 3-6 through 3-8.[4,6,13,20] The straight leg raise test was also discussed in several CPGs but was generally not recommended due to concerns about its validity, reliability, and interpretation.[6,10,11,13,19,20] For LBP with substantial neurologic involvement that did not improve with conservative management, advanced imaging such as MRI or CT was often recommended.[6,11,19,20] Findings from the 10 recent CPGs that were pertinent to diagnostic testing are summarized in Table 3-6.

Evaluating the Severity of Symptoms and Functional Limitations

Several CPGs noted the importance of assessing the severity of pain and other symptoms related to LBP, as well as evaluating the physical functional limitations encountered in activities of daily living as a result of LBP.[4,6,7,10,19,20] Although it was generally indicated that validated and standardized outcome measures should be used to accomplish this goal whenever possible, little specific guidance was offered by CPGs on this topic. For example, there were few recommendations related to selecting among the multitude of questionnaires available to assess symptoms and physical function related to LBP. Few CPGs specified an appropriate frequency for reassessment with these questionnaires. There was also little discussion about using these outcomes to determine whether the minimum clinically important difference (MCID) had been met at subsequent follow-ups to evaluate the success of the current clinical approach.

Identifying Risk Factors for Chronicity

Almost all CPGs recommended that clinicians should identify the presence of risk factors associated with a delayed recovery from LBP; the term *yellow flags* was often used to describe these risk factors.[4,6,10,11,13,19,23] Overall, 10 risk factors were identified among these CPGs, 7 of which were of a psychosocial nature. The most commonly identified risk factors for chronicity were emotional issues (e.g., anxiety, depression) and fear avoidance behavior (e.g., profound worry of aggravating LBP by doing normal activities), while the least common were prior LBP, substantial neurologic involvement, and severity of pain. Findings from the 10 recent CPGs that were pertinent to risk factors for chronicity are summarized in Table 3-7.

IMPLEMENTING GOAL-ORIENTED ASSESSMENT OF LOW BACK PAIN

A synthesis of recommendations from recent national CPGs suggests that a patient history and neurologic examination should be sufficient in the vast majority of patients with LBP.

Because there were more than 20 red flags proposed in these CPGs, an intake questionnaire could conceivably be devised to ask patients about each one, with clinicians asking appropriate follow-up questions based on those answers. A similar approach could also be taken to screening for specific causes of LBP such as systemic inflammatory, abdominal, genito-urinary, or cardiovascular disorders, in which symptoms are generally constant, neither aggravated by movement nor relieved with rest. Following the history, a brief neurologic examination of the L4, L5, and S1 dermatomes, myotomes, and DTRs could be sufficient to eliminate the possibility of rare but potentially serious or specific spinal pathology.

TABLE 3-6	**Recommendations About Diagnostic Testing Related to Low Back Pain**										
Country	Australia	Belgium	Europe (Acute)	Europe (Chronic)	Italy	New Zealand	Norway	United Kingdom	United States (1°)	United States (2°)	Count
Reference	4	19	10	11	20	7	13	18	6	21	
Diagnostic Testing (Indications)											
X-rays											
Red flags	X	X	X	X	X	X	X		X		8
Blood tests											
Red flags	X				X	X	X		X		5
MRI/CT											
Red flags	X	X	X	X	X	X	X	X	X		9
Neurologic involvement		X		X	X				X		4
EMG/NCV											
Neurologic involvement					X				X		2
None		X		X							2

1°, primary care; 2°, secondary care; CT, computed tomography; EMG, electromyography; LBP, low back pain; MRI, magnetic resonance imaging; NCV, nerve conduction velocity.

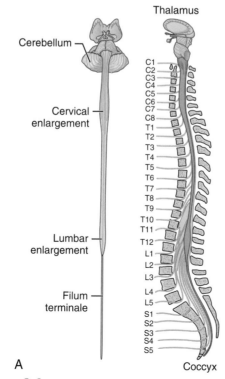

Figure 3-6 Spinal nerve roots (**A**) and their dermatomes (**B**).

Continued

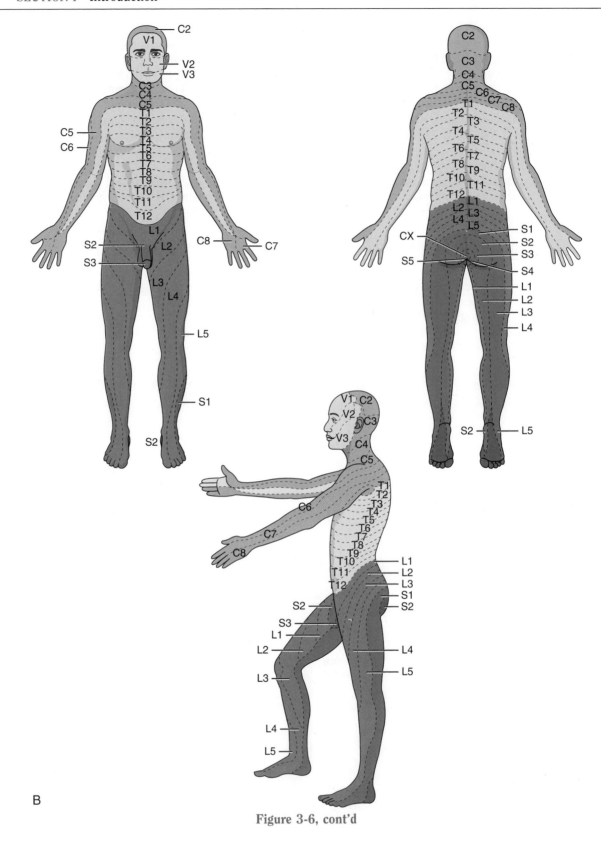

B

Figure 3-6, cont'd

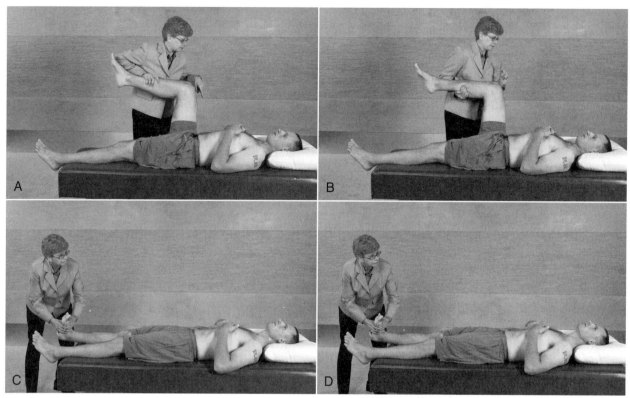

Figure 3-7 Lower extremity myotomes.

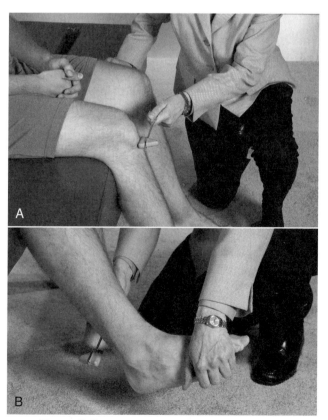

Figure 3-8 Lower extremity deep tendon reflexes.

It was reported that 99% of potentially serious pathology could be identified with this type of screening process.[11]

Should this assessment suggest that potentially serious spinal pathology or specific causes of LBP are present, diagnostic testing such as x-ray tests and blood tests, MRI/CT, or urgent surgical evaluation, depending on the nature of the pathology, were deemed appropriate. Whereas the management of LBP associated with serious spinal pathology was determined by these CPGs to be outside their scope, a synopsis could be informative for inquisitive clinicians in that it is clearly related and unlikely to become the focus of dedicated CPGs given its relative rarity.

For LBP with neurologic involvement, CPGs generally did not recommend any further assessment until conservative management had first been attempted. This was rarely defined in any detail, but might be interpreted as a minimum of four to six weeks of appropriate primary care management using one or more of the recommended interventions, with periodic reassessment to identify progression of neurologic signs and symptoms. Only in the event that such management failed was additional assessment with MRI or CT generally recommended. Even in such cases, however, it was suggested that since the goal of advanced imaging was to identify candidates for surgical or other more invasive interventions; those who are not interested in such management options may not wish to undergo presurgical assessment.

Despite the widespread use of diagnostic tests, few CPGs recommended electromyography or nerve conduction velocity testing, and none recommended discography, selective

			Europe	Europe		New		United	United	United	
Country	Australia	Belgium	(Acute)	(Chronic)	Italy	Zealand	Norway	Kingdom	States (1°)	States (2°)	Count
Reference	4	19	10	11	20	7	13	18	6	21	
Risk Factors for Chronicity											
Compensation issues	x	x	x	x		x			x		6
Emotional issues	x	x	x	x		x	x		x		7
Family problems	x					x	x				3
Fear avoidance behavior	x	x	x	x		x	x		x		7
Inappropriate beliefs	x	x	x	x		x	x				6
Neurologic involvement		x					x				2
Poor job satisfaction	x	x	x	x		x	x		x		7
Prior LBP		x				x					2
Severity of pain		x							x		2
Unrealistic treatment expectations	x	x	x	x		x	x				6

1°, primary care; 2°, secondary care; LBP, low back pain.

nerve root, facet joint, medial branch, or sacroiliac blocks for the assessment of LBP. This may be in part related to the practice of ordering such tests in patients who have marginal or otherwise unclear presentations of LBP that are not substantiated by concordant findings on advanced imaging, physical, and neurologic examination. The validity, reliability, and predictive value of diagnostic tests ordered under such conditions are often poor.

None of the CPGs reported that it was necessary, or even beneficial, for a clinician to attempt to identify the anatomic origins of LBP after having eliminated potentially serious spinal pathology, specific causes of LBP, and neurologic involvement.[6] It was even suggested that needlessly ordering diagnostic testing could independently increase the risk of chronicity.[22] In the context of LBP, it may be preferable for both clinicians and patients to accept that assessment is a more feasible objective than diagnosis, which implies a specific pathoanatomic cause that simply cannot be established for the vast majority of LBP.[22]

Whereas most CPGs suggested identifying patients with risk factors for chronicity, only one made any recommendations about what to do when these were identified.[7] Because many of the risk factors for chronicity are related to inappropriate beliefs and behaviors about LBP, clinicians may wish to recommend a combination of education and focused cognitive behavioral therapy to overcome these barriers.[7,10] Suggestions were also made to emphasize function over pain when measuring outcomes and to schedule more frequent reassessments to reinforce these messages.[7] Although clinically commendable, it is unclear whether implementing such an approach for patients deemed at high risk for development of CLBP would be feasible or cost effective on a population level. It should be noted that the presence of psychosocial risk factors does not eliminate the role of biologic factors in LBP.[13]

It was somewhat disappointing for CPGs to recommend that clinicians evaluate the severity of symptoms and functional limitations for LBP without offering some guidance on specific outcome measures. Numerous validated instruments are available to assess pain, including the visual analog scale (0-100 mm line) and numerical rating scales (whole numbers from 0 to 10).[24] Several instruments are also available to measure function specific to LBP, including the Roland Morris Disability Questionnaire and Oswestry Disability Index.[24] The MCID for those four instruments has been established for LBP and is generally 25%-35%.[24] Alternatively, a generic health instrument such as the short form 12 (SF-12) can also be used to evaluate physical function, with the added benefits of measuring mental function and yielding utility scores that can be used in health economic evaluations, such as the cost utility analyses that are currently lacking for LBP.[25,26]

Recommendations from 10 recent CPGs suggest that the assessment of patients with LBP should be goal oriented rather than focused on identifying appropriate indications for specific diagnostic testing. The important goals identified for the assessment of LBP include eliminating the possibility of very rare but potentially serious spinal pathology, ruling out rare but specific causes of LBP, identifying substantial neurologic involvement, evaluating the severity of symptoms and functional limitations, and acknowledging the presence of risk factors for chronicity. Accomplishing these goals should be centered on conducting a thorough patient history and neurologic examination. Diagnostic testing or advanced imaging such as MRI or CT should only be ordered when potentially serious spinal pathology, specific causes of LBP, or substantial neurologic involvement is suspected to identify candidates for focused surgical or medical interventions. Clinicians who adopt these recommendations must nevertheless continue to exercise clinical judgment and interpret what is in the best interest of the patients seeking care.

REFERENCES

1. Bigos S, Bowyer O, Braen G, et al. Acute low back problems in adults. Clinical Practice Guideline Number 14. AHCPR Pub. No. 95-0642. Rockville: US Department of Health and Human Services, Public Health Service, Agency for Health Care Policy and Research; 1994. Report no.: AHCPR Publication no. 95-0642.

2. Gozna E. For the Workplace Health Safety and Compensation Commission of New Brunswick. Guidelines for the diagnosis and treatment of low back pain. New Brunswick, Canada: WHSCC of New Brunswick; 2001.

3. Borkan J, Reis S, Werner S, et al. [Guidelines for treating low back pain in primary care. The Israeli Low Back Pain Guideline Group]. Harefuah 1996;130:145-151.

4. Australian Acute Musculoskeletal Pain Guidelines Group. Evidence-based management of acute musculoskeletal pain. Brisbane, Australia: Australian Academic Press Pty Ltd; 2003.

5. Staiger TO, Paauw DS, Deyo RA, et al. Imaging studies for acute low back pain. When and when not to order them. Postgrad Med 1999;105:161.

6. Chou R, Qaseem A, Snow V, et al. Diagnosis and treatment of low back pain: a joint clinical practice guideline from the American College of Physicians and the American Pain Society. Ann Intern Med 2007;147:478-491.

7. Accident Compensation Corporation (ACC), The National Health Committee. New Zealand Acute Low Back Pain Guide. Wellington, New Zealand: ACC; 1997.

8. Gilbert FJ, Grant AM, Gillan MGC, et al. Does early imaging influence management and improve outcome in patients with low back pain? A pragmatic randomised controlled trial. Health Technology Assessment 2004;8:1-131.

9. Jarvik JG, Hollingworth W, Martin B, et al. Rapid magnetic resonance imaging vs radiographs for patients with low back pain: a randomized controlled trial. JAMA 2003;289:2810-2818.

10. van Tulder M, Becker A, Bekkering T, et al. European guidelines for the management of acute nonspecific low back pain in primary care. Eur Spine J 2006;15:169-191.

11. Airaksinen O, Brox JI, Cedraschi C, et al. European guidelines for the management of chronic nonspecific low back pain. Eur Spine J 2006;15:192-300.

12. Bogduk N. Evidence-based clinical guidelines for the management of acute low back pain. Submitted to the Medical Health and Research Council of Australia, November 1999.

13. The Norwegian Back Pain Network, The Communication Unit. Acute low back pain: interdisciplinary clinical guidelines. Oslo, Norway: The Norwegian Back Pain Network; 2002.

14. Manchikanti L, Heavner JE, Racz GB, et al. Methods for evidence synthesis in interventional pain management. Pain Physician 2003;6:89-111.

15. Manchikanti L, Abdi S, Lucas LF. Evidence synthesis and development of guidelines in interventional pain management. Pain Physician 2005;8:73-86.

16. Chou R. Evidence-based medicine and the challenge of low back pain: where are we now? Pain Pract 2005;5:153-178.

17. Furlan AD, Pennick V, Bombardier C, et al. 2009 Updated method guidelines for systematic reviews in the Cochrane Back Review Group. Spine 2009;34:1929-1941.

18. National Institute for Health and Clinical Excellence (NICE). Low back pain: early management of persistent nonspecific low back pain. Report No.: NICE clinical guideline 88. London: National Institute of Health and Clinical Excellence; 2009.

19. Nielens H, van Zundert J, Mairiaux P, et al. Chronic low back pain. Vol. 48C. Brussels: KCE Reports; 2006.

20. Negrini S, Giovannoni S, Minozzi S, et al. Diagnostic therapeutic flow-charts for low back pain patients: the Italian clinical guidelines. Eura Medicophys 2006;42:151-170.

21. Chou R, Loeser JD, Owens DK, et al. Interventional therapies, surgery, and interdisciplinary rehabilitation for low back pain: an evidence-based clinical practice guideline from the American Pain Society. Spine 2009;34:1066-1077.

22. The Swedish Council on Technology Assessment in Health Care. Back pain neck pain an evidence based review summary and conclusions. Report No. 145; Stockholm, Sweden: SBU; 2000.

23. Guide to Physical Therapist Practice. Part 1: A description of patient/client management. Part 2: Preferred practice patterns. American Physical Therapy Association. Phys Ther 1997;77:1160-1656.

24. Ostelo RW, de Vet HC. Clinically important outcomes in low back pain. Best Pract Res Clin Rheumatol 2005;19:593-607.

25. Kolsi I, Delecrin J, Berthelot JM, et al. Efficacy of nerve root versus interspinous injections of glucocorticoids in the treatment of disk-related sciatica. A pilot, prospective, randomized, double-blind study. Joint Bone Spine 2000;67:113-118.

26. Johansson A, Hao J, Sjolund B. Local corticosteroid application blocks transmission in normal nociceptive C-fibres. Acta Anaesthesiol Scand 1990;34:335-338.

Note: Chapter 3 adapted from Dagenais S, Tricco AC, Haldeman S. Synthesis of recommendations for the assessment and management of low back pain from recent clinical practice guidelines. Spine J 2010;10(6):514-529.

CHAPTER 4

SIMON DAGENAIS
ANDREA C. TRICCO
SCOTT HALDEMAN

Management of Acute Low Back Pain

Many health care providers are routinely consulted for help with low back pain (LBP). LBP ranks as one of the top five reasons for seeking care and accounts for 5% of all visits to primary care providers (PCPs), doctors of chiropractic (DCs), and physical therapists (PTs).[1-5] Together, these health care providers are responsible for a large proportion of patient visits for LBP in primary care settings.[2,5,6] A sizeable number of those with LBP will also seek care in secondary care settings from both nonsurgical specialists such as neurologists, physiatrists, and rheumatologists, and surgical specialists such as orthopedic and neurologic spine surgeons.[7] Patients with LBP also seek care from allied health providers, including acupuncturists, naturopaths, and psychologists, among many others.[8]

Differences in the training, education, scope of practice, and clinical experience among these various types of providers has led to noted variations in practice patterns for the management of LBP.[9,10] Some of this variation is also attributable to the heterogeneous nature of patients with LBP, who may present with a variety of symptoms, including pain in the lumbosacral region, pain radiating into the lower extremity, muscle spasm, and limited range of motion, as well as numbness, tingling, or weakness in the thigh, leg, ankle, or foot. Only in very rare instances are such symptoms related to potentially serious spinal pathology or other specific causes of LBP that may benefit from medical or surgical interventions targeting specific anatomic structures.

Some patients with longstanding symptoms related to LBP may also benefit from one or more of the many treatment approaches that are available for this condition and whose evaluation and comparison form the basis for much of the discussion in this book. Indeed, it is often the management of chronic LBP (duration more than 12 weeks) that is often most perplexing to clinicians. This is understandable because chronic LBP results in growing frustration not only with the impact that persistent symptoms have on health and quality of life, but also with the cumulative despair that may follow repeated failed attempts to achieve satisfactory pain relief or improvement in disability with other interventions that have previously been tried.

By comparison, the management of acute LBP (i.e., duration less than 12 weeks) is simpler. Symptoms of a shorter duration are more likely to resolve at least temporarily,

whether spontaneously or following a successfully implemented management plan. Patients whose optimism has not yet been taxed too heavily by the passage of time may also be less recalcitrant to treatments for LBP in general. Because patient expectations about their outcomes may impact their prognosis, this important aspect of managing LBP should not be overlooked. There are also far fewer options that need to be considered for the management of acute LBP because a common requirement for more invasive treatment approaches is to first try conservative interventions, which is usually done during the acute phase of LBP when symptoms first appear.

Nevertheless, the current management of acute LBP is far from optimal. Although several clinical practice guidelines (CPGs) have been conducted on this topic in the past two decades, compliance with their recommendations by PCPs, DCs, PTs, and other clinicians involved in managing LBP is often reported as low.[11-26] Attempts to increase compliance with recommendations from CPGs among clinicians have reported mixed results.[15,27-30]

Barriers noted to the broader adoption of recommendations from CPGs by clinicians include a lack of understanding about how they are conducted, insufficient clarity to apply recommendations to specific patients, perceived inconsistencies among different CPGs, or disagreement by clinicians with specific recommendations from CPGs.[31] Methods for CPGs are not yet standardized and can differ considerably, which may impact the validity of their recommendations.[32,33] Previous reviews of CPGs related to LBP have reported that although many of their recommendations were similar, discrepancies were noted regarding the use of medication, spinal manipulation therapy (SMT), exercise, and patient education.[9,34] Flaws were also noted in their methodologic quality, and suggestions were made for improving future CPGs related to LBP to increase their adoption by clinicians.[34,35]

To foster an enhanced understanding of recommendations from evidence-based CPGs related to the management of LBP and evaluate any inconsistencies that may be present in these documents, a review and synthesis of recent CPGs was conducted.[36] Only CPGs sponsored by national organizations related to both the assessment and management of LBP and which had been published in English in the past 10 years were included. Although 10 such CPGs were identified for this synthesis of recommendations, only 6 pertained to the management of acute LBP.[1-3,37-39] Recommendations from CPGs about the use of specific interventions were dichotomized to "recommended" if there was strong, moderate, or limited evidence of efficacy (or similar wording), or "not recommended" if there was insufficient or conflicting evidence, or evidence against a particular intervention (or similar wording). When CPGs contained multiple recommendations about an intervention, the one contained in its summary was selected.

In addition, conclusions from recent high-quality systematic reviews (SRs) from the Cochrane Collaboration and those conducted by the American College of Physicians (ACP) and the American Pain Society (APS) in conjunction with their CPGs, were also summarized where appropriate. Interventions are presented according to their most likely setting, that is, primary care or secondary care. A distinction was often made in CPGs with respect to weaker opioid analgesics (e.g., codeine, tramadol) and stronger opioid analgesics (e.g., oxycodone, morphine); the former are grouped with primary care interventions, while the latter are discussed in secondary care interventions. Recommendations from the CPGs reviewed related to specific interventions encountered in primary care and secondary care for the management of acute LBP are summarized in Table 4-1.

PRIMARY CARE INTERVENTIONS

The most commonly discussed primary care interventions for the management of acute LBP were centered on patient education, medications, manual therapy, physical modalities, and other interventions. Each is briefly discussed here. Some of the primary care interventions that were generally recommended by CPGs for acute LBP are also illustrated in Figures 4-1 through 4-4.

Patient Education

Patient education was often one of the most highly recommended interventions for the management of acute LBP. All six CPGs recommended that clinicians should (1) tell their patients to remain active despite their LBP, (2) present their patients with brief education about the basic facts of LBP (e.g., unclear etiology, benign nature, favorable short-term prognosis), and (3) advocate against bed rest. Five of the CPGs recommended against prescribing back exercises for acute LBP and recommended that clinicians provide reassurance to patients with acute LBP (e.g., severity of symptoms does not reflect physical harm, function may improve before symptoms). Only two CPGs recommended back schools for acute LBP.

Brief Education

An SR conducted in 2008 by the Cochrane Collaboration on patient education for nonspecific acute LBP identified

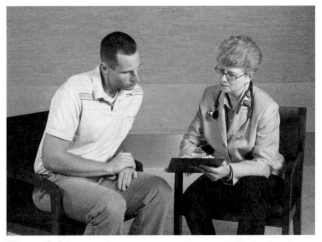

Figure 4-1 Generally recommended for acute low back pain: patient education.

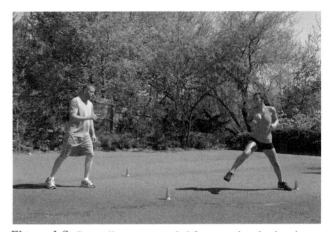

Figure 4-2 Generally recommended for acute low back pain: advice to remain active. (From Muscolino JE: Kinesiology: the skeletal system and muscle function, ed. 2. St. Louis, 2011, Elsevier.)

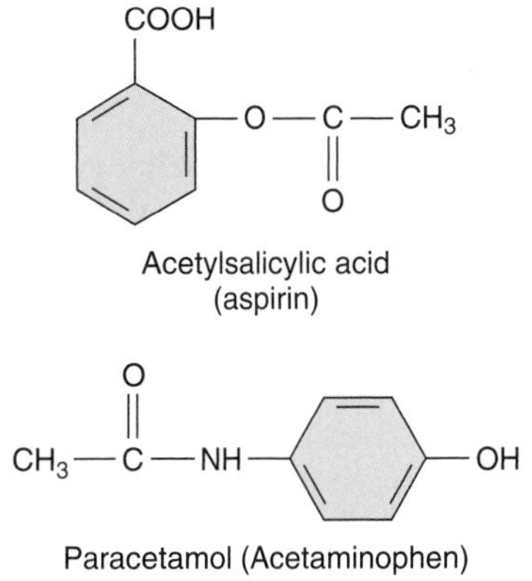

COOH

Acetylsalicylic acid
(aspirin)

Paracetamol (Acetaminophen)

Figure 4-3 Generally recommended for acute low back pain: simple analgesics. (Adapted from Wecker L: Brody's human pharmacology, ed. 5. Philadelphia, 2010, Elsevier.)

14 randomized controlled trials (RCTs).[40] This review found that a 2.5-hour individual patient education session was more effective than no intervention and was equally effective as noneducational interventions (i.e., SMT, physical therapy). However, shorter education sessions, such as

| TABLE 4-1 | Recommendations from Clinical Practice Guidelines About Management of Patients with Acute Low Back Pain |

Country	Australia	Europe	Italy	New Zealand	Norway	United States (1°)	Recommended
Reference	36	37	3	38	2	1	
Primary Care							
Education							
Advice to stay active	yes	yes	yes	yes	yes	yes	6
Back schools	no	no	yes	—	yes	no	2
Bed rest	no	no	no	no	no	no	0
Brief education on LBP	yes	yes	yes	yes	yes	yes	6
Back exercises	no	no	no	no	yes	no	1
Reassurance	yes	yes	yes	yes	yes	—	5
Medication							
Acetaminophen	no	yes	yes	yes	yes	yes	5
Muscle relaxants	no	yes	yes	no	yes	yes	4
NSAIDs	no	yes	yes	yes	yes	yes	5
Weaker opioid analgesics	no	yes	yes	—	yes	yes	4
Manual Therapy							
Massage	no	no	no	no	yes	no	1
SMT	no	yes	yes	yes	yes	yes	5
Physical Modalities							
Heat/cold	yes	—	no	no	no	yes*	2
TENS	no	no	no	no	—	no	0
Traction	no	no	no	no	no	—	0
Ultrasound	—	—	no	no	no	—	0
Other							
Acupuncture	no	—	no	no	no	no	0
Biofeedback	no	—	—	no	—	—	0
Lumbar supports	no	—	no	no	no	no	0
Secondary Care							
Medication							
Adjunctive analgesics	—	—	—	—	—	no	0
Stronger opioid analgesics	no	—	—	—	—	yes	1
Injections							
Epidural steroid injections	no	no	—	no	—	—	0
Facet injections	no	—	—	—	—	—	0
Soft tissue injections	no	—	—	—	—	—	0
Surgery							
Decompression surgery	—	—	no	yes	no	—	1
Fusion surgery	—	—	no	no	no	—	0
Other							
Behavioral therapy	no	no	—	—	yes	no	1
Multidisciplinary rehabilitation	no	yes	—	yes	—	no	2

*Only heat was recommended.
1°, primary care; LBP, low back pain; NSAIDs, nonsteroidal anti-inflammatory drugs; SMT, spinal manipulation therapy; TENS, transcutaneous electrical nerve stimulation.

written educational materials, were not more effective than no intervention.

Back Schools
An SR conducted in 1999 and updated in 2003 by the Cochrane Collaboration on back schools for nonspecific acute LBP included four RCTs.[41-43] The review reported conflicting evidence on the effectiveness of back schools for acute LBP. An SR conducted in 2006 by the APS and ACP on back schools for acute LBP identified three SRs on this topic, including the Cochrane SR described previously.[44] Those 3 SRs included 31 RCTs. This review concluded that

back schools are not effective for LBP of any duration (e.g., acute, chronic).

Medications

The medications most commonly discussed for acute LBP were acetaminophen, nonsteroidal anti-inflammatory drugs (NSAIDs), muscle relaxants, and opioid analgesics. Both acetaminophen and NSAIDs were recommended by five CPGs, whereas muscle relaxants and weaker opioids were each recommended by four CPGs. Conclusions from SRs on related topics follow.

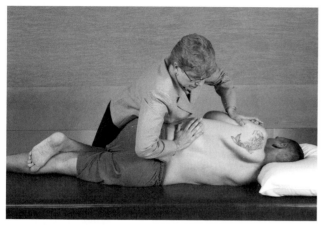

Figure 4-4 Generally recommended for acute low back pain: spinal manipulation.

Common Analgesics

An SR conducted in 2008 by the Cochrane Collaboration on NSAIDs reviewed 37 RCTs related to acute LBP.[45,46] This review concluded that NSAIDs are effective for global improvement in patients with acute LBP, although their effect is small. In addition, meta-analysis of RCTs showed that NSAIDs were more effective than placebo for acute LBP without sciatica, but resulted in more adverse events (AEs) than placebo. There was moderate evidence that NSAIDs are as effective as acetaminophen for pain relief and global improvement, but that they have more AEs than acetaminophen. There was no evidence that a specific type of NSAID is more effective than other NSAIDs.

Muscle Relaxants

An SR conducted in 2003 by the Cochrane Collaboration on muscle relaxants for nonspecific acute LBP included 23 RCTs.[47] The review concluded that there was strong evidence that muscle relaxants (nonbenzodiazepines) were more effective than placebo in short-term pain relief and overall improvement. However, muscle relaxants were also associated with more AEs than placebo, mostly related to the central nervous system. The evidence was less clear for use of benzodiazepines compared with placebo for acute LBP. There was strong evidence that muscle relaxants in combination with acetaminophen or NSAIDs were more effective than either one alone, but had more AEs than either one individually.

Opioid Analgesics

An SR conducted in 2007 by the Cochrane Collaboration examined opioids for chronic LBP but did not make any conclusions for acute LBP. An SR conducted in 2007 by the APS and ACP on medications for LBP concluded that opioid analgesics may be a reasonable treatment option but did not distinguish acute from chronic LBP. Another SR conducted in 2007 reviewed opioid analgesics for LBP.[48] This review concluded that opioid analgesics may be efficacious for short-term relief of acute or chronic LBP. However, a meta-analysis in that review reported no significant pain reduction for opioid analgesics when compared with placebo.

Manual Therapy

The manual therapy approaches most commonly discussed in the CPGs were SMT and massage. Although five CPGs recommended SMT for acute LBP, only one CPG recommended massage for acute LBP. Conclusions from SRs on related topics are discussed below.

Spinal Manipulation Therapy

An SR conducted in 2004 by the Cochrane Collaboration on SMT for acute LBP included 29 RCTs.[49] This review found evidence of short-term improvement in both pain and physical function when SMT was compared with traction, corset, bed rest, home care, topical gel, no treatment, diathermy, or minimal massage. In addition, SMT was as effective as common analgesics, physical modalities, exercises, or back school.

Massage

An SR conducted in 2008 by the Cochrane Collaboration on massage for nonspecific acute LBP included seven RCTs.[50,51] The review concluded that massage might be beneficial for patients with acute LBP if combined with exercise and delivered by a licensed therapist. An SR conducted in 2007 by the APS and ACP on massage for acute LBP identified two SRs on this topic, including the Cochrane SR described earlier.[44] This review concluded that there was not enough evidence to evaluate the efficacy of massage in acute LBP.

Physical Modalities

The physical modalities most commonly discussed in CPGs for acute LBP were superficial heat/cold, electrotherapy (e.g., transcutaneous electrical nerve stimulation), traction therapy, and ultrasound. The only physical modalities recommended by CPGs were superficial heat/cold, which were supported by two CPGs. None of the CPGs recommended electrotherapy, traction therapy, or ultrasound for acute LBP. Conclusions from SRs on related topics are discussed below.

Superficial Heat/Cold

An SR conducted in 2005 by the Cochrane Collaboration on superficial heat or cold for acute LBP included five RCTs for heat and one RCT for cold.[52] This review concluded that heat wraps were effective at reducing pain and disability for acute LBP, and that these effects may be enhanced when combined with exercise. Related to superficial cold, this Cochrane review concluded that there is insufficient evidence for cold therapy for LBP of any duration (e.g., acute, chronic). The review reported that there is conflicting evidence for heat versus cold therapy for LBP.

Electrotherapy

An SR conducted in 2006 by the APS and ACP on electrotherapy for acute LBP included three RCTs.[44] This review concluded that interferential therapy has not been shown to be beneficial for acute LBP.

Traction Therapy

An SR conducted in 2006 by the APS and ACP on traction therapy for acute LBP identified three SRs on this topic.[44] All of the SRs reported that there was no evidence or there was insufficient evidence supporting the use of traction therapy for acute LBP. This SR concluded that traction therapy has not been shown to be beneficial for acute LBP.

Other Interventions

The other interventions discussed among the CPGs for acute LBP were acupuncture, biofeedback, and lumbar supports (e.g., belts, braces, corsets). However, none of the CPGs recommended these interventions for acute LBP. Conclusions from SRs on related topics follow.

Acupuncture

An SR conducted in 2003 by the Cochrane Collaboration on acupuncture and dry needling for acute LBP included three RCTs.[53] This review found insufficient evidence to support the use of acupuncture and dry needling for acute LBP. An SR conducted in 2007 by the APS and ACP on acupuncture for acute LBP identified three SRs on this topic, including the Cochrane SR described earlier.[44] Two of these SRs were of high quality and concluded that there is insufficient evidence to support the use of acupuncture for acute LBP.

SECONDARY CARE INTERVENTIONS

The most commonly discussed secondary care interventions for the management of acute LBP included medications, injections, surgery, and other approaches. Each is briefly discussed here.

Medications

In addition to those reviewed earlier for primary care settings, medications discussed in CPGs for acute LBP included adjunctive analgesics (e.g., antidepressants, anticonvulsants), and stronger opioid analgesics. None of the CPGs recommended adjunctive analgesics for acute LBP, and only one CPG recommended stronger opioids for acute LBP. It should be noted that the recommendation in that particular CPG may have lacked specificity in that it combined both weaker and stronger opioid analgesics.

Injections

The different types of injections discussed among the CPGs for acute LBP included epidural steroid injections, facet injections, and soft tissue injections (e.g., trigger point injections, local anesthetic injections). None of the CPGs recommended these injection treatments for acute LBP.

Surgery

The two main surgical approaches applicable to the management of LBP are decompression surgery (e.g., laminectomy, discectomy) and fusion surgery (e.g., with or without surgical hardware, using autograft, allograft, or bone growth protein). Only one of the CPGs recommended decompression surgery for acute LBP, while none of the CPGs recommended fusion surgery for acute LBP.

Other Approaches

Other secondary care interventions discussed in the CPGs reviewed included behavioral therapy and multidisciplinary rehabilitation. Two of the CPGs recommended multidisciplinary rehabilitation for acute LBP, while only one CPG recommended behavioral therapy for acute LBP.

Options for managing symptoms of acute LBP included various primary and secondary care approaches such as patient education, medication, manual therapies, physical modalities, injections, surgery, and other interventions. The scope of interventions discussed in each CPG was slightly different, and it was unclear why certain approaches were included or excluded from their literature search and summary recommendations. A synthesis of management recommendations suggests that clinicians should educate patients with acute LBP about its etiology (e.g., unknown/nonspecific), prognosis (e.g., likely to improve within weeks with or without care), and recurrence (e.g., future occurrences are common), and recommend that the patient stay active despite discomfort associated with activities of daily living. For short-term symptomatic relief among those with acute LBP, acetaminophen, NSAIDs, and SMT are options. It was noted in some CPGs that trial and error would likely be required when managing LBP because not all patients respond to the same interventions.[37] Adopting these recommendations should provide satisfactory care for the vast majority of patients with LBP in primary care settings.

REFERENCES

1. Chou R, Qaseem A, Snow V, et al. Diagnosis and treatment of low back pain: a joint clinical practice guideline from the American College of Physicians and the American Pain Society. Ann Intern Med 2007;147:478-491.
2. The Norwegian Back Pain Network, The Communication Unit. Acute low back pain: interdisciplinary clinical guidelines. Oslo, Norway: The Norwegian Back Pain Network; 2002.
3. Negrini S, Giovannoni S, Minozzi S, et al. Diagnostic therapeutic flow-charts for low back pain patients: the Italian clinical guidelines. Eura Medicophys 2006;42:151-170.
4. Cote P, Cassidy JD, Carroll L. The treatment of neck and low back pain: who seeks care? Who goes where? Med Care 2001;39:956-967.
5. Lind BK, Lafferty WE, Tyree PT, et al. The role of alternative medical providers for the outpatient treatment of insured patients with back pain. Spine 2005;30:1454-1459.
6. Renfrew DL, Moore TE, Kathol MH, et al. Correct placement of epidural steroid injections: fluoroscopic guidance and contrast administration. AJNR Am J Neuroradiol 1991;12:1003-1007.
7. Flower RJ, Blackwell GJ. Anti-inflammatory steroids induce biosynthesis of a phospholipase A2 inhibitor which prevents prostaglandin generation. Nature 1979;278:456-459.

8. Haldeman S, Dagenais S. A supermarket approach to the evidence-informed management of chronic low back pain. Spine J 2008;8:1-7.

9. Koes BW, van Tulder MW, Ostelo R, et al. Clinical guidelines for the management of low back pain in primary care: an international comparison. Spine 2001;26:2504-2513.

10. Hasue M. Pain and the nerve root. An interdisciplinary approach. Spine 1993;18:2053-2058.

11. Furlan AD, Pennick V, Bombardier C, et al. 2009 Updated method guidelines for systematic reviews in the Cochrane Back Review Group. Spine 2009;34:1929-1941.

12. Webster BS, Courtney TK, Huang YH, et al. Survey of acute low back pain management by specialty group and practice experience. J Occup Environ Med 2006;48:723-732.

13. Walsh L, Menzies D, Chamberlain K, et al. Do occupational health assessments match guidelines for low back pain? Occup Med (Lond) 2008;58:485-489.

14. Somerville S, Hay E, Lewis M, et al. Content and outcome of usual primary care for back pain: a systematic review. Br J Gen Pract 2008;58:790.

15. Bishop PB, Wing PC. Knowledge transfer in family physicians managing patients with acute low back pain: a prospective randomized control trial. Spine J 2006;6:282-288.

16. Bishop PB, Wing PC. Compliance with clinical practice guidelines in family physicians managing worker's compensation board patients with acute lower back pain. Spine J 2003;3:442-450.

17. Gonzalez-Urzelai V, Palacio-Elua L, Lopez-de-Munain J. Routine primary care management of acute low back pain: adherence to clinical guidelines. Eur Spine J 2003;12:589-594.

18. Jackson JL, Browning R. Impact of national low back pain guidelines on clinical practice. South Med J 2005;98:139-143.

19. Hourcade S, Treves R. Computed tomography in low back pain and sciatica. A retrospective study of 132 patients in the Haute-Vienne district of France. Joint Bone Spine 2002;69:589-596.

20. Ammendolia C, Taylor JA, Pennick V, et al. Adherence to radiography guidelines for low back pain: a survey of chiropractic schools worldwide. J Manipulative Physiol Ther 2008;31:412-418.

21. Fullen BM, Maher T, Bury G, et al. Adherence of Irish general practitioners to European guidelines for acute low back pain: a prospective pilot study. Eur J Pain 2007;11:614-623.

22. Fritz JM, Cleland JA, Brennan GP. Does adherence to the guideline recommendation for active treatments improve the quality of care for patients with acute low back pain delivered by physical therapists? Med Care 2007;45:973-980.

23. Swinkels IC, van den Ende CH, van den BW, et al. Physiotherapy management of low back pain: does practice match the Dutch guidelines? Aust J Physiother 2005;51:35-41.

24. Strand LI, Kvale A, Raheim M, et al. Do Norwegian manual therapists provide management for patients with acute low back pain in accordance with clinical guidelines? Man Ther 2005;10:38-43.

25. Poitras S, Blais R, Swaine B, et al. Practice patterns of physiotherapists in the treatment of work-related back pain. J Eval Clin Pract 2007;13:412-421.

26. Poitras S, Blais R, Swaine B, et al. Management of work-related low back pain: a population-based survey of physical therapists. Phys Ther 2005;85:1168-1181.

27. Becker A, Leonhardt C, Kochen MM, et al. Effects of two guideline implementation strategies on patient outcomes in primary care: a cluster randomized controlled trial. Spine 2008;33:473-480.

28. Bekkering GE, Hendriks HJ, van Tulder MW, et al. Effect on the process of care of an active strategy to implement clinical guidelines on physiotherapy for low back pain: a cluster randomised controlled trial. Qual Saf Health Care 2005;14:107-112.

29. Bekkering GE, van Tulder MW, Hendriks EJ, et al. Implementation of clinical guidelines on physical therapy for patients with low back pain: randomized trial comparing patient outcomes after a standard and active implementation strategy. Phys Ther 2005;85:544-555.

30. Rao JK, Kroenke K, Mihaliak KA, et al. Can guidelines impact the ordering of magnetic resonance imaging studies by primary care providers for low back pain? Am J Manag Care 2002;8:27-35.

31. Cote AM, Durand MJ, Tousignant M, et al. Physiotherapists and use of low back pain guidelines: a qualitative study of the barriers and facilitators. J Occup Rehabil 2009;19:94-105.

32. Chou R. Evidence-based medicine and the challenge of low back pain: where are we now? Pain Pract 2005;5:153-178.

33. Manchikanti L. Evidence-based medicine, systematic reviews, and guidelines in interventional pain management, part I: introduction and general considerations. Pain Physician 2008;11:161-186.

34. van Tulder MW, Tuut M, Pennick V, et al. Quality of primary care guidelines for acute low back pain. Spine 2004;29:E357-E362.

35. Guide to Physical Therapist Practice. Part 1: A description of patient/client management. Part 2: Preferred practice patterns. American Physical Therapy Association. Phys Ther 1997;77:1160-1656.

36. Dagenais S, Tricco AC, Haldeman S. Synthesis of recommendations for the assessment and management of low back pain from recent clinical practice guidelines. Spine J 2010;10:514-529.

37. Australian Acute Musculoskeletal Pain Guidelines Group. Evidence-based management of acute musculoskeletal pain. Brisbane, Australia: Australian Academic Press Pty Ltd; 2003.

38. van Tulder M, Becker A, Bekkering T, et al. European guidelines for the management of acute nonspecific low back pain in primary care. Eur Spine J 2006;15:169-191.

39. Accident Compensation Corporation (ACC), The National Health Committee. New Zealand Acute Low Back Pain Guide. Wellington, New Zealand: ACC; 1997.

40. Engers A, Jellema P, Wensing M, et al. Individual patient education for low back pain. Cochrane Database Syst Rev 2008;(1):CD004057.

41. van Tulder MW, Esmail R, Bombardier C, et al. Back schools for non-specific low back pain. Cochrane Database of Systematic Reviews 2000;(2).

42. Heymans MW, van Tulder MW, Esmail R, et al. Back schools for nonspecific low back pain: a systematic review within the framework of the Cochrane Collaboration Back Review Group. Spine 2005;30:2153-2163.

43. Heymans MW, van Tulder MW, Esmail R, et al. Back schools for non-specific low-back pain. Cochrane Database of Systematic Reviews 2004;(4).

44. Chou R, Huffman LH. Nonpharmacologic therapies for acute and chronic low back pain: a review of the evidence for an American Pain Society/American College of Physicians clinical practice guideline. Ann Intern Med 2007;147:492-504.

45. Roelofs PD, Deyo RA, Koes BW, et al. Non-steroidal anti-inflammatory drugs for low back pain. Cochrane Database Syst Rev 2008;(1):CD000396.

46. van Tulder MW, Scholten RJ, Koes BW, et al. Nonsteroidal anti-inflammatory drugs for low back pain: a systematic review

within the framework of the Cochrane Collaboration Back Review Group. Spine 2000;25:2501-2513.

47. van Tulder MW, Touray T, Furlan AD, et al. Muscle relaxants for nonspecific low back pain: a systematic review within the framework of the Cochrane collaboration. Spine 2003;28:1978-1992.

48. Martell BA, O'Connor PG, Kerns RD, et al. Systematic review: opioid treatment for chronic back pain: prevalence, efficacy, and association with addiction. Ann Intern Med 2007;146: 116-127.

49. Assendelft WJ, Morton SC, Yu EI, et al. Spinal manipulative therapy for low back pain. Cochrane Database Syst Rev 2004;(1):CD000447.

50. Furlan AD, Brosseau L, Imamura M, et al. Massage for low-back pain: a systematic review within the framework of the Cochrane Collaboration Back Review Group. Spine 2002;27: 1896-1910.

51. Furlan AD, Imamura M, Dryden T, et al. Massage for low-back pain. Cochrane Database Syst Rev 2008;(4):CD001929.

52. French S, Cameron M, Walker B, et al. Superficial heat or cold for low back pain. The Cochrane Database of Systematic Reviews 2006;(1).

53. Furlan AD, van Tulder MW, Cherkin DC, et al. Acupuncture and dry-needling for low back pain. Cochrane Database Syst Rev 2005;(1):CD001351.

54. Bogduk N, Long DM. The anatomy of the so-called "articular nerves" and their relationship to facet denervation in the treatment of low-back pain. J Neurosurg 1979;51:172-177.

Note: Chapter 4 adapted from Dagenais S, Tricco AC, Haldeman S. Synthesis of recommendations for the assessment and management of low back pain from recent clinical practice guidelines. Spine J 2010;10(6):514-529.

EUGENE K. WAI
SEBASTIAN RODRIGUEZ-
    ELIZALDE
SIMON DAGENAIS
HAMILTON HALL

CHAPTER **5**

Physical Activity, Smoking Cessation, and Weight Loss

DESCRIPTION

Terminology and Subtypes

The World Health Organization has defined lifestyle as "a way of living based on identifiable patterns of behavior which are determined by the interplay between an individual's personal characteristics, social interactions, and socioeconomic and environmental living conditions."[1] To promote health and improve clinical outcomes in a variety of chronic conditions, including chronic low back pain (CLBP), health care providers increasingly recommend interventions aimed at addressing lifestyle.[2-4] Modifiable lifestyle risk factors are often nutritional or physiologic in nature, and interventions to address them commonly include general physical activity, smoking cessation, and weight loss. There are numerous types of interventions commonly used for modifiable lifestyle risk factors. For physical activity, these include walking and jogging, swimming, or cycling. For smoking cessation, these include "cold turkey," nicotine patch or gum, and group or cognitive behavioral approaches. For weight loss, these include calorie restriction, food-type restriction, and medically supervised diets.

History and Frequency of Use

Although health care providers have long sought to improve their patients' health through education and advice on general lifestyle modifications, this has generally depended on the availability of evidence to support an association between a risk factor and a particular health condition. The relationship between low back pain (LBP) and physical inactivity is likely complex because there is evidence suggesting that either too much or too little activity may be associated with LBP.[5] However, there exist numerous potential confounders as many studies on this topic have occurred in an occupational setting.

For example, although physical activity such as repetitive lifting or twisting has been associated with LBP, this was likely confounded by high job dissatisfaction and low education.[6-8] When examining recreational rather than occupational physical activity, many studies have reported that general physical fitness appears to lower the incidence or severity of LBP.[9,10] Several hypotheses have been offered for a possible association between LBP and smoking, including repeated microtrauma from chronic cough leading to disc herniations, reduced blood flow to the discs and vertebral bodies leading to early degeneration, and decreased bone mineral density leading to vertebral body or end plate injury.[11-13] Systematic reviews (SRs) have reported that 51% to 77% of epidemiologic studies found a positive association between smoking and LBP.[14-16] Although a causal link between obesity and LBP appears intuitive because of additional weight on load-bearing spinal elements and altered biomechanics leading to excessive wear and early degeneration, evidence to support such hypotheses is lacking. An SR of 65 epidemiologic studies reported that only 32% found a positive association between obesity and LBP.[17]

Little is currently known about the prevalence of lifestyle modification counseling among spine providers. A cross-sectional study of 52 consecutive patients presenting to an academic spine surgery clinic reported that despite an increased prevalence of morbid obesity (body mass index greater than 30) compared with the general population, less than 20% had received counseling about lifestyle modification from their primary care physicians.[18] It has been reported that chiropractors commonly offer preventive care services, including smoking cessation, weight-loss programs, fitness counseling, and stress management to their patients, including those with CLBP.[19]

Practitioner, Setting, and Availability

Physical activity, smoking cessation, and weight-loss programs may be self-administered or under the guidance of a physician, psychologist, therapist, physical therapist, or other health care provider. These interventions are typically administered in private practices, outpatient clinics, community health centers, or physical fitness centers, and are widely available throughout the United States.

Procedure

Physical Activity

According to the Centers for Disease Control and Prevention, regular moderate-intensity activity is sufficient to produce health benefits in those who are sedentary.[20] Health care providers should recommend that adults engage in 30 minutes of moderate-intensity activity 5 days per week, or 20 minutes of vigorous-intensity activity 3 days per week. Moderate-intensity activity burns 3.5 to 7 calories per minute and includes such activities as walking briskly, mowing the lawn, dancing, swimming for recreation, and bicycling (Figures 5-1 through 5-3). Vigorous-intensity activity burns greater than seven calories per minute and includes such activities as high-impact aerobic dancing, swimming continuous laps, or bicycling uphill. Regardless of intensity, patients should burn the recommended 1000 calories per week. To promote physical activity, patients need to be encouraged to set realistic personal goals, gradually increasing the length and intensity of activity, and varying the type of activities to remain interested and challenged.

Smoking Cessation

According to the American Cancer Society, smoking cessation involves four steps: (1) making the decision to quit; (2) setting a quit date and choosing a quit plan; (3) dealing with withdrawal; (4) staying "quit" (Figure 5-4).[21] The decision to quit smoking must originate from the patients, who are more likely to succeed if they: (1) are worried about tobacco-related disease; (2) believe they are able to quit; (3) believe that benefits outweigh risks; (4) know someone with smoking-related health problems. The quit date should occur within the next month to prepare appropriately and not delay much further, and might be selected for a special reason (e.g., birthday, anniversary, or Great American Smokeout, which occurs on the third Thursday in November) (Figure 5-5). Family and friends should be informed of the quit date, which may require modifying activities previously associated with smoking (e.g., coffee or alcohol use). Although

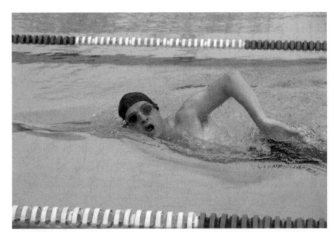

Figure 5-2 Moderate intensity physical activity: swimming. (© istockphoto.com/Darren Wise)

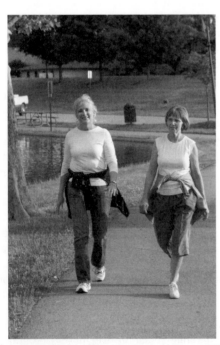

Figure 5-1 Moderate intensity physical activity: walking briskly. (© istockphoto.com/Gary Phillips)

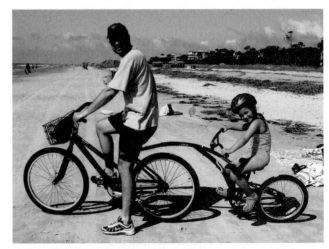

Figure 5-3 Moderate intensity physical activity: bicycling. (From Edelman CL, Mandle CL. Health promotion throughout the life span, ed 7. St Louis, 2010, Mosby.)

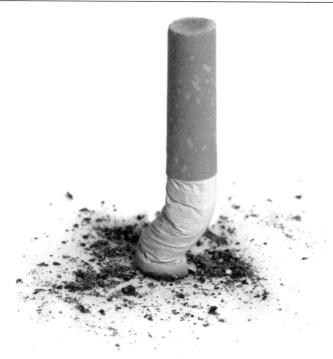

Figure 5-4 Smoking cessation steps: 1. Make the decision. 2. Set a quit date. 3. Deal with withdrawal. 4. Stay quit. (© www.istockphoto.com/Hermann Danzmayr.)

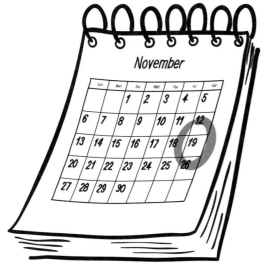

Figure 5-5 The great American smokeout, in the past, has taken place on the 3rd Thursday in November. It is a target date for smokers to use to quit the bad habit for good.

nicotine substitutes can reduce physical symptoms of withdrawal, they should be combined with a plan addressing psychological aspects of quitting, which are often hardest to overcome. Care must be taken to recognize and overcome rationalizations to resume smoking (e.g., "just one cigarette won't hurt"). Oral substitutes for cigarettes can be used,

including gum, candy, carrot sticks, or sunflower seeds; exercise and deep breathing may also help alleviate withdrawal symptoms. Small self-rewards for milestones achieved (e.g., one week, one month) can help stay motivated to quit. To prevent relapses, reasons for quitting should be reviewed periodically, emphasizing benefits already achieved and those still to come.

Weight Loss

According to the Weight-control Information Network at the National Institutes of Health, there are two main categories of weight-loss programs: nonclinical and clinical.[22] The former may be self-administered or performed with assistance from a weight-loss clinic, counselor, support group, book, or website. Nonclinical weight-loss programs should use educational materials written or reviewed by a physician or dietitian that address both healthy eating and exercise; programs neglecting the exercise component should be avoided (Figure 5-6). Although many commercial programs may promote proprietary foods, supplements, or products, these may be costly and will not teach participants about appropriate food selection to maintain long-term weight loss. Programs promoting specific formulas or foods for easy weight loss may offer short-term weight loss because of calorie restriction but should be avoided because they may not provide essential nutrients, do not teach healthy eating habits, and are not sustainable. Clinical weight-loss programs are administered by licensed health care providers including physicians, nurses, dietitians, or psychologists in a clinic or hospital setting. These programs may include nutrition education, physical activity, cognitive behavioral therapy (CBT), prescription weight loss drugs, or gastrointestinal surgery, depending on the desired weight-loss and health status.

Regulatory Status

Not applicable.

THEORY

Mechanisms of Action

Lifestyle interventions such as physical activity, smoking cessation, and weight loss have a wide range of effects on human health in general, which is likely an important determinant of CLBP. In addition to their general impact on the body, the specific aspects that may contribute to improving CLBP for each of these interventions is briefly described below.

Physical Activity

In general, exercises are used to strengthen muscles, increase soft tissue stability, restore range of movement, improve cardiovascular conditioning, increase proprioception, and reduce fear of movement. Engaging in physical activity through exercise programs is theorized to improve CLBP through multiple mechanisms, including improved conditioning and confidence for daily activities, release of endorphins,

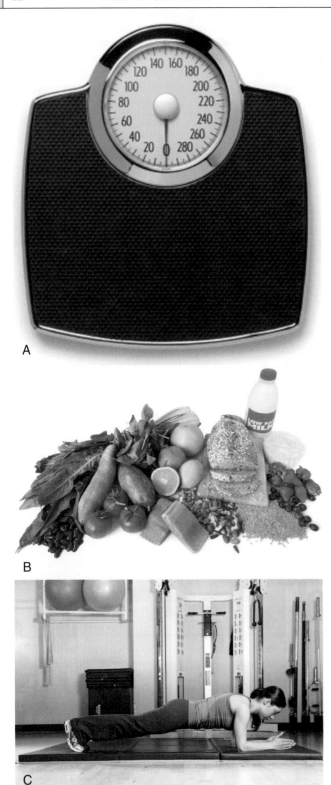

improved social interaction, reduced fear avoidance, and decreased generalized anxiety.[23-27] The warmth of the water in hydrotherapy has also been purported to reduce muscle pain.[28]

Disc metabolism may also be enhanced through repetitive exercise involving the spine's full active range of motion. Given that the absence of physical activity is known to reduce a healthy metabolism, it appears reasonable to believe that introducing exercise, such as lumbar stabilization exercise, may reverse such findings.[29] The association between biochemical abnormalities in the lumbar discs and CLBP has previously been documented.[30] Enhanced disc metabolism could improve repair and enhance reuptake of inflammatory and nociceptive mediators that may have migrated to an area of injury.

In some patients with particularly severe or prolonged CLBP, or psychological comorbidities such as anxiety or depression, maladaptive illness behavior may become established. This type of behavior may manifest itself as fear of engaging in any activity or movement that has previously been associated with symptoms of CLBP. As time passes, virtually all activities gain this association, leading to a generalized fear of movement in an attempt to minimize exacerbations. Engaging in supervised exercise therapy under the guidance of an experienced clinician able to gradually increase the type, dose, frequency, or intensity of movements can help break this cycle and demonstrate that not all movements or activities need be painful. This aspect is addressed further in other chapters of this text that discuss brief education, back schools, fear avoidance training, and functional restoration.

Smoking Cessation

Smoking cessation is thought to improve CLBP by decreasing exposure to the potentially harmful effects of smoking related to the lumbar spine. For example, it has been postulated that repeated microtrauma to the intervertebral discs from chronic coughing associated with long-term smoking can gradually lead to disc injury or herniation. Smoking is also thought to reduce blood flow to the discs, which already have a poor supply, as well as to the vertebral bodies.[31] These effects could eventually lead to accelerated or early degeneration from insufficient healing capacity and decreased bone mineral density. The time required to fully or partially reverse these effects and observe clinical improvement of CLBP after smoking cessation is currently unknown.

Weight Loss

Weight loss is thought to improve CLBP by decreasing exposure to the potentially harmful effects of obesity related to the lumbar spine (e.g., additional weight on load-bearing spinal elements and altered biomechanics leading to excessive wear and early degeneration).[17,32] It may also contribute to the improvement of CLBP by facilitating participation in general or back-specific exercises that may not be possible if a patient is overweight or obese. The time required to fully or partially reverse these effects and observe clinical improvements in CLBP after weight loss is currently unknown.

Figure 5-6 Weight loss programs (**A**) should emphasize both healthy eating (**B**) and increased exercise (**C**). (A © www.istockphoto.com/DNY59; **B**, © istockphoto.com/Robyn Mackenzie.)

Indication

Physical activity is indicated for all patients with CLBP. Smoking cessation is indicated for all patients with CLBP who are smokers. Weight loss is indicated for all patients with CLBP who have a body mass index greater than 30, high-risk waist circumference, and two or more risk factors related to obesity.[33] The included studies did not identify any factors related to the ideal patient for these interventions.[23,34-39] However, all studies noted issues related to motivation, which needs to be taken into consideration when recommending patient-driven lifestyle modifications. Prochaska and DiClemente[40] outlined five steps required to modify a person's lifestyle: (1) precontemplation, (2) contemplation, (3) determination, (4) action, and (5) maintenance. Specifically in regard to health issues, persistent lifestyle changes have generally been initiated when patients connect their lifestyle risk factor to the disease at hand (contemplation stage). Often these require a major disease event such as a heart attack. In the case of CLBP, the primary health care provider may be critical in helping patients establish this link as the first step toward motivating them toward change.

Assessment

Before receiving physical activity, smoking cessation, or weight loss counseling, patients should first be assessed for LBP using an evidence-based and goal-oriented approach focused on the patient history and neurologic examination, as discussed in Chapter 3. Additional diagnostic imaging or specific diagnostic testing is generally not required before initiating these interventions for CLBP. Certain questionnaires may be helpful to document the frequency of current physical activity, smoking, or caloric intake to establish a benchmark against which future outcomes can be compared.

EFFICACY

Evidence supporting the efficacy of these interventions for CLBP was summarized from recent clinical practice guidelines (CPGs), SRs, and randomized controlled trials (RCTs). Observational studies (OBSs) were also summarized where appropriate. Findings are summarized by study design for each intervention.

Clinical Practice Guidelines

Physical Activity

Four of the recent national CPGs on the management of CLBP have assessed and summarized the evidence to make specific recommendations about the efficacy of physical activity or advice to remain active, which implies some form of physical activity.

The CPG from Europe in 2004 found limited evidence that aerobic exercise was more effective than back school with respect to improvements in pain and function.[41] This CPG also found strong evidence that advice to remain active, when combined with brief education, is as effective as usual physical therapy or aerobic exercise with respect to improvements in function.[41]

The CPG from Italy in 2007 strongly recommended low impact aerobic exercise for the management of CLBP.[42]

The CPG from Belgium in 2006 found moderate-quality evidence to support the efficacy of aquatic therapy for the management of CLBP.[43] This CPG also recommended advice to remain active.[43]

The CPG from the United Kingdom in 2009 concluded that advice to remain active is likely to be beneficial.[44]

Smoking Cessation

None of the recent national CPGs on the management of CLBP have assessed and summarized the evidence to make specific recommendations about the efficacy of smoking cessation as an intervention for CLBP.

Weight Loss

None of the recent national CPGs on the management of CLBP have assessed and summarized the evidence to make specific recommendations about the efficacy of weight loss as an intervention for CLBP.

Findings from the above CPGs are summarized in Table 5-1.

Systematic Reviews

Physical Activity

Cochrane Collaboration. An SR was conducted in 2004 by the Cochrane Collaboration on all forms of exercise therapy

TABLE 5-1	Clinical Practice Guideline Recommendations on Physical Activity, Smoking Cessation, and Weight Loss for Chronic Low Back Pain		
Reference	Country	Conclusion*	
Physical Activity			
41	Europe	Limited evidence that aerobic exercise is more effective than back school Strong evidence that advice to remain active plus brief education is as effective as usual physical therapy or aerobic exercise	
42	Italy	Recommended low-impact aerobic exercise	
43	Belgium	Moderate-quality evidence to support efficacy of aquatic therapy Recommended advice to remain active	
44	United Kingdom	Advice to remain active is likely to be beneficial	

*No CPGs made specific recommendations about smoking cessation or weight loss as interventions for chronic low back pain.

for acute, subacute, and chronic LBP.[45] A total of 61 RCTs were identified, including 43 RCTs related to CLBP. Although results were generally favorable, this review combined all forms of exercise therapy, including stabilization, strengthening, stretching, McKenzie, aerobic, and others. As such, these conclusions are not specific to general physical activity as discussed in this chapter. This review identified three RCTs (five reports) that may be related to general physical activity for CLBP, which are discussed below.[23,35,38,46,47]

American Pain Society and American College of Physicians. An SR was conducted in 2007 by the American Pain Society and American College of Physicians Clinical Practice Guideline Committee on nonpharmacologic therapies for acute and chronic LBP.[48] That review identified seven SRs related to all forms of exercise and LBP, including the Cochrane Collaboration review mentioned previously.[45] Although results were generally favorable, this review combined all forms of exercise therapy, including stabilization, strengthening, stretching, McKenzie, aerobic, and others. As such, these conclusions are not specific to general physical activity as discussed in this chapter. This review did not identify any new RCTs.

Smoking Cessation

No recent, high-quality SRs were identified that reported specifically on the efficacy of smoking cessation as an intervention for LBP.

Weight Loss

No recent, high-quality SRs were identified that reported specifically on the efficacy of weight loss as an intervention for LBP.

Findings from the aforementioned SRs are summarized in Table 5-2.

Randomized Controlled Trials

Five RCTs and seven reports related to those studies were identified.[23,35,36,38,46,47,49] Their methods are summarized in Table 5-3. Their results are briefly described here and are summarized in Figures 5-7 and 5-8.

Physical Activity

An RCT conducted by Mannion and colleagues included CLBP patients without neurologic involvement, who had symptoms lasting longer than 3 months.[35,46] Participants were randomized to (1) an intervention consisting of low-impact aerobics classes, (2) a control consisting of active physical therapy (ergonomics, strengthening, coordination, and aerobics), and (3) a control consisting of trunk muscle conditioning devices. All three treatments included 1-hour sessions for 3 months. At the 12-month follow-up, pain scores (visual analogue scale [VAS]) improved similarly in all three groups (P values not reported). There were no significant differences in pain scores between groups. At 12 months' follow-up, disability scores (Roland Morris Disability Questionnaire [RMDQ]) improved in all three groups (P values not reported). The improvement in disability in the aerobics and muscle conditioning groups was significantly higher than

| TABLE 5-2 | Systematic Review Findings on Physical Activity, Smoking Cessation, and Weight Loss for Chronic Low Back Pain |

Reference	# RCTs in SR	#RCTs for CLBP	Conclusion
Physical Activity*			
45	61	43	Results were generally favorable but this review combined all forms of exercise therapy, including back-specific exercises discussed in other chapters. This conclusion is not specific to general physical activity as discussed in this chapter.
48	7	NR	Results were generally favorable but this review combined all forms of exercise therapy, including back-specific exercises discussed in other chapters. This conclusion is not specific to general physical activity as discussed in this chapter.

*No SRs were identified regarding smoking cessation or weight loss as interventions for chronic low back pain.
CLBP, chronic low back pain; NR, not reported; RCT, randomized controlled trial; SR, systematic review.

that of the physical therapy group. This study was considered of higher quality.

An RCT by Tritilanunt and colleagues[38] included CLBP patients with symptoms lasting longer than 3 months. Participants were randomized to either aerobic exercise (no further details provided) or a back flexion program for 12 weeks. After the treatment period, both groups saw a statistically significant improvement in pain scores (VAS). The aerobic exercise group had statistically significant improvement in pain compared to the back flexion group. This study was considered of lower quality.

An RCT conducted by Frost and colleagues[23,47] included CLBP patients without neurologic involvement, who had symptoms lasting longer than 6 months. Participants were randomized to an intervention consisting of a group circuit exercise class, motivation from a physical therapist, back school, and core exercise education, or to the control group, consisting of back school and core exercise education. The group circuit class included 1-hour sessions twice a week for four weeks, the back school included two 1.5-hour sessions, and core exercises were encouraged to be performed twice

TABLE 5-3	**Randomized Controlled Trials of Physical Activity for Chronic Low Back Pain**			
Reference	Indication	Intervention	Control (C1)	Control (C2)
35 46	CLBP without neurologic involvement, symptoms >3 months	Low-impact aerobics class 1 hr sessions × 3 mo PT n = 50	Active physical therapy (ergonomics, strengthening, coordination and aerobics) PT 1 hr sessions × 3 mo n = 49	Trunk muscle conditioning devices PT 1 hr sessions × 3 mo n = 49
38	CLBP, symptoms >3 months, neurologic involvement NR	Aerobic exercise (no further details provided) Practitioner not reported 12 wk n = 36	Back flexion program Practitioner not reported 12 wk n = 36	NA
47 23	CLBP without neurologic involvement, symptoms >6 months	Group circuit exercise class + motivation from PT + back school + taught core exercises PT 1 hr × 2 × 4 wk (Group circuit) 1.5 hr × 2 (back school) 2/day × 6 wk (exercises) n = 41	Back school + taught core exercises PT 1.5 hr × 2 (back school) 2/day × 6 wk (exercises) n = 40	NA
36	LBP, neurologic involvement NR, duration NR	Aquafitness class Trained pool volunteer 1-hr × 2 × 4 wk n = 56	Usual care on wait list n = 53	NA
49	CLBP with or without neurologic involvement, symptoms >8 weeks	Nordic walking Trained instructor 45 min × 2 × 8 wk Cointervention: pain medication n = 45	Unsupervised Nordic walking Trained instructor showed participants how to use the Nordic walker Home use as much as possible Cointervention: pain medication n = 46	Education about active living and exercise Maintained same level of physical activity Cointervention: pain medication n = 45

CLBP, chronic low back pain; LBP, low back pain; NA, not applicable; NR, not reported; PT, physical therapist.

daily for 6 weeks. At the 24-month follow-up, mean disability scores (Oswestry Disability Index [ODI]) significantly improved in the intervention group but not the control group. Disability scores were significantly better in the intervention group compared with the control group. Pain intensity was not measured in this study. This study was considered of higher quality.

An RCT by McIlveen and Robertson[36] included LBP patients, but the duration of symptoms was not reported. Participants were assigned to an intervention of aquafitness classes or a waiting list. The aquafitness classes included 1-hour sessions twice a week for four weeks. At the end of the treatment, the majority of participants in the intervention group reported improved pain scores (McGill Pain Questionnaire). A higher proportion of participants in the intervention reported improved pain scores (McGill Pain Questionnaire) compared with the controls (P values not reported). Almost all participants in the intervention group also reported improved disability scores (ODI), whereas less than half of

those in the control group reported improved disability (P values not reported).

An RCT by Hartvigsen and colleagues[49] included CLBP patients with or without neurologic involvement. In order to be included, participants had to experience symptoms for at least 8 weeks. Participants were randomized to one of three groups: (1) supervised Nordic walking with a trained instructor during two 45-minute sessions per week over 8 weeks, (2) instruction on how to Nordic walk and advice to continue Nordic walking at home as much as possible for 8 weeks, or (3) education about active living and exercise while maintaining the same levels of physical activity as the 4 previous weeks. After 52 weeks of follow-up, the supervised Nordic walking group experienced statistically significant improvement in pain and function versus baseline scores. However, participants in the other two groups did not experience statistically significant differences in pain or function after 52 weeks of follow-up compared with baseline scores. No statistically significant differences were observed

Review: Chronic low back pain and exercise
Comparison: 01 General exercise vs. active control (e.g., physical therapy, education, devices)
Outcome: 02 Disability at final follow-up

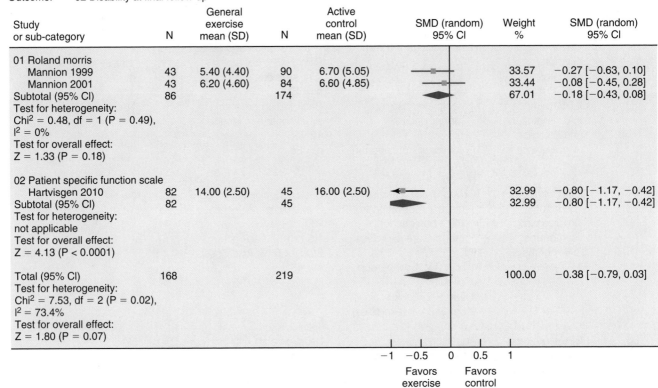

Figure 5-7 Physical activity for chronic low back pain: disability outcomes.

between the three groups after 52 weeks of follow-up regarding pain or function.

Smoking Cessation

No RCTs were identified that reported specifically on the efficacy of smoking cessation as an intervention for LBP.

Weight Loss

No RCTs were identified that reported specifically on the efficacy of weight loss as an intervention for LBP.

Observational Studies

Physical Activity

Sculco and colleagues[34] performed a two-phase study. The first phase involved a pseudo RCT comparing a home aerobic exercise physical activity program (walking or cycling) with a control group. There were no significant differences between groups in regard to overall pain as measured by the Brief Pain Inventory. The exercise group reported significantly lower "worst" pain scores as measured by VAS, which were 3.47 ± 2.00 (mean ± SD) for the physical activity group and 5.11 ± 2.80 for controls. The exercise group also had significantly less anger, depression, and total mood disturbance at the end of the intervention. The second phase involved encouraging all study participants to exercise; they were then assessed at 30 months. There was only a 57%

follow-up rate. Those patients who exercised routinely (including crossovers from the control group) had significantly less prescriptions for pain medication or physical therapy, and had improved work status. There were no differences in regard to office visits or epidural blocks between the two groups.

A pseudo RCT conducted by Sjogren and colleagues[37] included CLBP patients without neurologic involvement (duration of symptoms not reported). Participants were assigned to group exercise classes in water focusing on general strengthening, endurance, and trunk range of motion, or the same group exercise classes on land. The classes included 1-hour sessions twice a week for 6 weeks. After the treatment period, a significant improvement in mean pain scores (VAS) was observed in both groups. There was no significant difference in pain between the two groups.

SAFETY

Contraindications

Contraindications to lifestyle interventions include CLBP due to potentially serious spinal pathology such as fracture, cancer, infection, or cauda equina syndrome. It is unclear whether a specific subgroup of patients with CLBP could aggravate their symptoms by engaging in physical activity. A common exclusion criterion for studies involving physical

Review: Chronic low back pain and exercise
Comparison: 01 General exercise vs. active control (e.g., physical therapy, education, devices)
Outcome: 01 LBP at final follow-up

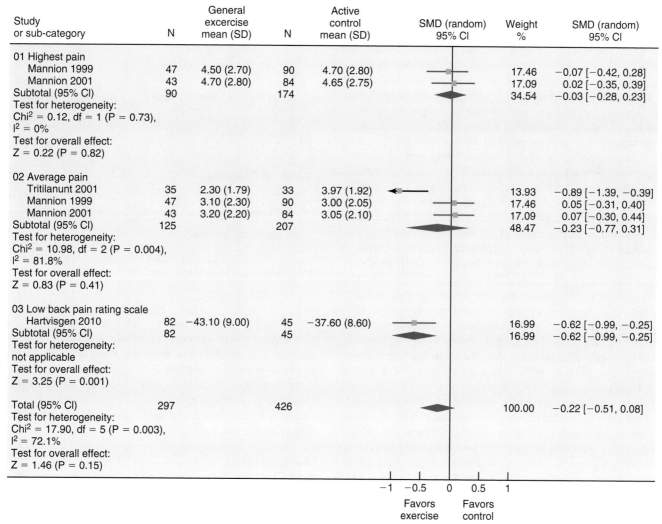

Study or sub-category	N	General excercise mean (SD)	N	Active control mean (SD)	SMD (random) 95% CI	Weight %	SMD (random) 95% CI
01 Highest pain							
Mannion 1999	47	4.50 (2.70)	90	4.70 (2.80)		17.46	−0.07 [−0.42, 0.28]
Mannion 2001	43	4.70 (2.80)	84	4.65 (2.75)		17.09	0.02 [−0.35, 0.39]
Subtotal (95% CI)	90		174			34.54	−0.03 [−0.28, 0.23]

Test for heterogeneity:
Chi² = 0.12, df = 1 (P = 0.73),
I² = 0%
Test for overall effect:
Z = 0.22 (P = 0.82)

02 Average pain							
Tritilanunt 2001	35	2.30 (1.79)	33	3.97 (1.92)		13.93	−0.89 [−1.39, −0.39]
Mannion 1999	47	3.10 (2.30)	90	3.00 (2.05)		17.46	0.05 [−0.31, 0.40]
Mannion 2001	43	3.20 (2.20)	84	3.05 (2.10)		17.09	0.07 [−0.30, 0.44]
Subtotal (95% CI)	125		207			48.47	−0.23 [−0.77, 0.31]

Test for heterogeneity:
Chi² = 10.98, df = 2 (P = 0.004),
I² = 81.8%
Test for overall effect:
Z = 0.83 (P = 0.41)

03 Low back pain rating scale							
Hartvigsen 2010	82	−43.10 (9.00)	45	−37.60 (8.60)		16.99	−0.62 [−0.99, −0.25]
Subtotal (95% CI)	82		45			16.99	−0.62 [−0.99, −0.25]

Test for heterogeneity:
not applicable
Test for overall effect:
Z = 3.25 (P = 0.001)

Total (95% CI)	297		426			100.00	−0.22 [−0.51, 0.08]

Test for heterogeneity:
Chi² = 17.90, df = 5 (P = 0.003),
I² = 72.1%
Test for overall effect:
Z = 1.46 (P = 0.15)

```
        −1   −0.5    0    0.5    1
           Favors     Favors
           exercise   control
```

Figure 5-8 Physical activity for chronic low back pain: pain outcomes.

activity is being medically unfit to participate. Some of the studies reviewed excluded participants with nerve root irritation or acute, severe symptoms.[23,34,35] However, evidence from a number of reviews suggests that staying active is beneficial for both acute LBP and sciatica.[50-52] It is unclear where the line needs to be drawn, if at all, between remaining active and engaging in a formal physical activity regimen; both are likely beneficial for common LBP.

Adverse Events

Lifestyle interventions are generally considered to be safe. None of the studies reviewed reported any adverse events associated with physical activity programs. However, some studies reported lack of participant compliance with the prescribed home exercise programs, which could potentially be related to exacerbation of symptoms experienced with this intervention. Such exacerbation of symptoms, if it does in fact occur, is likely short-lived and related to delayed onset

muscle soreness if the exercise is done too vigorously. As such, proper education on the concept of "hurt versus harm" is required before recommending lifestyle interventions involving physical activity. No serious adverse events have been reported with these interventions for CLBP. Cardiovascular events, such as a myocardial infarction, are rare but potentially serious adverse events that could be associated with physical activity undertaken by patients who are not medically fit due to comorbidities such as cardiopulmonary impairment.

COSTS

Fees and Third-Party Reimbursement

In the United States, counseling on lifestyle interventions such as physical activity, smoking cessation, and weight loss for CLBP can likely be delivered by a clinician in the context of an office or outpatient visit for a new patient using CPT codes 99201 (up to 10 minutes), 99202 (up to 20 minutes), or 99203 (up to 30 minutes). For an established patient, these can likely be provided during an office or outpatient visit using CPT codes 99211 (up to 5 minutes), 99212 (up to 10 minutes), or 99213 (up to 15 minutes). Although time is indicated for the various levels of service and can be a contributing component for selection of the level of office or outpatient visits, the overarching criteria for selection of the level of service should be based on medical necessity and the amount of history, examination, and medical decision making that was required and documented for that visit.

Alternatively, some of these interventions may also have more specific CPT codes. For example, smoking cessation counseling for CLBP can be delivered using CPT codes 99406 (up to 10 minutes) or 99407 (>10 minutes). For dietetic professional providers who perform counseling services for weight loss in management of CLBP, the services can be reported using CPT codes 97802 medical nutrition therapy (individual, initial visit, each 15 minutes), 97803 medical nutrition therapy (individual, subsequent visits, each 15 minutes), or 97804 medical nutrition therapy (group, each 30 minutes). If these services are provided by a physician, the appropriate level of evaluation and management codes (99201-99215) should be reported. If counseling on physical activity is provided by a physical therapist who supervises the exercise, it can be delivered using CPT code 97110 (therapeutic exercises, each 15 minutes).

These procedures are widely covered by other third-party payers such as health insurers and worker's compensation insurance. Although some payers continue to base their reimbursements on usual, customary, and reasonable payment methodology, the majority have developed reimbursement tables based on the Resource Based Relative Value Scale used by Medicare. Reimbursements by other third-party payers are generally higher than Medicare. Third-party payers will often reimburse a limited number of visits to licensed health care providers for physical activity, smoking cessation, and weight-loss interventions if they are prescribed by a physician and supported by adequate documentation deeming them medically necessary. Equipment or products required for those interventions are typically considered to be included in the procedure reported and are not separately reportable. Given the need to maintain the gains, if any, achieved in muscular function through physical activity, patients are often encouraged to continue this intervention beyond the initial period of supervised exercise therapy. The cost for membership in a private exercise facility is generally $50 to $100 per month. Some insurers in the United States also provide discounted membership fees to exercise facilities to their members to promote physical activity.

Typical fees reimbursed by Medicare in New York and California for these services are summarized in Table 5-4.

Cost Effectiveness

Evidence supporting the cost effectiveness of treatment protocols that compared these interventions, often in combination with one or more cointerventions, with control groups

TABLE 5-4	Medicare Fee Schedule for Related Services*	
CPT Code	New York City	Los Angeles
Office visits		
99201	$41	$44
99202	$70	$76
99203	$101	$109
99211	$20	$22
99212	$41	$44
99213	$68	$73
Smoking Cessation Counseling		
99406	$13	$15
99407	$26	$28
Nutritional Counseling		
97802	$30	$32
97803	$26	$28
97804	$13	
Supervised Exercise Therapy		
97110	$30	$32

*2010 Participating, nonfacility amount.

who received one or more other interventions, for either acute or chronic LBP, was identified from two SRs on this topic and is summarized below.[53,54] Although many of these study designs are unable to clearly identify the individual contribution of any intervention, their results provide some insight into the clinical and economic outcomes associated with these approaches.

Physical Activity

An RCT in the United Kingdom compared two approaches for patients with CLBP.[55] The active intervention was delivered by a physical therapist and consisted of a back school with education from a book and cassette, group education, advice to remain active, and CBT. Usual care was delivered by a general practitioner and included education from a book and cassette along with other interventions. Clinical outcomes after 15 months were similar between groups, in that both improved in pain, function, and utility. Direct medical costs associated with study and nonstudy interventions over 15 months were $47 higher in the active intervention group. Based on nonsignificant differences in utility, the incremental cost effectiveness ratio (ICER) of group training over brief education alone was $8650 per quality-adjusted life-year (QALY), well within the generally accepted threshold for cost utility analyses.

An RCT in the United States compared two approaches for patients with CLBP.[56] The naturopathic care group included acupuncture, exercise, dietary advice, and relaxation delivered by a naturopath. The control group included brief education from a naturopath given in 30-minute biweekly sessions over 3 months. Both groups also received an educational booklet, and voluntary crossover was offered to participants after 12 weeks. Clinical outcomes after 6 months favored the naturopathic care group for improvements in utility. Direct medical costs for study interventions over 6 months were $1469 in the naturopathic care group and $337 in the brief education group. Direct medical costs for nonstudy interventions over 6 months, including chiropractic, massage, physical therapy, pain medication, and other interventions, were $1203 lower in the naturopathic care group. Indirect productivity costs associated with lost work days were $1141 lower in the naturopathic care group. Authors concluded that naturopathic care was more cost effective than brief education.

An RCT in Finland compared three approaches for patients with acute LBP in an occupational health center.[32] The bed rest group was prescribed complete bed rest for 2 days, after which they were instructed to resume normal activities. The back exercise group received supervised exercise therapy by a physical therapist, including extension and lateral bending exercises every other hour. The active group received advice to remain active. Clinical outcomes after 12 weeks favored the active group for pain and function when compared to the bed rest group. Direct medical costs associated with study and nonstudy interventions over 12 weeks were $144 in the bed rest group, $165 in the back exercise group, and $123 in the active group. Direct medical costs associated with home help over 12 weeks were $90 in the bed rest group, $232 in the back exercise group, and $45 in the active group. Indirect productivity costs were not estimated, although the number of lost work days favored the active group. Authors concluded that if indirect productivity costs had been monetized, the active group would be favored.

An RCT in the United Kingdom compared two approaches for patients with subacute or chronic LBP.[57] The supervised exercise therapy group received up to eight sessions of stretching, strengthening, and aerobic exercises, and brief education on LBP. The usual care group received interventions prescribed by a general practitioner, including physical therapy in some cases. Clinical outcomes after 1 year favored the supervised exercise therapy group for improvement in pain, function, and utility. Direct medical costs associated with study and nonstudy interventions over 12 months were $145 in the supervised exercise therapy group and approximately $185 in the usual care group. Indirect productivity costs associated with lost work days over 12 months were approximately $456 in the supervised exercise therapy group and approximately $663 in the usual care group. Total costs (direct medical and indirect productivity) over 12 months were therefore approximately $601 in the supervised exercise therapy group and approximately $848 in the usual care group. These differences in costs were not statistically significant.

An RCT in Norway compared two approaches for patients sick-listed with CLBP.[58] The early intervention approach received advice to stay active and brief education. The control group received primary care as usual, which was not specified. Clinical outcomes after 1 year were similar between the two groups. Direct medical costs associated with the study intervention over 3 years were $303 higher in the early intervention group. Indirect productivity costs from lost work days were $3800 lower in the early intervention group, mostly due to a faster return to work within the first year of follow-up. Authors concluded that the benefits of the early intervention group exceed its costs.

An RCT in Norway compared three approaches for patients sick-listed with CLBP.[59] The supervised exercise therapy group received instruction on stabilization and strengthening exercise from a physical therapist. The conventional physical therapy group received one or more interventions including heat, ice, massage, stretching exercises, electrical muscle stimulation, or traction. The self-care group received instruction to walk. Participants in all groups received 3 sessions of 1 hour each week for 12 weeks (total 36 sessions). Clinical outcomes after 1 year reported that the supervised exercise therapy and conventional physical therapy groups had greater improvements in pain and function than the self-care group. Direct medical costs associated with the study interventions after 1 year were approximately $375 in the supervised exercise therapy group, approximately $584 in the conventional physical therapy group, and $0 in the self-care group. Indirect productivity costs associated with lost work days after 1 year were approximately $13,816 in the supervised exercise therapy group, approximately $12,062 in the conventional physical therapy group, and approximately $15,762 in the self-care group. Total costs (direct medical and indirect productivity) over 1 year were therefore approximately $14,191 in the supervised exercise therapy group, approximately $12,646 in the conventional physical therapy group, and approximately $15,762 in the self-care group. Authors concluded that both supervised exercise therapy and conventional physical therapy were cost saving when compared to self care.

An RCT in the United Kingdom compared two approaches for patients with acute LBP in primary care.[60] The brief pain management group included brief education, exercise, CBT, and general physical activity. The physical therapy group included spinal manipulation, mobilization, massage, back exercises, and brief education. Clinical outcomes after 1 year were similar between the two groups for function and quality of life, although the physical therapy group had marginally greater gains in utility. Direct medical costs for study and nonstudy interventions over 12 months were approximately $254 in the brief pain management group and approximately $354 in the physical therapy group. Indirect productivity costs were not reported in this study. Since the physical therapy group had marginally better clinical outcomes with greater costs, its ICER was estimated at approximately $3803 per QALY, well within the generally accepted threshold for cost utility analyses.

An RCT in The Netherlands compared two approaches for patients with CLBP.[61] The intensive training group included back school, and both individual and group supervised exercise therapy. The usual physical therapy group included interventions recommended in CPGs, which were not defined. Clinical outcomes after 1 year were similar between groups, which both improved in pain, function, and utility. Direct medical costs associated with study and nonstudy interventions over 1 year were approximately $1468 in the intensive training group and approximately $980 in the usual physical therapy group. Indirect productivity costs associated with lost work days over 1 year were approximately $3797 in the intensive training group and $3969 in the usual physical therapy group. Total costs (direct medical and indirect productivity) over 1 year were therefore approximately $5265 in the intensive training group and $4949 in the usual physical therapy group. Since the intensive training group had marginally better clinical outcomes with higher overall costs, its ICER was estimated at approximately $6957 per QALY, well within the generally accepted threshold for cost utility analyses.

An RCT in the United Kingdom compared four approaches for patients with subacute or chronic LBP.[62] The usual care from a general practitioner group included various unspecified interventions, brief education, and advice to remain active. The usual care from a general practitioner with exercise group included various unspecified interventions, individual, and group supervised exercise therapy classes. The usual care from a general practitioner with spinal manipulation group included various unspecified interventions and spinal manipulation. The usual care from a general practitioner with spinal manipulation and exercise group included various unspecified interventions, brief education, advice to remain active, group and individual supervised exercise therapy classes, and spinal manipulation. Clinical outcomes after 1 year were mostly similar, with improvement in pain, function, and utility, though greater improvement was reported for utility gains in the usual care with spinal manipulation and usual care with spinal manipulation and exercise groups. Direct medical costs associated with study and nonstudy interventions over 1 year were approximately $503 in the usual care group, $707 in the usual care with exercise group, $787 in the usual care with spinal manipulation group, and $685 in the usual care with spinal manipulation and exercise group. Indirect productivity costs were not reported. Because the usual care with spinal manipulation and exercise group had lower direct costs and greater gains in QALY than usual care with exercise or usual care with spinal manipulation, authors concluded that it was cost saving and dominated those two other choices; its ICER when compared to usual care was estimated at approximately $5509 per QALY, well within the generally accepted threshold for cost utility analyses.

The cost effectiveness of smoking cessation and weight loss for CLBP is currently unknown.

Findings from the above cost effectiveness analyses are summarized in Table 5-5.

Observational Study

A study compared health care charges for 20,332 employees at a large manufacturing company before and after smoking cessation for those with or without chronic conditions (arthritis, allergies, or CLBP).[63] Total medical charges among those with CLBP, arthritis, or allergies were significantly lower among former smokers, whether they had quit zero to four years ($4027) or five to nine years ago ($4050), compared with current smokers ($4208). Charges among current or former smokers were nevertheless significantly higher than among those who had never smoked ($3108). Authors concluded that health care providers should consider potential cost savings associated with health promotion such as smoking cessation among those with chronic conditions, including CLBP.

SUMMARY

Description

To promote health and improve clinical outcomes in a variety of medical conditions, including CLBP, health care providers increasingly recommend interventions aimed at improving lifestyle through physical activity (e.g., walking/jogging, swimming), smoking cessation (e.g., nicotine patch/gum, cognitive behavioral approaches), and weight loss (e.g., calorie restriction, medically supervised diets). Although these interventions are widely available throughout the United States, little is known regarding the prevalence of lifestyle modification counseling among spine providers. Chiropractors and physical therapists commonly offer preventive care services, including smoking cessation, weight-loss programs, fitness counseling, and stress management to their patients, including those with CLBP. Such interventions are typically administered in private practices or outpatient clinics.

Theory

In general, exercises are used to strengthen muscles, increase soft tissue stability, restore range of motion, improve cardiovascular conditioning, increase proprioception, and reduce fear of movement. Engaging in physical activity through exercise programs is theorized to improve CLBP through multiple mechanisms, including improved conditioning and confidence for daily activities, release of endorphins, improved social interaction, reduced fear avoidance, and decreased generalized anxiety. Disc metabolism may also be enhanced through repetitive exercise involving the spine's full active range of motion, improving repair, and enhancing reuptake of inflammatory and nociceptive mediators that may have migrated to an area of injury. It has been postulated that repeated microtrauma to the intervertebral discs from chronic coughing associated with long-term smoking can gradually lead to disc injury or herniation. Smoking is also thought to reduce blood flow to the discs, which already have a poor supply, as well as to the vertebral bodies, eventually leading to accelerated or early degeneration from insufficient healing capacity and decreased bone mineral density. Weight loss is thought to improve CLBP by decreasing exposure to the potentially harmful effects of obesity related to the lumbar spine, such as additional weight on load-bearing spinal elements and altered biomechanics leading to excessive wear and early degeneration. It may also contribute to improvement of CLBP by facilitating participation in general or back specific exercises that may not be possible if a patient is overweight or obese. Physical activity is indicated for all patients with CLBP. Smoking cessation is indicated for all patients with CLBP who are smokers. Weight loss is indicated for all patients with CLBP who have a body mass index greater than 30, high-risk waist circumference, and two or more risk factors related to obesity. Diagnostic imaging or other forms of advanced testing is generally not required before administering these interventions for CLBP.

TABLE 5-5	Cost Effectiveness and Cost Utility Analyses of Physical Activity, Smoking Cessation, and Weight Loss for Acute or Chronic Low Back Pain				
Reference Country Follow-up	Group	Direct Medical Costs	Indirect Productivity Costs	Total Costs	Conclusion
55 United Kingdom 15 months	1. Back school, education, CBT, advice to remain active 2. Usual care from general practitioner	1. $47 higher than group 2 2. NR	NR	NR	ICER of 1 over 2: $8650/QALY
56 United States 6 months	1. Naturopathic care (including exercise) 2. Control	1. $1469 2. $337	1. $1141 lower than group 2	NR	1. More cost effective than 2
32 Finland 12 weeks	1. Bed rest 2. Back exercise 3. Advice to remain active	1. $234 2. $397 3. $168	NR	Were not estimated	If indirect costs had been monetized, group 3 would be favored
57 United Kingdom 1 year	1. Supervised exercise therapy 2. Usual care	1. $145 2. $185	1. $456 2. $663	1. $601 2. $848	No significant difference
58 Norway 3 years	1. Early intervention (including advice to stay active) 2. Usual care	1. $303 higher than group 2	1. $3800 lower than group 2	NR	Benefits of early intervention exceed its cost
59 Norway 1 year	1. Supervised exercise therapy 2. Conventional physical therapy 3. Self-care	1. $375 2. $584 3. $0	1. $13,816 2. $12,062 3. $15,762	1. $14,191 2. $12,646 3. $15,762	Groups 1 and 2 were cost saving compared with group 3
60 United Kingdom 1 year	1. Brief pain management 2. Physical therapy	1. $254 2. $354	NR	NR	ICER of 1 over 2: $3803/QALY
61 The Netherlands 1 year	1. Intensive training 2. Usual physical therapy	1. $1468 2. $980	1. $3797 2. $3969	1. $5265 2. $4949	ICER of 1 over 2: $6957/QALY
62 United Kingdom 1 year	1. Usual care 2. Usual care + exercise 3. Usual care + SMT 4. Usual care + exercise + SMT	1. $503 2. $707 3. $787 4. $685	NR	NR	ICER of 4 over 1: $5509/QALY

CBT, cognitive behavioral therapy; ICER, incremental cost effectiveness ratio; NR, not reported; QALY, quality-adjusted life-year; SMT, spinal manipulation therapy.

Efficacy

Three recent CPGs make recommendations on physical activity for CLBP. One found limited evidence that aerobic exercise was more effective than back school with respect to improvements in pain and function, the second strongly recommended low impact aerobic exercise for CLBP, and the third reported moderate-quality evidence supporting aquatic therapy for CLBP. In addition, three of the recent national CPGs recommended advice to remain active for CLBP, which implies some form of physical activity. At least five RCTs examined the efficacy of general exercise for LBP, one reporting statistically significant improvement for aerobic exercise versus physical therapy and three reporting statistically significant functional improvement for general exercise versus other comparators. None of the recent national CPGs

on the management of CLBP provided recommendations about smoking cessation or weight loss. None of the identified SRs were specific to general exercise, smoking cessation, or weight loss for CLBP. No RCTs were identified for smoking cessation or weight loss for CLBP.

Safety

Contraindications to lifestyle interventions include CLBP due to potentially serious spinal pathology such as fracture, cancer, infection, or cauda equina syndrome. Lifestyle interventions are generally considered to be safe, yet muscle soreness may occur. Cardiovascular events may occur when patients who are not medically fit due to comorbidities such as cardiopulmonary impairment undertake physical activity.

Costs

Counseling on lifestyle interventions such as physical activity, smoking cessation, and weight loss for CLBP can likely be delivered by a clinician in the context of an outpatient visit. Medicare reimbursement for these visits ranges from $13 to $109. At least nine studies examined the cost effectiveness associated with general exercise for CLBP, the majority of which combined exercise with other interventions rendering it impossible to determine the contribution of exercise to the cost effectiveness. The cost effectiveness of smoking cessation and weight loss for CLBP is unknown.

Comments

Evidence from the CPGs, SRs, and RCTs reviewed suggest that general physical activity may be effective for individuals with CLBP. However, caution should be used as this conclusion is based on a small number of trials, many of which were of low quality. Also, many of the interventions were supervised exercise therapy and took place in a group setting. These factors may be important mediators for patient motivation and development of self-efficacy, in addition to any benefits derived from physical activity itself. There was no evidence uncovered as to the efficacy of smoking cessation or weight loss as interventions for CLBP. Given the possible causative link between CLBP and these modifiable lifestyle factors, and the known benefits of smoking cessation and weight loss on other health conditions, further research on the effectiveness of these interventions for CLBP is strongly encouraged.

CHAPTER REVIEW QUESTIONS

Answers are located on page 450.

1. Which of the following elements is not included in the World Health Organization definition of "lifestyle?"
   a. religious beliefs
   b. identifiable patterns of behavior
   c. social interactions
   d. environmental living conditions
2. Which of the following is not considered a modifiable lifestyle risk factor?
   a. nutritional
   b. psychological
   c. genetics
   d. environmental
3. Which of the following is not a theory explaining a possible association between smoking and low back pain?
   a. repeated microtrauma from chronic cough leading to disc herniation
   b. decreased lung capacity reducing ability to engage in physical activity
   c. reduced blood flow to the discs and vertebral bodies leading to early degeneration
   d. decreased bone mineral density leading to vertebral body or end plate injury

4. What is the proportion of epidemiologic studies that have reported a positive association between smoking and developing low back pain?
   a. 8% to 15%
   b. 29% to 44%
   c. 51% to 77%
   d. 81% to 89%
5. Guidelines generally recommend that adults should engage in physical activity for:
   a. 30 minutes at moderate intensity, 5 days per week
   b. 60 minutes at moderate intensity, 7 days per week
   c. 10 minutes at vigorous intensity 7 days per week
   d. 40 minutes at vigorous intensity 2 days per week
6. According to the American Cancer Society, which of the following is not one of the steps involved in smoking cessation?
   a. making the decision to quit
   b. setting a quit date and choosing a quit plan
   c. drinking less coffee and alcohol
   d. staying quit
7. Weight loss is generally indicated for patients with CLBP who have a body mass index greater than:
   a. 19
   b. 30
   c. 35
   d. 22
   e. 45

REFERENCES

1. Nutbeam D. Health Promotion Glossary. Geneva: World Health Organization; 1998.
2. Taylor MC, Dingle JL. Prevention of tobacco-caused disease. In: Canadian task force on periodic health examination. Canadian guide to clinical preventive health care. Ottawa: Public Health Agency of Canada; 1994. p. 500-511.
3. Lyons R, Langille L. Healthy lifestyle: strengthening the effectiveness of lifestyle approaches to improve health. Ottawa: Public Health Agency of Canada; 2000.
4. Beaulieu MD. Physical activity counselling. In: Canadian task force on periodic health examination. Canadian guide to clinical preventive health care. Ottawa: Public Health Agency of Canada; 1994. p. 560-569.
5. Kovacs FM, Llobera J, Abraira V, et al. Effectiveness and cost-effectiveness analysis of neuroreflexotherapy for subacute and chronic low back pain in routine general practice: a cluster randomized, controlled trial. Spine 2002;27:1149-1159.
6. Manchikanti L. Epidemiology of low back pain. Pain Physician 2000;3:167-192.
7. Hoogendoorn WE, van Poppel MN, Bongers PM, et al. Systematic review of psychosocial factors at work and private life as risk factors for back pain. Spine 2000;25:2114-2125.
8. Burdorf A, Sorock G. Positive and negative evidence of risk factors for back disorders. Scand J Work Environ Health 1997;23:243-256.
9. Suni JH, Oja P, Miilunpalo SI, et al. Health-related fitness test battery for adults: associations with perceived health, mobility, and back function and symptoms. Arch Phys Med Rehabil 1998;79:559-569.
10. Harreby M, Hesselsoe G, Kjer J, et al. Low back pain and physical exercise in leisure time in 38-year-old men and

women: a 25-year prospective cohort study of 640 school children. Eur Spine J 1997;6:181-186.

11. Kelsey JL, Greenberg RA, Hardy RJ, et al. Pregnancy and the syndrome of herniated lumbar intervertebral disc; an epidemiological study. Yale J Biol Med 1975;48:361-368.

12. Kauppila LI, Tallroth K. Postmortem angiographic findings for arteries supplying the lumbar spine: their relationship to low-back symptoms. J Spinal Disord 1993;6:124-129.

13. Hopper JL, Seeman E. The bone density of female twins discordant for tobacco use. N Engl J Med 1994;330:387-392.

14. Goldberg MS, Scott SC, Mayo NE. A review of the association between cigarette smoking and the development of nonspecific back pain and related outcomes. Spine 2000;25:995-1014.

15. Leboeuf-Yde C. Smoking and low back pain. A systematic literature review of 41 journal articles reporting 47 epidemiologic studies. Spine 1999;24:1463-1470.

16. Leboeuf-Yde C, Yashin A. Smoking and low back pain: is the association real? J Manipulative Physiol Ther 1995;18:457-463.

17. Leboeuf-Yde C. Body weight and low back pain. A systematic literature review of 56 journal articles reporting on 65 epidemiologic studies. Spine 2000;25:226-237.

18. Wai E, Gruszczynski A, Johnson G, et al. Modifiable lifestyle factors in patients presenting to a tertiary spine surgery clinic. J Bone Joint Surg Br 2008;90-B:118.

19. Hawk C, Long CR, Boulanger KT. Prevalence of nonmusculoskeletal complaints in chiropractic practice: report from a practice-based research program. J Manipulative Physiol Ther 2001;24:157-169.

20. Centers for Disease Control and Prevention. How active do adults need to be to gain some benefit? Atlanta, GA: Centers for Disease Control and Prevention; 2007. http://www.cdc.gov/physicalactivity/everyone/guidelines/index.html.

21. American Cancer Society. Guide to Quitting Smoking. American Cancer Society; 2006. http://www.cancer.org/docroot/PED/content/PED_10_13X_Guide_for_Quitting_Smoking.asp#How_to_Quit.

22. Weight-control information network. Weight loss for life. National Institutes of Health; 2006. Report No.: NIH Publication No. 04-3700.

23. Frost H, Klaber Moffett JA, Moser JS, et al. Randomised controlled trial for evaluation of fitness programme for patients with chronic low back pain. BMJ 1995;310:151-154.

24. Thoren P, Floras JS, Hoffmann P, et al. Endorphins and exercise: physiological mechanisms and clinical implications. Med Sci Sports Exerc 1990;22:417-428.

25. Langridge JC, Phillips D. Group hydrotherapy exercises for chronic back pain sufferers' introduction and monitoring. Physiotherapy 1988;74:269-272.

26. Liddle SD, Baxter GD, Gracey JH. Exercise and chronic low back pain: what works? Pain 2004;107:176-190.

27. Levine BA. Use of hydrotherapy in reduction of anxiety. Psychol Rep 1984;55:526.

28. Franchimont P, Juchmes J, Lecomte J. Hydrotherapy—mechanisms and indications. Pharmacol Ther 1983;20:79-93.

29. Mooney V, Verna J, Morris C. Clinical management of chronic, disabling low back syndromes. In: Morris C, editor. Low back syndromes: integrated clinical management. New York: McGraw-Hill; 2006.

30. Kitano T, Zerwekh J, Usui Y, et al. Biochemical changes associated with the symptomatic human intervertebral disk. Clin Orthop Relat Res 1993;Aug:372-377.

31. Loisel P, Lemaire J, Poitras S, et al. Cost-benefit and cost-effectiveness analysis of a disability prevention model for back pain management: a six year follow up study. Occupat Environ Med 2002;59:807-815.

32. Malmivaara A, Hakkinen U, Aro T, et al. The treatment of acute low back pain—bed rest, exercises, or ordinary activity? N Engl J Med 1995;332:351-355.

33. Practical Guide to the Identification, Evaluation, and Treatment of Overweight and Obesity in Adults. Bethesda, MD: National Institutes of Health; 2000. NIH Publication Number 00-4084. http://www.nhlbi.nih.gov/guidelines/obesity/prctgd_c.pdf.

34. Sculco AD, Paup DC, Fernhall B, et al. Effects of aerobic exercise on low back pain patients in treatment. Spine J 2001;1:95-101.

35. Mannion AF, Muntener M, Taimela S, et al. Comparison of three active therapies for chronic low back pain: results of a randomized clinical trial with one-year follow-up. Rheumatology (Oxford) 2001;40:772-778.

36. McIlveen B, Robertson VJ. A randomised controlled study of the outcome of hydrotherapy for subjects with low back or back and leg pain. Physiotherapy 1998;84:17-26.

37. Sjogren T, Long N, Storay I, et al. Group hydrotherapy versus group land-based treatment for chronic low back pain. Physiother Res Int 1997;2:212-222.

38. Tritilanunt T, Wajanavisit W. The efficacy of an aerobic exercise and health education program for treatment of chronic low back pain. J Med Assoc Thai 2001;84:528-533.

39. Iversen MD, Fossel AH, Katz JN. Enhancing function in older adults with chronic low back pain: a pilot study of endurance training. Arch Phys Med Rehabil 2003;84:1324-1331.

40. Prochaska JO, DiClemente CC. Transtheoretical therapy: toward a more integrative model of change. Psychotherapy: Theory Res Pract 1982;19:276-287.

41. Airaksinen O, Brox JI, Cedraschi C, et al. European guidelines for the management of chronic nonspecific low back pain. Eur Spine J 2006;15:192-300.

42. Negrini S, Giovannoni S, Minozzi S, et al. Diagnostic therapeutic flow-charts for low back pain patients: the Italian clinical guidelines. Eura Medicophys 2006;42:151-170.

43. Nielens H, van Zundert J, Mairiaux P, et al. Chronic low back pain, Vol. 48C. Brussels: KCE Reports; 2006.

44. National Institute for Health and Clinical Excellence (NICE). Low back pain: early management of persistent non-specific low back pain. Report No.: NICE clinical guideline 88. London: National Institute of Health and Clinical Excellence; 2009.

45. Hayden JA, van Tulder MW, Malmivaara A, et al. Exercise therapy for treatment of non-specific low back pain. Cochrane Database Syst Rev 2005;(3):CD000335.

46. Mannion AF, Muntener M, Taimela S, et al. A randomized clinical trial of three active therapies for chronic low back pain. Spine 1999;24:2435-2448.

47. Frost H, Lamb SE, Klaber Moffett JA, et al. A fitness programme for patients with chronic low back pain: 2-year follow-up of a randomised controlled trial. Pain 1998;75:273-279.

48. Chou R, Huffman LH. Nonpharmacologic therapies for acute and chronic low back pain: a review of the evidence for an American Pain Society/American College of Physicians clinical practice guideline. Ann Intern Med 2007;147:492-504.

49. Hartvigsen J, Morso L, Bendix T, Manniche C. Supervised and non-supervised Nordic walking in the treatment of chronic low back pain: a single blind randomized clinical trial. BMC Musculoskelet Disord 2010;11:30.

50. Waddell G, Burton A. Occupational health guidelines for the management of low back pain at work: evidence review. Occup Med 2001;51:124-135.

51. Waddell G, Feder G, Lewis M. Systematic reviews of bed rest and advice to stay active for acute low back pain. Br J Gen Pract 1997;47:647-652.

52. Hagen KB, Hilde G, Jamtvedt G, et al. Bed rest for acute low-back pain and sciatica. Cochrane Database Syst Rev 2004;(4):CD001254.

53. Dagenais S, Roffey DM, Wai EK, et al. Can cost utility evaluations inform decision making about interventions for low back pain? Spine J 2009;9:944-957.

54. van der Roer N, Goossens MEJB, Evers SMAA, et al. What is the most cost-effective treatment for patients with low back pain? A systematic review. Best Pract Res Clin Rheumatol 2005;19:671-684.

55. Johnson RE, Jones GT, Wiles NJ, et al. Active exercise, education, and cognitive behavioral therapy for persistent disabling low back pain: a randomized controlled trial. Spine 2007;32:1578-1585.

56. Herman PM, Szczurko O, Cooley K, et al. Cost-effectiveness of naturopathic care for chronic low back pain. Altern Ther Health Med 2008;14:32-39.

57. Moffett JK, Torgerson D, Bell-Syer S, et al. Randomised controlled trial of exercise for low back pain: clinical outcomes, costs, and preferences. BMJ 1999;319:279-283.

58. Molde Hagen E, Grasdal A, Eriksen HR. Does early intervention with a light mobilization program reduce long-term sick leave for low back pain: a 3-year follow-up study. Spine 2003;28:2309-2315.

59. Torstensen TA, Ljunggren AE, Meen HD, et al. Efficiency and costs of medical exercise therapy, conventional physiotherapy, and self-exercise in patients with chronic low back pain. A pragmatic, randomized, single-blinded, controlled trial with 1-year follow-up. Spine 1998;23:2616-2624.

60. Whitehurst DGT, Lewis M, Yao GL, et al. A brief pain management program compared with physical therapy for low back pain: results from an economic analysis alongside a randomized clinical trial. Arthrit Rheum 2007;57:466-473.

61. van der Roer N, van Tulder M, van Mechelen W, et al. Economic evaluation of an intensive group training protocol compared with usual care physiotherapy in patients with chronic low back pain. Spine 2008;33:445-451.

62. UK Beam Trial Team. United Kingdom back pain exercise and manipulation (UK BEAM) randomised trial: cost effectiveness of physical treatments for back pain in primary care. BMJ 2004;329:1377-1381.

63. Musich S, Faruzzi SD, Lu C, et al. Pattern of medical charges after quitting smoking among those with and without arthritis, allergies, or back pain. Am J Health Promot 2003;18:133-142.

BEN B. PRADHAN
JENS IVAR BROX
AAGE INDAHL

CHAPTER 6

Watchful Waiting and Brief Education

DESCRIPTION

Terminology and Subtypes

Watchful waiting, in the context of this chapter, is defined as minimal care through activity modification, education, and observation of the natural history of low back pain (LBP). It is passive in nature and does not include any interventions delivered by a health care provider to address specific symptoms (e.g., prescription medications, injections, supervised exercises, manual therapies). Watchful waiting does not indicate a complete absence of health care, and does not imply that symptoms are ignored by the patient. The decision to initiate watchful waiting may in fact be made by a health care provider after an initial consultation to rule out the possibility of potentially serious spinal pathology. This decision is often made in conjunction with the patient, and may represent an educated choice by those who have been informed of the relative efficacy, harms, and costs of available treatment options, and nevertheless select watchful waiting.

As a treatment philosophy, watchful waiting is very conservative and relies on giving the patient a chance to heal naturally without relying on external interventions. Watchful waiting can also include various patient-initiated comfort measures such as home heat or ice, postural modifications, lumbar supports (e.g., braces, belts) or over-the-counter topical analgesics. Self-care is encouraged to determine whether a patient can reduce his or her own symptoms through simple tactics before concluding that more invasive, costly, time-consuming, or potentially harmful interventions are warranted. Watchful waiting consists of the following types of approaches: watchfulness, waiting, reassurance, activity modification, and education. Most of these are tried in combination, and may be considered progressive steps in watchful waiting.

Brief education, on the other hand, usually consists of a single discussion with a health care provider. The content of this discussion varies, but typically includes basic education about the etiology of LBP, the expected prognosis of LBP, the treatment options available for LBP, tips for self-managing LBP, and circumstances in which to consider seeking additional care for LBP. Because watchful waiting also requires that clinicians educate their patients about why it may be an appropriate approach to managing LBP, the line between watchful waiting and brief education is often blurry. Advocates of watchful waiting often imply that brief education will be performed as part of this process without considering that brief education itself constitutes an intervention strategy for LBP. Although they are presented separately in this chapter, watchful waiting and brief education may in fact be synonymous depending on how they are implemented.

History and Frequency of Use

The management of LBP has undergone several paradigm shifts in the past century, from being mostly ignored to gradually being considered something of a nuisance. LBP was then attributed to newly discovered pain generators that could be eliminated with surgical interventions. After poor long-term results from those interventions, LBP was eventually deemed a condition whose etiology was complex but could nevertheless be addressed with prevention. When substantial sums were invested in workplace ergonomic modifications without noticeable improvement in LBP outcomes, it was proposed that LBP was a biopsychosocial illness involving physical, behavioral, occupational, and socioeconomic factors that could be addressed through behavioral approaches. That view largely prevails today, and common LBP is now widely considered a benign condition without any obvious anatomic cause that is self-limiting in the short term and is likely to recur, but can be managed with conservative approaches. Such statements are usually made with the caveat that LBP is occasionally associated with potentially serious spinal pathology or results in severe neurologic deficits, both of which may require more invasive interventions.

Given these changes in the broad understanding of LBP, it is not surprising that the advice given to patients by health care providers about LBP has changed markedly over the years, often resulting in contradictory messages, misconception, and confusion. The application of evidence-based medicine (EBM) to the management of LBP attempted to improve and clarify this situation. In the early 1990s, the Agency for Health Care Policy and Research (AHCPR), presently known as the Agency for Healthcare Research and Quality (AHRQ), assembled a multidisciplinary group of expert clinicians and researchers to develop clinical practice guidelines (CPGs) on the management of acute LBP in adults based on the best available scientific evidence.[1] It was proposed at the time that the first step in managing LBP was to conduct a basic diagnostic triage and group patients into one of three categories: (1) potentially serious spinal conditions (e.g., spinal fracture, spinal infection, spinal tumor, or cauda equina syndrome), (2) nerve root compression (e.g., sciatica, radiculopathy), and (3) nonspecific back symptoms. This triage was intended to be sequential and to unfold by process of elimination (e.g., after eliminating potentially serious spinal conditions and nerve root compression, it was assumed that the patient had nonspecific LBP). Although potentially serious spinal conditions required additional diagnostic testing, both nerve root compression and nonspecific LBP were deemed self-limiting in most cases and could improve without medical attention or with only conservative interventions. These recommendations were widely distributed in the United States, and this approach was slowly adopted by health care providers, after which watchful waiting became a more accepted option for LBP.

Traditional approaches based on the medical model of disease were contrasted with a biopsychosocial model of illness to reexamine success and failure in the management of LBP. This shift in thought regarding LBP inspired others to reconsider its management. For example, Indahl and colleagues began telling patients with LBP that light activity would not further injure their discs or other structures.[2] Following a clinical examination, brief education was given by a physiatrist, physical therapist, or nurse, who instructed patients that the worst thing they could do to their back was to be too careful. Any perceived link between emotions and chronic low back pain (CLBP) was simply attributed to increased tension in the muscles. Brief education has also been managed in the physical therapy setting.[3,4] Cherkin and colleagues evaluated the value of an educational booklet in patients with acute LBP, which was not effective in reducing symptoms, disability, or health care use.[5] Their findings challenged the value of purely educational approaches in reducing symptoms and costs of LBP when delivered solely with a booklet.

Practitioner, Setting, and Availability

A licensed health care provider trained in recognizing signs and symptoms of red flags associated with serious spinal pathology may administer this intervention. This may include a primary care physician, spine specialist, chiropractor, or physical therapist. The qualifications and training required for brief education varies considerably depending on the nature of the advice given. This intervention is widely available in the United States in a variety of private practice, clinic, or hospital settings.

Procedure

Watchful Waiting

Watchfulness. Waiting for symptoms of LBP to resolve does not mean ignoring telltale signs of something more serious, thus the term "watchful" waiting. If a health care provider is recommending watchful waiting for someone with LBP, a detailed medical history is critical. Certain conditions require urgent diagnosis and treatment (e.g., tumors, which usually cause slow, progressive pain, unless there is a pathologic fracture). Acute pain, in the back or leg, may also be caused by disc herniation, whereas paraspinal symptoms are usually muscular in origin. Most LBP is mechanical in nature (worse when loading or moving the back). Nonmechanical back pain, or pain during rest, usually indicates an inflammatory, infectious, or oncologic origin. There are also certain conditions that exhibit red flags, which can be detected with careful screening through history-taking and physical examination and need urgent diagnosis and appropriate treatment.

Waiting. It has been observed in several reports that the vast majority of acute LBP episodes resolve spontaneously with time (Figure 6-1). A preexisting active lifestyle has been shown to accelerate symptomatic recovery and to reduce chronic disability.[7] The routine use of passive treatment modalities is not recommended, because it might promote chronic pain behavior. Such interventions may be more appropriate for "subacute" pain. The *British Medical Journal* reported that increased stress from therapeutic exercises may be harmful in acute LBP based on a randomized clinical trial that was included in the Philadelphia Panel.[8]

Reassurance

Reassurance may help patients, decreasing their stress and anxiety, and thus reducing inappropriate pain behavior and encouraging proactive healthy behavior (Figure 6-2). Reassurance may be the first step of psychological treatment. Some authors recommend that in addition to the traditional examination of neurologic symptoms and signs, psychological factors should be considered at the initial visit for a

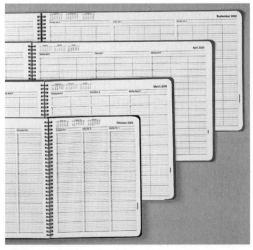

Figure 6-1 Watchful waiting requires patience and education. (Image courtesy of Deluxe for Business, Shoreview, MN.)

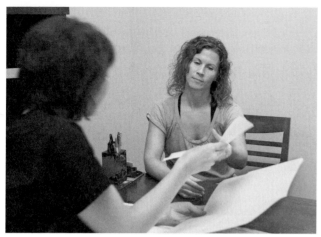

Figure 6-2 Reassurance is an important part of watchful waiting.

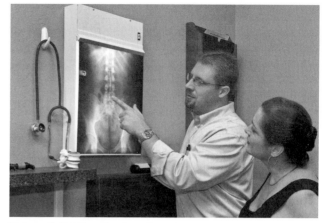

Figure 6-3 Education is an important component to managing low back pain. (© istockphoto.com/Richard Gaydos.)

patient with an episode of LBP. Reassurance usually consists of educating the patient that LBP is a common problem and that 90% of patients recover spontaneously in 4 to 6 weeks.[9] Patients also need to be reassured that complete pain relief usually occurs after, rather than before, resumption of normal activities and that they may return to work before obtaining complete pain relief; working despite some residual discomfort from LBP poses no threat and will not harm them.[10]

Activity Modification

Although severe LBP may necessitate rest or activity modification as tolerated by each patient, mandatory bed rest has not been shown to be beneficial in the overall course of acute back pain. If disabled by pain, bed rest may be recommended, but for no more than two days, because longer periods of bed rest can delay recovery.[10-12] The Philadelphia Panel found good evidence to encourage continuation of normal activities as an intervention for people with acute LBP.[8] The Institute for Clinical Systems Improvement (ICSI) also recommends that patients with acute LBP be advised to stay active and continue ordinary daily activities within the limits permitted by the pain. Patients may be advised to carefully introduce activities back into their day as they begin to recover.[10] Gradual stretches and regular walking are good ways to get back into action. Patients also need to be told to relax, because tension will only make their back feel worse. Patients should also be instructed to avoid activities that caused the onset or aggravation of symptoms, especially those that peripheralize (spread outward to the extremities) symptoms.

Education

Educating patients about LBP can help them take steps in their everyday lives that will help maintain back health (Figure 6-3). Although most studies point to the spontaneous resolution of the vast majority of episodes of LBP, there exists controversy in this area. For example, ICSI provides a slightly less optimistic outlook and states that most patients will experience partial improvement in 4 to 6 weeks and will have a recurrence of LBP in 12 months.[10] The long-term

course of LBP typically allows for a return to previous activities, although often with some pain. Employers are encouraged to develop and make available patient education materials concerning prevention of LBP and care of the healthy back. Topics that should be included are promotion of physical activity, smoking cessation, and weight control; these interventions are reviewed in Chapter 5. Emphasis should be on patient responsibility and self-care of acute LBP. Employer groups should also make available reasonable accommodations for modified duties or activities to allow early return to work and minimize the risk of prolonged disability. Education of frontline supervisors in occupational strategies to facilitate an early return to work and to prevent prolonged disabilities is recommended.[10]

Patients with CLBP often find that their symptoms wax and wane over time, and many of them have devised means of minimizing their symptoms. In the event that these methods are no longer effective, symptoms are worsening, physical function is interfering with their ability to conduct normal activities, sleep is deteriorating and is no longer restful, or quality of life has decreased markedly, it is reasonable to seek advice from a health care provider. Even those patients dedicated to watchful waiting may need to consult with a health care provider at some point to receive additional reassurance and advice on other approaches to managing their LBP.

Brief Education. Brief education encompasses many of the elements already described and attempts to achieve the same goals as back schools in a condensed time period. Brief education often consists of a single discussion with a health care professional, including physical therapists, primary care physicians, chiropractors, or behavioral health care providers. Follow-up sessions may also be held to reinforce some of the important messages or monitor changes in clinical presentation (Figure 6-4). Alternatively, brief education may also be delivered by a trained lay person (often someone who has personally experienced CLBP), or supplemented through a brochure or book, or in a moderated online discussion group.[13] Brief education often summarizes some of the basic information about LBP presented in lengthier back schools. Back schools are not standardized but generally encourage

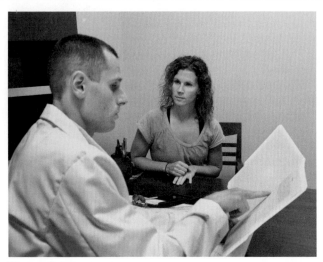

Figure 6-4 Reinforcement may be required to educate patients about low back pain.

self-management using heat, ice, over-the-counter analgesics, or relaxation techniques, provide advice to remain active despite the pain, and address common misconceptions about LBP (e.g., that diagnostic imaging is always required).

Regulatory status

Not applicable.

THEORY

Mechanism of Action

The principal mechanism of action involved in watchful waiting is allowing sufficient time for the body's natural healing mechanisms to repair the injured tissues at the root of CLBP, whatever they may be. Watchful waiting therefore depends on what is currently known about the natural history of LBP. Epidemiologic studies of LBP indicate that it is a common but benign condition of mostly unknown etiology that generally improves within a few weeks and disappears within a few months, although periodic recurrences are expected.[14] Such observations are based on population studies and cannot be extrapolated to every patient with LBP. Watchfulness is therefore necessary to identify rare but potentially serious spinal pathology that may be responsible for symptoms and may require urgent treatment. It is also important to identify rare nonspinal causes of LBP that may need to be addressed if the LBP is to improve.

An essential component of watchful waiting is continual reassurance, which is thought to decrease anxiety related to the LBP, and therefore minimize its negative impact on recovery and quality of life. Although temporary activity modification may occasionally be required for severe acute LBP, patients with CLBP need to be instructed to remain physically active and not attempt to favor their backs by avoiding activities perceived to aggravate symptoms. Educating patients, as stated previously, can help them take steps in their own everyday lives that will help maintain back health.

Nonspecific CLBP may have an association with an imprint of pain that exists in the central nervous system, specifically the spinal cord and the brain. Thus, patients who experience acute LBP – even if it fully resolves—may continue to have residual pain signals in the central nervous system. This makes it important to properly treat acute LBP, avoiding treatments that may unnecessarily aggravate the symptoms, and especially letting self-limiting episodes experience a natural recovery.

Indication

Watchful Waiting

This intervention is indicated for patients with nonspecific CLBP without red flags for serious spinal pathology who do not wish to seek any form of active care and understand the advantages and disadvantages of watchful waiting.

Brief Education

The ideal patient may be a young manual laborer who enjoys his or her job but has been out of work (for the first time) for less than 8 weeks due to LBP. Although these patients have a normal range of motion, they move carefully in an attempt to avoid pain, and their back muscles are tense and painful. Magnetic resonance imaging may have revealed a small disc protrusion, which is not believed to be the cause of pain or functional limitations. They may have tried medications, massage, and acupuncture, but these did not improve their symptoms.

Assessment

Before receiving watchful waiting or brief education, patients should first be assessed for LBP using an evidence-based and goal-oriented approach focused on the patient history and neurologic examination, as discussed in Chapter 3. Additional diagnostic imaging or specific diagnostic testing is generally not required before initiating these interventions for CLBP.

EFFICACY

Evidence supporting the efficacy of these interventions for CLBP was summarized from recent CPGs, systematic reviews (SRs), and randomized controlled trials (RCTs). Observational studies (OBSs) were also summarized where appropriate. Findings are summarized by study design for each intervention.

Clinical Practice Guidelines

Watchful waiting

None of the recent national CPGs on the management of CLBP have assessed and summarized the evidence to make specific recommendations about the efficacy of watchful waiting as a sole intervention for CLBP. However, many CPGs have included a discussion of related messages, i.e., diagnostic tests are rarely indicated for most patients with CLBP, many interventions have relatively small effects, and education and self-care should be encouraged to improve long-term outcomes.

Brief Education

Four of the recent national CPGs on the management of CLBP have assessed and summarized the evidence to make specific recommendations about the efficacy of brief education.

The CPG from Europe in 2004 found conflicting evidence that brief education delivered through Internet-based discussion groups is more effective than no intervention with respect to improvements in pain and function.[13] That CPG also found limited evidence that brief education is as effective as massage or acupuncture with respect to improvements in pain and function. That CPG also found moderate evidence that brief education combined with advice to remain active is more effective than usual care with respect to improvements in disability. That CPG also found moderate evidence that brief education encouraging self-care is more effective than usual care with respect to improvements in function, but not pain. That CPG also found strong evidence that brief education, when combined with advice to remain active, is as effective as usual physical therapy or aerobic exercise with respect to improvements in function. That CPG recommended brief education in the management of CLBP.

The CPG from Belgium in 2006 found moderate evidence that brief education is effective with respect to improvements in function and disability.[15] That CPG recommended brief education in the management of CLBP.

The CPG from the United States in 2007 found evidence of a moderate benefit for brief education in the management of CLBP.[16]

The CPG from the United Kingdom in 2009 reported that brief education alone is not sufficient for the management of CLBP.[17]

Findings from the above CPGs are summarized in Table 6-1.

| Systematic Reviews

Watchful Waiting

No recent, high-quality SRs were identified that reported specifically on the efficacy of watchful waiting as an intervention for LBP.

Brief Education

Cochrane Collaboration. An SR was conducted in 2008 by the Cochrane Collaboration on individual patient education for acute, subacute, and chronic nonspecific LBP.[18] A total of 24 RCTs were included. Of those, 14 included acute or subacute LBP patients, 4 included CLBP patients, and 6 included a mixed population.[2,19-40] This SR concluded that individual education was not effective compared with noneducational

| TABLE 6-1 | Clinical Practice Guideline Recommendations About Watchful Waiting and Brief Education for Chronic Low Back Pain* |

Reference	Country	Conclusion
Brief Education		
13	Europe	Recommended for management of CLBP
15	Belgium	Recommended for management of CLBP
16	United States	Evidence of moderate benefit
17	United Kingdom	Brief education alone is not sufficient

*No CPGs made recommendations about watchful waiting as an intervention for CLBP.
CLBP, chronic low back pain.

interventions for CLBP. In particular, written educational material is less effective than noneducational interventions.

Other. An SR was conducted in 2008 by Brox and colleagues on back schools, brief education, and fear avoidance training for CLBP.[41] A total of 23 RCTs were included, of which 12 pertained to brief education. This SR concluded that there is strong evidence that brief education leads to reduced sick leave and short-term disability versus usual care. However, there was strong evidence that brief education in the clinical setting did not reduce pain compared with usual care and limited evidence that brief education in the clinical setting did not reduce pain compared with back school or exercise. Furthermore, this SR concluded that there is conflicting evidence for certain types of brief education (e.g., back book, Internet discussion) versus comparators such as a waiting list, no intervention, massage, yoga, or exercise.

Findings from the above SRs are summarized in Table 6-2.

| Randomized Controlled Trials

Watchful Waiting

No RCTs were identified that reported specifically on the efficacy of watchful waiting as an intervention for LBP.

Brief Education

Eleven RCTs and 14 reports related to those studies were identified.[2,21,25,29,31,33,34,36,42-47] Their methods are summarized in Table 6-3. Their results are briefly described here.

An RCT conducted by Indahl and colleagues[2,42] included LBP patients at a spine clinic in Norway. Participants were patients with subacute or chronic (4 to 12 weeks) LBP who were referred to the clinic; excluded were pregnant women on sick leave for LBP and patients with LBP lasting longer than 12 weeks. The intervention group (initially, n = 463; 5-year follow-up, n = 245) were assigned to treatment consisting of an examination, information about reflex activation of spinal muscles, reassurance to reduce fear and sickness

TABLE 6-2   Systematic Review Findings on Watchful Waiting and Brief Education for Chronic Low Back Pain*

Reference	# RCTs in SR	#RCTs for CLBP	Conclusion
Brief Education			
18	24	4 chronic 6 mixed population	Brief education is not effective compared with noneducational interventions in CLBP.
41	12	12	Brief education in the clinical setting is not effective compared with usual care and does not reduce pain compared with back school or exercise. Conflicting evidence for certain types of brief education (e.g., back book, Internet discussion) versus comparators such as a waiting list, no intervention, massage, yoga, or exercise

*No SRs were identified about watchful waiting as an intervention for chronic low back pain.
CLBP, chronic low back pain; RCT, randomized controlled trial; SR, systematic review.

TABLE 6-3   Randomized Controlled Trials of Brief Education for Chronic Low Back Pain

Reference	Population	Intervention	Control (C1)	Control (C2)
2, 42	Subacute and CLBP, neurologic involvement NR, symptoms 4-12 weeks	Examination, information about reflex activation of spinal muscles, reassurance to reduce fear and sickness behavior, mini-back school, encouraged to set their own physical activity goals Physiatrist, nurse, PT 1 × 2-3 hr + 1 × 1-2 hr, reinforced after 3 mo and 1 yr, open door n = 463[2]; n = 245 for 5-year follow-up study[42]	Usual care n = 512[2]; n = 244 for 5-year follow-up study[42]	NA
43	LBP, neurologic involvement NR, duration of symptoms NR	Information on red flags, common causes of LBP, factors contributing to pain, exercise, and activity, biomechanics, stress management and problem solving, book and videotapes used for self-management, and exercises Lay person with LBP 2 hr × 4 in 4 wk n = 129	Usual care n = 126	NA
21, 44	LBP without neurologic involvement, duration NR	Examination and reassurance as described by Indahl,[2,42] stay active and home activity Physiatrist, PT 2 × 1-2 hr n = 220	Usual care GP n = 237	NA
36	LBP without neurologic involvement, duration NR	Educational book and video (self-care) Self-care n = 90	Traditional Chinese medical acupuncture Acupuncturists 10 visits in 10 weeks n = 94	Therapeutic massage Massage therapists 10 visits in 10 weeks n = 78
45	LBP without neurologic involvement, symptoms ≤90 consecutive days	Back pain e-mail discussion group + a book and videotape Physician, psychologist, PT Frequency, duration not defined n = 296	Subscription to a non–health-related magazine n = 284	NA

TABLE 6-3	Randomized Controlled Trials of Brief Education for Chronic Low Back Pain—cont'd			
Reference	Population	Intervention	Control (C1)	Control (C2)
29	LBP without neurologic involvement, duration NR	Examination and reassurance as described by Indahl,[2,42] assessment of function, instruction to activate deep stabilizing muscles, stay active Hospital outpatient and primary care Physiatrist, PT 2 × 0.5-1 hr n = 34	Examination and aerobic dance program modified for LBP patients PT 2-3 × 1 hr weekly for 15 weeks n = 30	Usual care GP, specialists if necessary n = 29
25, 46	LBP, neurologic involvement NR, symptoms >4 wks but <3 mos	Examination, information and reassurance as described by Indahl,[2,42] stay active, and home activity, confirmation by second physician Primary care, occupational medicine physician, physiatrist, PT 2 hr n = 56	Same + worksite visit by PT Primary care, occupational medicine, physician, physiatrist, PT 2 + 1 hr n = 51	Usual care GP, specialists if necessary n = 57
47	CLBP without neurologic involvement, symptoms >3 months	Internet-based pain management program with telephone support, discuss negative thoughts and beliefs, active coping, relaxation, stretching, exercises Psychologist and PT Active access for 8 weeks n = 22	Waiting list n = 29	NA
34	LBP without neurologic involvement, symptoms >12 weeks	Mailed self-care book* n = 30	Yoga Yoga instructor 12 weekly 75-min classes n = 36	Exercises (information, goal-setting, aerobic, strength, and flexibility exercises) PT 12 weekly 75-min classes n = 35
31	CLBP without neurologic involvement, current episode >12 weeks	Back book + back school PT 3 hr × 1 (back school) n = 60	Spinal stabilization exercises + back school PT 3 hr × 1 + 10 wk × 1 hr n = 121	Manual therapy + back school PT 3 hr × 1 + 10 wk × 1 hr n = 121
33	CLBP without neurologic involvement, symptoms >6 months	Information based on current knowledge of neurophysiology of pain PT 1 × 3 hr + homework (questions related to the education) daily for 2 weeks n = 31	Information in accordance with Swedish Back School 1 × 3 hr + homework (questions related to the education) daily for 2 weeks n = 27	

*Zelens design.
CLBP, chronic low back pain; GP, general practitioner; LBP, low back pain; NA, not applicable; NR, not reported; PT, physical therapist.

behavior, mini-back school, and encouragement to set their own physical activity goals. The control group (initially, n = 512; 5-year follow-up, 244) consisted of usual care. Pain and disability outcomes were not measured in this study. This study was considered of higher quality.

An RCT conducted by Von Korff and colleagues[43] included LBP patients in a primary care setting in the United States. Participants were eligible if they had a primary care visit for back pain and were aged 25 to 70 years. Those who were considered for back surgery, or were planning to disenroll from the health maintenance organization (HMO) at which the study was based were excluded. The intervention group (n = 129) was assigned to treatment consisting of four 2-hour sessions which provided information on red flags, common causes of LBP, factors contributing to pain, exercise and activity, biomechanics, stress management and problem-solving, book and videotapes used for self-management, as well as exercises over 4 weeks. The control group (n = 126) was assigned to usual care. At the 12-month follow-up, there was a reduction in pain intensity (scale 0-10) in both groups compared with baseline. In the intervention group, pain scores decreased from 5.35 ± 1.99 to 3.22 ± 2.03, and in the control group, they decreased from 5.66 ± 2.06 to 3.79 ± 2.35. The pain scores were not significantly different between the two groups at 12 months ($P = .19$). At the 12-month follow-up, disability scores (23-item Roland Morris Disability Questionnaire [RMDQ]) was reduced in both groups. In the intervention group, RMDQ scores decreased from 9.50 ± 6.11 to 5.75 ± 6.31, and in the control group, they decreased from 9.42 ± 6.45 to 6.75 ± 6.39. The difference between the groups at 12 months was not statistically significant ($P = .092$), but the trend was in favor of the intervention. This study was considered of lower quality.

An RCT by Molde Hagen and colleagues[21,44] included workers with subacute LBP in a rehabilitation department in Norway. Participants had to be sick-listed for 8 to 12 weeks for LBP with or without radiating pain and be aged 18 to 60 years. Exclusion criteria included pregnancy, recent low back trauma, cauda equina symptoms, cancer, osteoporosis, rheumatic low back disease, and ongoing treatment for LBP by another specialist. The intervention group (n = 220) was assigned to a program consisting of two sessions of 1 to 2 hours of an examination and reassurance as described by Indahl and colleagues,[2,42] advice to stay active, and encouragement of home activity. The control group (n = 237) was assigned to usual care. No pain and disability outcomes were measured. This study was considered of higher quality.

An RCT by Cherkin and colleagues[36] included workers with LBP in the United States. Participants were HMO enrollees who had a primary care visit for LBP, still had significant LBP, and were aged 20 to 70 years. Exclusion criteria included symptoms of sciatica, acupuncture or massage for LBP in the past year, back care from a specialist or complementary and alternative medicine provider, severe clotting disorders or anticoagulant therapy, cardiac pacemakers, underlying systemic or visceral disease, pregnancy, involvement with litigation or compensation claims for LBP, inability to speak English, severe or progressive neurologic deficits, lumbar surgery within the past three years, recent

vertebral fracture, serious comorbid conditions, and bothersomeness of LBP rated as less than 4 on a scale of 0 to 10. The intervention group (n = 90) was assigned to self-care with an educational book and video. The first control group (n = 94) was assigned to 10 sessions of traditional Chinese medical acupuncture over 10 weeks, and the second control group (n = 78) was assigned to 10 sessions of therapeutic massage over 10 weeks. At the 1-year follow-up, symptom bothersomeness was reduced in all three groups. Bothersomeness scores decreased from 6.1 (95% CI, 5.7-6.5) to 3.8 (95% CI, 3.1-4.5) in the intervention group; 6.2 (95% CI, 5.8-6.5) to 4.5 (95% CI, 3.8-5.2) in the acupuncture control group; 6.2 (95% CI, 5.8-6.6) to 3.2 (95% CI, 2.5-3.9) in the massage control group. The differences between the groups (adjusted for baseline values) were statistically significant ($P = .003$). At the 1-year follow-up, there were also improvements in disability in all three groups. RDQ scores decreased from 12.0 (95% CI, 10.9-13.0) to 6.4 (95% CI, 5.1-7.7) in the intervention group; 12.8 (95% CI, 11.7-13.8) to 8.0 (95% CI, 6.6-9.3) in the acupuncture control group; and 11.8 (95% CI, 10.8-12.7) to 6.8 (95% CI, 5.5-8.1) in the massage control group. The differences between the groups (adjusted for baseline values) were statistically significant ($P = .03$). Although the differences in symptom bothersomeness and disability between the massage and acupuncture groups were statistically significant, the improvements in the self-care intervention over the acupuncture control was not statistically significant. This study was considered of higher quality.

An RCT was conducted by Lorig and colleagues[45] on LBP patients recruited through the Internet, workplaces, and public service announcements. Participants had at least one outpatient visit for back pain in the past year, no red flags (back pain with unintended weight loss, pain not improved with rest, back pain secondary to significant trauma, acute onset of urinary retention or overflow incontinence, loss of anal sphincter tone or fecal incontinence, saddle anesthesia, or global or progressive motor weakness in the lower limbs), access to a computer and an e-mail account, and residence in the United States. Exclusion criteria included back pain that had continued for over 90 consecutive days and continued to cause major activity intolerance, planned back surgery, receiving disability insurance payments for back pain, inability to understand and write English, pregnancy, back pain due to systemic disease, comorbid conditions that limited functional ability, and terminal illness. The intervention group (n = 296) was assigned to a back pain e-mail discussion group, and received a book and videotape. The control group (n = 284) was assigned to a subscription to a non–health-related magazine. After 12 months, improvements in pain (visual numeric scale, 0-10) were greater in the intervention group compared with the control ($P = .002$). The mean change (standard deviation [SD]) in the intervention group was −1.50 (2.64) compared with −1.02 (2.60) in the control group. Disability (RDQ) also improved during this time, with greater improvements in the intervention group ($P \le .001$). The mean change (SD) in the intervention group was −2.77 (4.68) compared with −1.51 (4.97) in the control group. This study was considered of lower quality.

An RCT conducted by Storheim[29] included nonspecific LBP patients, with duration of symptoms unspecified. Participants were randomized to three groups: (1) intervention, consisting of an examination and reassurance as described by Indahl,[2,42] assessment of function, instruction to activate deep stabilizing muscles, and advice to stay active; (2) a control group consisting of examination and aerobic dance program modified for LBP patients; and (3) a control group consisting of usual care. The first intervention consisted of two 0.5- to 1-hour sessions with a hospital outpatient and primary care physiatrist, and a physical therapist. After the treatment period, there were improvements in pain scores (visual analog scale [VAS] 0-100) in all three groups, with the largest improvement in the intervention group (P values not reported). There were no statistically significant differences in pain between groups. After the treatment period, there were improvements in disability (RMDQ) in all three groups, with the largest improvement in the intervention group (P values not reported). The improvement in disability in the intervention group was significantly higher than in the usual care control group. There were no other significant differences between groups. This study was considered of higher quality.

An RCT conducted by Karjalainen and colleagues[25,46] included occupational LBP patients with symptoms of more than 4 weeks but less than 3 months. Participants were randomized to three groups: (1) examination, information, and reassurance as described by Indahl,[2,42] advice for staying active and home activity, and confirmation by a second physician (mini-intervention); (2) the same intervention as the first group, with a worksite visit by a physical therapist; and (3) usual care. The interventions consisted of a 2-hour session with a primary care physician, occupational medicine physician, physiatrist, and physical therapist. The worksite visit was 1 hour. After 24 months, there was a modest reduction in mean pain scores (0-10 scale) in all groups (P values not reported). There were no significant differences in pain between the mini-intervention group or the worksite visit group and the usual care control group. After 24 months, there were reductions in disability (Oswestry Disability Index [ODI]) in the worksite visit group and the usual care group, but not the mini-intervention group (P values not reported). There were no significant differences in disability between the mini-intervention group or the worksite visit group and the usual care control group. This study was considered of higher quality.

An RCT conducted by Buhrman and colleagues[47] included CLBP patients without neurologic involvement with symptoms lasting longer than 3 months. Participants were assigned to either an intervention consisting of an Internet-based pain management program with telephone support, discussion of negative thoughts and beliefs, active coping, relaxation, stretching, and exercises, or to a control group, consisting of being on a waiting list. Intervention participants had access to the program for 8 weeks and were treated by a psychologist and a physical therapist. At the 3-month follow-up, there was little change in mean pain scores (pain diary, Multidimensional Pain Index) in the intervention group (P values not reported), and a decrease in the control group.

The difference between the two groups was not statistically significant. Disability was not measured in this study. This study was considered of lower quality.

An RCT conducted by Sherman and colleagues[34] included LBP patients without neurologic involvement, with symptoms lasting longer than 12 weeks. Participants were randomized to three groups: (1) intervention, consisting of a mailed self-care book; (2) the first control, consisting of yoga classes; and (3) the second control, consisting of exercises (information, goal-setting, aerobic, strength, and flexibility exercises). The yoga and exercise groups had 75-minute classes once a week for 12 weeks. Twenty-six weeks after randomization, mean pain scores (bothersomeness) decreased for all three groups, with the largest reduction in the yoga group and the smallest reduction in the book group (P values not reported). The pain reduction in the yoga group was significantly higher than the book or exercise groups. There was no statistically significant different when comparing the book and exercise groups. Disability scores (RMDQ) also decreased in all three groups with the largest reduction in the yoga group and the smallest reduction in the book group (P values not reported). The improvement in disability in the yoga and exercise groups was significantly greater when compared with the book group. This study was considered of higher quality.

An RCT conducted by Goldby and colleagues[31] included CLBP patients without neurologic involvement, with a current episode lasting longer than 12 weeks. Participants were randomized to three groups: (1) an education intervention consisting of a back book and back school; (2) spinal stabilization exercises and back school; and (3) manual therapy and back school. The back school included one 3-hour session, and the manual therapy and spinal stabilization exercises were provided for 1 hour a week for 10 weeks. At the 24-month follow-up, mean pain scores (0-100 scale) significantly improved for the spinal stabilization and manual therapy groups, but worsened for the education group (not statistically significant). At the 24-month follow-up, mean disability scores (ODI) improved for all groups, with significant reductions in scores for the spinal stabilization and manual therapy groups, but not the education group. There were no significant differences between groups for pain or disability. This study was considered of lower quality.

An RCT conducted by Moseley and colleagues[33] included CLBP patients without neurologic involvement, with symptoms lasting longer than 6 months. Participants were assigned to either (1) information based on current knowledge of neurophysiology of pain or (2) information in accordance with Swedish Back School. Both programs included one 3-hour session along with homework daily for 2 weeks. After the treatment programs, there were no statistically significant changes in pain (VAS) in either group, and there was no significant difference between the groups. After the treatment programs, there was a small reduction in disability (RMDQ) in the neurophysiology education group and a small increase in the back school group (P values not reported). The difference in disability between groups was statistically significant in favor of the neurophysiology education group. This study was considered of higher quality.

SAFETY

Contraindications

Watchful Waiting

Contraindications to watchful waiting include CLBP due to potentially serious spinal pathology such as fracture, cancer, infection, or cauda equina syndrome, or other rare but specific causes of LBP. Watchful waiting is perhaps least likely to be successful in patients who exhibit psychosocial or other characteristics generally associated with a poor prognosis. These include psychological problems such as anxiety, stress, or depression, a previous history of LBP, poor job satisfaction, increased disability scores in standardized measurements, frequent lifting and postural stress, obesity, smoking, and poor general health.[48-50]

Brief Education

Contraindications to brief education include CLBP due to potentially serious spinal pathology such as fracture, cancer, infection, or cauda equina syndrome, or other rare but specific causes of LBP.

Adverse Events

Watchful Waiting

Watchful waiting is generally considered a safe intervention. A potential adverse event associated with watchful waiting is that symptoms may worsen, which could bring on psychological distress, anxiety, or depression if not addressed appropriately. No serious adverse events have been reported with this intervention for CLBP.

Brief Education

The CPG from Europe in 2004 determined that the safety of brief educational interventions in the treatment of CLBP (>3 months) is unknown.[13]

COSTS

Fees and Third-Party Reimbursement

In the United States, both watchful waiting and brief education for CLBP can likely be delivered by a clinician in the context of an office or outpatient visit for a new patient using CPT codes 99201 (up to 10 minutes), 99202 (up to 20 minutes), or 99203 (up to 30 minutes). For an established patient, watchful waiting and brief education for CLBP can likely be provided during an office or outpatient visit using CPT codes 99211 (up to 5 minutes), 99212 (up to 10 minutes), or 99213 (up to 15 minutes). Although time is indicated for the various levels of service and can be a contributing component for selection of the level of office/outpatient visits, the overarching criteria for selection of the level of service should be based on medical necessity and the amount of history, examination, and medical decision making that was required and documented for that visit.

TABLE 6-4	Medicare Fee Schedule for Related Services	
CPT Code	New York	California
99201	$41	$44
99202	$70	$76
99203	$101	$109
99211	$20	$22
99212	$41	$44
99213	$68	$73

2010 Participating, nonfacility amount.

These procedures are widely covered by other third-party payers such as health insurers and worker's compensation insurance. Although some payers continue to base their reimbursements on usual, customary, and reasonable payment methodology, the majority have developed reimbursement tables based on the Resource Based Relative Value Scale used by Medicare. Reimbursements by other third-party payers are generally much higher than by Medicare.

Typical fees reimbursed by Medicare in New York and California for these services are summarized in Table 6-4.

Cost Effectiveness

Evidence supporting the cost effectiveness of treatment protocols that compared these interventions, often in combination with one or more cointerventions, with control groups who received one or more other interventions, for either acute or chronic LBP, was identified from two SRs on this topic and is summarized in the following paragraphs.[51,52] Although many of these study designs are unable to clearly identify the individual contribution of any intervention, their results provide some insight into the clinical and economic outcomes associated with these approaches.

Watchful Waiting

No cost effectiveness analyses or cost utility analyses were identified which evaluated the cost effectiveness of watchful waiting as an intervention for LBP.

Brief Education

An RCT in the United States compared three approaches for patients with acute LBP presenting to an HMO. The physical therapy group received nine visits centered on the McKenzie method. The chiropractic group received nine visits of spinal manipulation. The brief education group received only an educational booklet. Clinical outcomes after 3 months reported greater improvement in pain for the physical therapy and chiropractic groups. Direct medical costs associated with study and nonstudy interventions provided by the HMO over 2 years were $437 in the physical therapy group, $429 in the chiropractic group, and $153 in the brief education group. Indirect productivity costs were not reported.

An RCT trial in Norway compared three approaches for patients with CLBP.[53] Participants received either: (1) a light multidisciplinary program consisting of education, fear avoidance training, and advice to remain active given by a physical therapist, nurse, and psychologist; (2) an extensive multidisciplinary program consisting of daily group sessions with cognitive behavioral therapy (CBT), education, fear avoidance training, and strengthening and stabilization exercises for 4 weeks; or (3) usual care by a general practitioner and possibly a physical therapist or chiropractor. Direct medical costs for the light and extensive multidisciplinary programs were estimated by dividing the total clinic costs for 1 year by the number of patients treated; direct costs were therefore assumed to be equal in both groups, regardless of large differences in time spent by clinic staff with patients in each group. Indirect productivity costs associated with lost work time were evaluated over 24 months. A limited cost benefit analysis for male participants only reported that the light multidisciplinary program would yield average savings of approximately $19,544 per patient over two years, and was therefore cost effective compared with usual care.

An RCT in the United Kingdom compared two approaches for patients with CLBP.[54] The active intervention was delivered by a physical therapist and consisted of a back school with education from a book and cassette, group education, advice to remain active, and CBT. Usual care was delivered by a general practitioner and included education from a book and cassette along with other interventions. Clinical outcomes after 15 months were similar between groups, as both improved in pain, function, and utility. Direct medical costs associated with study and non-study interventions over 15 months were $47 higher in the active intervention group. Based on nonsignificant differences in utility, the incremental cost effectiveness ratio (ICER) of group training over brief education alone was $8650 per quality-adjusted life-year (QALY), well within the generally accepted threshold for cost utility analyses.

An RCT in Finland compared three approaches for patients with subacute LBP treated in primary health care centers.[25] The three approaches were a minimal intervention group centered on brief education by a physician, a worksite visit group centered on education by a physician, nurse, physical therapist, and work supervisor, and a group that included an educational leaflet along with usual care from a general practitioner and a physical therapist as needed.[25] Clinical outcomes measured over 24 months were similar among the three groups, although differences were noted in favor of the minimal intervention group in days on sick leave when compared with usual care. Direct medical costs associated with the study interventions over 24 months were approximately $577 lower in the minimal intervention group and approximately $507 lower in the worksite visit group than in the usual care group. Total costs attributable to LBP (direct medical and indirect productivity) over 24 months were approximately $4626 in the minimal intervention group, approximately $5928 in the worksite visit group, and approximately $9417 in the usual care group. Total costs were lower in the minimal intervention group when compared with usual care, but differences between the minimal intervention and worksite visit group were not statistically significant.

An RCT in Finland compared two approaches for patients with CLBP in the rehabilitation unit of an orthopedic hospital.[55] One group received brief education by a physician and an education booklet. The other group received mobilization, stretching, and stabilization exercises from a manual therapist, as well as an educational booklet. Clinical outcomes after 12 months were mostly similar between the two groups, although slightly greater improvements were noted in pain and function in the manual therapist group. Direct medical costs associated with study and nonstudy interventions over 12 months were $431 in the brief education group and $470 in the manual therapist group. Indirect productivity costs from lost work days over 12 months were $2450 in the brief education group and $1848 in the manual therapist group. Total costs (direct medical and indirect productivity) over 12 months were therefore $2881 in the brief education group and $2318 in the manual therapist group. Total costs decreased in both groups when compared with historical health utilization and lost work days before having enrolled in the study, but cost differences between the groups were not significant.

An RCT in the United States compared two approaches for patients with CLBP.[56] The naturopathic care group included acupuncture, exercise, dietary advice, and relaxation delivered by a naturopath. The control group included brief education from a naturopath given in 30-minute, biweekly sessions over 3 months. Both groups also received an educational booklet, and voluntary crossover was offered to participants after 12 weeks. Clinical outcomes after 6 months favored the naturopathic care group for improvements in utility. Direct medical costs for study interventions over 6 months were $1469 in the naturopathic care group and $337 in the brief education group. Direct medical costs for nonstudy interventions over 6 months, including chiropractic, massage, physical therapy, pain medication, and other interventions, were $1203 lower in the naturopathic care group. Indirect productivity costs associated with lost work days were $1141 lower in the naturopathic care group. Authors concluded that naturopathic care was more cost effective than brief education.

A cluster RCT in The Netherlands compared two approaches for patients with subacute LBP presenting to 60 general practitioners in 41 offices.[57] The brief education approach was centered on CBT and discussion of psychosocial prognostic factors related to LBP, including fear avoidance beliefs. Usual care included interventions that were not specified. Clinical outcomes after 12 months were largely similar between the two groups. Direct medical costs for study and nonstudy interventions over 12 months were approximately $207 in the brief education group and approximately $202 in the usual care group. Indirect productivity costs associated with absenteeism for both paid and unpaid work over 12 months were approximately $575 in the brief education group and approximately $1059 in the usual care group. Total costs (direct medical and indirect productivity) were therefore approximately $782 in the brief education group and approximately $1261 in the usual care group. The brief education group therefore achieved similar clinical outcomes with lower costs.

An RCT in the United Kingdom compared three approaches for patients with CLBP.[58] The individual physical therapy approach included a maximum of 12 sessions with spinal manipulation, mobilization, massage, home exercises, and brief education. The spinal stabilization approach included a maximum of eight sessions with abdominal and multifidus exercises. The pain management approach included a maximum of eight sessions with education, exercises, CBT, and fear avoidance training. Clinical outcomes after 18 months were similar for all groups, with improvements noted in pain, function, and utility. Direct medical costs for study and nonstudy interventions paid by the National Health Service over 18 months were approximately $872 for individual physical therapy, approximately $698 for spinal stabilization, and approximately $304 for pain management. Indirect productivity costs were not reported. Over 18 months, the three groups experienced gains in QALY of 0.99, 0.90, and 1.00, respectively. By virtue of having lower direct medical costs and greater gains in utility, the pain management approach was reported to dominate over both individual physical therapy and spinal stabilization.

An RCT in the United States compared three approaches for patients with CLBP.[36] The traditional Chinese medicine (TCM) group received needle acupuncture with electrical or manual stimulation of needles, and possibly moxibustion; manual therapy was not permitted. The massage group received a variety of techniques, although acupressure was not permitted. The brief education group received education about LBP from a book and videos. Clinical outcomes after 12 months favored the massage group over the TCM group for improvement in both pain and function; medication use was also lowest in the massage group. Direct medical costs associated with study interventions over 12 months were $352 in the TCM group, $377 in the massage group, and $50 in the brief education group. Direct medical costs associated with nonstudy interventions including provider visits, medication use, and diagnostic imaging over 12 months were $252 in the TCM group, $139 in the massage group, and $200 in the brief education group. Total direct medical costs for both study and nonstudy interventions over 12 months were therefore $604 in the TCM group, $516 in the massage group, and $250 in the brief education group. Indirect productivity costs were not reported. Authors concluded that although cost differences between groups were not significant, massage appeared to be more effective than TCM.

An RCT in the United States compared two approaches for patients with acute LBP.[59] The first group received care according to the classification of symptoms and examination findings by a physical therapist, including possibly spinal manipulation, mobilization, traction therapy, and flexion, extension, strengthening, or stabilization exercises. The other group received brief education and general exercise from a physical therapist according to recommendations from CPGs, which were not specified. Clinical outcomes after 1 year favored the therapy according to classification group for improvement in function, although no differences were noted in the short form 36 (SF-36). Direct medical costs associated with study interventions over 1 year were $604 in the therapy according to classification group and $682 in the CPG-recommended care group; direct costs for all interventions over 1 year were $883 and $1160, respectively. Indirect productivity costs were not reported, although fewer participants

in the therapy according to classification group had missed work due to LBP after 12 months.

An RCT in the United Kingdom compared two approaches for patients with subacute or chronic LBP.[60] The supervised exercise therapy group received up to eight sessions of stretching, strengthening, and aerobic exercises, and brief education on LBP. The usual care group received interventions prescribed by a general practitioner, including physical therapy in some cases. Clinical outcomes after 1 year favored the supervised exercise therapy group for improvement in pain, function, and utility. Direct medical costs associated with study and nonstudy interventions over 12 months were $145 in the supervised exercise therapy group and approximately $185 in the usual care group. Indirect productivity costs associated with lost work days over 12 months were approximately $456 in the supervised exercise therapy group and approximately $663 in the usual care group. Total costs (direct medical and indirect productivity) over 12 months were therefore approximately $621 in the supervised exercise therapy group and approximately $848 in the usual care group. These differences in costs were not statistically significant.

An RCT in Norway compared two approaches for patients sick-listed with CLBP.[44] The early intervention approach received advice to stay active and brief education. The control group received primary care as usual, which was not specified. Clinical outcomes after 1 year were similar between the two groups. Direct medical costs associated with the study intervention over 3 years were $303 higher in the early intervention group. Indirect productivity costs from lost work days were $3800 lower in the early intervention group, mostly due to a faster return to work within the first year of follow-up. Authors concluded that the benefits of the early intervention group exceeded its costs.

An RCT in Sweden compared three approaches for patients sick-listed with acute LBP.[61] The manual therapy group received spinal manipulation, mobilization, assisted stretching, and exercises. The intensive training group received supervised exercise therapy with a physical therapist, including general and stabilization exercises. The usual care group received various interventions from a general practitioner, including common analgesics and brief education. Clinical outcomes were not reported. Direct medical costs associated with study interventions over 1 year including provider visits, diagnostic testing, and surgery (if needed) were approximately $1054 in the manual therapy group, approximately $1123 in the intensive training group, and approximately $404 in the usual care group. Indirect productivity costs associated with lost work days were approximately $6163 in the manual therapy group, approximately $5557 in the intensive training group, and approximately $7072 in the usual care group. Total costs (direct medical and indirect productivity) over 1 year were therefore approximately $7217 in the manual therapy group, approximately $6680 in the intensive training group, and approximately $7476 in the usual care group. Cost differences between groups were not significantly different.

An RCT in the United Kingdom compared two physical therapy approaches for patients with subacute or chronic

LBP.[62] The minimal physical therapy group received brief education. The standard physical therapy group included education, mobilization, massage, stretching, exercise, heat, or ice. Clinical outcomes after one year were similar between the two groups. Direct medical costs for study and nonstudy interventions over one year were approximately $376 in the minimal physical therapy group and approximately $486 in the standard physical therapy group. Indirect productivity costs were approximately $1305 in the minimal physical therapy group and approximately $856 in the standard physical therapy group, but these were excluded from the analysis. Since the standard physical therapy group had marginally better clinical outcomes with higher direct medical costs, its ICER was estimated at approximately $5538 per QALY, well within the generally accepted threshold for cost utility analyses.

An RCT in the United Kingdom compared two approaches for patients with acute LBP.[63] The brief pain management group included education, general exercise, and CBT. The physical therapy group included mobilization, spinal manipulation, massage, back exercise, and brief education. Clinical outcomes after 1 year were similar between the two groups. Direct medical costs for study and nonstudy interventions over 1 year were approximately $254 in the brief pain management group and approximately $354 in the physical therapy group. Indirect productivity costs were not considered. Since the physical therapy group had marginally better clinical outcomes with higher direct costs, its ICER was estimated at approximately $4710 per QALY, well within the generally accepted threshold for cost utility analyses.

An RCT in the United Kingdom compared four approaches for patients with subacute or chronic LBP.[64] The usual care from a general practitioner group included various unspecified interventions, brief education, and advice to remain active. The usual care from a general practitioner with exercise group included various unspecified interventions, and individual and group supervised exercise therapy classes. The usual care from a general practitioner with spinal manipulation group included various unspecified interventions and spinal manipulation. The usual care from a general practitioner with spinal manipulation and exercise group included various unspecified interventions, brief education, advice to remain active, individual and group supervised exercise therapy classes, and spinal manipulation. Clinical outcomes after 1 year were mostly similar, with improvement in pain, function, and utility, although greater improvement was reported for utility gains in the usual care with spinal manipulation and usual care with spinal manipulation and exercise groups. Direct medical costs associated with study and nonstudy interventions over one year were approximately $503 in the usual care group, approximately $707 in the usual care with exercise group, approximately $787 in the usual care with spinal manipulation group, and approximately $685 in the usual care with spinal manipulation and exercise group. Indirect productivity costs were not reported. Since the usual care with spinal manipulation and exercise group had lower direct medical costs and greater gains in QALY than usual care with exercise or usual care with spinal manipulation, authors concluded that it was cost saving and dominated

those two other choices; its ICER when compared with usual care was estimated at approximately $5509 per QALY, well within the generally accepted threshold for cost utility analyses.

Findings from the aforementioned cost effectiveness analyses are summarized in Table 6-5.

SUMMARY

Description

Watchful waiting can be defined as minimal care through activity modification, education, and observation of the natural history of LBP. It is passive in nature and does not include any interventions delivered by a health care provider to address specific symptoms. Watchful waiting can include patient-initiated comfort measures (e.g., home heat or ice, over-the-counter topical analgesics), watchfulness, waiting, reassurance, activity modification, and education. Watchful waiting does not indicate a complete absence of health care, and does not imply that symptoms are ignored by the patient. If a health care provider is recommending watchful waiting for someone with LBP, a detailed medical history will be obtained. Because watchful waiting requires education, it is often synonymous with brief education. These interventions are available throughout the United States in hospitals, private practices, and clinics. Licensed health care providers, including primary care physicians, spine specialists, chiropractors, physical therapists, and those trained in recognizing signs and symptoms of red flags associated with serious spinal pathology, can initiate watchful waiting and education.

Theory

The principal mechanism of action involved in watchful waiting or brief education is allowing sufficient time for the natural history of CLBP to occur, with gradual improvements over time. Epidemiologic studies of LBP indicate it is a common but benign condition of mostly unknown etiology that generally improves within a few weeks and disappears within a few months, although periodic recurrences are expected. Watchfulness is necessary to monitor development of rare but potentially serious spinal pathology and nonspinal causes of LBP that may need to be addressed. An essential component of watchful waiting is continual reassurance, which is thought to decrease anxiety related to the LBP, and therefore minimize its negative impact on recovery and quality of life. This intervention is indicated for patients with nonspecific CLBP. Diagnostic imaging or other forms of advanced testing is generally not required before administering this intervention for CLBP.

Efficacy

None of the recent national CPGs provide recommendations related specifically to watchful waiting for CLBP. However, four recent national CPGs provide recommendations on brief education for CLBP, two recommending it, one reporting

TABLE 6-5 | **Cost Effectiveness and Cost Utility Analyses of Watchful Waiting and Brief Education for Acute or Chronic Low Back Pain**

Ref Country Follow-up	Group	Direct Costs	Indirect Costs	Total Costs	Conclusion
United States 2 years	1. PT 2. chiropractic 3. brief education	1. $437 2. $429 3. $153	NR	NR	No conclusion as to cost effectiveness
53 Norway 2 years	1. light multidisciplinary program (including fear avoidance training) 2. extensive multidisciplinary program (including fear avoidance training) 3. usual care	NR	NR	NR	Group 1: average savings of $19,544/patient over 2 years
54 United Kingdom 15 months	1. back school, education, CBT 2. usual care from GP	1. $47 higher than group 2 2. NR	NR	NR	ICER of 1 over 2: $8650/QALY
25 Finland 2 years	1. minimal intervention (including brief education) 2. worksite visit (including education) 3. usual care	1. $577 lower than group 3 2. $507 lower than group 3	NR	1. $4626 2. $5928 3. $9417	No significant difference between groups 1 and 2
55 Finland 1 year	1. brief education by physician 2. treatment by manual therapist + booklet	1. $431 2. $470	1. $2450 2. $1848	1. $2881 2. $2318	No significant difference
56 United States 6 months	1. naturopathic care 2. control	1. $1469 2. $337	1. $1141 lower than group 2	NR	1. more cost effective than 2
57 The Netherlands 1 year	1. brief education approach (including fear avoidance training) 2. usual care	1. $207 2. $202	1. $575 2. $1059	1. $782 2. $1261	Group 1 achieved similar clinical outcomes with lower costs
58 United Kingdom 18 months	1. individual PT 2. spinal stabilization 3. pain management (including fear avoidance training)	1. $872 2. $698 3. $304	NR	NR	Gains in QALY: 1. 0.99 2. 0.90 3. 1.00 Group 3 reported to dominate other interventions
36 United States 1 year	1. TCM 2. massage 3. brief education	1. $604 2. $516 3. $250	NR	NR	No significant difference
59 United States 1 year	1. care according to classification of symptoms 2. brief education + general exercise	1. $883 2. $1160	NR	NR	No conclusion as to cost effectiveness
60 United Kingdom 1 year	1. supervised exercise therapy 2. usual care	1. $145 2. $185	1. $456 2. $663	1. $601 2. $848	No significant difference
44 Norway 3 years	1. early intervention 2. usual care	1. $303 higher than group 2	1. $3800 lower than group 2	NR	Benefits of early intervention exceed its cost

TABLE 6-5	Cost Effectiveness and Cost Utility Analyses of Watchful Waiting and Brief Education for Acute or Chronic Low Back Pain—cont'd				
Ref Country Follow-up	Group	Direct Costs	Indirect Costs	Total Costs	Conclusion
61 Sweden 1 year	1. manual therapy 2. intensive training 3. usual care (inc. brief education)	1. $1054 2. $1123 3. 404	1. $6163 2. $5557 3. $7072	1. $7217 2. $6680 3. $7476	No significant difference
62 United Kingdom 1 year	1. minimal PT 2. standard PT	1. $376 2. $486	1. $1305 2. $856 (excluded from analysis)	NR	ICER of 2 over 1: $5538/QALY
63 United Kingdom 1 year	1. brief pain management 2. PT	1. $254 2. $354	NR	NR	ICER of 1 over 2: $4710/QALY
64 United Kingdom 1 year	1. usual care 2. usual care + exercise 3. usual care + SMT 4. usual care + exercise + SMT	1. $503 2. $707 3. $787 4. $685	NR	NR	ICER of 4 over 1: $5509/QALY

CBT, cognitive behavioral therapy; GP, general practitioner; ICER, incremental cost effectiveness ratio; NR, not reported; PT, physical therapy; QALY, quality-adjusted life-year; SMT, spinal manipulation therapy; TCM, traditional Chinese medicine.

moderate benefit of brief education for CLBP, and the fourth reporting that this intervention is not sufficient on its own for CLBP. An SR conducted by the Cochrane Collaboration concluded that individual education is not effective compared with noneducational interventions for CLBP. Another SR concluded that brief education leads to reduced sick leave and short-term disability versus usual care; however, conflicting evidence was observed for certain types of brief education (e.g., back book, Internet discussion) versus comparators (e.g., waiting list, no intervention). At least nine RCTs assessed the efficacy of brief education for pain and functional improvement among patients with CLBP. Two RCTs observed that brief education was superior to comparators in terms of pain relief and two other RCTs reported statistically significant pain relief for brief education versus other comparators. However, one RCT found that yoga and exercise were superior to brief education and another RCT reported that spinal manipulation and manual therapy were superior to brief education for CLBP.

Safety

Contraindications to watchful waiting include CLBP due to potentially serious spinal pathology such as fracture, cancer, infection, or cauda equina syndrome. Watchful waiting is generally considered a safe intervention. A potential adverse event associated with watchful waiting is that symptoms may worsen, which could bring on psychological distress, anxiety, or depression if not addressed appropriately.

Costs

A clinician usually delivers watchful waiting for CLBP during outpatient visits. Medicare reimbursement for such visits ranged from $20 to $109. The cost effectiveness of watchful waiting is unknown. At least 16 RCTs examined the cost effectiveness associated with brief education for CLBP, the majority of which combine brief education with other interventions, rendering it impossible to determine the contribution of this intervention to the cost effectiveness.

Comments

Evidence from the CPGs, SRs, and RCTs reviewed was unable to support the efficacy of watchful waiting as a specific intervention for CLBP. However, this evidence suggested that brief education might be effective for some patients with CLBP, yet it may not be effective on its own or as effective as other conservative treatment for LBP. It appears that brief education can be recommended in the clinical setting but that the effectiveness of brief education when given as a booklet or Internet communication is not supported by current evidence.

The mixed results reported in the studies reviewed could, in part, be explained by their many methodologic differences. For example, some of these studies were conducted in patients who had been on sick leave due to CLBP for a minimum of 8 to 12 weeks. Given the inevitable delays that likely occurred from the onset of LBP until sick leave registration, these interventions may have occurred later than would otherwise be ideal. Other differences were also noted in the nature of the interventions studied. Brief education may have consisted of a consultation that included a clinical examination and advice given by a health professional, or a booklet given without much human interaction. The lack of communication with a health care professional may have influenced the patients' expectations and satisfaction. Conversely, participation in an active group or repeated consultation with a health care professional might also enhance positive expectations and increase the possible non-specific (i.e., placebo) effect.

CHAPTER REVIEW QUESTIONS

Answers are located on page 450.

1. Which of the following is not considered a component of watchful waiting?
   a. never seeking care from a health care provider
   b. rest
   c. education
   d. avoiding aggravating factors

2. On which treatment philosophy is the watchful waiting approach based?
   a. complementary and alternative medicine
   b. traditional healing methods
   c. scientific evidence from epidemiologic and clinical studies
   d. technologically advanced medical interventions

3. When should a patient with LBP consult with a health care provider?
   a. when a prolonged period of self-care is no longer effective
   b. when symptoms worsen and prevent normal activities
   c. when they develop difficulty controlling their bowel or bladder
   d. all of the above

4. Which of the following are characteristics of the ideal patient for brief education?
   a. manual laborer
   b. first episode of low back pain
   c. back pain of less than 8 weeks' duration
   d. all of the above

5. True or false: watchful waiting has been shown to be cost effective.

6. True or false: watchful waiting is based on epidemiologic research showing that acute LBP usually resolves within a few weeks.

7. True or false: watchful waiting and brief education are closely related.

REFERENCES

1. Bigos S, Bowyer O, Braen G, et al. Acute low back pain problems in adults. Clinical Practice Guideline Number 14. AHCPR Pub. No. 95-0642. Rockville: US Department of Health and Human Services, Public Health Service, Agency for Health Care Policy and Research; 1994. Report no.: AHCPR Publication no. 95-0642.

2. Indahl A, Velund L, Reikeraas O. Good prognosis for low back pain when left untampered. A randomized clinical trial. Spine 1995;20:473-477.

3. Frost H, Lamb SE, Doll HA, et al. Randomised controlled trial of physiotherapy compared with advice for low back pain. BMJ 2004;329:708.

4. Rivero-Arias O, Gray A, Frost H, et al. Cost-utility analysis of physiotherapy treatment compared with physiotherapy advice in low back pain. Spine 2006;31:1381-1387.

5. Cherkin DC, Deyo RA, Battie M, et al. A comparison of physical therapy, chiropractic manipulation, and provision of an educational booklet for the treatment of patients with low back pain. N Engl J Med 1998;339:1021-1029.

6. Keller A, Brox JI, Gunderson R, et al. Trunk muscle strength, cross-sectional area, and density in patients with chronic low back pain randomized to lumbar fusion or cognitive intervention and exercises. Spine 2004;29:3-8.

7. Yue JJ, Patwardhan AV, White AP. Acute low back pain: orthopaedic knowledge update. In: Spivak JM, Connolly PJ, editors. Spine. 3rd ed. Rosemont, Ill: American Academy of Orthopaedic Surgeons; 2006.

8. Philadelphia Panel evidence-based clinical practice guidelines on selected rehabilitation interventions for low back pain. Phys Ther 2001;81:1641-1674.

9. Work Loss Data Institute. Low back—lumbar & thoracic (acute & chronic). Corpus Christi, TX: Work Loss Data Institute; 2006.

10. Institute for Clinical Systems Improvement (ICSI). Adult low back pain. Institute for Clinical Systems Improvement; 2006. p. 1-65. http://www.guideline.gov/summary/summary.aspx?doc_id=9863&nbr=005287&string=adult+AND+low+AND+back+AND+pain.

11. Hagen KB, Hilde G, Jamtvedt G, et al. The Cochrane review of advice to stay active as a single treatment for low back pain and sciatica. Spine 2002;27:1736-1741.

12. Vroomen PC, de Krom MC, Wilmink JT, et al. Lack of effectiveness of bed rest for sciatica. N Engl J Med 1999;340:418-423.

13. Airaksinen O, Brox JI, Cedraschi C, et al. European guidelines for the management of chronic nonspecific low back pain. Eur Spine J 2006;15(Suppl 2):192-300.

14. Mitchell RI, Carmen GM. The functional restoration approach to the treatment of chronic pain in patients with soft tissue and back injuries. Spine 1994;19:633-642.

15. Nielens H, van Zundert J, Mairiaux P, et al. Chronic low back pain. Vol. 48C. Brussels: KCE Reports; 2006.

16. Chou R, Qaseem A, Snow V, et al. Diagnosis and treatment of low back pain: a joint clinical practice guideline from the American College of Physicians and the American Pain Society. Ann Intern Med 2007;147:478-491.

17. National Institute for Health and Clinical Excellence (NICE). Low back pain: early management of persistent nonspecific low back pain. Report No.: NICE clinical guideline 88. London: National Institute of Health and Clinical Excellence; 2009.

18. Engers A, Jellema P, Wensing M, et al. Individual patient education for low back pain. Cochrane Database Syst Rev 2008;(1):CD004057.

19. Burton AK, Waddell G, Burtt R, et al. Patient educational material in the management of low back pain in primary care. Bull Hosp Jt Dis, 1996;55:138-141.

20. Deyo RA, Diehl AK, Rosenthal M. Reducing roentgenography use. Can patient expectations be altered? Arch Intern Med 1987;147:141-145.

21. Hagen EM, Eriksen HR, Ursin H. Does early intervention with a light mobilization program reduce long-term sick leave for low back pain? Spine 2000;25:1973-1976.

22. Hazard RG, Reid S, Haugh LD, et al. A controlled trial of an educational pamphlet to prevent disability after occupational low back injury. Spine 2000;25:1419-1423.

23. Hurley DA, Minder PM, McDonough SM, et al. Interferential therapy electrode placement technique in acute low back pain: a preliminary investigation. Arch Phys Med Rehabil 2001;82:485-493.

24. Jellema P, van der Windt DA, van der Horst HE, et al. Should treatment of (sub)acute low back pain be aimed at psychosocial prognostic factors? Cluster randomised clinical trial in general practice. BMJ 2005;331:84.

25. Karjalainen K, Malmivaara A, Mutanen P, et al. Mini-intervention for subacute low back pain: two-year follow-up and modifiers of effectiveness. Spine 2004;29:1069-1076.

26. Linton SJ, Andersson T. Can chronic disability be prevented? A randomized trial of a cognitive-behavior intervention and two forms of information for patients with spinal pain. Spine 2000;25:2825-2831.

27. Mayer JM, Ralph L, Look M, et al. Treating acute low back pain with continuous low-level heat wrap therapy and/or exercise: a randomized controlled trial. Spine J 2005;5:395-403.

28. Roberts L, Little P, Chapman J, et al. The back home trial: general practitioner-supported leaflets may change back pain behavior. Spine 2002;27:1821-1828.

29. Storheim K, Brox JI, Holm I, et al. Intensive group training versus cognitive intervention in subacute low back pain: short-term results of a single-blind randomized controlled trial. J Rehabil Med 2003;35:132-140.

30. Wand BM, Bird C, McAuley JH, et al. Early intervention for the management of acute low back pain: a single-blind randomized controlled trial of biopsychosocial education, manual therapy, and exercise. Spine 2004;29:2350-2356.

31. Goldby LJ, Moore AP, Doust J, et al. A randomized controlled trial investigating the efficiency of musculoskeletal physiotherapy on chronic low back disorder. Spine 2006;31:1083-1093.

32. Hurri H. The Swedish back school in chronic low back pain. Part I. Benefits. Scand J Rehabil Med 1989;21:33-40.

33. Moseley GL, Nicholas MK, Hodges PW. A randomized controlled trial of intensive neurophysiology education in chronic low back pain. Clin J Pain 2004;20:324-330.

34. Sherman KJ, Cherkin DC, Erro J, et al. Comparing yoga, exercise, and a self-care book for chronic low back pain: a randomized, controlled trial. Ann Intern Med 2005;143:849-856.

35. Cherkin DC, Deyo RA, Street JH, et al. Pitfalls of patient education. Limited success of a program for back pain in primary care. Spine 1996;21:345-355.

36. Cherkin DC, Eisenberg D, Sherman KJ, et al. Randomized trial comparing traditional Chinese medical acupuncture, therapeutic massage, and self-care education for chronic low back pain. Arch Intern Med 2001;161:1081-1088.

37. Frost H, Lamb SE, Doll HA, et al. Randomised controlled trial of physiotherapy compared with advice for low back pain. BMJ 2004;329:708.

38. Jackson L. Maximizing treatment adherence among back-pain patients: an experimental study of the effects of physician-related cues in written medical messages. Health Communication 1994;6:173-191.

39. Little P, Roberts L, Blowers H, et al. Should we give detailed advice and information booklets to patients with back pain? A randomized controlled factorial trial of a self-management booklet and doctor advice to take exercise for back pain. Spine 2001;26:2065-2072.

40. Roland M, Dixon M. Randomized controlled trial of an educational booklet for patients presenting with back pain in general practice. J R Coll Gen Pract 1989;39:244-246.

41. Brox JI, Storheim K, Grotle M, et al. Systematic review of back schools, brief education, and fear-avoidance training for chronic low back pain. Spine J 2008;8:948-958.

42. Indahl A, Haldorsen EH, Holm S, et al. Five-year follow-up study of a controlled clinical trial using light mobilization and an informative approach to low back pain. Spine 1998;23:2625-2630.

43. Von Korff M, Moore JE, Lorig K, et al. A randomized trial of a lay person-led self-management group intervention for back pain patients in primary care. Spine 1998;23:2608-2615.

44. Molde Hagen E, Grasdal A, Eriksen HR. Does early intervention with a light mobilization program reduce long-term sick leave for low back pain: a 3-year follow-up study. Spine 2003;28:2309-2315.

45. Lorig KR, Laurent DD, Deyo RA, et al. Can a back pain e-mail discussion group improve health status and lower health care costs? A randomized study. Arch Intern Med 2002;162:792-796.

46. Karjalainen K, Malmivaara A, Pohjolainen T, et al. Mini-intervention for subacute low back pain: a randomized controlled trial. Spine 2003;28:533-540.

47. Buhrman M, Faltenhag S, Strom L, et al. Controlled trial of Internet-based treatment with telephone support for chronic back pain. Pain 2004;111:368-377.

48. Heliovaara M. Risk factors for low back pain and sciatica. Ann Med 1989;21:257-264.

49. Linton SJ. Occupational psychological factors increase the risk for back pain: a systematic review. J Occup Rehabil 2001;11:53-66.

50. Shaw WS, Pransky G, Fitzgerald TE. Early prognosis for low back disability: intervention strategies for health care providers. Disabil Rehabil 2001;23:815-828.

51. Dagenais S, Roffey DM, Wai EK, et al. Can cost utility evaluations inform decision making about interventions for low back pain? Spine J 2009;9:944-957.

52. van der Roer N, Goossens MEJB, Evers SMAA, et al. What is the most cost-effective treatment for patients with low back pain? A systematic review. Best Pract Res Clin Rheumatol 2005;19:671-684.

53. Skouen JS, Grasdal AL, Haldorsen EM, et al. Relative cost-effectiveness of extensive and light multidisciplinary treatment programs versus treatment as usual for patients with chronic low back pain on long-term sick leave: randomized controlled study. Spine 2002;27:901-909.

54. Johnson RE, Jones GT, Wiles NJ, et al. Active exercise, education, and cognitive behavioral therapy for persistent disabling low back pain: a randomized controlled trial. Spine 2007;32:1578-1585.

55. Niemisto L, Lahtinen-Suopanki T, Rissanen P, et al. A randomized trial of combined manipulation, stabilizing exercises, and physician consultation compared to physician consultation alone for chronic low back pain. Spine 2003;28:2185-2191.

56. Herman PM, Szczurko O, Cooley K, et al. Cost-effectiveness of naturopathic care for chronic low back pain. Alt Ther Health Med 2008;14:32-39.

57. Jellema P, van der Roer N, van der Windt DAWM, et al. Low back pain in general practice: cost-effectiveness of a minimal psychosocial intervention versus usual care. Eur Spine J 2007;16:1812-1821.

58. Critchley DJ, Ratcliffe J, Noonan S, et al. Effectiveness and cost-effectiveness of three types of physiotherapy used to reduce chronic low back pain disability: a pragmatic randomized trial with economic evaluation. Spine 2007;32:1474-1481.

59. Fritz JM, Delitto A, Erhard RE. Comparison of classification-based physical therapy with therapy based on clinical practice guidelines for patients with acute low back pain: a randomized clinical trial. Spine 2003;28:1363-1371.

60. Moffett JK, Torgerson D, Bell-Syer S, et al. Randomised controlled trial of exercise for low back pain: clinical outcomes, costs, and preferences. BMJ 1999;319:279-283.

61. Seferlis T, Lindholm L, Nemeth G. Cost-minimisation analysis of three conservative treatment programmes in 180 patients sick-listed for acute low-back pain. Scand J Prim Health Care 2000;18:53-57.

62. Rivero-Arias O, Gray A, Frost H, et al. Cost-utility analysis of physiotherapy treatment compared with physiotherapy advice in low back pain. Spine 2006;31:1381-1387.

63. Whitehurst DGT, Lewis M, Yao GL, et al. A brief pain management program compared with physical therapy for low back pain: results from an economic analysis alongside a randomized clinical trial. Arthritis Rheumatism 2007;57:466-473.

64. UK Beam Trial Team. United Kingdom back pain exercise and manipulation (UK BEAM) randomised trial: cost effectiveness of physical treatments for back pain in primary care. BMJ 2004;329:1381.

JENS IVAR BROX
KJERSTI STORHEIM
MARGRETH GROTLE
TORILL HELENE TVEITO
AAGE INDAHL
HEGE R. ERIKSEN

CHAPTER **7**

Back Schools and Fear Avoidance Training

DESCRIPTION

Terminology and Subtypes

Back schools can be defined as interventions that include group education about low back pain (LBP), appropriate self-management of LBP, training about how to live and how to adapt activities of daily living while coping with LBP, and recommendations for general and back-specific exercises.[1] Fear avoidance training, on the other hand, is intended for individual patients with chronic low back pain (CLBP) and harmful or inappropriate beliefs or behaviors about their pain. Although the two types of training are reviewed in this chapter as distinct interventions, there is considerable overlap among modern back schools based on cognitive behavioral therapy (CBT) methods and fear avoidance training programs founded on similar concepts. Categorizing these interventions is intended to increase homogeneity among the studies reviewed and to improve the precision of recommendations concerning these interventions.

History and Frequency of Use

The Swedish Back School was introduced by Zachrisson-Forssell in 1969 based on her knowledge about the intervertebral disc, spinal anatomy and physiology, and ergonomics.[2-3] Patients attending back schools were initially taught how to protect spinal structures during daily activities; education about back-specific exercises were later added to the program.[4] Back schools were eventually incorporated into comprehensive multidisciplinary programs for CLBP.[5] The use of education grew after the Scottish spine surgeon Gordon Waddell proposed a new theoretical framework for the treatment of LBP based on his observations that the natural history and epidemiology of LBP suggest that it is benign and self-limiting, and that patients needed to be informed of these facts in order to recover.[6]

Lethem and colleagues[7] introduced the model of fear avoidance in 1983, and a questionnaire for measuring this concept was published by Waddell and colleagues[8] a decade later. The central concept of this model is that behavior, for

some patients with CLBP, is driven largely by fear of pain. This concept was further outlined by Vlaeyen and Linton[9] in 2000, who postulated that confrontation and avoidance are the two extreme responses that patients can exhibit to this fear of pain. Whereas the former leads to gradual reduction of fear over time and eventual recovery, the latter perpetuates and exacerbates this fear, which may generate a phobic state in patients with CLBP. Several studies have shown that physical performance and self-reported disability cannot solely be explained by sensory and biomedical parameters, and that they are also associated with cognitive and behavioral aspects of pain.[10-14] Behavior that is believed to be caused by fear of movement is commonly observed among persons with CLBP who have been told or experienced that the "wrong movement" might cause a serious problem and should be avoided, which may increase their risk for prolonged disability.[12,15]

It is difficult to estimate frequency of use for back schools among those with LBP. However, it has been reported that the number of back schools operating in Sweden in 1984 was approximately 300, with 1000 specialized pain clinics operating in the United States in 1986, more than 40 such clinics in the United Kingdom in 1987, and in excess of 70 specialized clinics in The Netherlands in 1992.[16] The use of some form of education in the management and prevention of LBP is now common, and most conservative treatment approaches include some discussion about minimizing biomechanical risk factors and improving lifting techniques.[17]

The association between biomechanical risk factors and lifting techniques is a persistent myth, and prospective studies have not found that interventions aimed to improve ergonomics have reduced the risk for LBP. Modern back schools educate patients about the knowledge gained from these studies and generally do not educate patients about perceived correct lifting techniques (Figure 7-1). Modern back schools in fact expose patients to performing activities that were previously not recommended, such as jumping and bending their backs while lifting. However, this approach is controversial among professionals and may contribute to the divergent results from trials evaluating the effectiveness of

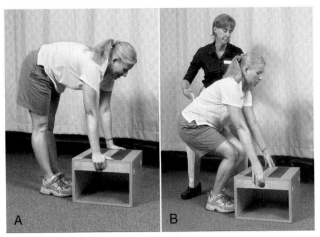

Figure 7-1 Modern back schools generally do not educate patients about so-called correct lifting techniques. (Courtesy of Dewey Neild. From Pagliarulo MA. Introduction to physical therapy, ed 3. St Louis, 2006, Mosby.)

back schools, which represent a heterogeneous intervention that cannot easily be studied.

Practitioner, Setting, and Availability

Many health care providers, including physical therapists, physicians, occupational therapists, and chiropractors, may deliver basic back school interventions with additional content-specific training. A trained mental health professional such as a psychologist or psychiatrist may be required for advanced fear avoidance training. These interventions occur in occupational settings or private practices of health care providers. These interventions are widely available in the United States, mostly in larger cities.

Procedure

In back schools, education is generally given about the anatomy of the spine, including structures that are commonly thought to be involved in the etiology of LBP. Methods for diagnosing LBP may be discussed, as may be spinal biomechanics and important concepts related to pain in general.[18-20] Information is also given about the epidemiology of LBP, its general prognosis over short and extended periods, and the strong possibility of recurrence. Appropriate management options for LBP may be described, including advice on how to live with LBP and adapt activities of daily living if necessary. Education about general and back-specific exercises is also provided; some back schools may include supervised exercise in their curriculum. Back schools are typically given by a physical therapist, or other health care provider with specialized training, to small groups of 8 to 12 participants. They may be delivered in an occupational setting or in a clinical setting as part of a spinal multidisciplinary rehabilitation program and often require multiple sessions given over a few weeks.[18-19]

Fear avoidance training is usually given to individuals with CLBP identified as having behavioral risk factors for further chronicity. It is often delivered in secondary care settings by physical therapists with advanced training, behavioral specialists, or nonsurgical spine specialists. Fear avoidance training includes much of the same basic education about LBP, but focuses more on overcoming behavioral barriers to recovery through graded activities of daily living and exercises. This intervention is named after the concept of fear avoidance, or *kinesiophobia*, which involves avoidance of common activities due to fear that they will exacerbate symptoms. Propensity for fear avoidance in patients with chronic pain can be assessed by validated questionnaires, including the Tampa Scale for Kinesiophobia (TSK) or the Fear Avoidance Beliefs Questionnaire (FABQ).[8,21,22]

Regulatory Status

Not applicable.

THEORY

Mechanism of Action

The word *doctor* comes from the Latin word *docere*, which means teacher. This etymology underscores the importance of education and communication in the doctor-patient relationship. Although most consultations with a health care provider contain some element of education, this aspect is rarely the focus of the encounter, which often centers on establishing a diagnosis and prescribing an intervention. The time allotted to patient education during a typical visit is therefore minimized in favor of what are perceived as the other, more crucial components of the encounter. However, when dealing with a complex disorder such as CLBP that is poorly understood by patients and surrounded by misinformation, education should become the focus of clinical encounters. Education should be provided about the diagnosis and prognosis of LBP, appropriate use of diagnostic and therapeutic interventions, and advice on how to manage symptoms at home by remaining active.

Education can then serve to minimize fears that patients may have about CLBP, prevent them from requesting inappropriate interventions that could cause them unnecessary harm, and provide them with the tools necessary to manage symptoms themselves when they arise. It is essential to reassure patients that the severity of pain does not by itself indicate the presence of any physical harm. When educating patients about CLBP, clinicians should encourage positive thoughts and actions, discourage impediments to recovery, and outline realistic treatment goals and expectations. These aspects are especially important if education was not provided at the onset of LBP or misinformation was provided, leading to the pursuit of ineffective therapies that may have further discouraged the patient about the prospects for their recovery.

Providers should not assume that adequate and correct education about LBP has already been provided by another clinician, regardless of how long symptoms have been present. Patients with CLBP often fail to discuss their fears

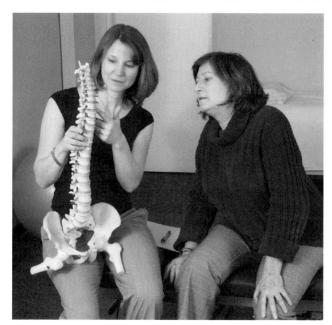

Figure 7-2 Clinicians should not assume that adequate and correct education about low back pain has already been provided by someone else, even for patients with chronic symptoms. (© istockphoto.com/Eliza Snow)

with health care providers unless asked directly because they do not want to receive unfavorable answers to their questions, dislike further questioning by health care providers about this topic, or worry that their fears will be belittled. This should be considered when providers are explaining the results of any diagnostic tests. Although clinicians appreciate that negative test results that indicate a lack of serious pathology, patients may perceive such tests as having failed to identify the cause of their pain. Clinicians must therefore carefully explain how these results should in fact reassure the patient about the absence of serious pathology (Figure 7-2).

Classic back schools teach about spinal anatomy and ergonomics to encourage protection of the spinal structures, although the impact of this information on patients' fear has not been addressed. Cherkin and colleagues[23] reported that although patient knowledge about the spine was improved following attendance in back schools, the effect on pain and disability was sparse compared with other treatments in patients with acute LBP. Behavior that derives from fear avoidance is inhibitory and may contribute to chronicity and even learned helplessness.[25] At present, we do not know whether this inhibition leads to a gradual development of depression, with its low psychomotor level in all dimensions. Although automated movements are unconscious, they may be brought to conscious analysis and observation in patients with CLBP, which can occupy more brain capacity and reduce physical performance.

If CLBP is perceived by patients as a threatening situation, anxiety will give priority to thoughts and information related to their fear. The cognitive activation theory of stress attempts to explain how pain leads to neurophysiologic activation and has proposed that a stress alarm occurs when there is a discrepancy between what is expected and what is experienced

by the individual.[26] Although the discrepancy is not an immediate threat to their health, a sustained state of related anxiety may lead to CLBP through established pathophysiologic responses. The challenge in patients with CLBP is to balance information and expectancies regarding spinal structures and the adoption of pain behavior. A positive response outcome expectancy (e.g., coping) may reduce the stress response whereas negative response outcome expectancy (e.g., hopelessness) may increase the risk for sustained activation. Interventions such as back school and fear avoidance may improve CLBP by increasing knowledge, which decreases false expectations, lending to fewer instances of discrepancies in their experience.

Indication

These interventions are used mainly for nonspecific mechanical CLBP and have not been evaluated for patients with serious somatic or psychiatric comorbidities that may require concurrent psychological or psychiatric care. The use of CBT and medications for CLBP is discussed elsewhere in this text (i.e., Sections 4 and 8). The ideal CLBP patients for each of these interventions are briefly described here, based on the authors' clinical experience.

Back Schools

The ideal patient for this approach may be middle aged, suffers from yearly recurrent episodes of moderate LBP, has been out of work for short periods yearly, reports that sitting and standing for more than half an hour is not comfortable, avoids lifting, is comfortable while walking but avoids jogging or more rigorous physical activities, and though medication and spinal manipulation therapy (SMT) may have relieved symptoms for short periods, they do not prevent recurrences.

Fear Avoidance Training

The ideal patient for this approach has moderate-to-severe pain, is unable to participate in ordinary physical activity, and has been told to avoid bending, jumping, lifting, and playing golf and tennis. Clinical examination reveals that all movements are painful and limited, although neurologic examination has not shown any signs of nerve root involvement; magnetic resonance imaging may have revealed disc degeneration and bulging of the two lower segments. A comprehensive examination reveals that the patient has poor physical tests and high scores on fear avoidance beliefs for physical activity. Standard conservative care has not been helpful and the patient is considered a potential candidate for spinal fusion.

Assessment

Before attending back schools or receiving fear avoidance training, patients should first be assessed for LBP using an evidence-based and goal-oriented approach focused on the patient history and neurologic examination, as discussed in Chapter 3. Additional diagnostic imaging or specific diagnostic testing is generally not required before initiating these interventions for CLBP. Certain questionnaires (e.g., TSK, FABQ) may help identify subsets of patients with CLBP who

Fear Avoidance Beliefs Questionnaire

Here are some of the things that other patients have told us about their pain. For each statement please circle any number from 0 to 6 to say how much physical activities such as bending, lifting, walking or driving affect or would affect your back pain.

	Completely disagree	Unsure			Completely agree
1. My pain was caused by physical activity	0	1 2	3	4 5	6
2. Physical activity makes my pain worse	0	1 2	3	4 5	6
3. Physical activity might harm my back	0	1 2	3	4 5	6
4. I should not do physical activities which (might) make my pain worse	0	1 2	3	4 5	6
5. I cannot do physical activities which (might) make my pain worse	0	1 2	3	4 5	6

The following statements are about how your normal work affects or would affect your back pain.

	Completely disagree	Unsure			Completely agree
6. My pain was caused by my work or by an accident at work	0	1 2	3	4 5	6
7. My work aggravated my pain	0	1 2	3	4 5	6
8. I have a claim for compensation for my pain	0	1 2	3	4 5	6
9. My work is too heavy for me	0	1 2	3	4 5	6
10. My work makes or would make my pain worse	0	1 2	3	4 5	6
11. My work might harm my back	0	1 2	3	4 5	6
12. I should not do my normal work with my present pain	0	1 2	3	4 5	6
13. I cannot do my normal work with my present pain	0	1 2	3	4 5	6
14. I cannot do my normal work till my pain is treated	0	1 2	3	4 5	6
15. I do not think that I will be back to my normal work within 3 months	0	1 2	3	4 5	6
16. I do not think that I will ever be able to go back to that work	0	1 2	3	4 5	6

Figure 7-3 Fear Avoidance Beliefs Questionnaire. (Reproduced with permission from Waddell G, et al. A Fear Avoidance Beliefs Questionnaire [FABQ] and the role of fear avoidance beliefs in chronic low back pain and disability. Pain 1993;52;157-168.)

may benefit from specific interventions aimed at addressing those issues (e.g., fear avoidance training) (Figure 7-3).

EFFICACY

Evidence supporting the efficacy of these interventions for CLBP have been summarized from recent clinical practice guidelines (CPGs), systematic reviews (SRs), and randomized controlled trials (RCTs). Observational studies (OBSs) are also summarized where appropriate. Findings are summarized by study design for each intervention in the following paragraphs.

Clinical Practice Guidelines

Back Schools

Two recent national CPGs on the management of CLBP have assessed and summarized the evidence to make specific recommendations about the efficacy of back schools.

The CPG from Europe in 2004 found conflicting evidence to support back schools when compared with undefined placebo interventions with respect to improvements in pain, function, and return to work.[27] That CPG also found moderate evidence that back schools are more effective than brief education, exercise, or SMT with respect to improvements in pain and function, both in the short term and in the long term.

TABLE 7-1	Clinical Practice Guideline Recommendations On Back Schools and Fear Avoidance Training for Chronic Low Back Pain*	
Reference	Country	Conclusion
Back Schools		
27	Europe	Consider as possible option for short-term improvement of CLBP
28	Belgium	Low-quality evidence of effectiveness

*No CPGs made specific recommendations about fear avoidance training as an intervention for CLBP.

CLBP, chronic low back pain; CPG, clinical practice guideline.

That CPG concluded that back schools should be considered as one possible option for short-term improvement of CLBP.

The CPG from Belgium in 2006 found low-quality evidence as to the effectiveness of back schools for CLBP.[28]

Fear Avoidance Training

None of the recent national CPGs on the management of CLBP have assessed and summarized the evidence to make specific recommendations about the efficacy of fear avoidance training.

Findings from the aforementioned CPGs are summarized in Table 7-1.

Systematic Reviews

Back Schools

Cochrane Collaboration. An SR was conducted in 1999 and updated in 2003 by the Cochrane Collaboration on back schools for nonspecific low back pain.[29-31] A total of 19 RCTs were identified, including 12 studies of CLBP patients, 4 studies of acute/subacute LBP patients, and 3 of mixed populations.[4,18,20,32-47] The authors concluded that the methodologic quality of studies was low, and there is conflicting evidence on the effectiveness of back schools for acute/subacute LBP. However, moderate evidence exists for the effectiveness of back schools compared with other treatments for pain and functional status in the short and intermediate term among patients with CLBP. Furthermore, there is moderate evidence that back schools in an occupational setting are more effective than other treatments, placebo, or waiting list controls for pain, functional status, and return to work in the short and intermediate term for patients with CLBP. This review did not discuss results specific to radicular or axial pain.

American Pain Society and American College of Physicians. An SR was conducted in 2006 by the American Pain Society and American College of Physicians CPG committee on nonpharmacologic therapies for acute and chronic LBP.[48] That review identified three SRs on back schools,[30,31,49,50] including the Cochrane review previously described. The three SRs included 31 unique trials. The review found the conclusions of the SRs were consistent, that back schools have not been shown to be effective in acute, subacute, or chronic LBP. However, some benefits were observed in trials of back schools in occupational settings and in more intensive programs based on the original Swedish Back School.

Other. Brox and colleagues conducted an SR in 2008 examining back schools, brief education, and fear avoidance training for CLBP.[51] A total of 23 RCTs were included, of which 8 pertained to back schools. This SR concluded that there is conflicting evidence for back schools related to pain and disability improvement compared with waiting list, no intervention, and placebo. This SR also concluded that there was limited evidence for back schools related to pain and disability improvement versus usual care, exercise, or a cognitive behavioral back school.

Fear Avoidance Training

Cochrane Collaboration. Not available.

American Pain Society and American College of Physicians. Not available.

Other Systematic Reviews. In an SR published in 2008[51] on fear avoidance training in CLBP (>12 weeks), three RCTs in four reports were included.[24,52-54] RCTs involving fear avoidance training as a separate intervention or as part of a rehabilitation program were included. Based on one large high-quality trial, the authors of the SR concluded that there is limited evidence for the effectiveness of fear avoidance training in primary care and physical therapy compared with usual care.[52] Based on the other two trials, there is moderate evidence that fear avoidance training in a rehabilitation program is not more effective than spinal fusion.

Another review identified one RCT that found fear avoidance training in a rehabilitation program was more effective than usual care in reducing disability in acute LBP patients with high fear avoidance beliefs, but counterproductive for patients with low fear avoidance beliefs.[55-56]

Findings from the above SRs are summarized in Table 7-2.

Randomized Controlled Trials

Relevant RCTs were identified from the SRs summarized above, although not all were included. An electronic search of medical databases was also conducted to identify additional RCTs not previously summarized in SRs. Studies in which a majority of participants had symptoms for less than 12 weeks were excluded, as were studies related to CLBP with a specific etiology (e.g., spondylolisthesis or postoperative pain). Back schools were included when given to groups of patients by a paramedical or physical therapist (PT) or medical specialist and when the back schools constituted the main part of the intervention. Fear avoidance training was included when the training was a separate intervention or part of a rehabilitation program. In addition, pain-related fear and beliefs about avoidance behavior were measured before and after the intervention. Two authors independently assessed the methodologic quality of each study using 10 criteria proposed by the Cochrane Back Review Group (CBRG), awarding 1 point for each condition (5 or more was considered of higher quality).[57]

TABLE 7-2	Systematic Review Findings on Back Schools and Fear Avoidance Training for Chronic Low Back Pain		
Reference	# RCTs in SR	#RCTs for CLBP	Conclusion
Back Schools			
29-31	19	12 chronic, 3 mixed	Back schools are effective compared with other treatments for pain and functional status and return-to-work in short term for patients with CLBP
48	31	NR	Back schools are not effective in CLBP. Some benefits observed in occupational settings
Fear Avoidance Training			
51	3	NR	Limited evidence for the effectiveness of fear avoidance training compared with usual care; may be considered as an alternative to spinal fusion

CLBP, chronic low back pain; NR, not reported; RCT, randomized controlled trial; SR, systematic review.

Back Schools

Seven RCTs and eight study reports related to those RCTs were identified.[4,18-20,35,37-38,58] Their methods are summarized in Table 7-3. Their results are briefly described here.

Klaber Moffett and colleagues[4] performed an RCT including CLBP patients from a hospital outpatient orthopedic clinic in the United Kingdom. In order to be included, participants had to be between ages 18 and 67 and have LBP lasting longer than 6 months. Those who had a history of spinal surgery, concurrent physical therapy treatments, and evidence of underlying disease, such as fracture, ankylosing spondylitis, or multiple myeloma, were excluded. Two patients who were unable to understand the treatment program and complete the questionnaires were also excluded. A total of 92 patients were enrolled; 40 participants in the intervention and 38 in the control groups were included in analysis. Participants in the intervention group received three 1.5-hour sessions in 1 week of Swedish Back School with exercise with a PT and occupational therapist (OT), while the control group received three 0.5-hour sessions in 1 week of the same exercises used in the intervention group. The control groups also received handouts of exercises and back care leaflets. After 16 weeks, a larger decrease in pain scores (visual analog scale [VAS]) compared with baseline were observed among the Swedish Back School group, but the difference was not statistically significant. After 16 weeks, there was also a decrease in functional disability scores (Oswestry

Disability Index [ODI]) compared with baseline among the Swedish Back School participants, while scores among the exercise-only group remained similar compared with baseline. However, this difference was not statistically significant. This study was considered of higher quality.

Hurri[35] conducted an RCT of female employees with CLBP in Finland. Participants with idiopathic LBP lasting at least 12 months and with LBP present on at least 1 day each week during the preceding month and/or activity of daily living (ADL) limitations were included. Those with rheumatoid arthritis or other systemic connective tissue disease or a history of back surgery were excluded. A total of 204 females were enrolled; 95 in the intervention group and 93 in the control group were included in analysis. The intervention included 1-hour sessions of Swedish Back School 6 times in 3 weeks and there was no intervention in the control group, but control participants received written materials of the back school. Pain was measured using a VAS and the Low Back Pain Index. After 12 months, there was a statistically significant improvement in VAS pain scores in the intervention group but not the control group compared with baseline. With the Low Back Pain Index, there were significant improvements in pain scores at 12 months compared with baseline in both intervention and control groups. There were no significant changes in functional status (ODI) at 12 months compared with baseline in either group. There were no significant differences between the two groups in pain or functional status. This study was considered of lower quality.

Keijsers and colleagues[18] conducted an RCT of CLBP patients recruited through a local newspaper. Participants with LBP lasting longer than 6 months were included. Excluded patients were those with medical contraindications suggesting a need for medical and surgical treatment or inability to participate in aerobic exercise or relaxation training, high or very high scores on a scale of rigidity, distress and self satisfaction (Dutch Personality Questionnaire), and high or very high score on a psychopathology scale (Short Dutch Minnesota Multiphase Personality Inventory). A total of 40 participants were enrolled into the intervention group, while 18 were enrolled into the control group. The intervention consisted of the Maastricht Back School, with seven 2.5-hour lessons with a refresher lesson after 8 weeks, and the control participants were put on a waiting list. Of the 40 participants in the intervention group, 30 completed the back school. After 8 weeks, there was a decrease in mean pain scores (VAS) compared with baseline for both the intervention group (38.86 to 28.86) and the control group (41.47 to 31.88). However, there were no statistically significant differences between the groups. After 8 weeks, there were no improvements in daily activities compared with baseline (West Haven-Yale Multidimensional Pain Inventory [WHYMPI]) and no significant differences between the groups. This study was considered of lower quality.

Another RCT by Keijsers and colleagues[38] included participants in a primary care setting who had LBP lasting at least 2 months and up to 3 years, while excluding patients who were eligible for medical or surgical treatment or unable to participate in an exercise program or relaxation training. A total of 90 patients were included, with 13

TABLE 7-3	Randomized Controlled Trials of Back Schools for Chronic Low Back Pain			
Reference	Indication	Intervention	Control (C1)	Control (C2)
4	CLBP, neurologic involvement NR, symptoms >6 months	Swedish Back School including exercises PT and occupational therapist 3 × 1.5 hr in 1 wk n = NR (92 total) n analyzed = 40	Exercises and a back care leaflet PT 3 × 0.5 hr in 1 wk n = NR (92 total) n analyzed = 38	NA
35	CLBP without neurologic involvement, symptoms >12 months	Swedish Back School including exercises PT and physician 6 × 1 hr in 3 wk + 2 classes after 6 mo n = NR (204 total) n analyzed = 95	No intervention n = NR (204 total) n analyzed = 93	NA
18	CLBP, neurologic involvement NR, symptoms >6 months	Maastricht Back School including training of skills Hospital PT and invited lecturers* 7 × 2.5 hr + 1 class after 8 wk n = 40	Waiting list n = 18	NA
38	LBP, neurologic involvement NR, symptoms >2 months to max of 3 yr	Maastricht Back School including training of skills Hospital PT and invited lecturers* 7 × 2.5 hr + 1 class after 8 wk n = NR (90 total)	Waiting list n = NR (90 total)	NA
37	LBP, neurologic involvement NR, duration of symptoms NR	Back school in groups of 10-12 people Hospital PT and physical education instructor 4 × 1.5 hr in 2 wk + 1 class after 2 mo n = 46	Flexion and extension exercises in groups of 10-12 people 24 × 3/4 hr; 2 times weekly for 3 mo n = 46	No intervention n = 50
20, 58	LBP, neurologic involvement NR, duration of symptoms NR	Back school including practical training and exercises PT 20 × 1 hr (20 min education + 40 min practical training and exercises) for 13 wk n = 43, 5 dropouts	No intervention n = 38, 3 dropouts	NA
19	LBP, secondary prophylaxis, neurologic involvement NR, duration of symptoms NR	Swedish Back School including exercises (2 hr exam + home exercises twice daily) Physician and PT 4 × 2 hr (0.5 hr education + 1.5 hr exercises) for 4 wk n = 98 (70 completed all treatments)	Cognitive behavioral-based back school including simulation of workplace tasks and a graded exercise program 4 × 2 hr (0.5 hr education + 1.5 hr exercises) for 4 wk n = 98 (75 completed all treatments)	Usual care (Dutch guidelines) 16 × 1 hr for 8 wk n = 103

*Invited lecturers from psychology, pedagogy, neurology, orthopedics, rehabilitation medicine, and occupational therapy.
CLBP, chronic low back pain; LBP, low back pain; NA, not applicable; NR, not reported; PT, physical therapist.

dropouts. The intervention consisted of the Maastricht Back School, with seven 2.5-hour lessons with a refresher lesson after 6 months, and the control participants were put on a waiting list. At 6 months, there were no statistically significant differences in mean pain scores (VAS) or functional status (WHYMPI) in the intervention or control groups compared with baseline. There were also no statistically significant differences between the two groups. This study was considered of lower quality.

An RCT by Donchin and colleagues[37] included employees of a university hospital in Israel who had at least three annual episodes of LBP. A total of 142 participants were enrolled. The intervention group (n = 46) consisted of a back school in groups of 10 to 12 people with four 1.5-hour sessions in a 2-week period and one session after 2 months. There were two control groups. The first control group (n = 46) was assigned to 45-minute sessions of flexion and extension exercises biweekly for 3 months in groups of 10 to 12; the second control group (n = 50) was a waiting list. After 12 months, the incidence of LBP episodes (mean number of painful months during follow-up) in the intervention group (7.3) was not significantly different from the waiting list control group (7.4). The exercise control group had significantly less episodes (4.5) than the intervention or waiting list control groups. This study was considered of lower quality.

An RCT by Lonn and colleagues[20,58] included LBP patients recruited through local advertisements and referrals from health care professionals. Patients aged 18 to 50 years who had experienced at least one episode of LBP in the past year and had finished treatment and sick leave were included for secondary prevention. Those with previous surgical procedures for LBP, who were pregnant, had specific rheumatologic diseases, spondylolisthesis, spinal tumor, spinal fracture, drug or alcohol abuse, or documented mental illness were excluded. Forty-three participants (5 dropouts) were included in the intervention group, and 38 participants (3 dropouts) were included in the control group. The intervention consisted of twenty 1-hour sessions of a back school including practical training and exercises (20 min education + 40 min practical training and exercises) for 13 weeks. There was no intervention for the control group. After 12 months, the mean pain score was significantly reduced in the intervention group compared with baseline from 3.5 (95% CI, 2.9-4.0) to 2.2 (95% CI, 1.5-2.8). A significant reduction was also observed in the control group, from 4.0 (95% CI, 3.4-4.7) to 3.3 (95% CI, 2.6-4.0). The difference in pain scores between the two groups was also statistically significant ($P < .05$), but not after correction for baseline values ($P = .06$). After 12 months, the mean functional score (VAS on daily activities) significantly improved in the intervention group compared with baseline from 4.7 (95% CI, 4.1-5.3) to 6.7 (95% CI, 6.0-7.5). The improvement in the control group from 4.1 (95% CI, 2.4-4.7) to 5.2 (95% CI, 4.4-6.0) was not statistically significant. The improvement in the intervention group was significantly different than that in the control group ($P < .01$), even after correction for baseline values ($P < .05$). This study was considered of higher quality.

An RCT by Heymans and colleagues[19] included employees aged 18 to 65 years, sick-listed for LBP in the Netherlands. Those who were able to complete questionnaires in Dutch were included, while those who were sick-listed less than a month before the current sick-leave episode for LBP, those who were pregnant, those with specific pathology, or those with juridical conflict at work were excluded. The intervention group (n = 98) was assigned to four 2-hour sessions of a Swedish Back School including exercises for 4 weeks. The first control group (n = 98) was assigned to four 2-hour sessions of cognitive behavioral-based back school including simulation of workplace tasks and a graded exercise program for 4 weeks. The second control group was assigned to standard care based on Dutch guidelines, with sixteen 1-hour sessions for 8 weeks. After 6 months, mean pain scores (VAS) decreased in all groups compared with baseline, from 6.5 ± 1.6 to 3.9 ± 0.4 for the Swedish Back School group, from 6.8 ± 1.7 to 3.5 ± 0.3 for the cognitive behavioral-based back school group, and from 6.5 ± 2.0 to 4.0 ± 0.3 for the standard care group. There were no statistically significant difference in pain scores between the Swedish Back School group and the two control groups. After 6 months, mean functional scores (Roland Morris Disability Questionnaire [RMDQ]) did not improve compared with baseline, from 8.1 ± 3.9 to 7.8 ± 0.6 for the Swedish Back School group, from 7.9 ± 3.9 to 6.9 ± 0.6 for the cognitive behavioral-based back school group, and from 9.8 ± 5.0 to 7.9 ± 0.6 for the standard care group. There were no statistically significant difference in functional status scores between the Swedish Back School group and the two control groups. This study was considered of higher quality.

Fear Avoidance Training

The methods for five high-quality RCTs and six study reports related to those RCTs are summarized in Table 7-4.[24,52-54,59,60] Their results are briefly described below.

In an RCT conducted by Brox and colleagues[24,54] on patients with CLBP in a hospital setting in Norway, participants were eligible if they were aged 25 to 60 years, had pain lasting at least 1 year, had a score of 30 or greater on the ODI, and had degeneration at L4-L5 or L5-S1 (spondylosis) on plain radiographs. Exclusion criteria included widespread myofascial pain, spinal stenosis with reduced walking distance and neurologic signs, recurrent disc herniation or lateral recess stenosis with clinical signs of radiculopathy, inflammatory disease, previous spinal fracture, previous spine surgery, pelvic pain, generalized disc degeneration on plain radiographic examination, ongoing somatic or psychiatric disease that excluded either one or both treatment alternatives, registered medical abuse, and reluctance to accept one or both of the study treatments. The intervention group (n = 37, two lost to follow-up) was assigned to 3 weeks of cognitive intervention (information, reassurance, exposure) and exercises (general and stabilizing), whereas the control group (n = 27, one lost to follow-up) was assigned to instrumented lumbar fusion with postoperative advice by a PT and exercises after 3 months. After 1 year of follow-up, mean back pain scores (VAS) decreased in both groups compared with baseline. In the intervention group, mean pain scores decreased from 64.1 ± 13.7 to 48.7 ± 24.0. In the control group, scores decreased from 62.1 ± 14.5 to 39.4 ± 25.5. The

TABLE 7-4	Randomized Controlled Trials of Fear Avoidance Training for Chronic Low Back Pain		
Reference	Indication	Intervention	Control (C1)
54 24	CLBP without neurologic involvement, symptoms >1 yr	Cognitive intervention (information, reassurance, exposure) and exercises (general and stabilizing) Hospital physiatrist, PT, lay person 1 wk at hospital + 2 wk at home + 2 wk at hospital, ~25 hr/wk n = 37	Instrumented lumbar fusion L4-L5 and/or L5-S1 + postoperative advice by PT + exercises after 3 months Orthopedic or neurosurgeon n = 27
53 24	CLBP with neurologic involvement, symptoms >1 yr	Cognitive intervention (information, reassurance, exposure) and exercises (general and stabilizing) Hospital physiatrist, PT, lay person 1 wk at hospital + 2 wk at home + 2 wk at hospital, ~25 hr/wk n = 29 (1 lost to follow-up)	Instrumented lumbar fusion L4-L5 and/or L5-S1 + postoperative advice by PT + exercises after 3 months Orthopedic or neurosurgeon n = 31 (2 lost to follow-up)
59*	CLBP, neurologic involvement NR, symptoms >6 months	Exposure to fear-eliciting situations, individually tailored, embedded in a comprehensive behavioral program Practitioner not specified 3 weeks n = 4	Graded activity using the operant principles described by Fordyce and Lindstrom, embedded in a comprehensive behavioral program Practitioner not specified 3 weeks n = 4
60*	CLBP without neurologic involvement, symptoms >6 months	Exposure to fear-eliciting situations, individually tailored, embedded in a comprehensive behavioral program Practitioner not specified 3 weeks n = 6	Graded activity using the operant principles described by Fordyce, embedded in a comprehensive behavioral program Practitioner not specified 3 weeks n = 6
52	LBP, neurologic involvement NR, duration of symptoms NR	Two visits to psychologist and PT, respectively Primary care psychologist PT 1-2 × 4 over 35 days n = 119	Usual care n = 121

*Crossover design.
CLBP, chronic low back pain; LBP, low back pain; NR, not reported; PT, physical therapist.

mean difference between groups was not statistically significant. After one year of follow-up, mean disability scores (ODI) also decreased in both groups compared with baseline. In the intervention group, ODI scores decreased from 43.0 ± 13.0 to 29.7 ± 19.6, and in the control group, scores decreased from 42.0 ± 11.0 to 26.4 ± 16.4. The mean difference in disability between the two groups was not statistically significant. This study was considered of higher quality.

In another RCT by Brox and colleagues[24,54] in patients with CLBP in a hospital setting in Norway, the study protocol was similar to the previous RCT except that patients with previous surgery for disc herniation were recruited. Participants were eligible if they were aged 25 to 60 years, had pain lasting at least 1 year after previous surgery for disc herniation, had a score of 30 or greater on the ODI, and had degeneration at L4-L5 or L5-S1 (spondylosis) on plain radiographs. Exclusion criteria included widespread myofascial pain, spinal stenosis with reduced walking distance and neurologic signs, recurrent disc herniation or lateral recess stenosis with clinical signs of radiculopathy, inflammatory disease, previous spinal fracture, pelvic pain, generalized disc degeneration on plain radiographic examination, ongoing somatic or psychiatric disease that excluded either one or both treatment alternatives, registered medical abuse, and reluctance to accept one or both of the study treatments. The intervention group (n = 29, one lost to follow-up) was assigned to 3 weeks of cognitive intervention (information, reassurance, exposure) and exercises (general and stabilizing), whereas the control group (n = 31, two lost to follow-up) was assigned to instrumented lumbar fusion with postoperative advice by a PT and exercises after 3 months. After one year of follow-up, mean back pain scores (VAS) decreased in both groups compared with baseline. In the intervention group, mean pain scores decreased from 64.7 (interquartile range 11.1) to 49.5 (20.0). In the control group, scores decreased from 64.6 (15.4) to 50.7 (27.3). The mean difference between groups was not statistically significant. After 1 year of follow-up, mean disability scores (ODI) also decreased in both groups compared with baseline. In the intervention group, the mean difference in ODI scores between baseline and 1 year of follow-up was 12.6 (95% CI, 6.0-19.2; $P < .001$), and in the control group, the mean difference was 8.9 (95% CI, 1.3-18.5; $P < .023$). The mean difference in disability between the two groups was not statistically significant. This study was considered of higher quality.

An RCT with a crossover design was conducted by Vlaeyen and colleagues[59] on CLBP patients at a rehabilitation center in The Netherlands. Participants had CLBP lasting longer than 6 months, were aged 18 to 65 years, were referred to the rehabilitation center for outpatient behavioral rehabilitation, reported fear of movement/reinjury (TSK score >40), and had a discrepancy between objective medical findings and pain complaints. Exclusion criteria included illiteracy, pregnancy, alcohol or drug abuse, and serious psychopathology (based on Dutch norms for the Symptom Checklist [SCL]-90). Four consecutive participants meeting eligibility criteria were included in the study. The intervention consisted of three weeks of individually tailored exposure to fear-eliciting situations embedded in a comprehensive behavioral program. The control consisted of 3 weeks of graded activity using the operant principles of Fordyce and Lindstrom, embedded in a comprehensive behavioral program. After the end of both treatments (63 days), there was a decrease in pain disability (Pain Cognition List [PCL] and RMDQ) after the intervention treatment, but not after the control treatment. Pain intensity was not measured. This study was considered of higher quality.

Another RCT with a crossover design was conducted by Vlaeyen and colleagues[60] on CLBP patients at a rehabilitation center in the Netherlands. Participants had CLBP lasting longer than 6 months, were aged 18 to 65 years, were referred to the rehabilitation center for outpatient behavioral rehabilitation, reported fear of movement/reinjury (TSK score ≥40), and had a discrepancy between objective medical findings and pain complaints. Exclusion criteria included illiteracy, pregnancy, alcohol or drug abuse, and serious psychopathology (based on Dutch norms for the SCL-90). Six consecutive participants meeting eligibility criteria were included in the study. The intervention consisted of 3 weeks of individually tailored exposure to fear-eliciting situations embedded in a comprehensive behavioral program. The control consisted of 3 weeks of graded activity using the operant principles of Fordyce, embedded in a comprehensive behavioral program. After the end of both treatments, the intervention was associated with statistically significant pain reduction, but the control group was not. One patient became almost pain-free after the intervention. After the end of both treatments, the intervention was also associated with a clinically relevant reduction (based on predefined criteria) in disability

scores (RMDQ) compared with baseline, but the control group was not. The improvement in functional status was sustained after 12 months. This study was considered of higher quality.

An RCT conducted by Von Korff and colleagues[52] included LBP patients in a primary care setting in the United States. Participants were eligible if they had a primary care visit for back pain and reported at least 7 activity limitations on the RMDQ during their assessment. Those who were considered for back surgery, were being managed by a PT or psychologist for LBP, and were planning to disenroll from a health maintenance organization where the study was based were excluded. The intervention group (n = 119) was assigned to four visits with a psychologist or PT over 35 days, whereas the control group (n = 121) was assigned to usual care. After 24 months, there was a modest reduction in average pain intensity (0-10 scale) in both groups compared with baseline. Pain scores decreased from 5.7 ± 1.8 to 4.3 ± 2.1 in the intervention group and from 5.8 ± 1.8 to 4.6 ± 2.5 in the control group. The difference between the two groups after 24 months was not statistically significant ($P = .115$) compared with baseline, but the mean difference over the entire follow-up period (2, 6, 12, 24 months) was statistically significant (overall $P < .0012$). At the 24-month follow-up, there was also a reduction in disability scores (RMDQ) compared with baseline. Disability scores decreased from 12.3 ± 5.5 to 8.1 ± 6.5 in the intervention group, and decreased from 11.4 ± 5.7 to 9.1 ± 7.2 in the control group. The difference between the two groups was statistically significant ($P = .0078$) at this follow-up time compared with baseline. This study was considered of higher quality.

Observational Studies

Back Schools

Lankhorst and colleagues[32] performed a nonrandomized controlled trial on CLBP patients in a primary care setting in the Netherlands. Participants with idiopathic LBP lasting longer than 6 months and not responding to conventional physical therapy were included. Those with inflammatory or other specific spinal disorders, abnormal reflexes, sensory loss, significant muscle weakness, scoliosis of more than 15 degrees, or spondylolisthesis of more than 1 cm were excluded. A total of 48 consecutive patients were enrolled; analysis included 21 participants in the intervention group and 22 participants in the control group. The intervention involved four sessions of Swedish Back School for 45 minutes each over a 2-week period. The control involved four sessions with detuned short-wave applications over a 2-week period. At 12 months, there were no significant changes in pain (10-point scale) or functional capacity (10-point scale) in either group compared with baseline. There were no significant differences between the two groups in pain or functional capacity.

Fear Avoidance Training

A replicated single-case experimental study was conducted by de Jong and colleagues[61] on patients with CLBP at a rehabilitation center in The Netherlands. Participants had

CLBP lasting longer than 6 months, were aged 18 to 65 years, were referred to the rehabilitation center for outpatient behavioral rehabilitation, reported fear of movement/reinjury (TSK score ≥40), and had a discrepancy between objective medical findings and pain complaints. Exclusion criteria included illiteracy, pregnancy, alcohol or drug abuse, and serious psychopathology (based on Dutch norms for the SCL-90). Six consecutive participants meeting eligibility criteria were included in the study. The intervention consisted of education, followed by 24 hours of individually tailored exposure to fear-eliciting situations embedded in a comprehensive behavioral program over 6 weeks. The control also consisted of education, but was followed by 32 hours of graded activity using the operant principles of Fordyce and Lindstrom, embedded in a comprehensive behavioral program over 8 weeks. After 6 months of follow-up, a statistically significant reduction in pain intensity occurred in the intervention group compared with baseline. No significant reductions were observed in the control group. After 6 months of follow-up, mean pain disability scores based on the RMDQ decreased in both groups compared with baseline, and the differences exceeded the predefined criterion of 5 as clinically relevant. In the intervention group, RMDQ scores decreased from a mean of 15 to 2, while in the control group, they decreased from 16 to 6. This study was considered of higher quality.

SAFETY

Contraindications

Contraindications to back schools and fear avoidance training include CLBP due to potentially serious spinal pathology such as fracture, cancer, infection, or cauda equina syndrome.

Adverse Events

Back schools and fear avoidance training are generally considered to be safe interventions. A clinical trial of back schools with 47 participants reported 6 cases of transient exacerbation of symptoms.[47] No serious adverse events have been reported with these interventions for CLBP. The CPG from Europe in 2004 reported that the safety of back schools for CLBP is currently unknown.[27]

COSTS

Fees and Third-Party Reimbursement

Back Schools

In the United States, back schools for CLBP are typically delivered in group settings outside the context of an outpatient visit that can be billed by a licensed health care provider. Many third-party payers have policies which indicate that this service will not be reimbursed as the service is considered to be not medically necessary, unproven, or ineffective for patients with acute LBP. Participants or their employers may be required to directly contribute a fee (e.g., $50 to $100) to the person or organization operating the back school. CPT code 97535 may be used if the patient receives direct one-on-one contact by the health care provider who instructs the patient in self-care and home management activities (e.g., ADLs) and compensatory training, meal preparation, safety procedures, and instructions in use of assistive technology devices/adaptive equipment; this CPT code is reported in 15-minute increments. It is recommended that preauthorization be obtained from the insurance carrier. Based on the third-party payers queried, it appears that third-party payers may pay for this procedure and it is considered medically necessary when it requires the professional skills of a provider, is designed to address specific needs of the patient, and must be part of an active treatment plan directed at a specific outcome. If the insurance carrier denies payment of the claim, a letter of appeal can be sent to the insurance carrier, requesting review of the claim based on medical necessity.

Fear Avoidance Training

In the United States, fear avoidance training involves a collaboration among different types of health care providers, each of whom can bill separately for their services. For the behavioral health specialist, fear avoidance training in an outpatient setting can be delivered using CPT codes for individual psychotherapy. CPT codes used to report insight-oriented, behavior-modifying, and/or supportive individual psychotherapy are 90804 (20 to 30 minutes), 90806 (45 to 50 minutes), 90808 (75 to 80 minutes), 90805 (20 to 30 minutes with additional evaluation and management), 90807 (45 to 50 minutes with additional evaluation and management), and 90809 (75 to 80 minutes with additional evaluation and management). For the PT, fear avoidance training in an outpatient setting can be delivered using CPT codes 97110 (therapeutic exercises, each 15 minutes) and 97530 (therapeutic activities, each 15 minutes). These procedures are widely covered by other third-party payers such as health insurers and worker's compensation insurance. Although some payers continue to base their reimbursements on usual, customary, and reasonable payment methodology, the majority have developed reimbursement tables based on the Resource Based Relative Value Scale used by Medicare. Reimbursements by other third-party payers are generally higher than Medicare.

Typical fees reimbursed by Medicare in New York and California for these services are summarized in Table 7-5.

Cost Effectiveness

Evidence supporting the cost effectiveness of treatment protocols that compared these interventions, often in combination with one or more cointerventions, with control groups who received one or more other interventions, for either acute or chronic LBP, was identified from two SRs on this topic and is summarized here.[62,63] Although many of these study designs are unable to clearly identify the individual contribution of any intervention, their results provide some

TABLE 7-5	Medicare Fee Schedule for Related Services	
CPT Code	New York	California
Back Schools		
97535	$32	$34
Fear Avoidance Training		
90804	$65	$69
90805	$74	$78
90806	$90	$95
90807	$103	$109
90808	$132	$139
90809	$146	$154
97110	$30	$32
97530	$32	$35

2010 Participating, nonfacility amount.

insight into the clinical and economic outcomes associated with these approaches.

Back Schools

An RCT in the United Kingdom compared two approaches for patients with CLBP.[64] The active intervention was delivered by a PT and consisted of a back school with education from a book and cassette, group education, advice to remain active, and CBT. Usual care was delivered by a general practitioner (GP) and included education from a book and cassette along with other interventions. Clinical outcomes after 15 months were similar between groups, in that both improved in pain, function, and utility. Direct medical costs associated with study and nonstudy interventions over 15 months were $47 higher in the active intervention group. Based on nonsignificant differences in utility, the incremental cost effectiveness ratio (ICER) of group training over brief education alone was $8650 per quality-adjusted life-year (QALY), well within the generally accepted threshold for cost utility analyses.

An RCT in Canada compared four approaches for occupational CLBP.[65] The four groups compared were usual care, a clinical intervention centered on back school and possible multidisciplinary rehabilitation, an occupational intervention centered on ergonomics, and a combination of the clinical and occupational interventions (termed the *Sherbrooke model*). Clinical outcomes were not reported. Direct medical costs associated with study interventions over a mean 6.4 years were approximately $6502 in the usual care group, approximately $4663 in the clinical intervention group, approximately $2334 in the occupational intervention group, and approximately $5055 in the combined clinical and occupational group. Indirect productivity costs associated with lost work days and disability pensions over a mean 6.4 years were approximately $15,992 in the usual care group, approximately $6831 in the clinical intervention group, approximately $8718 in the occupational intervention group, and approximately $4801 in the combined clinical and occupational group. Total costs (direct medical and indirect productivity) over a mean 6.4 years were therefore approximately

$22,494 in the usual care group, approximately $11,494 in the clinical intervention group, approximately $11,052 in the occupational intervention group, and approximately $9856 in the combined clinical and occupational group. Authors concluded that a nonsignificant trend was noted toward cost benefit and cost effectiveness for the three study interventions compared with usual care.

An RCT from Canada compared two approaches for patients who had been injured at work and subsequently suffered from CLBP.[66] The functional restoration group included CBT, fear avoidance training, education, biofeedback, group counseling, and strengthening and stretching exercises. The usual care group could receive a variety of interventions, including physical therapy, acupuncture, back school, SMT, medication, or supervised exercise therapy. Clinical outcomes were not reported. Direct medical costs associated with the study intervention were $2507 higher in the functional restoration group. Indirect productivity costs associated with lost work days were $3172 lower in the functional restoration group. Total costs for interventions, lost work days, and disability pensions were $7068 lower in the functional restoration group. These differences were not statistically significant.

An RCT in the Netherlands compared two approaches for patients with CLBP.[67] The intensive training group included back school, and both individual and group supervised exercise therapy. The usual physical therapy group included interventions recommended in CPGs, which were not defined. Clinical outcomes after 1 year were similar between groups, which both improved in pain, function, and utility. Direct medical costs associated with study and nonstudy interventions over 1 year were approximately $1468 in the intensive training group and approximately $980 in the usual physical therapy group. Indirect productivity costs associated with lost work days over 1 year were approximately $3797 in the intensive training group and approximately $3969 in the usual physical therapy group. Total costs (direct medical and indirect productivity) over 1 year were therefore approximately $5265 in the intensive training group and approximately $4949 in the usual physical therapy group. Because the intensive training group had marginally better clinical outcomes with higher overall costs, its ICER was estimated at approximately $6957 per QALY, well within the generally accepted threshold for cost utility analyses.

Fear Avoidance Training

An RCT in Norway compared three approaches for patients with CLBP.[68] Participants received either a light multidisciplinary program consisting of education, fear avoidance training, and advice to remain active given by a PT, nurse, and psychologist, an extensive multidisciplinary program consisting of daily group sessions with CBT, education, fear avoidance training, and strengthening and stabilization exercises for 4 weeks, or usual care by a GP and possibly a PT or chiropractor. Direct medical costs for the light and extensive multidisciplinary programs were estimated by dividing the total clinic costs for one year by the number of patients treated; direct medical costs were therefore assumed to be equal in both groups, regardless of large differences in time spent by clinic staff with patients in each group. Indirect productivity costs associated with lost work time were evaluated over 24 months. A limited cost benefit analysis for male participants only reported that the light multidisciplinary program would yield average savings of approximately $19,544 per patient over 2 years, and was therefore cost-effective compared with usual care.

A cluster RCT in the Netherlands compared two approaches for patients with subacute LBP presenting to 60 GPs in 41 offices.[69] The brief education approach was centered on CBT and discussion of psychosocial prognostic factors related to LBP, including fear avoidance beliefs. Usual care included interventions that were not specified. Clinical outcomes after 12 months were largely similar between the two groups. Direct medical costs for study and nonstudy interventions over 12 months were approximately $207 in the brief education group and approximately $202 in the usual care group. Indirect productivity costs associated with absenteeism for both paid and unpaid work over 12 months were approximately $575 in the brief education group and approximately $1059 in the usual care group. Total costs (direct medical and indirect productivity) were therefore approximately $782 in the brief education group and approximately $1261 in the usual care group. The brief education group therefore achieved similar clinical outcomes with lower costs.

An RCT in the United Kingdom compared three approaches for patients with CLBP.[70] The individual physical therapy approach included a maximum of 12 sessions with SMT, mobilization, massage, home exercises, and brief education. The spinal stabilization approach included a maximum of eight sessions with abdominal and multifidus exercises. The pain management approach included a maximum of eight sessions with education, exercises, CBT, and fear avoidance training. Clinical outcomes after 18 months were similar for all groups, with improvements noted in pain, function, and utility. Direct medical costs for study and nonstudy interventions paid by the National Health Service over 18 months were approximately $872 for individual physical therapy, approximately $698 for spinal stabilization, and approximately $304 for pain management. Indirect productivity costs were not reported. Over 18 months, the three groups experienced gains in QALY of 0.99, 0.90, and 1.00, respectively. By virtue of having lower direct medical costs and greater gains in utility, the pain management approach was reported to dominate over both individual physical therapy and spinal stabilization.

An RCT from the Netherlands compared three behavioral approaches in patients with CLBP.[1] The first behavioral intervention included CBT, fear avoidance training, and relaxation. The second behavioral intervention included CBT, fear avoidance training, and group discussion. The third behavioral intervention included fear avoidance training after a 10-week waiting period. Clinical outcomes after 1 year reported no difference in utility scores or global assessment of change between groups. Direct medical costs associated with study interventions after 1 year were $9196 in the relaxation group, $8607 in the group discussion group, and $8795 in the delayed fear avoidance training group.

Direct medical costs associated with nonstudy interventions after 1 year were $1088 in the relaxation group, $575 in the group discussion group, and $651 in the delayed fear avoidance training group. Direct medical costs associated with non–health care expenditures after 1 year were $2316 in the relaxation group, $1544 in the group discussion group, and $1641 in the delayed fear avoidance training group. Indirect productivity costs associated with lost work days after 1 year were $6522 in the relaxation group, $5938 in the group discussion group, and $8213 in the delayed fear avoidance training group. Total costs (direct medical and indirect productivity) over 1 year were therefore $19,122 in the relaxation group, $16,664 in the group discussion group, and $19,300 in the delayed fear avoidance training group. Authors concluded that neither behavioral intervention was cost effective when compared with fear avoidance training alone.

Findings from the aforementioned cost effectiveness analyses are summarized in Table 7-6.

SUMMARY

Description

Back schools are interventions that include group education about LBP, appropriate self-management of LBP, training about how to live with LBP and adapt activities of daily living if necessary, as well as recommended general and back-specific exercises. Fear avoidance training is intended for individual patients with CLBP and harmful or inappropriate beliefs or behaviors about their pain. There is overlap between modern back schools based on CBT principles and fear avoidance training. Back schools were introduced in 1969 and fear avoidance training in 1983. Both are widely available in the United States and are usually conducted in occupational settings or private practitioner practices. Many health care providers deliver basic back school interventions with additional content-specific training, including PTs, physicians, OTs, and chiropractors. A trained mental health professional such as a psychologist or psychiatrist may be required for advanced fear avoidance training.

Theory

Classic back schools teach about spinal anatomy and ergonomics to encourage protection of the spinal structures, although the impact of this information on fear avoidance behavior has not been addressed. Behavior that derives from fear avoidance is inhibitory and may contribute to chronicity and even learned helplessness. However, it is unclear whether this inhibition leads to a gradual development of depression, with its low psychomotor level in all dimensions. If CLBP is viewed as a threatening situation, anxious persons will give priority to thoughts and information related to their fear. The cognitive activation theory of stress attempts to explain how pain leads to neurophysiologic activation and has proposed that a stress alarm occurs when there is a discrepancy between what is expected and what is experienced by the individual.

| TABLE 7-6 | **Cost Effectiveness and Cost Utility Analyses of Back Schools and Fear Avoidance Training for Acute or Chronic Low Back Pain** |

Ref Country Follow-up	Group	Direct Medical Costs	Indirect Productivity Costs	Total Costs	Conclusion
Back Schools					
64 United Kingdom 15 months	1. back school, education, CBT 2. usual care from GP	1. $47 higher than group 2 2. NR	NR	NR	ICER of 1. over 2: $8650/QALY
65 Canada 6.4 years	1. usual care 2. back school + multidisciplinary rehabilitation 3. occupational intervention (ergonomics) 4. combined 2. and 3.	1. $6502 2. $4663 3. $2334 4. $5055	1. $15,992 2. $6831 3. $8718 4. $4801	1. $22,494 2. $11,494 3. $11,052 4. $9856	No significant difference
66 Canada NR	1. functional restoration (including back school) 2. usual care	1. $2507 higher than group 2 2. NR	1. $3172 lower than group 2 for lost work days 2. NR	1. $7068 lower than group 2 (lost work days + disability pensions 	No significant difference
67 The Netherlands 1 year	1. intensive training group (including back school) 2. usual PT group	1. $1468 2. $980	1. $3797 2. $3969	1. $5265 2. $4949	ICER of 1. over 2: $6957/QALY
Fear Avoidance Training					
68 Norway 2 years	1. light multidisciplinary program (including fear avoidance training) 2. extensive multidisciplinary program (including fear avoidance training) 3. usual care	NR	NR	NR	Group 1: average savings of $19,544/patient over 2 years
69 The Netherlands 1 year	1. brief education approach (including fear avoidance training) 2. usual care	1. $207 2. $202	1. $575 2. $1059	1. $782 2. $1261	Group 1 achieved similar clinical outcomes with lower costs
70 United Kingdom 18 months	1. individual PT 2. spinal stabilization 3. pain management (including fear avoidance training)	1. $872 2. $698 3. $304	NR	NR	Gains in QALY: 1. 0.99 2. 0.90 3. 1.00 Group 3 reported to dominate other interventions
1 The Netherlands 1 year	1. CBT + fear avoidance training + relaxation 2. CBT + fear avoidance training + group discussion 3. fear avoidance training after 10 weeks	1. $12,600 2. $10,726 3. $11,087	1. $6522 2. $5938 3. $8213	1. $19,122 2. $16,664 3. $19,300	No significant difference

CBT, cognitive behavioral therapy; GP, general practitioner; ICER, incremental cost effectiveness ratio; NR, not reported; PT, physical therapy; QALY, quality-adjusted life-year.

Although the discrepancy is not an immediate threat to their health, a sustained state of related anxiety may lead to CLBP through established pathophysiologic responses. Interventions such as back school and fear avoidance training may improve CLBP by increasing knowledge, which in turn decreases false expectations, lending to fewer instances of discrepancies in experience. The indication for back schools and fear avoidance training is mechanical, nonspecific CLBP. Diagnostic imaging or other forms of advanced testing is generally not required before administering these interventions for CLBP.

Efficacy

One recent CPG concluded that back schools are an option for short-term improvement of CLBP and another CPG found low-quality evidence as to the effectiveness of back schools for CLBP. Four SRs consistently found that back schools are not effective in acute, subacute, or chronic LBP. One SR found conflicting evidence supporting back schools compared with other comparators (e.g., waiting list, placebo). At least seven RCTs assessed the efficacy of back school, only one of which found statistically significant differences in pain versus comparators. None of the recent national CPGs provided recommendations on fear avoidance training for CLBP. Two SRs found that fear avoidance training in a rehabilitation program was more effective than usual care.

Safety

Contraindications to back schools and fear avoidance training include CLBP due to potentially serious spinal pathology such as fracture, cancer, infection, or cauda equina syndrome. Back schools and fear avoidance training are generally considered to be safe interventions.

Costs

Back schools for CLBP are typically delivered in group settings outside the context of an outpatient visit that can be billed by a licensed health care provider. This generally indicates that third-party payers will not reimburse this service. Participants or their employers may be required to directly contribute a fee (e.g., $50 to $100) to the person or organization operating the back school. In the United States, fear avoidance training involves collaboration among different types of health care providers, each of whom can bill separately for their services. Medicare reimbursement varies according to the type of therapist and duration of the session, and ranges from $30 to $154. At least four studies examined the cost effectiveness of back schools for CLBP, yet the individual contribution of back schools could not be determined because they were only one component of the interventions studied. At least four studies examined the cost effectiveness of fear avoidance training for CLBP, one of which concluded that fear avoidance training alone was cost effective versus comparators that combined fear avoidance training with other treatments.

Comments

Evidence from the CPGs, SRs, and RCTs reviewed is somewhat mixed regarding the efficacy of back schools and fear avoidance training for pain relief and disability improvement among patients with CLBP. These mixed results could, in part, be explained by differences in clinical protocols and methodologic challenges inherent to these studies. For example, blinding of the therapist and patient is impossible in all the interventions included. It is therefore uncertain whether observed differences between study groups could be attributed to the intervention, positive (placebo) or negative (nocebo) expectations, or the provider's communication skills, empathy, or other factors.[71] Differences in results reported between study groups were often small and generally fell within the theoretical measurement error of the outcome measure; their statistical significance is therefore of doubtful clinical relevance. The improvements noted within study groups from baseline to the final follow-up were often larger than any differences noted between the groups.

More research was identified on back schools than fear avoidance training, which is expected because back schools have been in existence longer and therefore subjected to more evaluation. Given the increasing importance of integrating both behavioral approaches and exercise therapy into the management of CLBP, further research on fear avoidance training is warranted to clarify its potential role as an intervention for this condition. Future studies could evaluate the addition of different forms of fear avoidance training to usual care to increase our understanding of the most appropriate indications, educational content, number of sessions required, and ideal mix of health care providers for this intervention.

Although studies evaluating the cost effectiveness of interventions that included components of back schools have been conducted, the individual contribution of back schools themselves could not be determined because of the comparators used in those studies. Future studies could attempt to determine the relative cost effectiveness of brief education by a physician or a PT (or both) compared with more involved educational approaches such as back schools.

CHAPTER REVIEW QUESTIONS

Answers are located on page 450.

1. What are the two extreme responses to fear of pain?
   a. confrontation and avoidance
   b. avoidance and panic
   c. aggression and retreat
   d. anger and acceptance
2. Give a brief definition of back schools.
   a. Back schools are an intervention consisting of group training, medication, and injections
   b. Back schools are an intervention consisting of massage, acupuncture, and education
   c. Back schools are an intervention consisting of group education, training, and exercises
   d. Back schools are an intervention consisting of relaxation training and surgery

3. Which of the following is not a commonly reported reason that patients with LBP fail to discuss their fears with health care providers?
   a. fear of receiving unfavorable answers to their questions
   b. worry that their fears will be belittled
   c. providers do not typically ask patients about fears related to their LBP
   d. none of the above

4. Who introduced the Swedish Back School?
   a. Mai Zetterling
   b. Jenny Tschernichin-Larsson
   c. Marianne Zachrisson-Forssell
   d. Anni-Frid Lyngstad

5. True or false: Back schools were introduced before fear avoidance training.

6. True or false: Modern back schools based on the principles of CBT share a common scientific underpinning with fear avoidance training programs.

▍ REFERENCES

1. Goossens ME, Rutten-Van Molken MP, Kole-Snijders AM, et al. Health economic assessment of behavioural rehabilitation in chronic low back pain: a randomised clinical trial. Health Econ 1998;7:39-51.
2. Forssell MZ. The Swedish Back School. Physiotherapy 1980;66:112-114.
3. Nachemson A, Elfstrom G. Intravital dynamic pressure measurements in lumbar discs. A study of common movements, maneuvers and exercises. Scand J Rehabil Med Suppl 1970;1:1-40.
4. Klaber Moffett JA, Chase SM, et al. A controlled, prospective study to evaluate the effectiveness of a back school in the relief of chronic low back pain. Spine 1986;11:120-122.
5. Harkapaa K, Jarvikoski A, Mellin G, et al. A controlled study on the outcome of inpatient and outpatient treatment of low back pain. Part I. Pain, disability, compliance, and reported treatment benefits three months after treatment. Scand J Rehabil Med 1989;21:81-89.
6. Waddell G. 1987 Volvo award in clinical sciences. A new clinical model for the treatment of low-back pain. Spine 1987;12:632-644.
7. Lethem J, Slade PD, Troup JD, et al. Outline of a fear avoidance model of exaggerated pain perception–I. Behav Res Ther 1983;21:401-408.
8. Waddell G, Newton M, Henderson I, et al. A Fear Avoidance Beliefs Questionnaire (FABQ) and the role of fear avoidance beliefs in chronic low back pain and disability. Pain 1993;52:157-168.
9. Vlaeyen JW, Linton SJ. Fear avoidance and its consequences in chronic musculoskeletal pain: a state of the art. Pain 2000;85:317-332.
10. Keller A, Johansen JG, Hellesnes J, et al. Predictors of isokinetic back muscle strength in patients with low back pain. Spine 1999;24:275-280.
11. Brox JI, Brevik JI, Ljunggren AE, et al. Influence of anthropometric and psychological variables pain and disability on isometric endurance of shoulder abduction in patients with rotator tendinosis of the shoulder. Scand J Rehabil Med 1996;28:193-200.
12. Vlaeyen JW, Kole-Snijders AM, Boeren RG, et al. Fear of movement/(re)injury in chronic low back pain and its relation to behavioral performance. Pain 1995;62:363-372.
13. Al-Obaidi SM, Nelson RM, Al-Awadhi S, et al. The role of anticipation and fear of pain in the persistence of avoidance behavior in patients with chronic low back pain. Spine 2000;25:1126-1131.
14. Moseley GL. Evidence for a direct relationship between cognitive and physical change during an education intervention in people with chronic low back pain. Eur J Pain 2004;8:39-45.
15. Crombez G, Vlaeyen JW, Heuts PH, et al. Pain-related fear is more disabling than pain itself: evidence on the role of pain-related fear in chronic back pain disability. Pain 1999;80:329-339.
16. Koes BW, van Tulder MW, van der Windt WM, et al. The efficacy of back schools: a review of randomized clinical trials. J Clin Epidemiol 1994;47:851-862.
17. Indahl A, Haldorsen EH, Holm S, et al. Five-year follow-up study of a controlled clinical trial using light mobilization and an informative approach to low back pain. Spine 1998;23:2625-2630.
18. Keijsers JF, Groenman NH, Gerards FM, et al. A back school in The Netherlands: evaluating the results. Patient Educ Couns 1989;14:31-44.
19. Heymans MW, de Vet HC, Bongers PM, et al. The effectiveness of high-intensity versus low-intensity back schools in an occupational setting: a pragmatic randomized controlled trial. Spine 2006;31:1075-1082.
20. Lonn JH, Glomsrod B, Soukup MG, et al. Active back school: prophylactic management for low back pain. A randomized, controlled, 1-year follow-up study. Spine 1999;24:865-871.
21. Kori SH, Miller RP, Todd DD. Kinesiophobia: a new view of chronic pain behavior. Pain Management 1990;3:35-43.
22. Grotle M, Vollestad NK, Veierod MB, et al. Fear avoidance beliefs and distress in relation to disability in acute and chronic low back pain. Pain 2004;112:343-352.
23. Cherkin DC, Deyo RA, Street JH, et al. Pitfalls of patient education. Limited success of a program for back pain in primary care. Spine 1996;21:345-355.
24. Keller A, Brox JI, Gunderson R, et al. Trunk muscle strength, cross-sectional area, and density in patients with chronic low back pain randomized to lumbar fusion or cognitive intervention and exercises. Spine 2004;29:3-8.
25. Ursin H. Press stop to start: the role of inhibition for choice and health. Psychoneuroendocrinology 2005;30:1059-1065.
26. Eriksen HR, Murison R, Pensgaard AM, et al. Cognitive activation theory of stress (CATS): from fish brains to the Olympics. Psychoneuroendocrinology 2005;30:933-938.
27. Airaksinen O, Brox JI, Cedraschi C, et al. European guidelines for the management of chronic nonspecific low back pain. Eur Spine J 2006;15:192-300.
28. Nielens H, van Zundert J, Mairiaux P, et al. Chronic low back pain, Vol. 48C. Brussels: KCE Reports; 2006.
29. van Tulder MW, Esmail R, Bombardier C, et al. Back schools for non-specific low back pain. Cochrane Database of Systematic Reviews 2000;(2).
30. Heymans MW, van Tulder MW, Esmail R, et al. Back schools for nonspecific low back pain: a systematic review within the framework of the Cochrane Collaboration Back Review Group. Spine 2005;30:2153-2163.

31. Heymans MW, van Tulder MW, Esmail R, et al. Back schools for non-specific low-back pain. Cochrane Database of Systematic Reviews 2004;(4).

32. Lankhorst GJ, Van de Stadt RJ, Vogelaar TW, et al. The effect of the Swedish Back School in chronic idiopathic low back pain. A prospective controlled study. Scand J Rehabil Med 1983;15:141-145.

33. Postacchini F, Facchinici M, Palieri P. Efficacy of various forms of conservative treatment in low back pain: a comparative study. Neuro-orthopedics 1988;6:28-35.

34. Hellinger J, Linke R, Heller H. A biophysical explanation for Nd:YAG percutaneous laser disc decompression success. J Clin Laser Med Surg 2001;19:235-238.

35. Hurri H. The Swedish back school in chronic low back pain. Part I. Benefits. Scand J Rehabil Med 1989;21:33-40.

36. Linton SJ, Bradley LA, Jensen I, et al. The secondary prevention of low back pain: a controlled study with follow-up. Pain 1989;36:197-207.

37. Donchin M, Woolf O, Kaplan L, et al. Secondary prevention of low-back pain. A clinical trial. Spine 1990;15:1317-1320.

38. Keijsers J, Steenbakkers M, Meertens RM, et al. The efficacy of the back school: a randomized trial. Arthritis Care Res 1990;3:204-209.

39. Dalichau S, Perrey RM, Solbach T, et al. Erfahrungen bei der Durchfuhrung eines berufsbezogenen Rückenschulmodells in Baugewerbe. Arbeitsmedizin 1998;48:72-80.

40. Penttinen J, Nevala-Puranen N, Airaksinen O, et al. Randomized controlled trial of back school with and without peer support. J Occup Rehabil 2002;12:21-29.

41. Bergquist-Ullman M, Larsson U. Acute low back pain in industry. A controlled prospective study with special reference to therapy and confounding factors. Acta Orthop Scand 1977;(170):1-117.

42. Lindequist S, Lundberg B, Wikmark R, et al. Information and regime at low back pain. Scand J Rehabil Med 1984;16:113-116.

43. Indahl A, Velund L, Reikeraas O. Good prognosis for low back pain when left untampered. A randomized clinical trial. Spine 1995;20:473-477.

44. Leclaire R, Esdaile JM, Suissa S, et al. Back school in a first episode of compensated acute low back pain: a clinical trial to assess efficacy and prevent relapse. Arch Phys Med Rehabil 1996;77:673-679.

45. Berwick DM, Budman S, Feldstein M. No clinical effect of back schools in an HMO. A randomized prospective trial. Spine 1989;14:338-344.

46. Herzog W, Conway PJ, Willcox BJ. Effects of different treatment modalities on gait symmetry and clinical measures for sacroiliac joint patients. J Manipulative Physiol Ther 1991;14:104-109.

47. Hsieh CY, Adams AH, Tobis J, et al. Effectiveness of four conservative treatments for subacute low back pain: a randomized clinical trial. Spine 2002;27:1142-1148.

48. Chou R, Huffman LH. Nonpharmacologic therapies for acute and chronic low back pain: a review of the evidence for an American Pain Society/American College of Physicians clinical practice guideline. Ann Intern Med 2007;147:492-504.

49. Elders LA, van der Beek AJ, Burdorf A. Return to work after sickness absence due to back disorders—a systematic review on intervention strategies. Int Arch Occup Environ Health 2000;73:339-348.

50. Maier-Riehle B, Harter M. The effects of back schools—a meta-analysis. Int J Rehabil Res 2001;24:199-206.

51. Brox JI, Storheim K, Grotle M, et al. Systematic review of back schools, brief education, and fear avoidance training for chronic low back pain. Spine J 2008;8:948-958.

52. Von Korff M, Balderson BH, Saunders K, et al. A trial of an activating intervention for chronic back pain in primary care and physical therapy settings. Pain 2005;113:323-330.

53. Brox JI, Reikeras O, Nygaard O, et al. Lumbar instrumented fusion compared with cognitive intervention and exercises in patients with chronic back pain after previous surgery for disc herniation: a prospective randomized controlled study. Pain 2006;122:145-155.

54. Brox JI, Sorensen R, Friis A, et al. Randomized clinical trial of lumbar instrumented fusion and cognitive intervention and exercises in patients with chronic low back pain and disc degeneration. Spine 2003;28:1913-1921.

55. Leeuw M, Goossens ME, Linton SJ, et al. The fear avoidance model of musculoskeletal pain: current state of scientific evidence. J Behav Med 2007;30:77-94.

56. George SZ, Fritz JM, Bialosky JE, et al. The effect of a fear avoidance-based physical therapy intervention for patients with acute low back pain: results of a randomized clinical trial. Spine 2003;28:2551-2560.

57. van Tulder MW, Assendelft WJ, Koes BW, et al. Method guidelines for systematic reviews in the Cochrane Collaboration Back Review Group for Spinal Disorders. Spine 1997;22:2323-2330.

58. Glomsrod B, Lonn JH, Soukup MG, et al. "Active back school" prophylactic management for low back pain: three-year follow-up of a randomized, controlled trial. J Rehabil Med 2001;33:26-30.

59. Vlaeyen JW, de Jong J, Geilen M, et al. Graded exposure in vivo in the treatment of pain-related fear: a replicated single-case experimental design in four patients with chronic low back pain. Behav Res Ther 2001;39:151-166.

60. Vlaeyen JW, de Jong J, Geilen M, et al. The treatment of fear of movement/(re)injury in chronic low back pain: further evidence on the effectiveness of exposure in vivo. Clin J Pain 2002;18:251-261.

61. de Jong JR, Vlaeyen JW, Onghena P, et al. Fear of movement/(re)injury in chronic low back pain: education or exposure in vivo as mediator to fear reduction? Clin J Pain 2005;21:9-17.

62. Dagenais S, Roffey DM, Wai EK, et al. Can cost utility evaluations inform decision making about interventions for low back pain? Spine J 2009;9:944-957.

63. van der Roer N, Goossens MEJB, Evers SMAA, et al. What is the most cost-effective treatment for patients with low back pain? A systematic review. Best Pract Res Clin Rheumatol 2005;19:671-684.

64. Johnson RE, Jones GT, Wiles NJ, et al. Active exercise, education, and cognitive behavioral therapy for persistent disabling low back pain: a randomized controlled trial. Spine 2007;32:1578-1585.

65. Loisel P, Lemaire J, Poitras S, et al. Cost-benefit and cost-effectiveness analysis of a disability prevention model for back pain management: a six year follow up study. Occupat Environ Med 2002;59:807-815.

66. Mitchell RI, Carmen GM. The functional restoration approach to the treatment of chronic pain in patients with soft tissue and back injuries. Spine 1994;19:633-642.

67. van der Roer N, van Tulder M, van Mechelen W, et al. Economic evaluation of an intensive group training protocol compared with usual care physiotherapy in patients with chronic low back pain. Spine 2008;33:445-451.

68. Skouen JS, Grasdal AL, Haldorsen EM, et al. Relative cost-effectiveness of extensive and light multidisciplinary treatment programs versus treatment as usual for patients with chronic low back pain on long-term sick leave: randomized controlled study. Spine 2002;27:901-909.

69. Jellema P, van der Roer N, van der Windt DAWM, et al. Low back pain in general practice: cost-effectiveness of a minimal psychosocial intervention versus usual care. Eur Spine J 2007;16:1812-1821.

70. Critchley DJ, Ratcliffe J, Noonan S, et al. Effectiveness and cost-effectiveness of three types of physiotherapy used to reduce chronic low back pain disability: a pragmatic randomized trial with economic evaluation. Spine 2007;32: 1474-1481.

71. Thompson GW. The placebo effect and health. New York: Prometheus Books; 2005.

SIMON DAGENAIS
JOHN MAYER

CHAPTER 8

Lumbar Stabilization Exercise

DESCRIPTION

Terminology and Subtypes

Exercise, loosely translated from Greek, means "freed movement" and describes a wide range of physical activities. Therapeutic exercise indicates that the purpose of the exercise is for the treatment of a specific medical condition rather than recreation. The main types of therapeutic exercise for low back pain (LBP) include (1) general physical activity (e.g., advice to remain active); (2) aerobic (e.g., brisk walking, cycling); (3) aquatic (e.g., swimming, exercise classes in a pool); (4) directional preference (e.g., McKenzie); (5) flexibility (e.g., stretching, yoga, Pilates); (6) proprioceptive/coordination (e.g., wobble board, stability ball); (7) stabilization (e.g., targeting abdominal and trunk muscles); and (8) strengthening (e.g., lifting weights).[1] This chapter focuses exclusively on stabilization exercises for chronic LBP (CLBP).

Therapeutic exercise for individuals with LBP has evolved over time. Recently, there has been a focus on exercises that aim to maintain stability in the lumbar spine.[2] This type of exercise approach has been termed lumbar stabilization, core stabilization, or segmental stabilization. Although no formal definition of lumbar stabilization exercise (LSE) exists, this approach is generally aimed at improving the neuromuscular control, strength, and endurance of muscles central to maintaining dynamic and static spinal and trunk stability. Several groups of muscles are targeted through LSEs, particularly the transversus abdominis (TrA), lumbar multifidus, and other paraspinal, abdominal, diaphragmatic, and pelvic musculature (Figure 8-1).

Although the LSE program developed by Richardson and Jull is the most widely studied, numerous other LSE programs are available through physical therapists, exercise physiologists, personal trainers, Pilates instructors, yoga teachers, or other health personnel involved in the management of LBP with therapeutic exercise.

History and Frequency of Use

In the 1980s, Bergmark undertook a mechanical engineering approach to the study of the lumbar spine.[3] His goal was to assess the role of the trunk musculature in providing stabilization for the lumbar spine and measure the specific forces applied to the spine by different muscles to understand the biomechanical "rationale" for the complex anatomic features of the lumbar spine. Using a mechanical modeling approach, musculature acting on the lumbar spine was divided into two groups: local and global. The global musculature (e.g., erector spinae, rectus abdominis) was thought to transfer load between the thoracic spine and pelvis. The local musculature (e.g., multifidus) consists of muscles that act directly on the lumbar spine and are attached to the lumbar vertebrae. Functionally, the global musculature was thought to balance the outer loads on the body, enabling the local system to maintain force control within the lumbar spine and center postural activity at a range within the load tolerance of the spinal structures.

Panjabi then proposed a basis for understanding spinal stability, injury, dysfunction, and recovery by asserting that there are three interdependent subsystems that function to stabilize the spine: passive, active, and neural.[4] The passive subsystem includes the vertebrae, intervertebral discs, ligaments, zygapophyseal joints, and passive components of the associated musculotendinous structures. The active subsystem comprises the musculotendinous units attached to, or influencing, the spinal column.[4] The neural subsystem includes sensory receptors in the spinal structures, their central connections, and cortical and subcortical control centers. These three subsystems are interdependent and work together to maintain spinal stability and intervertebral motion. For example, an injury or breakdown in the passive subsystem, such as a fracture, disc herniation, or disc degeneration, may decrease the inherent stability of the spine and alter segmental motion patterns. Enhancement of the neural and active subsystems could potentially help compensate for this loss and partially restore stability.

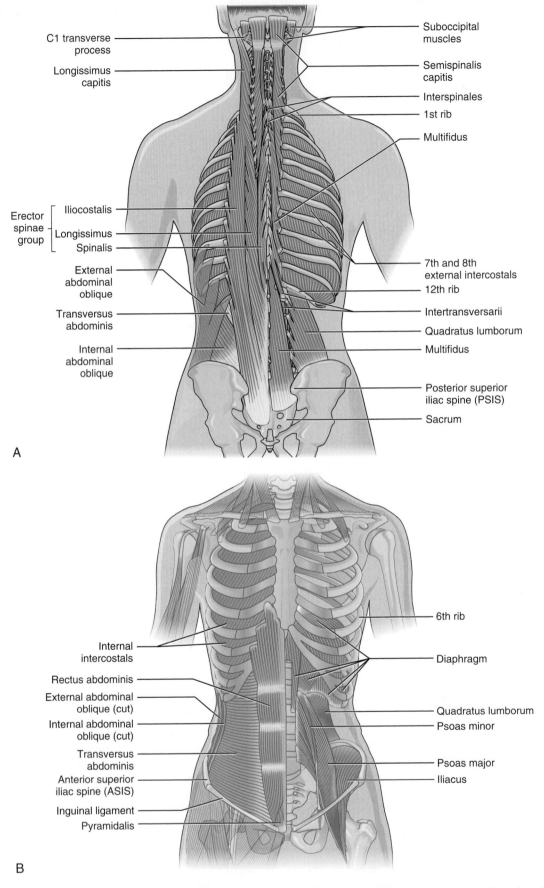

C1 transverse process

Longissimus capitis

Suboccipital muscles

Semispinalis capitis

Interspinales

1st rib

Multifidus

Erector spinae group
- Iliocostalis
- Longissimus
- Spinalis

External abdominal oblique

Transversus abdominis

Internal abdominal oblique

7th and 8th external intercostals

12th rib

Intertransversarii

Quadratus lumborum

Multifidus

Posterior superior iliac spine (PSIS)

Sacrum

A

Internal intercostals

Rectus abdominis

External abdominal oblique (cut)

Internal abdominal oblique (cut)

Transversus abdominis

Anterior superior iliac spine (ASIS)

Inguinal ligament

Pyramidalis

6th rib

Diaphragm

Quadratus lumborum

Psoas minor

Psoas major

Iliacus

B

Figure 8-1 Several groups of muscles in the trunk and pelvis are targeted with lumbar stabilization exercises. **A,** Posterior view. **B,** Anterior view.

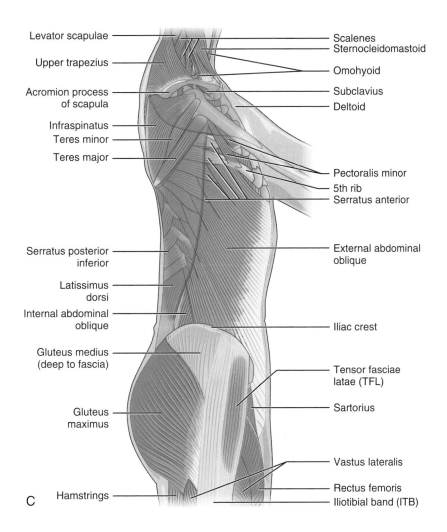

Levator scapulae
Upper trapezius
Acromion process of scapula
Infraspinatus
Teres minor
Teres major
Serratus posterior inferior
Latissimus dorsi
Internal abdominal oblique
Gluteus medius (deep to fascia)
Gluteus maximus
Hamstrings

Scalenes
Sternocleidomastoid
Omohyoid
Subclavius
Deltoid
Pectoralis minor
5th rib
Serratus anterior
External abdominal oblique
Iliac crest
Tensor fasciae latae (TFL)
Sartorius
Vastus lateralis
Rectus femoris
Iliotibial band (ITB)

C

Figure 8-1, cont'd C, Lateral view. (Modified from Muscolino JE. The muscle and bone palpation manual with trigger points, referral patterns, and stretching. St Louis, 2009, Mosby.)

A number of authors have assessed the role and activation patterns of trunk musculature as they relate to spinal stability. Cresswell and colleagues[5-7] conducted a series of studies on intra-abdominal pressure and activation of trunk muscula-ture. They reported that intra-abdominal pressure was increased during functional tasks by muscles that did not create a significant flexion movement of the lumbar spine (particularly the TrA and diaphragm), and activation of the TrA was correlated with changes in intra-abdominal pressure. It was also discovered that abdominal wall muscles were activated before the erector spinae if ventral loading of the trunk was expected, and concurrently with the erector spinae in unexpected ventral loading. This finding suggested that abdominal musculature may play a role in enhancing spinal stability during trunk motion or loading.

Hodges and Richardson[8] further pursued this line of research by studying activation patterns of trunk musculature with alteration of spinal posture by movement of an upper limb. In those without LBP, the TrA was the first muscle activated, contracting before upper limb movement regardless of direction of motion. This suggested that the TrA provides stability for the lumbar spine in anticipation of perturbations of posture. In individuals with LBP, however, the contraction of the TrA was significantly delayed, indicat-ing a potential for decreased spinal stability and fundamental problems with motor control. Similar findings were noted in later studies on the effects of lower extremity motion in those with and without LBP.[9,10]

There have also been several studies on the lumbar mul-tifidi in those with LBP. In 1994, Hides and colleagues[11] reported finding significant ipsilateral atrophy in the lumbar multifidi of individuals with unilateral LBP, whereas they noted very little asymmetry in these muscles in a control group of subjects without LBP. Patients with acute, first-episode LBP who were treated with usual medical manage-ment had limited recovery of multifidus muscle mass after 10 weeks, whereas those treated with a specific exercise program had greater recovery of multifidus muscle mass.[12] On the basis of these conceptual models, Richardson and Jull[2] described a specific exercise program to train co-contraction of the deep trunk muscles, particularly the TrA and lumbar multifidi, to enhance spinal stability in individuals with LBP. This treatment program has been the basis for a large number of further clinical studies and other publications and for what is commonly used in "core stability" programs.[12-25]

Other authors, and particularly Stuart McGill, have addressed additional aspects of stabilization training to emphasize broader and more integrative approaches and effects.[21,26,27] Early studies on the effects of these exercise programs indicated that they may have substantial benefit in the treatment of individuals with first-time acute LBP or with specific structural abnormalities in the spine.[13,16] In clinical practice, these programs are applied to a wide range of patients with LBP, although the popularity of these treatment programs is difficult to quantify. The number of recent studies conducted on this topic, along with the publication of a recent systematic review (SR) of stabilization exercises on LBP, suggest that these programs are increasingly popular.[26,28-31]

Practitioner, Setting, and Availability

Because this type of exercise is used to treat CLBP, it must be prescribed and monitored by licensed clinicians such as physicians, chiropractors, or physical therapists. The actual treatment, however, can be carried out under the supervision of athletic trainers, exercise physiologists, or personal trainers who report periodically to the prescribing clinician. Lumbar stabilization exercise protocols could also be self-administered at fitness facilities without a health care provider, although this is not recommended for CLBP. Various training and certification courses are offered to clinicians for lumbar stabilization exercise protocols. Despite the lack of regulation, any person delivering exercise therapy should be well versed in the basic principles and practice of exercise testing and prescription for the general population and the particular condition being treated. The typical settings for lumbar stabilization programs are outpatient treatment centers, health and fitness facilities, and athletic training centers under the supervision of trained personnel. Because little or no equipment is required, LSEs are suitable outside of health care settings. Home exercise may be more appropriate during latter stages of rehabilitation after a formal, supervised exercise program has been completed in a medical or fitness facility. This treatment is readily available throughout the United States. Education in training techniques is available through a variety of organizations and medical societies offering postgraduate or continuing medical education, and formal training may be variably present in the primary curriculum of schools of physical therapy, among others.

Procedure

The exercise program of Richardson and Jull[2] addressing the TrA and multifidi is described in detail in their text, and formal training in this program is generally administered by a physical therapist. The initial aim of this program is to achieve isometric co-contraction of the local muscles of the trunk, with activation of the TrA and multifidi being considered the "basic functional unit of a movement skill."[2] Patients are instructed to draw in the lower abdominal wall while simultaneously contracting the multifidi isometrically. A number of techniques were proposed to facilitate the learning of this particular motor skill, including visual correction, specific verbal instructions, manual facilitation, and use of a pressure biofeedback unit; specific postures are also advocated to assist in motor learning. A strong emphasis is placed on the accurate performance of the maneuvers, and the patients are progressed into functional positions while maintaining muscle activation. Exercises can be advanced when the patient is able to maintain 10 isometric "holds" for 10 seconds without fatiguing. In their study using this training protocol, O'Sullivan and colleagues[13] noted that, for some subjects, it took 4 to 5 weeks of training just to obtain an accurate pattern of isometric co-contraction of these muscles. This program has been modified by other investigators, and many have described progression through functional programs that incorporate previously painful motion patterns. A variety of exercises have been developed over the years to promote trunk stabilization (e.g., Figures 8-2 and 8-3), some of which can be performed with exercise equipment such as Swiss balls (e.g., Figures 8-4 and 8-5).

Additional methods of facilitation, including the use of ultrasound, educational pamphlets, and video demonstrations, have also been applied.[23-25] Reflecting the nonstandardized and generally multifactorial nature of many physical

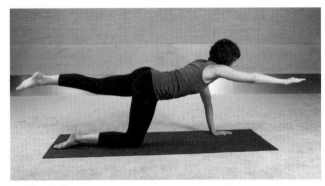

Figure 8-2 Example of trunk and lumbar stabilization exercise performed on the floor.

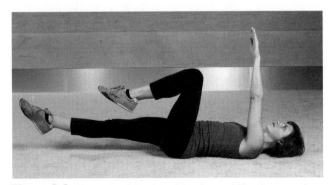

Figure 8-3 Example of trunk and lumbar stabilization exercise performed on the floor.

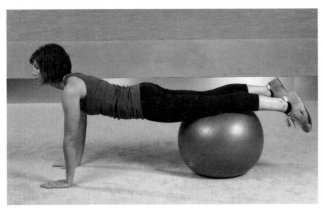

Figure 8-4 Example of trunk and stabilization exercise performed with a Swiss ball.

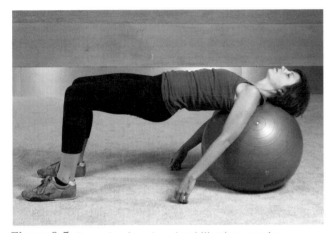

Figure 8-5 Example of trunk and stabilization exercise performed with a Swiss ball.

therapy treatments, studies have varied in their use of cointerventions such as manual therapy techniques, general conditioning, and varying degrees of physical and cognitive behavioral therapy. Settings also varied among studies that used either group classes or individual treatment approaches. It is difficult to describe a "typical" treatment course, but 6 to 12 sessions of LSE instruction are relatively common for a straightforward clinical scenario. However, many patients have a number of mitigating conditions that may affect the frequency and duration of care required.

Regulatory Status

Not applicable.

THEORY

Mechanism of Action

In general, exercises are used to strengthen muscles, increase soft tissue stability, restore range of movement, improve

cardiovascular conditioning, increase proprioception, and reduce fear of movement. The mechanism of action of LSE is currently unknown, but may be related to improving the neurophysiologic functioning of lumbar muscles and other muscles involved in stability to prevent continual re-injury or nociceptive input in the absence of true injury, or psychological mechanisms; each proposed theory is briefly described here.

Lumbar Stability

Lumbar stabilization exercises provide an opportunity to simultaneously exercise the passive, active, and neural subsystems of spinal stabilization proposed by Panjabi.[4] It has been suggested that injury to the vertebrae, intervertebral discs, ligaments, or zygapophyseal joints that comprise the passive subsystem could perhaps be compensated by enhancing the neural and active subsystems, thereby restoring lumbar stability. Lumbar stabilization exercise may also improve abdominal muscle strength and endurance, thereby compensating for decreased stability due to lumbar musculature injury. Improving function of abdominal muscles such as the TrA through LSE involving limb movements could also prevent spinal instability by compensating for injured lumbar muscles.[9,10] Lumbar stabilization exercise emphasizing co-contraction of the TrA and lumbar multifidi could also enhance spinal stability in individuals with LBP, thereby reducing their risk for reinjury.[2] When combined with dynamic and isometric intensive resistance training, LSE was associated with increased cross-sectional lumbar musculature.[32] Because these changes were not noted with LSE alone, they may be attributable to the progressive resistance exercises, or possibly an interaction effect of lumbar stabilization and strengthening.

Psychological Mechanisms

In some patients with particularly severe or prolonged CLBP, or CLBP with psychological comorbidities such as anxiety or depression, maladaptive illness behavior may become established. This type of behavior may manifest itself as fear of engaging in any activity or movement that has previously been associated with symptoms of CLBP. As time passes, virtually all activities gain this association, leading to a generalized fear of movement in an attempt to minimize exacerbations. Engaging in supervised exercise therapy under the guidance of an experienced clinician able to gradually increase the type, dose, frequency, or intensity of movements, can help break this cycle and demonstrate that not all movements or activities need be painful. This aspect is discussed further in other chapters of this text (e.g., Section 8—Behavioral Therapies), and is not specific to LSEs.

Indication

The use of LSEs has been recommended for nonspecific mechanical CLBP with or without specific anatomic abnormalities such as spondylolisthesis. Isometric exercise of the trunk musculature may be an appropriate consideration for any LBP beyond the acute stage. By extrapolating from Panjabi's model of spinal instability and the work of many of the authors previously discussed, there may be a rationale for using LSE in almost any patient with CLBP, including those with ongoing pain and a clearly definable structural source or those without correlative pathology identified on standard imaging.[4] This intervention may be most effectively applied in a patient who presents with a reproducible, mechanical pattern of lumbopelvic pain that follows a specific plane of movement or functional task. Often these patients demonstrate altered activation patterns of stabilizing musculature or poor endurance of core stabilizing musculature with testing.

With patients who have specific functional demands that are limited by CLBP, individualizing the progression of exercise through a task-specific approach designed to meet those physical demands may be the most effective application of LSE. More pragmatically, care of the patient with CLBP must include a thorough understanding of that individual and should follow the biopsychosocial model of chronic pain assessment and treatment. When treating individuals with substantial physical, social, or psychological barriers to functional recovery, LSE alone may not be sufficient to maximize improvement. In addressing overall function, the use of LSE training may be beneficial for individuals with CLBP, particularly in patients with clearly defined anatomic barriers to functional performance and well-managed social or psychological barriers to recovery. However, when those latter barriers become paramount, a multimodal behavioral modification approach to treatment should take precedence over unimodal LSE.

Assessment

Before receiving LSE training, patients should first be assessed for LBP using an evidence-based and goal-oriented approach focused on the patient history and neurologic examination, as discussed in Chapter 3. Additional diagnostic imaging or specific diagnostic testing is generally not required before initiating this intervention for CLBP. Nevertheless, several diagnostic tests are used clinically to apply the proper and safe dose of exercise, monitor progress throughout treatment, and document that the target muscles are being appropriately activated. These include a functional assessment of strength, flexibility, balance, endurance, and coordination, and potential assessment of lumbar muscle activity through real-time ultrasound and surface electromyography to allow a more precise prescription for LSE training.[12,33-35]

EFFICACY

Evidence supporting the efficacy of this intervention for CLBP was summarized from recent clinical practice guidelines (CPGs), SRs, and randomized controlled trials (RCTs). Findings are summarized by study design in the following paragraphs.

Clinical Practice Guidelines

None of the recent national CPGs on the management of CLBP have assessed and summarized the evidence to make specific recommendations about the efficacy of LSEs, though most have recommended therapeutic exercises in general for CLBP.

Systematic Reviews

Cochrane Collaboration

The Cochrane Collaboration conducted an SR in 2004 on all forms of exercise therapy for acute, subacute, and chronic LBP.[36] A total of 61 RCTs were identified, including 43 RCTs related to CLBP. Although results were generally favorable, this review combined all forms of exercise therapy, including stabilization, strengthening, stretching, McKenzie, aerobic, and others. As such, these conclusions were not specifically about the efficacy of LSEs for CLBP. This review identified two RCTs that may be related to LSEs for CLBP and one RCT related to LSES for acute LBP.[12,18,19] The RCTs examining CLBP are discussed below.

Other

Another review identified an additional RCT on LSE for CLBP that was not included in the Cochrane review; that RCT is also summarized below.[13,37] This SR did not make any conclusions specific to LSE for CLBP.

Another SR was conducted in 2008 on motor control exercise for persistent nonspecific LBP.[38] All of the 14 included RCTs examined patients whose LBP symptoms lasted for at least 6 weeks, with or without neurologic involvement. The number of RCTs specifically examining the effects of LSE for CLBP was not reported. Three of the included RCTs were also summarized in the reviews mentioned above.[13,24,25] This SR concluded that motor control exercise in general is effective in reducing pain and disability among patients with persistent LBP, but did not make any conclusions specific to LSE as defined in this chapter.

Findings from the aforementioned SRs are summarized in Table 8-1.

Randomized Controlled Trials

The methods for six RCTs of LSE for CLBP are summarized in Table 8-2.[13,18,19,23-25] Their results are briefly described here.

An RCT conducted by Cairns and colleagues[23] included LBP patients without neurologic involvement (duration of symptoms not reported). Participants were randomized to either the intervention group consisting of stabilization exercises or the control group consisting of conventional physical therapy. Manual therapy, modalities, education, and advice were also available to both groups. Both treatment programs included up to 12 half-hour sessions over 12 weeks. At the 12-month follow-up, disability scores were significantly reduced in both groups compared with baseline, however, there were no significant differences between groups. There were also reductions in pain in both groups (McGill Pain Questionnaire), although none of the reductions were

TABLE 8-1	Systematic Review Findings on Lumbar Stabilization Exercises for Chronic Low Back Pain		
Reference	#RCTs in SR	#RCTs for CLBP	Conclusion
36	61	43	Conclusions are not specific to LSE; the review combined all forms of exercise therapy
50	5	5	Conclusions are not specific to LSE; the review combined all forms of exercise therapy
38	14	14	Conclusions are not specific to LSE; the review combined all forms of exercise therapy

CLBP, chronic low back pain; LSE, lumbar stabilization exercise; RCT, randomized controlled trial; SR, systematic review.

TABLE 8-2	Randomized Controlled Trials of Lumbar Stabilization Exercises for Chronic Low Back Pain			
Reference	Indication	Intervention	Control (C1)	Control (C2)
23	LBP without neurologic involvement, duration of symptoms NR	Stabilization exercises + manual therapy, modalities, education, advice PT 0.5 hr × max 12 for 12 wk n = 47	Conventional physical therapy + manual therapy, modalities, education, advice PT 0.5 hr × max 12 for 12 wk n = 50	NA
24	CLBP without neurologic involvement, current episode >12 weeks	Spinal stabilization exercises + back school PT 3 hr × 1 + 10 wk × 1 hr n = 121	Manual therapy + back school PT 3 hr × 1 + 10 wk × 1 hr n = 121	Back book + back school PT 3 hr × 1 (back school) n = 60
25	CLBP without neurologic involvement, symptoms >3 months	Motor control (stabilization) exercise PT 12 sessions n = 80	SMT PT Up to 12 sessions n = 80	General exercise PT 1 hr × 12 n = 80
13	Isthmic spondylolysis or spondylolisthesis with or without neurologic involvement, symptoms >3 months	Stabilization exercise PT 15 min/day × 7 days × 10 wk Cointervention: NR n = 21	Control (general exercise) GP 0.5 hr × max 12 for 12 wk Cointervention: heat, massage, ultrasound, supervised exercise n = 21	NA
18	CLBP with or without neurologic involvement, symptoms >3 months	SMT + stabilization exercise Manual therapist 60 min evaluation, treatment, exercise × 4 over 4 wk Cointervention: education, reassurance n = 102	Control (education, reassurance) GP 2 sessions over 5 months Cointervention: activity limitations, exercise n = 102	NA
19	Subacute or chronic LBP without neurologic involvement, symptoms >6 wk	Stabilization exercise + biopressure PT 45-min × 1 day/wk × 6 wk + 10-15 min/day at home Cointervention: pain medication n = 22	Manual therapy (traction, stretching, MOB) PT 45-min × 1 day/wk × 6 wk Cointervention: pain medication, exercise n = 20	NA

CLBP, chronic low back pain; GP, general practitioner; LBP, low back pain; MOB, mobilization; NA, not applicable; NR, not reported; PT, physical therapist; SMT, spinal manipulation therapy.

statistically significant. The difference between groups was also not statistically significant. This study was considered of higher quality and also deemed clinically relevant to LSEs for CLBP.

An RCT conducted by Goldby and colleagues[24] included CLBP patients without neurologic involvement who had a current episode lasting longer than 12 weeks. Participants were randomized to three groups: (1) spinal stabilization exercises and back school; (2) manual therapy and back school; (3) an educational intervention consisting of a back book and back school. The back school included one 3-hour session, and the manual therapy and spinal stabilization exercises were provided for 1 hour a week for 10 weeks. At the 24-month follow-up, mean pain scores (0-100 scale) significantly improved for the spinal stabilization and manual therapy groups, but worsened for the education group (not statistically significant). At the 24-month follow-up, mean disability scores (Oswestry Disability Index) improved for all groups, with significant reductions in scores for the spinal stabilization and manual therapy groups, but not the education group. There were no significant differences between groups for pain or disability. This study was considered of lower quality.

An RCT conducted by Ferreira and colleagues[25] included LBP patients without neurologic involvement, who had symptoms lasting longer than 3 months. Participants were randomized to: (1) motor control (stabilization) exercises; (2) spinal manipulation therapy; or (3) general exercise. After 12 months, there were improvements in pain (visual analog scale) in all 3 groups (P values not reported). There were also improvements in disability (Roland Morris Disability Questionnaire) in all three groups (P values not reported). The differences in pain and disability between groups were not statistically significant. This study was considered of higher quality and also deemed clinically relevant to LSE for CLBP.

An RCT conducted by O'Sullivan and colleagues[13] included isthmic spondylolysis or spondylolisthesis patients with or without neurologic involvement. To be included, patients had to experience symptoms for at least 3 months. Participants were randomized to a stabilization exercise group or a control group over 10 weeks. Physical therapists administered the exercise therapy to those in the stabilization exercise group, while general practitioners followed participants in the control group. After 30 months, participants in the stabilization exercise group experienced statistically significant improvement in pain and disability compared with baseline scores. The control group did not experience statistically significant change compared with baseline. Furthermore, those in the stabilization exercise group experienced statistically significant improvement in pain and disability versus the control group.

An RCT conducted by Niemisto and colleagues[18] examined patients with CLBP with or without neurologic involvement. To be included, participants had to experience symptoms for at least 3 months. Participants were randomized to a treatment group receiving spinal manipulation and stabilization exercise from a manual therapist or to a physician's consultation group. After 1 year of follow-up, those in the spinal manipulation and stabilization exercise group experienced statistically significant improvement in pain and disability compared with those in the physician's consultation group. This study was considered of lower quality.

An RCT conducted by Rasmussen-Barr and colleagues[19] examined patients with subacute or chronic LBP. To be included, participants had to experience symptoms for more than 6 weeks and could not have signs of neurologic involvement. Participants were randomized to a stabilization exercise group or a manual therapy group that received traction, stretching, or mobilization. A physical therapist administered treatment to both groups. Individuals in the stabilization group met with the physical therapist for 45 minutes per week over 6 weeks and were encouraged to exercise at home. After 12 months of follow-up, the stabilization exercise group experienced statistically significant improvement in pain and disability compared with baseline scores. These differences were not observed in the manual therapy group. No statistically significant differences were observed between the two groups regarding pain and disability after 12 months of follow-up. This study was considered of lower quality.

SAFETY

Contraindications

Contraindications to LSE include spinal or medical conditions that preclude exercise for the trunk musculature, such as acute unstable spine injury, severe acute neurologic compromise, or cardiovascular instability. LSE should not be used in patients with any other structural lesions in the spine that may any other be adversely affected by exercise. As with other forms of back exercise, LSE is generally not recommended during acute flare-ups of CLBP when increased movement may temporarily worsen symptoms. Some of the RCTs reviewed on LSE for CLBP excluded patients with fracture, grade III or IV spondylolisthesis, malignancy, inflammatory arthropathies, pregnancy, significant neurologic loss, prior spine surgery, or other medical conditions that made them unsuitable for participation in therapeutic exercise.[23-25]

Adverse Events

No serious adverse events have been reported for LSE in the studies reviewed. However, minor adverse events were reported in a few cases. An RCT reported that 15 of 105 participants dropped out, including 6 who believed that the experimental treatment had aggravated their symptoms.[39] Another RCT reported that seven participants withdrew, including two with increased pain and one with dyspepsia.[40] Similarly, eight participants assigned to the exercise group dropped out of an RCT because of increased pain.[41] Four participants in another RCT experienced a sudden increase in pain.[42] Although two participants in another study withdrew due to disc prolapse, investigators indicated this was a preexisting condition and not related to LSE.[43] A Cochrane review on exercise therapy for LBP reported that only 26% of studies commented on adverse events, the majority of which reported mild effects such as increased pain and muscle soreness in a minority of participants.[36]

COSTS

Fees and Third-Party Reimbursement

In the United States, LSE that is supervised by a licensed health practitioner such as a physical therapist in an outpatient setting can be delivered using CPT codes 97110 (therapeutic exercises, each 15 minutes), 97112 (neuromuscular reeducation, each 15 minutes), or 97530 (therapeutic activities, each 15 minutes). The initial evaluation of lumbar function can be delivered using CPT codes 97001 (physical therapy initial evaluation) or 97750 (physical performance test or measurement, each 15 minutes). Periodic reevaluation of lumbar function can be delivered using CPT codes 97002 (physical therapy reevaluation) or 97750 (physical performance test or measurement, each 15 minutes).

These procedures are widely covered by other third-party payers such as health insurers and worker's compensation insurance. Although some payers continue to base their reimbursements on usual, customary, and reasonable payment methodology, the majority have developed reimbursement tables based on the Resource Based Relative Value Scale used by Medicare. Reimbursements by other third-party payers are generally higher than Medicare.

Third-party payers often reimburse a limited number of visits to licensed health care providers if they are prescribed by a physician and supported by adequate documentation deeming them medically necessary. Equipment or products required for those interventions are rarely typically considered inclusive in the procedure reported and are not separately reportable. Given the need to maintain the gains achieved in muscular function through lumbar stabilization, patients are often encouraged to continue this intervention beyond the initial period of supervised exercise therapy. The cost for membership in a private exercise facility is generally $50 to $100 per month. Some insurers in the United States also provide discounted membership fees to exercise facilities to their members to promote physical activity.

Typical fees reimbursed by Medicare in New York and California for these services are summarized in Table 8-3.

Cost Effectiveness

Evidence supporting the cost effectiveness of treatment protocols that compared these interventions, often in combination with one or more cointerventions, with control groups who received one or more other interventions, for either acute or chronic LBP, was identified from two SRs on this topic and is summarized here.[44,45] Although many of these study designs are unable to clearly identify the individual contribution of any intervention, their results provide some insight as to the clinical and economic outcomes associated with these approaches.

An RCT in Norway compared three approaches for patients with CLBP.[46] Participants received either: (1) a light multidisciplinary program consisting of education, fear avoidance training, and advice to remain active given by a physical therapist, nurse, and psychologist; (2) an extensive multidisciplinary program consisting of daily group sessions with cognitive behavioral therapy, education, fear avoidance training, and strengthening and stabilization exercises for 4 weeks; or (3) usual care by a general practitioner and possibly a physical therapist or chiropractor. Direct medical costs for the light and extensive multidisciplinary programs were estimated by dividing the total clinic costs for 1 year by the number of patients treated; direct costs were therefore assumed to be equal in both groups, regardless of large differences in time spent by clinic staff with patients in each group. Indirect productivity costs associated with lost work time were evaluated over 24 months. A limited cost-benefit analysis for male participants only reported that the light multidisciplinary program would yield average savings of approximately $19,544 per patient over 2 years, and was therefore cost effective compared with usual care.

An RCT in Finland compared two approaches for patients with CLBP in the rehabilitation unit of an orthopedic hospital.[18] One group received brief education by a physician and an education booklet. The other group received mobilization, stretching, and stabilization exercises from a manual therapist, as well as an educational booklet. Clinical outcomes after 12 months were mostly similar between the two groups, although slightly greater improvements were noted in pain and function in the manual therapist group. Direct medical costs associated with study and nonstudy interventions over 12 months were $431 in the brief education group and $470 in the manual therapist group. Indirect productivity costs from lost work days over 12 months were $2450 in the brief education group and $1848 in the manual therapist group. Total costs (direct medical and indirect productivity) over 12 months were therefore $2881 in the brief education group and $2318 in the manual therapist group. Total costs decreased in both groups when compared with historical health utilization and lost work days before having enrolled in the study, but cost differences between the groups were not significant.

An RCT in the United Kingdom compared three approaches for patients with CLBP.[47] The individual physical therapy approach included a maximum of 12 sessions with spinal manipulation, mobilization, massage, home exercises, and brief education. The spinal stabilization approach included a maximum of eight sessions with abdominal and multifidus exercises. The pain management approach included a maximum of eight sessions with

TABLE 8-3	Medicare Fee Schedule for Related Services	
CPT Code	New York	California
97001	$73	$78
97002	$40	$43
97110	$30	$32
97112	$31	$33
97530	$32	$35
97750	$21	$33

2010 Participating, nonfacility amount.

education, exercises, cognitive behavioral therapy, and fear avoidance training. Clinical outcomes after 18 months were similar for all groups, with improvements noted in pain, function, and utility. Direct medical costs for study and nonstudy interventions paid by the National Health Service over 18 months were approximately $872 for individual physical therapy, approximately $698 for spinal stabilization, and approximately $304 for pain management. Indirect productivity costs were not reported. Over 18 months, the three groups experienced gains in quality-adjusted life-years of 0.99, 0.90, and 1.00, respectively. By virtue of having lower direct medical costs and greater gains in utility, the pain management approach was reported to dominate over both individual physical therapy and spinal stabilization.

An RCT in the United States compared two approaches for patients with acute LBP.[48] The first group received care according to the classification of symptoms and examination findings by a physical therapist, including possibly spinal manipulation, mobilization, traction therapy, and flexion, extension, strengthening, or stabilization exercises. The second group received brief education and general exercise from a physical therapist according to recommendations from CPGs, which were not specified. Clinical outcomes after 1 year favored the therapy according to classification group for improvement in function, although no differences were noted in the SF-36. Direct medical costs associated with the study interventions over 1 year were $604 in the therapy according to classification group and $682 in the CPG recommended care group; direct medical costs for all interventions over 1 year were $883 and $1160, respectively. Indirect productivity costs associated with lost productivity were not reported, although fewer participants in the therapy according to classification group had missed work due to LBP after 12 months.

An RCT in Sweden compared three approaches for patients sick-listed with acute LBP.[49] The manual therapy group received spinal manipulation, mobilization, assisted stretching, and exercises. The intensive training group received supervised exercise therapy with a physical therapist, including general and stabilization exercises. The usual care group received various interventions from a general practitioner, including common analgesics and brief education. Clinical outcomes were not reported. Direct medical costs associated with study interventions over 1 year, including provider visits, diagnostic testing, and surgery (if needed), were approximately $1054 in the manual therapy group, approximately $1123 in the intensive training group, and approximately $404 in the usual care group. Indirect productivity costs associated with lost work days were approximately $6163 in the manual therapy group, approximately $5557 in the intensive training group, and approximately $7072 in the usual care group. Total costs (direct medical and indirect productivity) over 1 year were therefore approximately $7217 in the manual therapy group, approximately $6680 in the intensive training group, and approximately $7476 in the usual care group. Cost differences between groups were not significantly different.

Findings from the aforementioned cost effectiveness analyses are summarized in Table 8-4.

SUMMARY

Description

LSE is generally aimed at improving the neuromuscular control, strength, and endurance of muscles central to maintaining dynamic and static spinal and trunk stability. Stabilization is widely available across the United States. Because it is used to treat CLBP, it must be prescribed and monitored by licensed clinicians such as physicians, chiropractors, or physical therapists. The actual treatment, however, can be carried out under the supervision of athletic trainers, exercise physiologists, or personal trainers who report periodically to the prescribing clinician. The typical settings for lumbar stabilization programs are outpatient treatment centers, health and fitness facilities, and athletic training centers under the supervision of trained personnel. Home exercise may be more appropriate during latter stages of rehabilitation after a formal, supervised exercise program has been completed in a medical or fitness facility.

Theory

In general, therapeutic exercises for CLBP are used to strengthen muscles, increase soft tissue stability, restore range of movement, improve cardiovascular conditioning, increase proprioception, and reduce fear of movement. The specific mechanism of action of LSE for CLBP is currently unknown, but may be related to improving the neurophysiologic functioning of lumbar muscles and other muscles involved in stability. Disc metabolism could potentially be enhanced through repetitive exercise involving the spine's full active range of motion as performed in some LSEs, improving repair and enhancing reuptake of inflammatory and nociceptive mediators. In addition, in some patients with particularly severe or prolonged CLBP or psychological comorbidities such as anxiety or depression, maladaptive illness behavior may occur, leading to fear of engaging in any activity or movement previously associated with the CLBP. Engaging in any form of therapeutic exercise under the guidance of an experienced clinician, including LSE, could potentially help break this cycle and demonstrate that not all movements are painful. LSE is recommended for nonspecific mechanical CLBP with or without specific anatomic abnormalities such as spondylolisthesis. Diagnostic imaging or other forms of advanced testing are generally not required before administering LSEs for CLBP.

Efficacy

None of the recent national CPGs made recommendations specific to LSE for CLBP, though many recommended therapeutic exercises in general. Although three SRs were identified on exercise therapy for LBP, none made conclusions specific to LSE for CLBP. At least six RCTs examined the

TABLE 8-4	Cost Effectiveness and Cost Utility Analyses of Lumbar Stabilization Exercises for Acute or Chronic Low Back Pain				
Ref Country Follow-up	Group	Direct Costs	Indirect Costs	Total Costs	Conclusion
46 Norway 2 years	1. light multidisciplinary program 2. extensive multidisciplinary program (including stabilization exercises) 3. usual care	NR	NR	NR	Group 1: average savings of $19,544/patient over 2 years
18 Finland 1 year	1. brief education by physician 2. treatment by manual therapist (including stabilization exercises)	1. $431 2. $470	1. $2450 2. $1848	1. $2881 2. $2318	No significant difference
47 United Kingdom 18 months	1. individual physical therapy 2. spinal stabilization 3. pain management	1. $872 2. $698 3. $304	NR	NR	Gains in QALY: 1. 0.99 2. 0.90 3. 1.00 Group 3 reported to dominate other interventions
48 United States 1 year	1. care according to classification of symptoms (including stabilization exercises) 2. brief education + general exercise	1. $883 2. $1160	NR	NR	No conclusion as to cost effectiveness
49 Sweden 1 year	1. manual therapy 2. intensive training (including stabilization exercises) 3. usual care	1. $1054 2. $1123 3. 404	1. $6163 2. $5557 3. $7072	1. $7217 2. $6680 3. $7476	No significant difference

NR, not reported; QALY, quality-adjusted life-years.

efficacy of LSE for CLBP, with many reporting favorable outcomes and two reporting statistically significant improvement in pain and function versus comparators.

Safety

Contraindications to LSE include spinal or medical conditions that preclude exercise for the trunk musculature, such as acute unstable spine injury, severe acute neurologic compromise, or cardiovascular instability. LSE should not be used in patients with any other structural lesions in the spine that may be adversely affected by exercise. Adverse events are minor and self-limited and may include temporarily increased pain, muscle soreness, and dyspepsia.

Costs

The Medicare reimbursement for LSE in an outpatient setting that is supervised by licensed health practitioners (e.g., physical therapist) ranges from $21 to $78, depending on the duration and type of session (e.g., assessment, reevaluation). At least five studies have examined the costs associated with various forms of LSE for CLBP, yet the individual contribution of LSE to the overall cost effectiveness could not be determined because the RCTs also included other co-interventions along with LSE.

Comments

The evidence from the CPGs, SRs, and RCTs reviewed was unable to provide definitive recommendations about efficacy of LSE as an intervention for CLBP. Although the theory supporting this type of therapeutic exercise for CLBP appears sound, additional research is required to determine the optimal type and dose of LSE, as well as information is needed on the subset of patients with CLBP who is most likely to benefit. Studies on LSE have generally enrolled a heterogeneous group of subjects with nonspecific CLBP, and were thus unable to determine which subgroup of patients may be more responsive to LSE. Based on the proposed model of spinal instability, LSE is likely more applicable to a narrower rather than a broader group of patients with LCBP. Because most studies excluded patients with prior spinal surgery, the efficacy of LSE in this population is also unknown. Future studies focusing on this indication may be warranted.

Additional information is also required about the optimal setting for delivering this type of care, the most effective specific LSEs, as well as the effects of individual or group settings, supervised or unsupervised training, and the optimal dose, duration, frequency, and progression of LSE for CLBP. Future studies should also evaluate the potential benefits of specific LSEs that are more closely matched with the recreational and occupational demands of the rehabilitating individual, such as multiplanar functional core training. Although

LSE has historically focused on the activation patterns of the TrA and lumbar multifidi, physical demands in many patients may require a higher degree of coordinated muscle activation and control than would be obtainable through only isolated training of these muscles.[27]

CHAPTER REVIEW QUESTIONS

Answers are located on page 450.

1. Which of the following muscle groups are not targeted in lumbar stabilization exercises?
   a. deltoids
   b. transversus abdominis
   c. lumbar multifidi
   d. paraspinals
2. Which of the following descriptions correctly matches a subsystem with its corresponding components?
   a. neural subsystem—sensory receptors in spinal structures
   b. passive musculoskeletal subsystem—musculotendinous units attached to/influencing the spinal column
   c. active musculoskeletal subsystem—sensory receptors in spinal structures
   d. neural subsystem—vertebrae, intervertebral discs, ligaments, and z-joints
3. What was a major advancement in the development of lumbar stabilization for CLBP?
   a. Panjabi's discovery of a herniated disc
   b. Cresswell's mastering of the stabilization technique
   c. Bergmark's examination of the lumbar spine
   d. Richardson and Jull's collaboration with Hides
4. When were lumbar stabilization exercises first used to treat CLBP?
   a. 1950s
   b. 1960s
   c. 1970s
   d. 1980s
5. Which of the following is not one of the interdependent subsystems that function to stabilize the spine as proposed by Panjabi?
   a. passive
   b. active
   c. reactive
   d. neural
6. Who proposed the technique that stabilization is often associated with?
   a. Cresswell
   b. Richardson
   c. Panjabi
   d. Bergmark
7. What are some of the side effects associated with lumbar stabilization exercise?
   a. herniated disc
   b. tight tendons
   c. light-headedness
   d. muscle soreness

REFERENCES

1. Mooney V, Verna J, Morris C. Clinical management of chronic, disabling low back syndromes. In: Morris C, editor. Low back syndromes: integrated clinical management. New York: McGraw-Hill; 2006.
2. Richardson CA, Jull GA. Muscle control-pain control. What exercises would you prescribe? Man Ther 1995;1:2-10.
3. Bergmark A. Stability of the lumbar spine. A study in mechanical engineering. Acta Orthop Scand Suppl 1989;230:1-54.
4. Panjabi MM. The stabilizing system of the spine. Part I. Function, dysfunction, adaptation, and enhancement. J Spinal Disord 1992;5:383-389.
5. Cresswell AG, Grundstrom H, Thorstensson A. Observations on intra-abdominal pressure and patterns of abdominal intramuscular activity in man. Acta Physiol Scand 1992;144: 409-418.
6. Cresswell AG, Oddsson L, Thorstensson A. The influence of sudden perturbations on trunk muscle activity and intra-abdominal pressure while standing. Exp Brain Res 1994;98:336-341.
7. Cresswell AG, Thorstensson A. The role of the abdominal musculature in the elevation of the intra-abdominal pressure during specified tasks. Ergonomics 1989;32:1237-1246.
8. Hodges PW, Richardson CA. Inefficient muscular stabilization of the lumbar spine associated with low back pain. A motor control evaluation of transversus abdominis. Spine 1996;21: 2640-2650.
9. Hodges PW, Richardson CA. Contraction of the abdominal muscles associated with movement of the lower limb. Phys Ther 1997;77:132-142.
10. Hodges PW, Richardson CA. Delayed postural contraction of transversus abdominis in low back pain associated with movement of the lower limb. J Spinal Disord 1998;11:46-56.
11. Hides JA, Stokes MJ, Saide M, et al. Evidence of lumbar multifidus muscle wasting ipsilateral to symptoms in patients with acute/subacute low back pain. Spine 1994;19:165-172.
12. Hides JA, Richardson CA, Jull GA. Multifidus muscle recovery is not automatic after resolution of acute, first-episode low back pain. Spine 1996;21:2763-2769.
13. O'Sullivan PB, Phyty GD, Twomey LT, et al. Evaluation of specific stabilizing exercise in the treatment of chronic low back pain with radiologic diagnosis of spondylolysis or spondylolisthesis. Spine 1997;22:2959-2967.
14. O'Sullivan PB, Twomey L, Allison GT. Altered abdominal muscle recruitment in patients with chronic back pain following a specific exercise intervention. J Orthop Sports Phys Ther 1998;27:114-124.
15. Richardson C, Jull G, Hodges P, et al. Therapeutic exercise for spinal segmental stabilization in low back pain: scientific basis and clinical approach. London: Churchill Livingstone; 2003.
16. Hides JA, Jull GA, Richardson CA. Long-term effects of specific stabilizing exercises for first-episode low back pain. Spine 2001;26:E243-E248.
17. Moseley L. Combined physiotherapy and education is efficacious for chronic low back pain. Aust J Physiother 2002;48: 297-302.
18. Niemisto L, Lahtinen-Suopanki T, Rissanen P, et al. A randomized trial of combined manipulation, stabilizing exercises, and physician consultation compared to physician consultation alone for chronic low back pain. Spine 2003;28:2185-2191.
19. Rasmussen-Barr E, Nilsson-Wikmar L, Arvidsson I. Stabilizing training compared with manual treatment in subacute and chronic low-back pain. Man Ther 2003;8:233-241.

20. Whitman JM, Fritz JM, Childs JD. The influence of experience and specialty certifications on clinical outcomes for patients with low back pain treated within a standardized physical therapy management program. J Orthop Sports Phys Ther 2004;34:662-672.

21. Hicks GE, Fritz JM, Delitto A, et al. Preliminary development of a clinical prediction rule for determining which patients with low back pain will respond to a stabilization exercise program. Arch Phys Med Rehabil 2005;86:1753-1762.

22. Koumantakis GA, Watson PJ, Oldham JA. Trunk muscle stabilization training plus general exercise versus general exercise only: randomized controlled trial of patients with recurrent low back pain. Phys Ther 2005;85:209-225.

23. Cairns MC, Foster NE, Wright C. Randomized controlled trial of specific spinal stabilization exercises and conventional physiotherapy for recurrent low back pain. Spine 2006;31: E670-E681.

24. Goldby LJ, Moore AP, Doust J, et al. A randomized controlled trial investigating the efficiency of musculoskeletal physiotherapy on chronic low back disorder. Spine 2006;31:1083-1093.

25. Ferreira ML, Ferreira PH, Latimer J, et al. Comparison of general exercise, motor control exercise and spinal manipulative therapy for chronic low back pain: a randomized trial. Pain 2007;131:31-37.

26. McGill SM. Low back stability: from formal description to issues for performance and rehabilitation. Exerc Sport Sci Rev 2001;29:26-31.

27. Kavcic N, Grenier S, McGill SM. Determining the stabilizing role of individual torso muscles during rehabilitation exercises. Spine 2004;29:1254-1265.

28. Hodges PW. Core stability exercise in chronic low back pain. Orthop Clin North Am 2003;34:245-254.

29. Barr KP, Griggs M, Cadby T. Lumbar stabilization: core concepts and current literature, Part 1. Am J Phys Med Rehabil 2005;84:473-480.

30. Kibler WB, Press J, Sciascia A. The role of core stability in athletic function. Sports Med 2006;36:189-198.

31. Rackwitz B, de BR, Limm H, von GK, et al. Segmental stabilizing exercises and low back pain. What is the evidence? A systematic review of randomized controlled trials. Clin Rehabil, 2006;20:553-567.

32. Danneels L, Cools A, Vanderstraeten C, et al. The effects of three different training modalities on the cross-sectional area of the paravertebral muscles. Scand J Med Sci Sports 2001;11:335-341.

33. Risch S, Norvell N, Pollock M, et al. Lumbar strengthening in chronic low back pain patients. Physiologic and psychological benefits. Spine 1993;18:232-238.

34. Biering-Sorensen F. Physical measurements as risk indicators for low back trouble over a one-year period. Spine 1984;9: 106-119.

35. Sung P. Multifidi muscles median frequency before and after spinal stabilization exercises. Arch Phys Med Rehabil 2003;84:1313-1318.

36. Hayden JA, van Tulder MW, Malmivaara A, et al. Exercise therapy for treatment of nonspecific low back pain. Cochrane Database Syst Rev 2005;(3):CD000335.

37. Maher CG. Effective physical treatment for chronic low back pain. Orthop Clin North Am 2004;35:57-64.

38. Macedo LG, Maher CG, Latimer J, et al. Motor control exercise for persistent, nonspecific low back pain: a systematic review. Phys Ther 2009;89:9-25.

39. Manniche C, Hesselsoe G, Bentzen R, et al. Clinical trial of intensive muscle training for chronic low back pain. Lancet 1988;2:1473-1476.

40. Johannsen F, Remvig L, Kryger P, et al. Exercises for chronic low back pain: a clinical trial. J Orthop Sports Phys Ther 1995;22:52-59.

41. Hansen F, Bendix T, Jensen C, et al. Intensive, dynamic back-muscle exercises, conventional physiotherapy, or placebo-controlled treatment of low-back pain. Spine 1993;18:98-108.

42. Frost H, Lamb SE, Doll HA, et al. Randomised controlled trial of physiotherapy compared with advice for low back pain. BMJ 2004;329:708.

43. Kankaanpaa M, Taimela S, Airaksinen O, et al. The efficacy of active rehabilitation in chronic low back pain. Effect on pain intensity, self-experienced disability, and lumbar fatigability. Spine 1999;24:1034-1042.

44. Dagenais S, Roffey DM, Wai EK, et al. Can cost utility evaluations inform decision making about interventions for low back pain? Spine J 2009;9:944-957.

45. van der Roer N, Goossens MEJB, Evers SMAA, et al. What is the most cost-effective treatment for patients with low back pain? A systematic review. Best Pract Res Clin Rheumatol 2005;19:671-684.

46. Skouen JS, Grasdal AL, Haldorsen EM, et al. Relative cost-effectiveness of extensive and light multidisciplinary treatment programs versus treatment as usual for patients with chronic low back pain on long-term sick leave: randomized controlled study. Spine 2002;27:901-909.

47. Critchley DJ, Ratcliffe J, Noonan S, et al. Effectiveness and cost-effectiveness of three types of physiotherapy used to reduce chronic low back pain disability: a pragmatic randomized trial with economic evaluation. Spine 2007;32:1474-1481.

48. Fritz JM, Delitto A, Erhard RE. Comparison of classification-based physical therapy with therapy based on clinical practice guidelines for patients with acute low back pain: a randomized clinical trial. Spine 2003;28:1363-1371.

49. Seferlis T, Lindholm L, Nemeth G. Cost-minimisation analysis of three conservative treatment programmes in 180 patients sick-listed for acute low-back pain. Scand J Prim Health Care 2000;18:53-57.

50. Chibnall JT, Tait RC, Merys SC. Disability management of low back injuries by employer-retained physicians: ratings and costs. Am J Indust Med 2000;38:529-538.

CHAPTER 9

JOHN MAYER
VERT MOONEY
SIMON DAGENAIS

Lumbar Strengthening Exercise

DESCRIPTION

Terminology and Subtypes

Exercise, loosely translated from Greek, means "freed movement" and describes a wide range of physical activities. Therapeutic exercise indicates that the purpose of the exercise is for the treatment of a specific medical condition rather than recreation. The main types of therapeutic exercise relevant to chronic low back pain (CLBP) include (1) general physical activity as usual (e.g., advice to remain active), (2) aerobic (e.g., brisk walking, cycling), (3) aquatic (e.g., swimming, exercise classes in a pool), (4) directional preference (e.g., McKenzie), (5) flexibility (e.g., stretching, yoga, Pilates), (6) proprioceptive/coordination (e.g., wobble board, stability ball), (7) stabilization (e.g., targeting abdominal and trunk muscles), and (8) strengthening (e.g., lifting weights).[1] This chapter focuses exclusively on strengthening exercises of the lumbar extensors for CLBP.

Lumbar Extensors

The term *lumbar extensor* is used colloquially to refer to the erector spinae muscle group, which is comprised of the iliocostalis lumborum, longissimus thoracis, and spinalis thoracis. These three long, narrow muscles are positioned lateral to the multifidus, have a common origin on the upper iliac crest and lumbar aponeurosis, and each inserts on several ribs superiorly.[2] The erector spinae allow for vertebral rotation in the sagittal plane (e.g., lumbar extension) and posterior vertebral translation when muscles contract bilaterally.[3] The multifidus muscle is also involved with lumbar extension movements and is therefore a target of lumbar strengthening exercises. The fascicular arrangement of the multifidus suggests that this muscle assists the erector spinae group and acts on vertebral rotation in the sagittal plane without posterior translation. Both the multifidus and erector spinae are also capable of vertebral rotation in the coronal plane (e.g., lumbar lateral flexion) and transverse plane (e.g., axial rotation) with unilateral contraction.[4]

Strengthening Exercises

Strengthening exercises are also known as progressive resistance exercise (PRE), which is based on the principles of overload, specificity, reversibility, frequency, intensity, repetitions, volume, duration, and mode. Each of these concepts is briefly discussed here as it relates to lumbar extensor strengthening exercises.[5,6]

Overload

For PRE to result in continued increases in muscular strength and endurance, training must progressively overload the targeted musculature, that is, make muscles function beyond their current capacity by increasing the intensity and volume of exercises.[6] Overloading the intensity of exercise tends to produce gains in muscular strength, whereas overloading the volume of exercise tends to improve muscular endurance. Although important to achieve long-term goals, overload in intensity and volume should be gradual to avoid reinjury.[7]

Specificity

Specificity implies that the target muscle must be isolated during the prescribed exercises to achieve sufficient muscular activation.[6] Trunk extension is a compound movement of the hip, pelvis, and lumbar spine through the action of the lumbar extensors, gluteals, and hamstrings.[8] The relative contribution of individual muscle groups is unknown, but it is assumed that the larger gluteal and hamstring muscles generate the majority of the force.[9] Therefore it has been suggested that to enhance specificity for the lumbar extensors, torque production from the gluteals and hamstrings should be minimized.[8] This can be achieved through various types of equipment and techniques. The lumbar dynamometer, for example, incorporates restraint mechanisms to limit pelvic and hip rotation and maximize lumbar extension in the seated position.[10] Similarly, prone back extensions on Roman chairs or benches improve specificity and isolation of the lumbar extensors by aligning the pelvis on the device, internally rotating the hips, and accentuating lumbar lordosis.[11]

Reversibility

With all PRE training programs, much of the gains in muscular strength and endurance will be lost unless exercise is continued.[6] To prevent this reversibility, it is recommended that therapeutic exercises be carried out long term. Once substantial improvement has been achieved, it may be possible to maintain physiologic gains with a reduced training frequency that may be as low as once per month.[12]

Frequency

The optimal frequency for PRE varies based on initial physical condition, duration of injury, and therapeutic goals. Generally, a frequency of one to three sessions per week of PRE is recommended.[13] Patients who are most deconditioned may initially achieve gains with only one session per week, which must be gradually increased to exceed that improvement.[14,15] Studies have reported improvement in lumbar extensor strength in patients with CLBP who trained once per week; no differences were noted between two and three sessions per week.[16,17] Training frequency needs to also consider intensity and volume, because particularly challenging PRE sessions may require additional recovery time.[6] It is often suggested that patients allow for at least 48 hours between sessions.

Intensity

The intensity of PRE is related to both the amount of resistance used (e.g., weight) and the number of repetitions. To increase muscle strength, high-intensity PRE consisting of higher resistance and lower repetitions is generally prescribed, whereas low-intensity PRE with lower resistance and higher repetition is used to improve muscular endurance.[6] Depending on the therapeutic goals (e.g., strength vs. endurance), 6 to 25 repetitions at intensities of 30% to 85% of the theoretical maximum intensity can be used for PRE. In a randomized controlled trial (RCT) of PRE for CLBP, there were no differences in clinical outcomes between high- and low-intensity lumbar extensor strength training.[18]

Repetitions

In PRE, the number of repetitions is corollary to the amount of resistance: as resistance increases, repetitions decrease. Regardless of the number, each repetition of a particular exercise should be performed in a slow, controlled fashion. It has been suggested that, as a general rule, it should take two seconds for the concentric/shortening phase and four seconds for the eccentric/lengthening phase of a PRE.[19]

Volume

The volume of PRE refers to the number of sets performed at one time and is one of the elements that can be varied to maintain gains in strength and endurance once a certain level of resistance and repetitions can be comfortably achieved. Although the optimal volume of PRE is unknown, one to three sets of each exercise is typically recommended for each session.[13] For asymptomatic individuals, lumbar extensor strength gains achieved with one set of exercises were equal to those achieved with three sets when using a dynamometer.[19] However, in patients with CLBP, an RCT reported that clinical outcomes were maximized with an increased volume of prone back extension exercises on benches.[20]

Duration

In the context of PRE, duration refers to the total length of the exercise program and not the length of individual sessions. Clinical improvement can be seen after only a few weeks of a resistance training program due to changes in specific physical function, whereas long-term improvements are attributable to physiologic changes as a result of PRE.[6] A minimum of 10 to 12 weeks of PRE is generally required to achieve measurable physiologic changes (e.g., hypertrophy) in skeletal muscles.[6] However, compliance with any therapeutic exercise program tends to decrease over time and it can be challenging to maintain patient participation for that period once functional improvements are achieved and symptoms diminish.

Mode

Mode refers to the specific type of exercises and equipment used during PRE.[6] This can be defined according to muscular contractions, which are either isometric or dynamic. Isometric exercise implies that the targeted muscle contracts without changing its length, whereas dynamic exercise implies that the targeted muscle shortens (concentric phase) or lengthens (eccentric phase) while contracting, which also results in associated joint movement. The three categories of dynamic exercise are isotonic, variable resistance, and isokinetic.[6] Isotonic dynamic exercise involves muscular contraction against a fixed resistance providing constant tension (e.g., dumbbells). Variable resistance dynamic exercise involves a muscular contraction against variable resistance that attempts to mimic the strength curve of the targeted muscle (e.g., Nautilus). Isokinetic dynamic exercise involves muscular contraction at fixed speed (e.g., treadmill). The five main modes of lumbar extensor strengthening exercise protocols use (1) machines (Figure 9-1), (2) benches (Figure 9-2), (3) Roman chairs (Figure 9-3), (4) free weights (Figure 9-4), and (5) stability balls (Figure 9-5). The characteristics, advantages, and disadvantages of each are highlighted in Table 9-1.

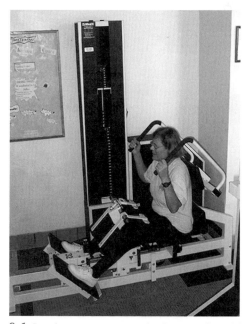

Figure 9-1 Lumbar extensor strengthening exercise with a machine.

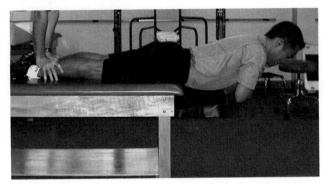

Figure 9-2 Lumbar extensor strengthening exercise with a bench.

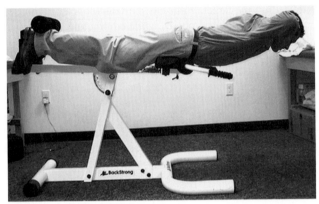

Figure 9-3 Lumbar extensor strengthening exercise with a variable-angle Roman chair.

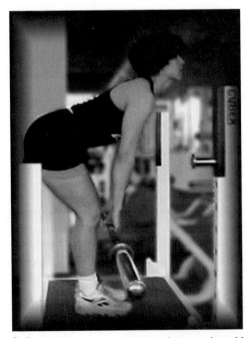

Figure 9-4 Lumbar extensor strengthening exercise with stiff-legged dead-lifts.

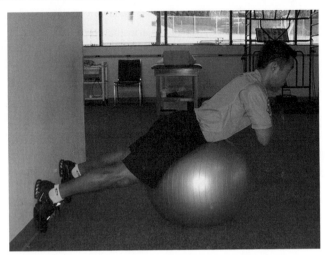

Figure 9-5 Lumbar extensor strengthening exercise with a stability ball.

History and Frequency of Use

Physical exercise has been used throughout human history. Hippocrates noted that lack of exercise led to atrophy, liability for disease, and quicker aging.[7] In 1865, Gustav Zander developed a technique named *medical mechanical therapy* using exercise equipment, including a device to strengthen the back extensors.[21] Although Zander described progressive exercise using equipment in the late 1800s, the idea did not receive much attention in the medical community for treating disease.[7] The first known treatment program for musculoskeletal care that can likely be characterized as therapeutic exercise was by Thomas De Lorme in 1945 for rehabilitation of injured or postsurgical joints.[22] The PREs were founded on the principles of weightlifters and bodybuilders using free weights (barbells and dumbbells) in a progressively demanding approach by increasing the amount of weight and number of repetitions. Today's athletic training programs continue to use these basic PRE principles. Exercise equipment specifically designed to treat CLBP by strengthening the lumbar extensors through PREs appeared in the late 1980s. Soon after this, protocols were published for isometric testing and dynamic variable resistance training on dynamometers that isolated the lumbar spine.[6,8] The availability of these measurement-based machines made it possible to more clearly define the dose of exercise during the treatment of CLBP. Although dynamometers and isokinetic machines effectively administer PREs to strengthen the lumbar extensors, the use of these machines for CLBP has been questioned because of their relatively high cost and inconvenience.[23,24] As a result, less costly protocols were developed including fixed-angle Roman chairs and benches, variable-angle Roman chairs (VARC), floor exercises, and stability balls. However, it is still unclear whether these options provide the overload stimulus necessary to elicit clinically meaningful gains in lumbar extensor strength.[25,26]

TABLE 9-1	Subtypes of Lumbar Extensor Strengthening Exercises					
Type	**Examples**	**Position/ Movement**	**PRE**	**Measurement**	**Advantages**	**Disadvantages**
Machines	Variable resistance dynamometers	Seated; isotonic (with or without variable resistance) Closed-chain exercise for both upper and lower body	Pin loaded weight stack, pneumatic, electronic/ cam system	Strength: isometric and dynamic strength tests over full ROM using machine's assessment mechanisms Endurance: isometric and dynamic tests over full ROM	Gradual/incremental progression of exercise load Standardized protocols for testing and training; loads in ranges necessary for patients Visual feedback of performance (computerized devices) High degree of isolation of lumbar spine improves force production from lumbar extensors Variable resistance allows for consistent load throughout ROM; safety	Relatively expensive ($6000-$8000 for noncomputerized machines) Large size Exercise in one plane or one direction only
Machines	Isokinetic	Standing or seated	Pin loaded weight stack Altering rate of motion	Strength and endurance: isokinetic measurement of workload over full ROM	Gradual/incremental progression of exercise load Standardized protocols for testing and training Loads in ranges necessary for patients Visual feedback of performance (computerized devices)	Torque overshoot Acceleration/ deceleration may lead to harmful impact forces Unnatural movement patterns No known commercial devices are currently manufactured
Benches and Roman chairs	Prone back extensions on bench; fixed-angle Roman chair; VARC	Prone Isotonic Closed chain for upper or lower body, but not both	Dependent on gravity's action on upper body or lower body Alter device angle (VARC) Alter hand position, hip rotation, lumbar posture Hand-held weights	Strength: dynamic strength tests (e.g., 1 repetition max) using external hand-held weights. Endurance: dynamic and isometric (e.g., Sorensen test)	All: simple Low cost Some isolation of lumbar spine VARC: able to accommodate loads in ranges necessary for patients Gradual progression of load Roman chairs: trunk exercise possible in more than one plane More natural movement pattern for lumbar musculature (compared with seated machines) Short learning curve for patients and administrators because of simplicity	Ability to provide the overload necessary to stimulate lumbar extension strength gains is unclear No safe or standardized protocols to assess strength Unable to accommodate loads required for patients without assistance from therapist (prone back extension on bench)

Continued

TABLE 9-1 | **Subtypes of Lumbar Extensor Strengthening Exercises—cont'd**

Type	Examples	Position/Movement	PRE	Measurement	Advantages	Disadvantages
Free weights	Barbells and plates: e.g., stiff-legged dead-lifts; good mornings	Standing Isotonic Closed-chain exercise for lower body	Dependent on gravity's action on upper body or lower body Increase load with metal barbells and plates	Strength: dynamic strength tests (e.g., 1 repetition max) using external hand-held weights Endurance: dynamic	Simple Relatively low cost Gradual progression of load	Potentially unsafe Awkward movements for patients Unable to accommodate loads necessary for patients Unable to standardize load (given the contribution of upper body mass) No isolation Not frequently used for clinical patients
Floor and stability balls	Floor back extension exercise (e.g., "cobra"); stability ball back extension exercise	Prone Isotonic or isometric Closed-chain exercise for upper and/or lower body	Dependent on gravity's action on upper or lower body Increase repetitions	Strength: NA Endurance: dynamic or isometric	Simple Low cost	Unlikely to provide overload stimulus for strength gains Restricted ROM Movement from neutral to extension only (prone floor exercises) Very few, if any, levels of progression within a small range of loads Loads related to progression are unknown or not standardized Labile surface of balls decreases safety

NA, not applicable; PRE, progressive resistance exercise; ROM, range of motion; VARC, variable-angle Roman chair.

Practitioner, Setting, and Availability

Because this type of exercise is used to treat CLBP, it must be prescribed and monitored by licensed clinicians such as physicians, chiropractors, or physical therapists. The actual treatment, however, can be carried out under the supervision of athletic trainers, exercise physiologists, or personal trainers who report periodically to the prescribing clinician. Lumbar strengthening exercise protocols could also be self-administered at fitness facilities without a health care provider, although this is not recommended for CLBP. Various

training and certification courses are offered to clinicians for lumbar strengthening exercise protocols. Despite the lack of regulation, any person delivering exercise therapy should be well versed in the basic principles and practice of exercise testing and prescription for the general population and the particular condition being treated. The typical settings for lumbar strengthening programs are outpatient treatment centers, health and fitness facilities, and athletic training centers under the supervision of trained personnel. There are several commercially available home exercise devices that appear to be suitable for unsupervised lumbar strengthening exercise outside of health care settings. Home exercise may be more appropriate during latter stages of rehabilitation after a formal, supervised exercise program has been completed in a medical or fitness facility. This treatment is readily available throughout the United States.

Procedure

Lumbar Extension Dynamometer

The lumbar dynamometer allows for dynamic exercise through a 72-degree arc in the sagittal plane, with an adjustable weight stack to provide resistance from 9 kg to 364 kg in 0.5-kg increments.[8] Variable resistance is accomplished through a cam with a flexion-extension ratio of 1.4:1. After securing the pelvic restraint mechanisms, the patient begins this exercise in the most flexed position that is pain free, and is instructed to extend their back into a position near terminal extension in a smooth, controlled manner, taking 2 seconds for the concentric phase (lifting the weight) and 4 seconds for the eccentric phase (lowering the weight). The supervising therapist typically provides encouragement to the patient to perform as many repetitions as possible. The machine itself also provides visual feedback on performance via a monitor that displays exercise load and position. When the patient is able to complete 20 or more repetitions with a particular resistance, the resistance is increased in 5% increments at the next training session.[1]

Variable-Angle Roman Chair

The VARC is similar to fixed-angle Roman chairs, except that the angle can be adjusted from 75 degrees (nearly vertical) to 0 degrees (parallel to the ground) in 15-degree increments.[26] Patients typically begin the training program at a low resistance level with an angle setting of 60 degrees with their hands positioned on their sternum. After achieving the correct positioning on the device, the patients start each repetition of dynamic exercise in the extended position and lower their trunk in a smooth, controlled fashion, completing the eccentric phase in 4 seconds. Next, patients raise their torso during the concentric phase in 2 seconds and are verbally encouraged by the supervising therapist to perform as many repetitions as possible. When patients complete 20 to 25 or more repetitions at one angle, resistance is increased. Gradual PRE is achieved by altering the angle setting and the subject's hand position.[25] Internally rotating the hips and accentuating lumbar intersegmental extension during lumbar extension further optimizes targeted muscle activity.[25]

Regulatory Status

Some of the more sophisticated lumbar extensor strengthening machines (e.g., lumbar dynamometer, isokinetic machines, VARCs) are defined as class I or II medical devices with the US Food and Drug Administration (FDA). Specifically, they are classified as 980.5370 (nonmeasuring exercise equipment) or 890.1925 (isokinetic testing and evaluation system). Other equipment used for lumbar extensor

strengthening (e.g., benches, floors, stability balls) is not regulated by the FDA.

THEORY

Mechanism of Action

In general, exercises are used to strengthen muscles, increase soft tissue stability, restore range of movement, improve cardiovascular conditioning, increase proprioception, and reduce fear of movement. The mechanism of action of lumbar extensor strengthening exercise is likely related to the physiologic effects of conditioning the lumbar muscles through PRE, enhancing the metabolic exchange of the lumbar discs through repetitive movement, as well as the psychological mechanisms involving kinesiophobia and locus of control; each is briefly described here.[1,16,18,27]

Conditioning Lumbar Musculature

The lumbar extensor muscles have long been considered the "weak link" in lower trunk function.[9] For patients with CLBP, the lumbar extensors have been described as weak, atrophied, and highly fatigable, displaying abnormal activation patterns and excessive fatty infiltration.[15,28-30] It is therefore reasonable to focus on conditioning these muscles through PREs to improve their physiologic and structural integrity. Reversal of muscular dysfunction and structural abnormalities has been documented in patients with CLBP following lumbar extensor strengthening exercises.[16,31] Both isolation and progressive overload of the lumbar extensors are necessary to achieve these benefits.

Lumbar extensor PREs on machines, benches, or Roman chairs likely provide sufficient isolation and overload to improve lumbar muscular strength and endurance.[9,20,26] Whether or not appropriate isolation and overload actually occur from low load floor exercise (e.g., lumbar stabilization) or stability ball exercise is currently unknown. In a recent study by Sung,[32] no change in the fatigue status of the lumbar multifidus was noted after a 4-week supervised stabilization exercise program. In another study, the effect of three different exercise-training modalities on the cross-sectional area of the lumbar extensor muscles of patients with CLBP was assessed.[33] Stabilization exercise alone was not sufficient to change lumbar muscle cross-sectional area but when combined with dynamic and isometric intensive resistance training, an increase in cross-sectional area of the musculature was noted.

Disc Metabolism

Disc metabolism could potentially be enhanced through repetitive exercise involving the spine's full active range of motion, as performed with lumbar extensor strengthening exercises. Given that the absence of physical activity is known to reduce a healthy metabolism, it appears reasonable to believe that introducing exercise such as lumbar extensor strengthening may reverse such findings.[1] The association between biochemical abnormalities in the lumbar discs and CLBP has previously been documented.[34] Enhanced disc metabolism could improve repair and enhance reuptake of inflammatory and nociceptive mediators that may have migrated to an area of injury.

Psychological Mechanisms

In some patients with particularly severe or prolonged CLBP, or psychological comorbidities such as anxiety or depression, maladaptive illness behavior may become established. This type of behavior may manifest itself as fear of engaging in any activity or movement that has previously been associated with symptoms of CLBP. As time passes, virtually all activities gain this association, leading to a generalized fear of movement in an attempt to minimize exacerbations. Engaging in any form of supervised exercise therapy under the guidance of an experienced clinician able to gradually increase the type, dose, frequency, or intensity of movements can help break this cycle and demonstrate that not all movements are painful. This aspect is discussed further in other chapters of this text (e.g., Section 8—Behavioral Therapies).

Indication

Lumbar extensor strengthening exercises are typically indicated for nonspecific CLBP of mechanical origin.[1] Although these exercises are likely most appropriate for those with CLBP who have suspected or demonstrated deficiencies in muscle strength, endurance, or coordination, they have been shown to be beneficial for those with wide ranges of muscular capacities at treatment onset.[35,36] Based on anecdotal experience, the ideal CLBP patient for this intervention is one who is in good general health, both physically and psychologically, and is willing to take responsibility for his or her own self-care by committing to an active exercise program. As is typical of any strenuous exercise activity, lumbar extensor strengthening exercise may be associated with some short-term discomfort. Thus, the recognition of long-term benefit by the patient and subsequent compliance to the program, despite the possibility of short-term discomfort, optimizes their chance for positive outcomes.

Assessment

Before initiating lumbar extensor strengthening exercises, patients should first be assessed for LBP using an evidence-based and goal-oriented approach focused on the patient history and neurologic examination, as discussed in Chapter 3. Additional diagnostic imaging or specific diagnostic testing is generally not required before initiating these interventions for CLBP. Nevertheless, several diagnostic tests are used clinically to apply the proper and safe dose of exercise, monitor progress throughout treatment, and document that the target muscles are being appropriately activated. These include standardized tests for isometric lumbar extension strength and endurance (e.g., Biering-Sorenson test) and assessment of lumbar muscle activity through real-time ultrasound and surface electromyography.[16,32,37,38] More technologically advanced options to assess lumbar muscle cross-sectional area, fatty infiltration, and activation patterns include magnetic resonance imaging and computed

tomography scanning.[15,39,40] It should be noted that these tests are typically reserved for research settings and are not typically required for clinical practice.

EFFICACY

Evidence supporting the efficacy of these interventions for CLBP was summarized from recent clinical practice guidelines (CPGs), systematic reviews (SRs), and RCTs. Observational studies (OBSs) were also summarized where appropriate. Findings are summarized by study design in the following section.

Clinical Practice Guidelines

None of the recent national CPGs on the management of CLBP have assessed and summarized the evidence to make specific recommendations about the efficacy of lumbar extensor strengthening exercises, though many recommended therapeutic exercise in general for CLBP.

Systematic Reviews

Cochrane Collaboration

The Cochrane Collaboration conducted an SR in 2004 on all forms of exercise therapy for acute, subacute, and chronic LBP.[41] A total of 61 RCTs were identified, including 43 RCTs related to CLBP. Although no specific recommendations were made about the efficacy of lumbar extensor strengthening exercises, the review included two relevant RCTs.[16,42] In addition, it is possible that lumbar extensor strengthening exercises may also have been performed in five more RCTs, although insufficient details are provided in the review to determine this conclusively.[42-46]

Other

Another SR on trunk-strengthening exercises in CLBP also did not provide conclusions that were specific to lumbar extensor exercises.[27] This review included three unique RCTs that may have performed this type of exercise.[20,47,48]

Another SR on the management of back pain identified one additional RCT on lumbar extensor strengthening exercises and one other RCT in which this type of exercise may have been performed.[49-51]

Findings from the aforementioned SRs are summarized in Table 9-2.

Randomized Controlled Trials

Eleven RCTs and 13 reports related to those studies were identified.[16,18,20,33,42,45-48,52-55] Their methods are summarized in Table 9-3. Their results are briefly described here.

An RCT conducted by Manniche and colleagues[20] included CLBP patients without neurologic involvement, who had symptoms lasting longer than 6 months, or had at least three episodes within the past 6 months. Participants were randomly assigned to high- or low-intensity exercise, or to control. Exercise groups consisted of isotonic prone back

TABLE 9-2	Systematic Review Findings on Lumbar Extensor Strengthening Exercises for Chronic Low Back Pain

Reference	# RCTs in SR	#RCTs for CLBP	Conclusion
41	61	43	Results for exercise therapy were generally favorable; however, no specific results were made to lumbar extensor strengthening exercises

CLBP, chronic low back pain; RCT, randomized controlled trial; SR, systematic review.

TABLE 9-3	Randomized Controlled Trials Included in Systematic Reviews

Reference	Indication	Intervention	Control (C1)	Control (C2)	Control (C3)	Control (C4)
20	LBP without neurologic involvement, symptoms >6 months or 3+ episodes in past 6 months	LES-high: isotonic prone back extension on bench—leg lift and trunk lift; latissimus pull down (plate-loaded cable machine) + hot packs; general flexibility exercises PT Up to 10 repetitions/set, up to 10 sets, 2-3×/wk, 3 months, PRE-increase reptitions and load n = 35	LES-low: same exercises as LES-high + hot packs; general flexibility exercises PT ⅕ of the exercise dose/session as intervention n = 35	Mild floor trunk exercises—isometric prone back extension, isometric trunk curl, dynamic trunk curl + hot packs; general flexibility exercises PT 1 hr (1 set, 10 repetitions/set) × 8 in 1 month; 2 months no treatment n = 35	NA	NA
48	CLBP without neurologic involvement, duration of symptoms NR	LES: isotonic prone back extension on bench (leg lift and trunk lift—performed to 0-degree lumbar extension) + latissimus pull down (plate-loaded cable machine) (up to 10 repetitions/set, up to 10 sets, 2×/wk, 3 months, PRE-increase repetitions and load) + abdominal crunch (50 repetitions/set, 1 set) + hot packs PT 1-1.5 hr × 2/wk × 3 months n = 31	LES-EXT: same as LES, except prone back extensions performed to greatest possible lumbar extension position + hot packs PT 1-1.5 hr × 2/wk × 3 months n = 31	NA	NA	NA
16	CLBP, with and without neurologic involvement, symptoms >1 year	LES: isolated lumbar extension machine, seated, isotonic (8-12 repetitions/set, 1 set, 1-2×/wk, 10 wk, PRE-increase load) PT 2/wk for 4 wk; 1/wk for 6 wk n = 31	No treatment, waiting list n = 23	NA	NA	NA

Continued

TABLE 9-3   Randomized Controlled Trials Included in Systematic Reviews—cont'd

Reference	Indication	Intervention	Control (C1)	Control (C2)	Control (C3)	Control (C4)
47	CLBP without neurologic involvement, symptoms >6 months	LES: lumbar extension, lumbar flexion, lateral flexion, and rotation machines, isotonic and isokinetic, seated and standing; latissimus pull down + bike (10 min) PT 10 repetitions/set, 1 set, 3×/wk, 8 wk, PRE-increase load n = 50	Lumbar stabilization and McKenzie-type extension exercises + home exercise with same movements PT 10 repetitions/set, 2-3 sets, 3×/wk, 8 wk + home exercise daily n = 50	SMT to lumbar spine PT 3×/wk, 8 wk n = 50	Passive therapies including hot packs, TENS, ultrasound PT 3×/wk, 8 wk n = 50	No treatment n = 50
46	CLBP without neurologic involvement, symptoms >3 months	LES: isolated lumbar extension, lumbar flexion, lateral flexion, and rotation machines, isotonic, seated (repetitions/set, NR; set, NR; PRE-increase load); flexibility and relaxation exercises; behavioral support; ergonomic advice; home back exercises PT 2×/wk, 12 wk n = 30	Weeks 1-8, no intervention; weeks 9-12, massage, thermal therapy PT 1 session/wk n = 24	NA	NA	NA
52 53 45	CLBP with or without neurologic involvement, symptoms >3 months	LES: isolated lumbar extension, lumbar flexion, lateral flexion, and rotation machines, isotonic, seated (repetitions/set—NR, set-NR, PRE-increase load); bike (5- 10 min); flexibility and relaxation exercises PT 1-hr sessions ×2/wk × 3 months n = 49	Individual physical therapy to improve functional capacity using unspecified strengthening, coordination, and aerobic exercise (30 min); ergonomic instruction; home exercise PT 1-hr sessions × 3 months n = 49	Group low impact aerobic classes— aerobics, flexibility exercise, trunk and leg muscle exercise; relaxation exercise 1-hr sessions × 3 months PT n = 50	NA	NA
42	LBP, without neurologic involvement, symptoms >6 months or intermittent for >2 years	LES: isolated lumbar extension machine, seated isotonic (1 set—up to 11 repetitions, PRE-increase load); resistance exercise for the abdominal and thigh muscles PT 1-2×/wk × 12 wk n = 30	Whole-body vibration exercise PT 1-2×/wk × 12 wk n = 30	NA	NA	NA

TABLE 9-3   **Randomized Controlled Trials Included in Systematic Reviews—cont'd**

Reference	Indication	Intervention	Control (C1)	Control (C2)	Control (C3)	Control (C4)
54	CLBP without neurologic involvement, symptoms >1 year and >3 months in last year	LES: isotonic prone back extension on bench (leg lift and trunk lift performed to 0-degree lumbar extension); latissimus pull down (plate-loaded cable machine); abdominal crunch (up to 10 repetitions/set, up to 10 sets, PRE-increase repetitions or load); bike (10 min); flexibility exercise (10 min) PT 1 hr × 2×/wk, 3 months n = 20	Group exercises emphasizing coordination, balance, and stability for the low back, shoulder, and hip (up to 40 repetitions/set, 1 set); warm-up including jogging (10 min); flexibility exercise (10 min) PT 1 hr × 2×/wk, 3 months n = 20	NA	NA	NA
33	CLBP, neurologic involvement NR, symptoms >3 months	LES-DYN: isotonic prone back extension on bench-leg lift and trunk lift; leg lift floor exercise (15-18 repetitions/set, volume NR; maintain 70% of 1 repetition max; PRE-increase repetitions and load); lumbar stabilization floor exercises PT 3/wk × 10 wk n = 20	LES-STATIC: same as LES-DYN, except alternate between isotonic and isometric exercise PT 3/wk × 10 wk n = 20	Lumbar stabilization floor exercises PT 3/wk × 10 wk n = 19	NA	NA
18	LBP, without neurologic involvement, symptoms >12 wk (continuous or recurrent)	LES-HIGH (high-intensity training): isolated lumbar extension machine, seated, isotonic (10-20 repetitions/set, 1 set, start at 35% peak strength, PRE-increase load) PT 1-2×/wk × 12 wk n = 41	LES-LOW (low intensity training): isolated lumbar extension machine, seated, isotonic (10–20 repetitions/set, 1 set, start at 20% peak strength, PRE-none) PT 1- 2×/wk × 12 wk n = 40	NA	NA	NA
55	CLBP with neurologic involvement, symptom duration NR	LES: isolated lumbar extension machine, isotonic, seated (repetitions NR, 1 set, PRE-increase load); aerobic exercise; limb-strengthening exercise PT Frequency NR, 12 wk n = 40	Home-based lumbar conditioning exercise Self-care 12 wk n = 40	NA	NA	NA

CLBP, chronic low back pain; LBP, low back pain; LES, lumbar extensor strengthening; NA, not applicable; NR, not reported; PRE, progressive resistance exercise; PT, physical therapist; SMT, spinal manipulation therapy; TENS, transcutaneous electrical nerve stimulation.

extension exercises on a bench and latissimus pull down exercises (plate-loaded cable machine); the high-intensity group performed five times as many sets as the low-intensity group. The control group performed light floor exercises. Cointerventions for all groups consisted of thermotherapy and massage. Treatment was administered 2 to 3 times per week for 10 weeks. At the 1 year follow-up, pain and disability (Low Back Pain Rating Scale composite score) improved in all three groups compared with before treatment (P values not reported). There were no statistically significant differences between groups at this follow-up.

In another RCT by Manniche and colleagues,[48] individuals with CLBP without neurologic involvement who had surgery for lumbar disc protrusion were randomly assigned to receive intensive dynamic back extensor exercise with or without hyperextension. Back extensor exercises were similar to those used by the high-intensity group in the previous study.[20] The hyperextension group performed dynamic exercise to terminal lumbar extension, whereas the other group stopped at the neutral lumbar position. Cointerventions for both groups were hot packs and abdominal crunches. Treatment was administered twice a week for 3 months. Outcomes (including pain and disability) were assessed with the LBP rating scale composite score. At 15 months, there was an improvement in the LBP rating scale composite score in both groups compared with before treatment (P values not reported), but the difference between groups was not statistically significant.

In an RCT by Risch and colleagues,[16] individuals with CLBP with or without neurologic involvement and with symptoms lasting longer than 1 year were randomized to receive lumbar extensor strengthening exercise or control. The lumbar strengthening group performed isolated lumbar extensor PREs on a variable resistance dynamometer machine 1 to 2 times per week for 10 weeks. The control group was wait-listed and received no intervention. At 10 weeks, the lumbar strengthening exercise group displayed improvements in pain intensity (West Haven-Yale Multidimensional Pain Inventory) compared with before treatment (P values not reported). The improvement was significantly greater than that of the control group. This study was considered of lower quality.

In an RCT by Timm,[47] individuals with CLBP without neurologic involvement who had symptoms lasting longer than 6 months and had one-level L5 laminectomy, were randomly assigned to: (1) lumbar strengthening exercise; (2) lumbar stabilization and extension range of motion exercise; (3) spinal manipulation; (4) passive modalities including hot packs, transcutaneous electrical nerve stimulation, and ultrasound; or (5) no treatment control. The lumbar strengthening exercise group performed lumbar extensor PREs on isokinetic and isotonic machines. Cointerventions for the strengthening exercise group included lumbar flexion and rotation, latissimus dorsi PREs on machines, and bike exercise. Treatments were administered 3 times per week for 8 weeks. At 8 weeks, improvements in disability (Oswestry Disability Index [ODI]) were observed in all groups, with the largest improvements in the lumbar extensor and stabilization exercise groups. The improvements in disability for the

lumbar extensor exercise and stabilization exercise groups were significantly greater than the spinal manipulation, passive modalities, and control groups.

In an RCT by Kankaanpaa and colleagues,[46] individuals with CLBP without neurologic involvement who had symptoms lasting longer than 3 months were randomly assigned to lumbar strengthening exercise or control. The lumbar strengthening exercise group performed isolated lumbar extensor PREs on machines twice a week for 12 weeks. Cointerventions for this group included lumbar flexion, lateral flexion, and rotation PREs on machines, flexibility and relaxation exercises, behavioral support, ergonomic advice, and home back exercises. The control group received no intervention for 9 weeks and massage and thermotherapy for 3 weeks. At 12 months, there was a statistically significant improvement in pain (visual analog scale [VAS]) and disability (Pain Disability Index [PDI]) scores in the lumbar strengthening group compared with baseline, but not in the control group. The improvements in each outcome were significantly greater for the lumbar strengthening group than for control. This study was considered of lower quality.

In an RCT by Mannion and colleagues,[45,52,53] individuals with CLBP with or without neurologic involvement with symptoms lasting longer than 3 months were randomly assigned to lumbar strengthening exercise along with cointerventions, physical therapy, or aerobic exercise. The lumbar strengthening exercise group performed isolated lumbar extensor strengthening PREs as described by Kankaanpaa and colleagues,[46] along with cointerventions consisting of lumbar flexion, lateral flexion, and rotation PREs on machines; as well as bicycle, flexibility, and relaxation exercises. The physical therapy group performed individual physical therapy to improve functional capacity using unspecified strengthening, coordination, and aerobic exercise, along with ergonomic instruction and home exercise. The aerobic exercise group performed low-impact aerobics classes. Interventions were administered twice a week for 3 months. At 12 months, pain scores (VAS) improved similarly in all three groups (P values not reported). There were no significant differences in pain scores between groups. At 12 months, disability scores (Roland Morris Disability Questionnaire [RMDQ]) improved in all three groups (P values not reported). The improvement in disability in the aerobics and muscle conditioning groups was significantly higher than that of the physical therapy group. This study was considered of higher quality.

In an RCT by Rittweger and colleagues,[42] individuals with CLBP without neurologic involvement were randomly assigned to lumbar strengthening exercise or vibration therapy. The lumbar strengthening exercise group performed isolated lumbar extensor PREs on a variable resistance lumbar dynamometer machine as described by Risch and colleagues,[16] along with cointerventions of resistance exercise for the abdominal and thigh muscles. Interventions were administered 1 to 2 times per week for 12 weeks. At 12 weeks, pain scores (VAS) improved significantly in both groups, but there were no significant differences between groups. At 6 months, disability scores (PDI) also improved in both groups, but without significant difference between groups. This study was considered of lower quality.

In an RCT by Johannsen and colleagues,[54] individuals with CLBP for at least 1 year without neurologic involvement and who had symptoms lasting longer than 3 months in the past year were randomly assigned to receive lumbar strengthening exercise or the control group. The lumbar strengthening exercise group performed prone back extension exercises as described by Manniche and colleagues.[20] Cointerventions included abdominal crunch exercises. The control group performed group exercises emphasizing balance and stability for the low back, shoulders, and hips. Cointerventions for both groups included flexibility and bike exercise. Treatments were administered twice a week for 3 months. At 6 months, there was a significant improvement in pain scores (0-8 scale) in both groups. There was also a significant improvement in disability scores (0-12 scale) in both groups. However, there were no significant differences between the groups for either outcome. This study was considered of lower quality.

In an RCT by Danneels and colleagues,[33] individuals with CLBP lasting longer than 3 months were randomly assigned to dynamic lumbar strengthening exercises with and without isometric contractions combined with lumbar stabilization exercise or lumbar stabilization exercise alone. The lumbar strengthening exercise groups performed prone back extension exercises as described by Manniche and colleagues[20] with or without alternating isometric contractions at terminal extension. Interventions were administered for 10 weeks at 3 sessions a week. Pain and disability outcomes were not measured in this study.

In an RCT by Helmhout and colleagues,[18] individuals with LBP without neurologic involvement, who had continuous or recurrent symptoms for longer than 12 weeks, were assigned to high- or low-intensity lumbar strengthening exercise. Both groups performed isolated lumbar extensor strengthening exercises on machines 1 to 2 times per week for 12 weeks. The high-intensity group performed PREs by increasing exercise load, whereas the low-intensity group performed the same low load (20% peak strength from baseline measurement) throughout the entire exercise program. At 9 months, there was a greater proportion of participants in both groups reporting improved pain compared with baseline (P values not reported). There was also an improvement in disability scores (RMDQ, ODI) in both groups (P values not reported). There were no significant differences between the groups in pain intensity or disability.

In an RCT by Choi and colleagues,[55] individuals with CLBP with neurologic involvement and who had undergone lumbar discectomy were randomly assigned to lumbar extensor strengthening exercise or home exercise. The lumbar extensor strengthening group performed isolated lumbar extensor PREs on a variable resistance lumbar dynamometer machine as described by Risch and colleagues,[16] along with cointerventions of aerobic and limb-strengthening exercise for 12 weeks at an unspecified frequency. At 12 months, there was a significant improvement in pain (VAS) in both groups, but there was no difference between the groups. At 12 weeks

(after treatment period), disability (ODI) was improved in both groups but there were no significant differences between the groups. Disability was not measured at the 12-month follow-up.

SAFETY

Contraindications

Contraindications to lumbar strengthening exercises are those relevant to any PRE training as outlined by the American College of Sport Medicine.[56] These include unstable angina, systolic blood pressure ≥160 mm Hg, diastolic blood pressure ≥ 100 mm Hg, uncontrolled dysrhythmia, recent history of untreated congestive heart failure, severe stenotic or regurgitant valvular disease, hypertrophic cardiomyopathy, poor left ventricular function, and angina or ischemia at low workloads (<5 to 6 metabolic equivalent of task [METs]). Other contraindications for CLBP include spinal fracture, infection, dislocation, or tumor.

Osteoporosis is frequently listed as an exclusion criterion for participants in RCTs of lumbar extensor strengthening exercises, presumably under the assumption that overload could result in fractures. However, studies have demonstrated that lumbar training with PRE significantly improved lumbar vertebral body bone density after heart and lung transplantation.[57,58] It is therefore possible that spinal osteoporosis could in fact be improved with a gradual, controlled, and measured increase in resistance using isolated lumbar extensor strengthening exercises. An observational study reported that lumbar strength training with PRE on machines was safe and improved functional capacity in older adults with CLBP.[59]

Noncompliance is probably the most significant predictor of negative outcomes for lumbar strengthening exercise. This treatment requires active patient participation for many exercise sessions, lasting from several weeks to a few months. Thus, motivation and willingness to participate for an extended period of time are necessary to gain the physiologic benefit of improved function by way of an active exercise program. Predictors of negative outcome for other conservative therapies for CLBP (e.g., yellow flags) are also likely to apply to this intervention.

Adverse Events

Performance of intensive lumbar extensor strengthening exercise may result in delayed onset muscle soreness (DOMS) of the lumbar muscles.[60] DOMS occurs as a consequence of unfamiliar strenuous physical activity, especially during the first few days or weeks of performance. Typically, symptoms of lumbar DOMS include a mild increase in pain and stiffness, which peaks at approximately 24 to 72 hours after initial exercise sessions and rapidly attenuates.[61] This is a normal response to vigorous exercise and is not associated with any long-term adverse events when exercise is appropriately administered under supervision. Temporary effects, including increased LBP and dizziness, were reported in 3 of the 11 RCTs reviewed.[20,48,54]

Every physical activity is associated with some risk of rare adverse events. Intensive lumbar extensor strengthening exercise performed under load is associated with a small risk of musculoskeletal injury, including lumbar disc herniation and fracture. Individuals with cardiovascular disease may also be at risk of cardiovascular adverse events during strenuous exercise.

TABLE 9-4	Medicare Fee Schedule for Related Services	
CPT Code	New York	California
97001	$73	$78
97002	$40	$43
97110	$30	$32
97112	$31	$33
97530	$32	$35
97750	$21	$33

2010 Participating, nonfacility amount.

COSTS

Fees and Third-Party Reimbursement

In the United States, lumbar strengthening exercise that is supervised by a licensed health practitioner such as a physical therapist in an outpatient setting can be delivered using CPT codes 97110 (therapeutic exercises, each 15 minutes), 97112 (neuromuscular reeducation, each 15 minutes), or 97530 (therapeutic activities, each 15 minutes). The initial evaluation of lumbar function can be delivered using CPT codes 97001 (physical therapy initial evaluation) or 97750 (physical performance test or measurement, each 15 minutes). Periodic reevaluation of lumbar function can be delivered using CPT codes 97002 (physical therapy reevaluation) or 97750 (physical performance test or measurement, each 15 minutes).

These procedures are widely covered by other third-party payers such as health insurers and worker's compensation insurance. Although some payers continue to base their reimbursements on usual, customary, and reasonable payment methodology, the majority have developed reimbursement tables based on the Resource Based Relative Value Scale used by Medicare. Reimbursements by other third-party payers are generally higher than Medicare.

Third-party payers will often reimburse a limited number of visits to licensed health care providers if they are prescribed by a physician and supported by adequate documentation deeming them medically necessary. Equipment or products required for those interventions are rarely typically considered inclusive in the procedure reported and are not separately reportable. Given the need to maintain the gains achieved in muscular function through lumbar strengthening, patients are often encouraged to continue this intervention beyond the initial period of supervised exercise therapy. The cost for membership in a private exercise facility is generally $50 to $100 per month. Some insurers in the United States also provide discounted membership fees to exercise facilities to their members to promote physical activity.

Typical fees reimbursed by Medicare in New York and California for these services are summarized in Table 9-4.

Cost Effectiveness

Evidence supporting the cost effectiveness of treatment protocols that compared these interventions, often in combination with one or more co-interventions, with control groups who received one or more other interventions, for either acute or chronic LBP, was identified from two SRs on this topic and is summarized in the following paragraphs.[62,63] Although many of these study designs are unable to clearly identify the individual contribution of any intervention, their results provide some insight as to the clinical and economic outcomes associated with these approaches.

An RCT in Norway compared three approaches for patients with CLBP.[64] Participants received either a light multidisciplinary program consisting of education, fear avoidance training, and advice to remain active given by a physical therapist, nurse, and psychologist, an extensive multidisciplinary program consisting of daily group sessions with cognitive behavioral therapy, education, fear avoidance training, and strengthening and stabilization exercises for 4 weeks, or usual care by a general practitioner and possibly a physical therapist or chiropractor. Direct medical costs for the light and extensive multidisciplinary programs were estimated by dividing the total clinic costs for 1 year by the number of patients treated; direct costs were therefore assumed to be equal in both groups, regardless of large differences in time spent by clinic staff with patients in each group. Indirect productivity costs associated with lost work time were evaluated over 24 months. A limited cost-benefit analysis for male participants only reported that the light multidisciplinary program would yield average savings of approximately $19,544 per patient over 2 years, and was therefore cost effective compared with usual care.

An RCT in the United States compared two approaches for patients with acute LBP.[65] The first group received care according to the classification of symptoms and examination findings by a physical therapist, including possibly spinal manipulation; mobilization; traction therapy; and flexion, extension, strengthening, or stabilization exercises. The second group received brief education and general exercise from a physical therapist according to recommendations from CPGs, which were not specified. Clinical outcomes after 1 year favored the therapy according to classification group for improvement in function, although no differences were noted in the SF-36. Direct medical costs associated with the study interventions over 1 year were $604 in the therapy according to classification group and $682 in the CPG recommended care group; direct costs for all interventions over 1 year were $883 and $1160, respectively. Indirect productivity costs associated with lost productivity were not reported, although fewer participants in the therapy according to classification group had missed work due to LBP after 12 months.

An RCT in Finland compared three approaches for patients with acute LBP in an occupational health center.[66] The bed rest group was prescribed complete bed rest for two days, after which they were instructed to resume normal activities. The back exercise group received supervised exercise therapy by a physical therapist, including extension and lateral bending exercises every other hour. The active group received advice to remain active. Clinical outcomes after 12 weeks favored the active group for pain and function when compared with the bed rest group. Direct medical costs associated with study and nonstudy interventions over 12 weeks were $144 in the bed rest group, $165 in the back exercise group, and $123 in the active group. Direct medical costs associated with home help over 12 weeks were $90 in the bed rest group, $232 in the back exercise group, and $45 in active group. Indirect productivity costs were not estimated, although the number of lost work days favored the active group. Authors concluded that if indirect productivity costs had been monetized, the active group would be favored.

An RCT from Canada compared two approaches for patients who had been injured at work and subsequently suffered from CLBP.[67] The functional restoration group included cognitive behavioral therapy, fear avoidance training, education, biofeedback, and group counseling, as well as strengthening and stretching exercises. The usual care group could receive a variety of interventions, including physical therapy, acupuncture, back school, spinal manipulation, medication, or supervised exercise therapy. Clinical outcomes were not reported. Direct medical costs associated with the study interventions were $2507 higher in the functional restoration group. Indirect productivity costs associated with lost work days were $3172 lower in the functional restoration group. Total costs for interventions, lost work days, and disability pensions were $7068 lower in the functional restoration group. These differences were not statistically significant.

In an RCT in the United Kingdom researchers compared two approaches for patients with subacute or chronic LBP.[68] The supervised exercise therapy group received up to eight sessions of stretching, strengthening, and aerobic exercises, and brief education on LBP. The usual care group received interventions prescribed by a general practitioner, including physical therapy in some cases. Clinical outcomes after 1 year favored the supervised exercise therapy group for improvement in pain, function, and utility. Direct medical costs associated with study and nonstudy interventions over 12 months were $145 in the supervised exercise therapy group and approximately $185 in the usual care group. Indirect productivity costs associated with lost work days over 12 months were approximately $456 in the supervised exercise therapy group and approximately $663 in the usual care group. Total costs (direct medical and indirect productivity) over 12 months were therefore approximately $621 in the supervised exercise therapy group and approximately $848 in the usual care group. These differences in costs were not statistically significant.

Findings from the aforementioned cost effectiveness analyses are summarized in Table 9-5.

SUMMARY

Description

The term *lumbar extensor* is used colloquially to refer to the erector spinae muscle group, which is comprised of the iliocostalis lumborum, longissimus thoracis, and spinalis thoracis. The lumbar multifidus muscle is also a target of lumbar extensor strengthening exercise. Strengthening exercise is also known as PRE, which is based on the principles of overload (i.e., making muscles function beyond their current capacity by increasing the intensity and volume of exercises), specificity (i.e., isolating the targeted muscle), reversibility (i.e., long-term commitment to exercise program), frequency (i.e., number of sessions per week), intensity (i.e., amount of resistance and number of repetitions), repetitions, volume (i.e., number of sets performed at one time), duration (i.e., total length of exercise program), and mode (i.e., specific type of exercise and equipment used). Lumbar extensor strengthening is widely available across the United States. Because it is used to treat CLBP, it must be prescribed and monitored by licensed clinicians such as physicians, chiropractors, or physical therapists. The actual treatment, however, can be carried out under the supervision of athletic trainers, exercise physiologists, or personal trainers who report periodically to the prescribing clinician. The typical settings for lumbar strengthening programs are outpatient treatment centers, health and fitness facilities, and athletic training centers under the supervision of trained personnel. There are several commercially available home exercise devices that appear to be suitable for unsupervised lumbar strengthening exercise outside of health care settings. Home exercise may be more appropriate during latter stages of rehabilitation after a formal, supervised exercise program has been completed in a medical or fitness facility.

Theory

In general, exercises are used to strengthen muscles, increase soft tissue stability, restore range of movement, improve cardiovascular conditioning, increase proprioception, and reduce fear of movement. The mechanism of action of lumbar extensor strengthening exercise is likely related to the physiologic effects of conditioning the lumbar muscles through PRE. Disc metabolism may also be enhanced through repetitive exercise involving the spine's full active range of motion, improving repair and enhancing reuptake of inflammatory and nociceptive mediators. In addition, in some patients with particularly severe or prolonged CLBP or psychological comorbidities such as anxiety or depression, maladaptive illness behavior may occur, leading to fear of engaging in any activity or movement previously associated with the CLBP. Engaging in supervised exercise therapy under the guidance of an experienced clinician can help break this cycle and demonstrate that not all movements or activities need be painful. Lumbar extensor strengthening exercises are typically indicated for nonspecific CLBP of mechanical origin. Diagnostic imaging or other forms of advanced testing

| TABLE 9-5 | Cost Effectiveness and Cost Utility Analyses on Lumbar Extensor Strengthening Exercises for Acute or Chronic Low Back Pain |

Ref Country Follow-up	Group	Direct Costs	Indirect Costs	Total Costs	Conclusion
64 Norway 2 years	1. light multidisciplinary program 2. extensive multidisciplinary program (inc. strengthening exercises) 3. usual care	NR	NR	NR	Group 1: average savings of $19,544/ patient over 2 years
65 United States 1 year	1. care according to classification of symptoms 2. brief education + general exercise	1. $883 2. $1160	NR	NR	No conclusion as to cost effectiveness
66 Finland 12 weeks	1. bed rest 2. back exercise 3. advice to remain active	1. $234 2. $397 3. $168	NR	Were not estimated	If indirect costs had been monetized, group 3 would be favored
67 Canada NR	1. functional restoration (including strengthening exercises) 2. usual care	1. $2507 higher than group 2 2. NR	1. $3172 lower than group 2 for lost work days 2. NR	1. $7068 lower than group 2 (lost work days + disability pensions)	No significant difference
68 United Kingdom 1 year	1. supervised exercise therapy 2. usual care	1. $145 2. $185	1. $456 2. $663	1. $601 2. $848	No significant difference

NR, not reported.

are generally not required before administering lumbar extensor strengthening exercises for CLBP.

Efficacy

None of the recent national CPGs provide specific recommendations for managing CLBP with lumbar extensor strengthening exercises, though most recommended therapeutic exercises in general. SRs were also not identified specifically on lumbar extensor strengthening exercises for CLBP, though SRs on therapeutic exercises for LBP generally reported favorable outcomes. Eleven RCTs reported generally favorable short- and long-term results with lumbar extensor strengthening exercises for CLBP. Improvements were generally noted for both pain and physical function when compared with other forms of exercise or other conservative therapies.

Safety

Contraindications to lumbar strengthening exercise include angina, systolic blood pressure ≥160 mm Hg, diastolic blood pressure ≥100 mm Hg, uncontrolled dysrhythmia,

recent history of untreated congestive heart failure, severe stenotic or regurgitant valvular disease, hypertrophic cardiomyopathy, poor left ventricular function, angina or ischemia at low workloads (<5 to 6 METs), spinal fracture, infection, dislocation, and tumor. Adverse events include delayed onset muscle soreness, increase in pain, and stiffness. Intensive lumbar extensor strengthening exercise performed under load is associated with a small risk of musculoskeletal injury, including lumbar disc herniation and fracture. Individuals with cardiovascular disease may also be at risk of cardiovascular adverse events during strenuous exercise.

Costs

The Medicare reimbursement for treatment with lumbar strengthening exercise in an outpatient setting by licensed health practitioners (e.g., physical therapists) ranges from $21 to $78, depending on the duration and type of session (e.g., assessment, reevaluation). At least five studies examined the cost effectiveness of lumbar strengthening exercise for CLBP, yet the individual contribution of lumbar strengthening exercise to the overall cost effectiveness could not be determined because the RCTs examined many other interventions at the same time.

Comments

Evidence from the CPGs and SRs reviewed generally did not make any recommendations specifically about lumbar extensor strengthening exercises for CLBP. However, summary findings on back exercises for CLBP were mostly positive. The RCTs reviewed reported favorable short- and long-term results with lumbar extensor strengthening exercises for CLBP. Improvements were noted for both pain and physical function when this intervention was compared with other forms of exercise or other conservative therapies. The relative efficacy of the various subtypes of back exercises for the treatment of CLBP, however, has not been assessed in RCTs.

Well-designed and conducted RCTs with larger sample sizes, well-defined patient groups, and long-term outcomes are needed to assess the efficacy of lumbar extensor strengthening exercise for CLBP versus other interventions. Of particular interest are RCTs comparing different exercise programs, administered alone or alongside other interventions, with or without supervision from a health care professional.

Future research is needed to develop and test classification systems to distinguish responders from nonresponders regarding lumbar extensor strengthening exercise for CLBP. The optimal dose of strengthening exercise needs to be clarified, including exercise intensity, frequency, volume, and duration. Similarly, the optimal mode needs to be established (e.g., costly machines vs. low-cost options), and supervised vs. unsupervised exercise programs. Future studies on the mechanisms of action of lumbar strengthening exercise would be useful to determine if tissue loading, repetitive movement, psychological factors, or a combination of these is responsible for the intervention's beneficial effects.

CHAPTER REVIEW QUESTIONS

Answers are located on page 450.

1. Which of the following is not a subcategory of therapeutic exercise?
   a. aerobic
   b. aquatic
   c. stabilization
   d. mindful breathing
2. Which of the following is not a subtype of lumbar strengthening exercise protocols?
   a. benches and Roman chairs
   b. aquatic
   c. free weights
   d. floor and stability balls
3. How many weeks of resistance training are required to achieve physiologic changes in skeletal structure?
   a. 2-4
   b. 4-6
   c. 8-10
   d. 10-12

4. Which of the following descriptions of dynamic exercise is correct?
   a. isotonic exercise is muscle contraction at fixed length
   b. isotonic exercise is muscle contraction at fixed resistance
   c. isokinetic exercise is muscle contraction at fixed length
   d. isokinetic exercise is muscle contraction at fixed resistance
5. Which of the following are contraindications to lumbar strengthening exercises?
   a. post exercise muscle soreness
   b. unstable angina
   c. lack of motivation
   d. shortness of breath after vigorous running
6. Which of the following is not associated with the mechanism of action for lumbar extensor strengthening?
   a. strengthening muscles
   b. increasing tendon stability
   c. increasing fear avoidance behavior
   d. restoring collagen in the joint
7. What was a major advancement in the development of lumbar extensor strengthening for CLBP?
   a. Hippocrates' rejection of superstition
   b. Thomas De Lorme's mastering of lumbar extensor strengthening technique
   c. Bergmark's Roman chair invention
   d. Zander's development of the medical mechanical therapy technique
8. What are some of the side effects associated with lumbar extensor strengthening?
   a. herniated disc
   b. tight tendons
   c. muscle soreness
   d. light-headedness

REFERENCES

1. Mooney V, Verna J, Morris C. Clinical management of chronic, disabling low back syndromes. In: Morris C, editor. Low back syndromes: integrated clinical management. New York: McGraw-Hill; 2006.
2. Bogduk N. A reappraisal of the anatomy of the human lumbar erector spinae. J Anat 1980;131:525-540.
3. MacIntosh J, Bogduk N. The attachments of the lumbar erector spinae. Spine 1991;16:783-792.
4. Bogduk N, Twomey L. Clinical anatomy of the lumbar spine. New York: Churchill Livingstone; 1990.
5. American College of Sports Medicine. ACSM's resource manual for guidelines for exercise testing and prescription. New York: Lippincott Williams & Wilkins; 2005.
6. Pollock M, Graves J, Carpenter D, et al. Muscle. In: Hochschuler S, Guyer R, Cotler H, editors. Rehabilitation of the spine: science and practice. St. Louis: Mosby; 1993.
7. Mooney V. The unguarded moment. A surgeon's discovery of the barriers to the prescription of inexpensive, effective health care in the form of therapeutic exercise. New York: Vantage Press; 2007.

8. Graves J, Pollock M, Carpenter D, et al. Quantitative assessment of full range-of-motion isometric lumbar extension strength. Spine 1990;15:289-294.

9. Pollock M, Leggett S, Graves J, et al. Effect of resistance training on lumbar extension strength. Am J Sports Med 1989;17:624-629.

10. Graves J, Webb D, Pollock M, et al. Pelvic stabilization during resistance training: its effect on the development of lumbar extension strength. Arch Phys Med Rehabil 1994;75:210-215.

11. Mayer J, Verna J, Manini T, et al. Electromyographic activity of the trunk extensor muscles: effect of varying hip position and lumbar posture during Roman chair exercise. Arch Phys Med Rehabil 2002;83:1543-1546.

12. Tucci J, Carpenter D, Pollock M, et al. Effect of reduced frequency of training and detraining on lumbar extension strength. Spine 1992;17:1497-1501.

13. American College of Sports Medicine. ACSM's guidelines for exercise testing and prescription. New York: Lippincott Williams & Wilkins; 2005.

14. Kumar S, Dufresne R, Van Schoor T. Human trunk strength profile in flexion and extension. Spine 1995;20:160-168.

15. Mooney V, Gulick J, Perlman M, et al. Relationships between myoelectric activity, strength, and MRI of the lumbar extensor muscles in back pain patients and normal subjects. J Spinal Disord 1997;10:348-356.

16. Risch S, Norvell N, Pollock M, et al. Lumbar strengthening in chronic low back pain patients. Physiologic and psychological benefits. Spine 1993;18:232-238.

17. Rainville J, Jouve C, Hartigan C, et al. Comparison of short- and long-term outcomes for aggressive spine rehabilitation delivered two versus three times per week. Spine J 2002;2:402-407.

18. Helmhout P, Harts C, Staal J, et al. Comparison of a high-intensity and a low-intensity lumbar extensor training program as minimal intervention treatment in low back pain: a randomized trial. Eur Spine J 2004;13:537-547.

19. Graves J, Pollock M, Foster D, et al. Effect of training frequency and specificity on isometric lumbar extension strength. Spine 1990;15:504-509.

20. Manniche C, Lundberg E, Christiansen I, et al. Intensive dynamic back exercises for chronic low back pain: a clinical trial. Pain 1991;47:53-63.

21. Zander G. OM Medico-Mekaniska Instituteti Stockholm. J Nord Medical Archive 1872;Band IV(9).

22. De Lorme T. Restoration of muscle power by heavy-resistance exercises. J Bone Joint Surg Am 1945;27:645-667.

23. Alaranta H, Hurri H, Heliovaara M, et al. Non-dynamometric trunk performance tests: reliability and normative data. Scand J Rehabil Med 1994;26:211-215.

24. Ostelo R, de Vet H, Waddell G, et al. Rehabilitation following first-time lumbar disc surgery: a systematic review within the framework of the Cochrane collaboration. Spine 2003;28:209-218.

25. Mayer J, Graves J, Robertson V, et al. Electromyographic activity of the lumbar extensor muscles: effect of angle and hand position during Roman chair exercise. Arch Phys Med Rehabil 1999;80:751-755.

26. Verna J, Mayer J, Mooney V, et al. Back extension endurance and strength: effect of variable angle Roman chair exercise training. Spine 2002;27:1772-1777.

27. Slade S, Keating J. Trunk-strengthening exercises for chronic low back pain: a systematic review. J Manipulative Physiol Ther 2006;29:163-173.

28. Cassisi J, Robinson M, O'Conner P, et al. Trunk strength and lumbar paraspinal muscle activity during isometric exercise in chronic low back pain patients and controls. Spine 1993;18:245-251.

29. Hakkinen A, Kuukkanen T, Tarvainen U, et al. Trunk muscle strength in flexion, extension, and axial rotation in patients managed with lumbar disc herniation surgery and in healthy control subjects. Spine 2003;28:1068-1073.

30. Kankaanpaa M, Taimela S, Laaksonen D, et al. Back and hip extensor fatigability in chronic low back pain patients and controls. Arch Phys Med Rehabil 1998;79:412-417.

31. Parkkola R, Kujala U, Rytokoski U. Response of the trunk muscles to training assessed by magnetic resonance imaging and muscle strength. Eur J Appl Physiol 1992;65:383-387.

32. Sung P. Multifidi muscles median frequency before and after spinal stabilization exercises. Arch Phys Med Rehabil 2003;84:1313-1318.

33. Danneels L, Cools A, Vanderstraeten C, et al. The effects of three different training modalities on the cross-sectional area of the paravertebral muscles. Scand J Med Sci Sports 2001;11:335-341.

34. Kitano T, Zerwekh J, Usui Y, et al. Biochemical changes associated with the symptomatic human intervertebral disk. Clin Orthop Relat Res 1993;Aug:372-377.

35. Leggett S, Mooney V, Matheson L, et al. Restorative exercise for clinical low back pain: a prospective two-center study with 1-year follow-up. Spine 1999;24:889-898.

36. Nelson B, O'Reilly E, Miller M, et al. The clinical effects of intensive, specific exercise on chronic low back pain: a controlled study of 895 consecutive patients with 1-year follow up. Orthopedics 1995;18:971-981.

37. Biering-Sorensen F. Physical measurements as risk indicators for low back trouble over a one-year period. Spine 1984;9:106-119.

38. Hides JA, Richardson CA, Jull GA. Multifidus muscle recovery is not automatic after resolution of acute, first-episode low back pain. Spine 1996;21:2763-2769.

39. Flicker P, Fleckenstein J, Ferry K, et al. Lumbar muscle usage in chronic low back pain. Spine 1993;18:582-586.

40. Danneels L, Vanderstraeten G, Cambier D, et al. CT imaging of trunk muscles in chronic low back pain patients and healthy control subjects. Eur Spine J 2000;9:266-272.

41. Hayden JA, van Tulder MW, Malmivaara A, et al. Exercise therapy for treatment of nonspecific low back pain. Cochrane Database Syst Rev 2005;(3):CD000335.

42. Rittweger J, Just K, Kautzsch K, et al. Treatment of chronic lower back pain with lumbar extension and whole-body vibration exercise: a randomized controlled trial. Spine 2002;27(17):1829-1834.

43. Chok B, Lee R, Latimer J, et al. Endurance training of the trunk extensor muscles in people with subacute pain. Phys Ther 1999;79:1032-1042.

44. Hansen F, Bendix T, Jensen C, et al. Intensive, dynamic back-muscle exercises, conventional physiotherapy, or placebo-controlled treatment of low-back pain. Spine 1993;18:98-108.

45. Mannion A, Taimela S, Muntener M, et al. Active therapy for chronic low back pain part 1. Effects on back muscle activation, fatigability, and strength. Spine 2001;26:897-908.

46. Kankaanpaa M, Taimela S, Airaksinen O, et al. The efficacy of active rehabilitation in chronic low back pain. Effect on pain intensity, self-experienced disability, and lumbar fatigability. Spine 1999;24:1034-1042.

47. Timm KE. A randomized-control study of active and passive treatments for chronic low back pain following L5 laminectomy. J Orthop Sports Phys Ther 1994;20:276-286.

48. Manniche C, Asmussen K, Lauritsen B, et al. Intensive dynamic back exercises with or without hyperextension in chronic back pain after surgery for lumbar disc protrusion. A clinical trial. Spine 1993;18:560-567.

49. Quittan M. Management of back pain. Disabil Rehabil 2002;24:423-434.

50. Graves JE, Pollock ML, Foster D, et al. Effect of training frequency and specificity on isometric lumbar extension strength. Spine 1990;15:504-509.

51. Manniche C, Hesselsoe G, Bentzen R, et al. Clinical trial of intensive muscle training for chronic low back pain. Lancet 1988;2:1473-1476.

52. Mannion AF, Muntener M, Taimela S. Comparison of three active therapies for chronic low back pain: results of a randomized clinical trial with one-year follow-up. Rheumatology (Oxford) 2001;40:772-778.

53. Mannion AF, Muntener M, Taimela S, et al. A randomized clinical trial of three active therapies for chronic low back pain. Spine 1999;24:2435-2448.

54. Johannsen F, Remvig L, Kryger P, et al. Exercises for chronic low back pain: a clinical trial. J Orthop Sports Phys Ther 1995;22:52-59.

55. Choi G, Raiturker P, Kim M, et al. The effect of early isolated lumbar extension exercise program for patients with herniated disc undergoing lumbar discectomy. Neurosurgery 2005;57: 764-772.

56. Pollock M, Franklin B, Balady G, et al. AHA Science Advisory. Resistance exercise in individuals with and without cardiovascular disease: benefits, rationale, safety, and prescription: an advisory from the Committee on Exercise, Rehabilitation, and Prevention, Council on Clinical Cardiology, American Heart Association; Position paper endorsed by the American College of Sports Medicine. Circulation 2000;101:828-833.

57. Braith R, Conner JA, Fulton M, et al. Comparison of alendronate vs alendronate plus mechanical loading as prophylaxis for osteoporosis in lung transplant recipients: a pilot study. J Heart Lung Transplant 2007;26132-26137.

58. Braith R, Mills R, Welsch M, et al. Resistance exercise training restores bone mineral density in heart transplant recipients. J Am Coll Cardiol 1996;28:1471-1477.

59. Holmes B, Leggett S, Mooney V, et al. Comparison of female geriatric lumbar-extension strength: asymptotic versus chronic low back pain patients and their response to active rehabilitation. J Spinal Disord 1996;9:17-22.

60. Mayer J, Mooney V, Matheson L, et al. Continuous low-level heat wrap therapy for the prevention and early phase treatment of delayed onset muscle soreness of the low back: a randomized controlled trial. Arch Phys Med Rehabil 2006;87: 1310-1317.

61. Szymanski D. Recommendations for the avoidance of delayed-onset muscle soreness. Strength Cond J 2001;23:7-13.

62. Dagenais S, Roffey DM, Wai EK, et al. Can cost utility evaluations inform decision making about interventions for low back pain? Spine J 2009;9:944-957.

63. van der Roer N, Goossens MEJB, Evers SMAA, et al. What is the most cost-effective treatment for patients with low back pain? A systematic review. Best Pract Res Clin Rheumatol 2005;19:671-684.

64. Skouen JS, Grasdal AL, Haldorsen EM, et al. Relative cost-effectiveness of extensive and light multidisciplinary treatment programs versus treatment as usual for patients with chronic low back pain on long-term sick leave: randomized controlled study. Spine (Phila Pa 1976) 2002;27:901-909.

65. Fritz JM, Delitto A, Erhard RE. Comparison of classification-based physical therapy with therapy based on clinical practice guidelines for patients with acute low back pain: a randomized clinical trial. Spine 2003;28:1363-1371.

66. Malmivaara A, Hakkinen U, Aro T, et al. The treatment of acute low back pain—bed rest, exercises, or ordinary activity? N Engl J Med 1995;332:351-355.

67. Mitchell RI, Carmen GM. The functional restoration approach to the treatment of chronic pain in patients with soft tissue and back injuries. Spine 1994;19:633-642.

68. Moffett JK, Torgerson D, Bell-Syer S, et al. Randomised controlled trial of exercise for low back pain: clinical outcomes, costs, and preferences. BMJ 1999;319:279-283.

CHAPTER 10

STEPHEN MAY
RONALD DONELSON

McKenzie Method

DESCRIPTION

Terminology and Subtypes

Exercise, loosely translated from Greek, means "freed movement" and describes a wide range of physical activities. Therapeutic exercise indicates that the purpose of the exercise is for the treatment of a specific medical condition rather than recreation. The main types of therapeutic exercise relevant to chronic low back pain (CLBP) include (1) general physical activity (e.g., advice to remain active), (2) aerobic (e.g., brisk walking, cycling), (3) aquatic (e.g., swimming, exercise classes in a pool), (4) directional preference (e.g., McKenzie), (5) flexibility (e.g., stretching, yoga, Pilates), (6) proprioceptive/coordination (e.g., wobble board, stability ball), (7) stabilization (e.g., targeting abdominal and trunk muscles), and (8) strengthening (e.g., lifting weights).[1] The management section of this chapter focuses exclusively on directional preference exercises related to the McKenzie method, which are determined through the McKenzie assessment process.

The McKenzie method is a comprehensive approach to spinal pain, including CLBP, which includes both an assessment and an intervention consisting primarily of directional preference exercises. The goal of the McKenzie assessment is to classify patients with CLBP according to the type of therapy to which they are most likely to respond. Because it combines assessment and intervention, the McKenzie method is commonly referred to as *mechanical diagnosis and therapy* (MDT).[2] One of the principal tenets of MDT is centralization, which refers to the sequential and lasting abolition of distal referred symptoms, as well as subsequent abolition of any remaining spinal pain in response to a single direction of repeated movements or sustained postures.

Because the direction that can achieve centralization can differ among patients with CLBP, the McKenzie assessment attempts to uncover a patient's directional preference. Directional preference refers to a particular direction of lumbosacral movement or sustained posture that results in centralization or a decrease in pain while returning range of motion to normal.[3] The opposite of centralization is peripheralization, which can occur if distal referred symptoms increase in response to a particular repeated movement or sustained posture.[4] Whereas centralization should be encouraged, peripheralization should be avoided. Many clinicians use only the intervention component of the McKenzie method, without the McKenzie method of assessment. It is preferable in such instances to identify the intervention descriptively (e.g., repeated prone lumbar extension) rather than referring to them as McKenzie exercises, which denotes a paired assessment and matched intervention approach. This point is very important in light of the frequency with which the McKenzie method has mistakenly been reduced and equated with lumbar extension exercises.

According to MDT, patients may be classified into one of three mechanical syndromes: derangement, dysfunction, or postural.[5,6] Derangement syndrome is the most common, and indicates that centralization can be achieved with directional preference movements. Dysfunction syndrome is found only in patients with chronic symptoms and is characterized by intermittent pain produced only at end-range in a single direction of restricted movement. Adherent nerve root is a particular type of dysfunction that typically follows an episode of radicular pain after which pain can be elicited when the nerve root and its adhering scar tissue are stretched. Postural syndrome is likewise intermittent, but pain is typically midline or symmetrical, produced only by sustained slouched sitting, and subsequently abolished by posture correction (restoring the lumbar lordosis); it is typically not seen in CLBP. The minority of patients who cannot be classified into one of these three syndromes would be termed *other*.

History and Frequency of Use

In 1958, a patient with low back pain (LBP)-related leg symptoms presented to a physical therapy clinic in Wellington, New Zealand, and inadvertently lay prone in substantial lumbar extension for a prolonged time (approximately 10 minutes), after which he reported to the clinician (Robin McKenzie) that his leg had not felt this good for weeks (Figure 10-1). Surprised and intrigued by this event, McKenzie began experimenting with sustained and repeated movements of the lumbar spine for various spinal symptoms, including LBP. This fortuitous encounter led to the development of MDT. In his own words: "Everything I know I learnt from my patients. I did not set out to develop a McKenzie method. It evolved spontaneously over time as a result of clinical observation."[7]

Throughout many years, McKenzie observed patterns of pain response to particular positions and movements and developed a system to classify many spinal pain problems based on those findings. McKenzie was the first clinician to systematically demonstrate the benefits of having patients

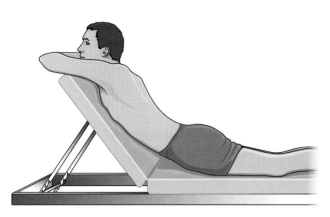

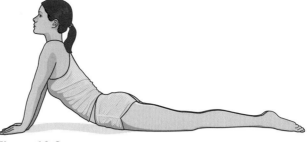

Figure 10-2 Common directional preference exercise used in the McKenzie method.

Figure 10-1 A patient who inadvertently lay prone in substantial lumbar extension for a prolonged time reported to Robin McKenzie that his leg pain was much improved.

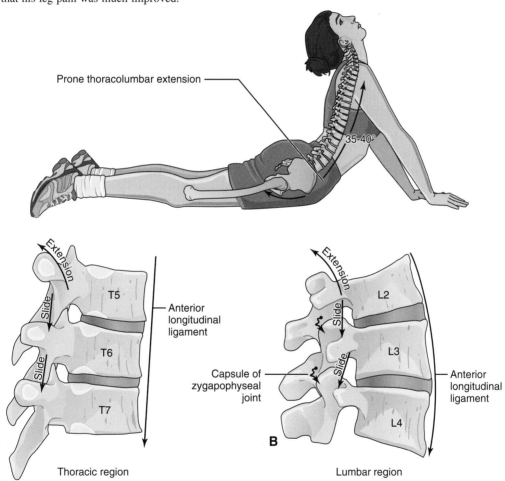

Figure 10-3 The impact of directional preference exercises on specific lumbar spine anatomic structures is not known. (From Neumann DA: Kinesiology of the musculoskeletal system: foundations for physical rehabilitation. St. Louis, 2010, Mosby.)

perform repeated lumbar movements and sustained postures, both to end-range. As long as each direction of lumbar movement was tested repetitively to end-range, McKenzie observed that a single direction would very commonly elicit centralization. A common directional preference exercise for those whose symptoms decrease in extension is shown in Figures 10-2 through 10-4. Treatment with MDT also includes strict

temporary posture modifications to avoid loading the lumbar spine opposite to the direction of preference for any length of time.

The overall objective of the McKenzie method is patient self-management and includes educating patients about three components: (1) beneficial effects of specific positions and end-range movements, and the aggravating effects of the

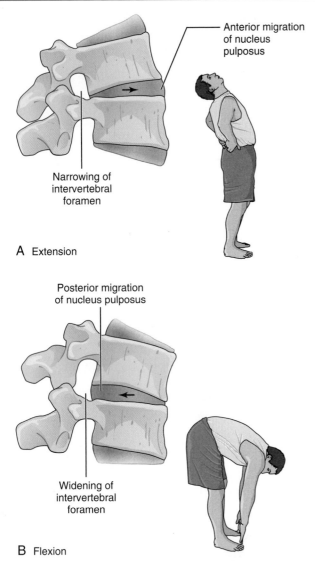

Figure 10-4 The impact of directional preference exercises on specific lumbar spine anatomic structures is not known. (Modified from Mansfield PJ: *Essentials of kinesiology for the physical therapy assistant.* St. Louis, 2008, Mosby.)

opposite movements and postures; (2) maintaining the reduction and abolition of symptoms; and (3) restoring full function to the lumbar spine without symptom recurrence. McKenzie authored several books aimed at helping patients manage their own LBP and neck pain, and these books have been sold worldwide for more than 25 years; companion textbooks for clinicians are also available.[8-10] Research into the McKenzie method began in 1990 when the first diagnostic reliability study, randomized controlled trial (RCT), and study of the concept of centralization were published.[11-13] Since then, numerous studies have been published every year on the reliability and prognostic validity of the McKenzie assessment, as well as the efficacy of McKenzie method interventions.

Practitioner, Setting, and Availability

Treatment with the McKenzie method is offered through a variety of providers involved in spine care, including physical therapists, chiropractors, and physicians who receive additional training on this approach. The qualification of McKenzie method clinicians is structured, internationally standardized, and educationally validated. Four postgraduate courses and a credentialing examination complete basic training, and for those who wish to pursue more advanced studies, a course, clinical mentorship, and examination are required to be recognized as a McKenzie Diplomat. In seeking competent McKenzie method clinicians for patient referral and research purposes, it is wise to first inquire about their educational credentials for assurance that the all important assessment and classification processes will be performed thoroughly and reliably. Typically, clinicians trained in the McKenzie method can be found in many inpatient and outpatient settings, departments in hospitals, and in private practice. The availability of certified McKenzie method practitioners can be verified with a Web-based database for areas of the United States, Canada, and other countries (www.mckenziemdt.org). The number of spine practitioners who may recommend specific components of the McKenzie method, such as directional preference exercise, far outnumbers those practitioners who are certified in the entire approach.

Procedure

The aim of the assessment is to classify patients into one of three possible mechanical syndromes. The proportion of patients who could be classified has been generally high, with a mean of 87% across five studies.[7,11,14-16] For example, 83% of 607 patients were classified in one of the mechanical syndromes, with 78% classified as derangement.[17] Pain centralization, a hallmark of the derangement syndrome, has been reported in 52% of 325 CLBP patients.[4] Directional preference was elicited in 74% of subjects in an RCT, of which 53% had symptoms duration greater than 7 weeks.[18]

Management According to Classification

For derangement syndrome, the aim of MDT is to rapidly centralize, decrease, and eventually abolish all symptoms and restore all lumbar movement. For dysfunction syndrome, eliminating the symptoms requires treatment aimed at intentionally reproducing the symptoms at end-range as an indicator that the short, painful structure is being adequately stretched so it can heal, lengthen, and become pain-free over time. For postural syndrome, the pain is eliminated simply by improving posture to avoid prolonged tensile stress on normal structures. This is done through educating patients in posture correction while they experience the beneficial effects on their pain.

Within each syndrome, MDT findings dictate further treatment considerations. For example, although two patients might both be classified as derangement, one may experience centralization with extension exercises and the other with flexion exercises. Their prescribed directional preference exercises and postures will therefore obviously be opposite. It should be noted that there is no generic prescription of standardized McKenzie method exercises, and no specific benefit can be expected by simply cycling through all possible exercises and postures repeatedly. An important aspect of the McKenzie method is self-management, with the clinician serving primarily as the assessor, classifier, and educator. With the clinician's guidance and through their own experiential education, patients quickly and easily become empowered in how to first eliminate their own pain and then to become proactive with these same strategies to prevent its return.

For a minority of patients with CLBP, completely eliminating pain may require more end-range force than they are able to generate themselves. In these cases, clinicians can provide manual pressure at end-range, or deliver spinal mobilization or manipulation in the patient's direction of preference. Brief and minimal forces are often all that is needed to gain the desired effect of centralization and pain elimination, after which most patients can self-manage using end-range exercises under the clinicians' guidance and education, with no further need for clinician-generated manual forces.

Regulatory Status

Not applicable.

THEORY

Mechanism of Action

In general, exercises are used to strengthen muscles, increase soft tissue stability, restore range of movement, improve cardiovascular conditioning, increase proprioception, and reduce fear of movement. Most McKenzie method exercises are intended to directly and promptly diminish and eliminate patients' symptoms by providing beneficial and corrective mechanical directional end-range loads to the underlying pain generator.[18] The anatomic means by which these rapid pain changes occur is addressed in an article by Wetzel and Donelson.[19] Treatment with the McKenzie method may also provide psychological mechanism–related benefits.

Psychological Mechanisms

In some patients with particularly severe or prolonged CLBP, or psychological comorbidities such as anxiety or depression, maladaptive illness behavior may become established. This type of behavior may manifest itself as fear of engaging in any activity or movement that has previously been associated with symptoms of CLBP. As time passes, virtually all activities gain this association, leading to a generalized fear of movement in an attempt to minimize exacerbations. Engaging in any form of supervised exercise therapy under the guidance of an experienced clinician able to gradually increase the type, dose, frequency, or intensity of movements can help break this cycle and demonstrate that not all movements or activities need be painful. This aspect is discussed further in other chapters of this text (e.g., Section 8—Behavioral Therapies).

Indication

This intervention is generally indicated for patients with non-specific mechanical CLBP, recurrent LBP, and those classified as centralizers following MDT.

Mechanical Low Back Pain

Patients who may be responsive to the McKenzie method are those whose symptoms are affected by changes in postures and activities (e.g., pain made worse by sitting and bending, but better with walking or moving). Such a history is often indicative of a directional preference for extension, which can be confirmed during the repeated end-range testing of the physical examination. Such mechanical responsiveness to changes in posture and activity has been commonly reported.[12,20-23]

Recurrent Low Back Pain

Patients who report recurring LBP are routinely found to have a directional preference, are centralizers, and are therefore ideal treatment candidates. Furthermore, even if a patient has responded to some other form of treatment for past LBP but is frustrated with recurrences and in need of further treatment, they are often pleased with the ability to self-manage their pain with this intervention.

Centralizers

At least six studies have reported on the favorable prognosis for patients who were categorized as centralizers if treatment is directed by the patients' directional preference.[13,24-28] A systematic review (SR) similarly concluded that centralization, when elicited, predicts a high probability of a good treatment outcome, again as long as treatment is guided by the assessment findings.[4] These patients might be considered the most ideal patients to experience an excellent treatment response with this approach. Initial clues for potentially responsive patients emerge during the history taking and then are confirmed with the repeated end-range movement portion of the physical testing.

Assessment

Before initiating the McKenzie method, patients should first be assessed for LBP using an evidence-based and goal-oriented approach focused on the patient history and neurologic examination, as discussed in Chapter 3. The standardized McKenzie method assessment also includes an examination in which responses to repeated lumbar movements are noted to enable the clinician to make a provisional classification of the patient's condition. Additional diagnostic imaging or specific diagnostic testing is generally not required before initiating this intervention for CLBP. To prescribe the appropriate directional preference exercises consistent with the principle of management according to classification, patients must first be assessed according to MDT, which may also bring awareness of atypical or nonmechanical pain responses that may alert clinicians to the possibility of serious spinal pathology related to CLBP (e.g., red flags).[2] Assessment using MDT generally involves observing the effects of repeated and sustained postures on patient-reported symptoms to identify specific directional preference.

EFFICACY

Evidence supporting the efficacy of this intervention for CLBP was summarized from recent clinical practice guidelines (CPGs), SRs, and RCTs. Observational studies (OBSs) were also summarized where appropriate. Findings are summarized in the following discussion by study design.

Clinical Practice Guidelines

None of the recent national CPGs on the management of CLBP have assessed and summarized the evidence to make specific recommendations about the efficacy of the McKenzie method using both the assessment and subsequent management.

The CPG from Europe in 2004 found limited evidence that one component of directional preference exercises (i.e., lumbar flexion exercise), when evaluated as a sole intervention outside of the McKenzie method context, was less effective than aerobic exercises with respect to short-term improvements in pain.[29] That CPG also found conflicting evidence regarding the efficacy of trunk flexion exercises when compared with trunk extension exercises. However, these findings are not directly applicable to the McKenzie method that encompasses both the assessment and management components described above.

Other Clinical Practice Guidelines

An older national CPG from Denmark in 1999 mentioned the assessment component of the McKenzie method.[30] That CPG found moderate evidence to support the use of the McKenzie method assessment as a diagnostic tool and prognostic indicator. That CPG also found limited evidence to support the use of the McKenzie method management component.

Three other non-national CPGs on the management of CLBP have also reported on the McKenzie method. The CPG from the United Kingdom Chartered Society of Physiotherapy in 2006 found weak scientific evidence to support the management component of the McKenzie method.[31] The CPG from the Philadelphia Panel on Selected Rehabilitation Interventions in 2001 found evidence of clinically important benefit to support therapeutic exercise.[32] The CPG from Quebec in 2006 found evidence that the management component of the McKenzie method was as effective as strengthening exercises with respect to improvements in pain and function.[33]

Findings from the aforementioned CPGs are summarized in Table 10-1.

Systematic Reviews

Cochrane Collaboration

The Cochrane Collaboration conducted an SR in 2004 on all forms of exercise therapy for acute, subacute, and chronic LBP.[34] A total of 61 RCTs were identified, including 43 RCTs

TABLE 10-1	Clinical Practice Guideline Recommendations on the McKenzie Method for Chronic Low Back Pain	
Reference	Country	Conclusion
29	Europe	Flexion exercise as an isolated component outside of the McKenzie method was less effective than aerobic exercises Conflicting evidence regarding the efficacy of trunk flexion exercises compared with trunk extension exercises when evaluated outside the McKenzie method
30	Denmark	Moderate evidence as a diagnostic tool and prognostic indicator Moderate evidence as an intervention
31	United Kingdom	Weak evidence to support the management component of the McKenzie method
32	United States	Clinically important benefit demonstrated for therapeutic exercise in general for pain and function
33	Canada	Management component of the McKenzie method was as effective as strengthening exercises

related to CLBP. Although results were generally favorable, this review combined all forms of exercise therapy, including stabilization, strengthening, stretching, directional preference, aerobic, and others. As such, these conclusions are not specific to the McKenzie method as discussed in this chapter and pertain only to isolated components (i.e., directional preference exercise). This review identified five RCTs related to the McKenzie method for acute, subacute, and chronic LBP, which are discussed in the section on RCTs that follows.[12,35-39]

American Pain Society and American College of Physicians

The American Pain Society and American College of Physicians CPG committee conducted an SR in 2007 on nonpharmacologic therapies for acute and chronic LBP.[40] That review identified two SRs related to McKenzie exercise, and both were considered of higher quality (based on the Oxman scale).[41,42] One found no clear difference between the McKenzie method and other types of exercise.[42] The other SR found that the McKenzie method was more effective than other interventions on short-term pain and disability, but no difference in effectiveness was observed for intermediate-term disability.[41] These SRs included eight additional RCTs related to the McKenzie method.[43-50] This SR did not make any conclusions specific to exercises used in the McKenzie method.

Other

Two SRs related to the McKenzie method have thus far been conducted.[41,42] Their conclusions were similar and indicated there was limited evidence with respect to CLBP.

Another SR examined the evidence regarding the effectiveness of physical therapy–directed exercise interventions after patients had been classified using symptom response methods.[51] This included mixed duration LBP (some chronic, but mostly subacute). Four of five of the included studies were related to the McKenzie method. All articles scored six or more by physiotherapy evidence database (PEDro) rating (suggesting high methodologic quality), and four of five found that a directed exercise program implemented according to patient response was significantly better than control or comparison groups. The authors noted a positive trend, but few studies have investigated this phenomenon. One unique RCT was identified in this study that was not included in the aforementioned reviews.[18] A recent SR on unloaded movement facilitation exercise in CLBP identified another unique RCT related to the McKenzie method.[52,53]

Findings from the SRs are summarized in Table 10-2.

Randomized Controlled Trials

An RCT conducted by Petersen and colleagues[36] included patients with LBP with or without leg pain who had symptoms lasting longer than 8 weeks. Participants were randomized to either the McKenzie method or strengthening exercises for 8 months in an outpatient clinic and 2 months at home. At the 8-month follow-up, there was a decrease in pain scores (Manniche) in the McKenzie group, but only a small decrease in the training group (P values not reported). The difference in pain between the two groups was not statistically significant. There was also a decrease in disability scores (Manniche) in both groups (P values not reported). The difference in disability between the two groups was not statistically significant. This study was considered of lower quality.

An RCT conducted by Long and colleagues[18] included patients with LBP with or without neurologic involvement (duration of symptoms not reported). Participants were assigned 6 sessions over 2 weeks of (1) McKenzie method, (2) opposite directional preference exercises, or (3) active nonspecific exercises. After the treatment period, there was a significant reduction in pain scores (visual analog score, 0-10) in all three groups. The difference in pain between groups was statistically significant, with the largest improvement in the McKenzie group. There was also a significant reduction in disability scores (Roland Morris Disability Questionnaire) in all three groups. The difference in disability between groups was borderline nonsignificant, with the largest improvement in the McKenzie group.

TABLE 10-2	Systematic Review Findings on the McKenzie Method for Chronic Low Back Pain		
Reference	#RCTs in SR	#RCTs for CLBP	Conclusion
34	61	43	Conclusions are not specific to the McKenzie method as the review combined all forms of exercise therapy
40	NR	NR	No difference between McKenzie and other forms of exercise McKenzie more effective than other interventions on short-term pain and disability
51	5	NR	Participants classified according to directional preference method had significantly better outcomes than controls
41	5	NR	Limited evidence about CLBP, but overall short-term effect size for pain and physical function
42	11	NR	Insufficient evidence about CLBP

CLBP, chronic low back pain; NR, not reported; RCT, randomized controlled trial; SR, systematic review.

An RCT by Miller and colleagues[53] included patients with CLBP and symptoms lasting longer than 7 weeks. Participants were randomized to either the McKenzie method or stabilization exercises for 6 weeks. After the treatment period, there was a statistically significant reduction in pain scores (Short-form McGill Pain Questionnaire) in the McKenzie group but not in the stabilization group. The difference in pain between groups was not statistically significant. There was no significant change in disability (Functional Status Questionnaire) in either group, and there were no significant differences between groups (Table 10-3).

Comments

Three RCTs were identified that were relevant to CLBP, of which two involved patients with nonspecific CLBP.[37,54] Although no significant differences between the study groups were reported in those two RCTs, this can be anticipated when clinicians must follow study protocols in which participants who are not appropriate candidates for the McKenzie method must nevertheless receive directional preference

TABLE 10-3	Randomized Controlled Trials of the McKenzie Method for Chronic Low Back Pain			
Reference	Indication	Intervention	Control (C1)	Control (C2)
36	LBP, with or without leg pain, symptoms >8 wk	McKenzie PT 8 mo + 2 mo at home n = 132	Strengthening exercises PT 8 mo + 2 mo at home n = 128	NA
18	LBP with or without neurologic involvement, duration of symptoms NR	McKenzie + education PT 6 sessions × 2 wk n = 80	Opposite DP exercises + education PT 6 sessions × 2 wk n = 69	Active nonspecific + education PT 6 sessions × 2 wk n = 80
53	CLBP, neurologic involvement not reported, symptoms >7 wk	McKenzie PT 6 wk n = 15	Stabilization exercises PT 6 wk n = 15	

CLBP, chronic low back pain; DR, directional preference; LBP, low back pain; NA, not applicable; NR, not reported; PT, physical therapist.

exercises specified in a study protocol. Results from those RCTs are therefore not applicable to the combined McKenzie method assessment and management according to classification as described in this chapter.

Observational Studies

Centralization Studies

An SR concluded that centralization is not only a common clinical occurrence with LBP but, with proper training, it can be reliably detected and has important prognostic and management implications.[4] Its occurrence was consistently associated with good prognosis across six studies and it can be used to guide appropriate exercise or manual therapy prescription. The study concluded that centralization should be routinely monitored during spinal assessment and be used to guide treatment strategies. A recent review concluded that only changes in pain location and/or intensity with repeated spinal movement testing or in response to treatment supported the use of symptomatic responses to guide management.[54]

Centralization and Psychosocial Factors

Two studies have demonstrated that centralization is a more important predictor of outcomes than fear avoidance and work-related issues in terms of long-term pain, disability, and a range of other health-related outcomes.[28,55] Conversely, failure to change the pain location during the baseline assessment (noncentralization) has been shown to be a strong predictor of poor outcomes and a predictor of a poor behavioral response to spine pain.[28] When noncentralization was found, for example, the patient was 9 times more likely to have nonorganic signs, 13 times more likely to have overt pain behaviors, 3 times more likely to have fear of work, and 2 times more likely to have somatization.[56] Given these findings, to prevent the development of CLBP, the presence of noncentralization during a baseline McKenzie assessment in more acute LBP suggests that additional psychosocial screening may be useful.

Reliability Studies

To have clinical utility, it is imperative that examination findings interpreted by different clinicians have high inter-examiner reliability (e.g., kappa values). Although several SRs of reliability studies have been published recently, only one attempted to differentiate basic methods of physical examination.[57] There would appear at first to be conflicting evidence regarding reliability of the McKenzie classification system from four studies, three of which are considered of higher quality. Two high-quality studies reported high reliability (kappa >0.85), but the third reported low reliability (kappa, 0.26).[7,14,15] However, clinicians involved in this latter study had little or no previous experience with the McKenzie method and errors could have resulted from this inexperience. In contrast, the first two studies used trained and experienced McKenzie method clinicians to classify patients according to the MDT system, producing quite high kappa values of 0.7/0.96 and 1.00/0.89.[7,14] A fourth study that also used trained McKenzie method clinicians likewise showed moderately high kappa values of 0.6/0.7.[3]

SAFETY

Contraindications

The assessment component of the McKenzie method may be contraindicated in patients with CLBP associated with severe spinal instability, trauma, or fracture that may be aggravated by movements of the lumbosacral spine toward the end-ranges of motion. However, this assessment may also serve to identify patients with potentially serious spinal pathology who may need to be referred for additional testing. The treatment component of the McKenzie method is contraindicated in patients with serious spinal pathology such as fracture, infection, cancer, or cauda equina syndrome.

Adverse Events

Treatment of CLBP using the McKenzie method is generally regarded as a safe intervention. None of the studies reviewed reported any serious adverse events. Although the exercises prescribed may temporarily increase pain or other symptoms, this is an expected reaction to mechanical loading according to directional preference, and it will subside.

It has been reported that failure to alter symptom distribution (noncentralization) is a strong predictor of negative outcomes and poor behavioral responses to interventions for LBP.[28,56]

COSTS

Fees and Third-Party Reimbursement

Presently, there are no CPT codes specific to the McKenzie method. In the United States, treatment with the McKenzie method that is supervised by a licensed health care practitioner such as a physical therapist in an outpatient setting can be delivered using CPT codes 97110 (therapeutic exercises, each 15 minutes), 97112 (neuromuscular reeducation, each 15 minutes), or 97530 (therapeutic activities, each 15 minutes). The initial evaluation of lumbar function can be delivered using CPT codes 97001 (physical therapy initial evaluation) or 97750 (physical performance test or measurement, each 15 minutes). Periodic reevaluation of lumbar function can be delivered using CPT codes 97002 (physical therapy reevaluation) or 97750 (physical performance test or measurement, each 15 minutes).

These procedures are widely covered by other third-party payers such as health insurers and worker's compensation insurance. Although some payers continue to base their reimbursements on usual, customary, and reasonable payment methodology, the majority have developed reimbursement tables based on the Resource Based Relative Value Scale used by Medicare. Reimbursements by other third-party payers are generally higher than Medicare.

Third-party payers will often reimburse a limited number of visits to licensed health care providers if they are prescribed by a physician and supported by adequate documentation deeming them medically necessary. Equipment or products required for those interventions are rarely typically considered inclusive in the procedure reported and are not separately reportable. Given the need to maintain the gains achieved in muscular function through the McKenzie method, patients are often encouraged to continue this intervention beyond the initial period of supervised exercise therapy. The cost for membership in a private exercise facility is generally $50 to $100 per month. Some insurers in the United States also provide discounted membership fees to exercise facilities to their members to promote physical activity.

Typical fees reimbursed by Medicare in New York and California for these services are summarized in Table 10-4.

TABLE 10-4	Medicare Fee Schedule for Related Services	
CPT Code	New York	California
97001	$73	$78
97002	$40	$43
97110	$30	$32
97112	$31	$33
97530	$32	$35
97750	$21	$33

2010 Participating, nonfacility amount.

Cost Effectiveness

Evidence supporting the cost effectiveness of treatment protocols that compared these interventions, often in combination with one or more cointerventions, with control groups who received one or more other interventions, for either acute or chronic LBP, was identified from two SRs on this topic and is summarized here.[58,59] Although many of these study designs are unable to clearly identify the individual contribution of any intervention, their results provide some insight as to the clinical and economic outcomes associated with these approaches.

An RCT in the United States compared three approaches for patients with acute LBP presenting to a health maintenance organization (HMO).[37] The physical therapy group received nine visits centered on the McKenzie method. The chiropractic group received nine visits of spinal manipulation. The brief education group received only an educational booklet. Clinical outcomes after 3 months reported greater improvement in pain for the physical therapy and chiropractic groups. Direct medical costs associated with study and nonstudy interventions provided by the HMO over 2 years were $437 in the physical therapy group, $429 in the chiropractic group, and $153 in the brief education group. Indirect productivity costs were not reported.

An RCT in the United States compared two approaches for patients with acute LBP.[60] The first group received care according to the classification of symptoms and examination findings by a physical therapist, including possibly spinal manipulation; mobilization; traction therapy; and flexion, extension, strengthening, or stabilization exercises. The second group received brief education and general exercise from a physical therapist according to recommendations from CPGs, which were not specified. Clinical outcomes after 1 year favored the therapy according to classification group for improvement in function, although no differences were noted (short form-36). Direct medical costs associated with the study interventions over 1 year were $604 in the therapy according to classification group and $682 in the CPG recommended care group; direct medical costs for all interventions over 1 year were $883 and $1160, respectively. Indirect productivity costs associated with lost productivity were not reported, although fewer participants in the therapy according to classification group had missed work due to LBP after 12 months.

TABLE 10-5	Cost Effectiveness and Cost Utility Analyses on the McKenzie Method for Acute or Chronic Low Back Pain					
Ref Country Follow-up	Group	Direct Medical Costs	Indirect Productivity Costs	Total Costs	Conclusion
37 United States 2 years	1. PT centered on McKenzie 2. chiropractic 3. brief education	1. $437 2. $429 3. $153	NR	NR	No conclusion as to cost effectiveness
60 United States 1 year	1. care according to classification of symptoms (including flexion extension) 2. brief education + general exercise	1. $883 2. $1160	NR	NR	No conclusion as to cost effectiveness
61	1. McKenzie method 2. CBT (i.e., Solution Finding approach)	1. $362 2. $347	1. $1085 2. $890	1. $1447 2. $1237	McKenzie method was cost effective ($2184/QALY)

CBT, cognitive behavioral therapy; NR, not reported; PT, physical therapy; QALY, quality-adjusted life-year.

Other

A cost-effectiveness analysis was conducted alongside a recent RCT to compare a cognitive behavioral therapy-based psychosocial intervention (i.e., Solution Finding approach) to the McKenzie method for LBP or neck pain using quality-adjusted life years (QALYs) as the outcome measure.[61] Two-thirds of participants (67%) had chronic symptoms, that is, pain for 3 months or more. The direct medical costs associated with the McKenzie group were slightly higher than those in the control group ($362 vs. $347), as were the indirect productivity costs ($1085 vs. $890) and total costs from a societal perspective ($1447 vs. $1237). However, the gain in QALYs over 12 months was also greater in the McKenzie group (0.726 vs. 0.692), resulting in a cost per incremental QALY of $2184, suggesting that the McKenzie approach was in fact cost effective.

Findings from the aforementioned cost effectiveness analyses are summarized in Table 10-5.

SUMMARY

Description

The McKenzie method is a comprehensive approach to CLBP that includes both an assessment and an intervention consisting primarily of directional preference exercises. The goals of the McKenzie assessment are to classify patients as having one of three mechanical syndromes (derangement, dysfunction, postural) and uncover a patient's directional preference. Directional preference refers to a particular direction of lumbosacral movement or sustained posture that results in centralization or decreased symptoms and returns range of motion to normal. The opposite of centralization is peripheralization, which can occur if distal referred symptoms increase in response to a particular repeated movement or sustained posture. The McKenzie intervention encourages centralization and attempts to avoid peripheralization. A physical therapist developed the McKenzie program in the

1960s. Treatment with the McKenzie method is offered in many inpatient and outpatient settings by a variety of providers, including physical therapists, chiropractors, and physicians who receive additional training on this approach.

Theory

In general, exercises are used to strengthen muscles, increase soft tissue stability, restore range of movement, improve cardiovascular conditioning, increase proprioception, and reduce fear of movement. Most McKenzie method exercises are intended to directly and promptly diminish and eliminate patients' symptoms by providing beneficial and corrective mechanical directional end-range loads to the underlying pain generator. In addition, in some patients with particularly severe or prolonged CLBP or psychological comorbidities such as anxiety or depression, maladaptive illness behavior may occur, leading to fear of engaging in any activity or movement previously associated with the CLBP. Engaging in any form of supervised exercise therapy under the guidance of an experienced clinician can help break this cycle and demonstrate that not all movements or activities need be painful. McKenzie exercise is generally indicated for patients with nonspecific mechanical CLBP, recurrent LBP, and those classified as centralizers following assessment. Diagnostic imaging or other forms of advanced testing is generally not required before administering the McKenzie method for CLBP.

Efficacy

None of the recent national CPGs make recommendations specific to the McKenzie method for CLBP. One CPG found limited evidence that flexion exercise, when studied as an isolated component outside the McKenzie method, was less effective than aerobic exercises with respect to short-term improvements in pain. There was also conflicting evidence regarding the efficacy of trunk flexion exercises compared with trunk extension exercises when evaluated as sole interventions rather than components of the McKenzie method. Two other CPGs reported limited or weak evidence supporting the McKenzie method for CLBP; one found clinically important benefits supporting therapeutic exercise, and another found that the McKenzie method was as effective as strengthening exercises for pain and functional improvement. Two SRs made conclusions about the McKenzie method for CLBP; one found no difference between the McKenzie method and other forms of exercise, while the other found that the McKenzie method was more effective than other interventions on short-term pain and disability. At least three RCTs assessed the efficacy of the McKenzie method versus other forms of exercise, all finding no statistically significant differences in pain or function between study groups.

Safety

The assessment component of the McKenzie method may be contraindicated in patients with CLBP associated with severe spinal instability, trauma, or fracture that may be aggravated by movements of the lumbosacral spine towards the end-ranges of motion. The treatment component of the McKenzie method is contraindicated in patients with serious spinal pathology such as fracture, infection, cancer, or cauda equina syndrome. Treatment of CLBP using the McKenzie method is generally regarded as a safe intervention. Although the exercises prescribed may temporarily increase pain or other symptoms, this is an expected reaction to mechanical loading according to directional preference, and it will subside.

Costs

The Medicare reimbursement for treatment with the McKenzie method in an outpatient setting by licensed health care practitioners (e.g., physical therapists) ranges from $21 to $78, depending on the duration and type of session (e.g., assessment, reevaluation). Three studies examining the cost effectiveness of extension exercises as part of treatment regimens also involving other cointerventions were identified, though no conclusions could be made as to the cost effectiveness of this approach.

Comments

Evidence from the CPGs, SRs, and RCTs reviewed reported somewhat mixed results supporting the efficacy of directional preference exercises loosely based on the McKenzie method approach for CLBP. However, such studies may not be representative of results that could be reported by studies assessing the efficacy of the combined McKenzie method of assessment and management based on classification. Nevertheless, some studies do support the McKenzie method of assessment as a potentially useful tool for classifying an often amorphous group of patients with CLBP into distinct subgroups with different treatment needs. Studies in this area need to shift away from studying patients with so-called nonspecific CLBP by identifying subgroups of patients most likely to respond to a particular intervention. Studies that have taken this approach in the past have demonstrated far more promising results than studies that have simply randomized participants with nonspecific CLBP to interventions that may not benefit them.

CHAPTER REVIEW QUESTIONS

Answers are located on page 450.
1. Which of the following components is included in the pattern of pain response called centralization?
   a. sequential and lasting abolition of spinal pain
   b. response to a single direction
   c. repeated movements or sustained posture
   d. all of the above
2. Which of the following is not a mechanical syndrome into which patients may be classified with the McKenzie assessment method?
   a. proprioceptive
   b. derangement
   c. dysfunction
   d. postural
3. When did the McKenzie method originate?
   a. 1938
   b. 1948
   c. 1958
   d. 1968
4. True or false: Peripheralization is encouraged in the McKenzie method.
5. Which of the following health care providers may deliver the McKenzie method with appropriate training?
   a. general practitioner
   b. chiropractor
   c. physical therapist
   d. all of the above
6. True or false: The McKenzie method includes both an assessment and an intervention.

REFERENCES

1. Mooney V, Verna J, Morris C. Clinical management of chronic, disabling low back syndromes. In: Morris C, editor. Low back syndromes: integrated clinical management. New York: McGraw-Hill; 2006.
2. McKenzie R, May S. The lumbar spine mechanical diagnosis and therapy. 2nd ed. Waikanae, New Zealand: Spinal Publications; 2003.
3. Kilpikoski S, Airaksinen O, Kankaanpaa M, et al. Interexaminer reliability of low back pain assessment using the McKenzie method. Spine 2002;27:E207-E214.
4. Aina A, May S, Clare H. The centralization phenomenon of spinal symptoms—a systematic review. Man Ther 2004;9: 134-143.
5. Moffett JK, Torgerson D, Bell-Syer S, et al. Randomised controlled trial of exercise for low back pain: clinical outcomes, costs, and preferences. BMJ 1999;319:279-283.
6. Seferlis T, Lindholm L, Nemeth G. Cost-minimisation analysis of three conservative treatment programmes in 180 patients sick-listed for acute low-back pain. Scand J Prim Health Care 2000;18:53-57.

7. Clare HA, Adams R, Maher CG. Reliability of McKenzie classification of patients with cervical or lumbar pain. J Manipulative Physiol Ther 2005;28:122-127.

8. McKenzie RA. The lumbar spine: mechanical diagnosis and therapy. Waikanae, New Zealand: Spinal Publications; 1981.

9. McKenzie R, May S. The human extremities: mechanical diagnosis and therapy. Waikanae, New Zealand: Spinal Publications; 2000.

10. McKenzie RA. The cervical and thoracic spine. Mechanical diagnosis and therapy. Waikanae, New Zealand: Spinal Publications; 1990.

11. Kilby J, Stigant M, Roberts A. The reliability of back pain assessment by physiotherapists, using a "McKenzie algorithm." Physiotherapy 1990;76:579-583.

12. Stankovic R, Johnell O. Conservative treatment of acute low-back pain. A prospective randomized trial: McKenzie method of treatment versus patient education in "mini back school." Spine 1990;15:120-123.

13. Donelson R, Silva G, Murphy K. Centralization phenomenon. Its usefulness in evaluating and treating referred pain. Spine 1990;15:211-213.

14. Razmjou H, Kramer JF, Yamada R. Intertester reliability of the McKenzie evaluation in assessing patients with mechanical low-back pain. J Orthop Sports Phys Ther 2000;30:368-383.

15. Riddle DL, Rothstein JM. Intertester reliability of McKenzie's classifications of the syndrome types present in patients with low back pain. Spine 1993;18:1333-1344.

16. Clare HA. Evaluation of the McKenzie method. Sydney, Australia: University of Sydney; 2005.

17. May S. Classification by McKenzie mechanical syndromes: a survey of McKenzie-trained faculty. J Manipulative Physiol Ther 2006;29:637-642.

18. Long A, Donelson R, Fung T. Does it matter which exercise? A randomized control trial of exercise for low back pain. Spine 2004;29:2593-2602.

19. Wetzel FT, Donelson R. The role of repeated end-range/pain response assessment in the management of symptomatic lumbar discs. Spine J 2003;3:146-154.

20. Boissonnault W, Fabio RP. Pain profile of patients with low back pain referred to physical therapy. J Orthop Sports Phys Ther 1996;24:180-191.

21. Pengel LH, Refshauge KM, Maher CG. Responsiveness of pain, disability, and physical impairment outcomes in patients with low back pain. Spine 2004;29:879-883.

22. van Deursen LL, Patijn J, Durinck JR, et al. Sitting and low back pain: the positive effect of rotary dynamic stimuli during prolonged sitting. Eur Spine J 1999;8:187-193.

23. Van Deursen L, Snijders C, Patijn J. Influence of daily life activities on pain in patients with low back pain. J Orthopaedic Med 2002;24:74-76.

24. Long AL. The centralization phenomenon. Its usefulness as a predictor or outcome in conservative treatment of chronic law back pain (a pilot study). Spine 1995;20:2513-2520.

25. Karas R, McIntosh G, Hall H, et al. The relationship between nonorganic signs and centralization of symptoms in the prediction of return to work for patients with low back pain. Phys Ther 1997;77:354-360.

26. Sufka A, Hauger B, Trenary M, et al. Centralization of low back pain and perceived functional outcome. J Orthop Sports Phys Ther 1998;27:205-212.

27. Werneke M, Hart DL, Cook D. A descriptive study of the centralization phenomenon. A prospective analysis. Spine 1999;24:676-683.

28. Werneke M, Hart DL. Centralization phenomenon as a prognostic factor for chronic low back pain and disability. Spine 2001;26:758-764.

29. Airaksinen O, Brox JI, Cedraschi C, et al. European guidelines for the management of chronic nonspecific low back pain. Eur Spine J 2006;15:192-300.

30. Statens institut for medicinsk teknologivurdering. Low-back pain: frequency, management, and prevention from an HTA perspective. Denmark: Danish Institute for Health Technology Assessment; 1999.

31. Rossignol M, Arsenault B. Clinique des Lombalgies Interdisciplinaire en Premiere Ligne. Guide de pratique. Quebec, Canada: Reseau provincial de recherche en adaptation et en readaptation du Quebec (REPAR/FRSQ); 2006.

32. Philadelphia Panel. Evidence-based clinical practice guidelines on selected rehabilitation interventions for low back pain. Phys Ther 2001;81:1641-1674.

33. Mercer C, Jackson A, Hettinga D, et al. Clinical guidelines for the physiotherapy management of persistent low back pain, Part 1: exercise. London: Charted Society of Physiotherapy; 2006.

34. Hayden JA, van Tulder MW, Malmivaara A, et al. Exercise therapy for treatment of nonspecific low back pain. Cochrane Database Syst Rev 2005;(3):CD000335.

35. Buswell L. Low back pain: a comparison of two treatment programmes. N Z J Physiother 1982;10:13-17.

36. Petersen T, Kryger P, Ekdahl C, et al. The effect of McKenzie therapy as compared with that of intensive strengthening training for the treatment of patients with subacute or chronic low back pain: a randomized controlled trial. Spine 2002;27:1702-1709.

37. Cherkin DC, Deyo RA, Battie M, et al. A comparison of physical therapy, chiropractic manipulation, and provision of an educational booklet for the treatment of patients with low back pain. N Engl J Med 1998;339:1021-1029.

38. Delitto A, Cibulka M, Erhard R, et al. Evidence for use of an extension-mobilization category in acute low back pain: a prescriptive validation pilot study. Phys Ther 1993;73:216-222.

39. Underwood MR, Morgan J. The use of a back class teaching extension exercises in the treatment of acute low back pain in primary care. Fam Pract 1998;15:9-15.

40. Chou R, Huffman LH. Nonpharmacologic therapies for acute and chronic low back pain: a review of the evidence for an American Pain Society/American College of Physicians clinical practice guideline. Ann Intern Med 2007;147:492-504.

41. Clare HA, Adams R, Maher CG. A systematic review of efficacy of McKenzie therapy for spinal pain. Aust J Physiother 2004;50:209-216.

42. Machado LA, de Souza MS, Ferreira PH, et al. The McKenzie method for low back pain: a systematic review of the literature with a meta-analysis approach. Spine 2006;31:E254-E262.

43. Roberts A. The conservative treatment of low back pain. Nottingham: University Hospital; 1990.

44. Gillan MG, Ross JC, McLean IP, et al. The natural history of trunk list, its associated disability and the influence of McKenzie management. Eur Spine J 1998;7:480-483.

45. Kjellman G, Oberg B. A randomized clinical trial comparing general exercise, McKenzie treatment and a control group in patients with neck pain. J Rehabil Med 2002;34:183-190.

46. Schenk R, Jozefczyk C, Kopf A. A randomised trial comparing interventions in patients with lumbar posterior derangement. J Manual Manipulative Ther 2003;11:95-102.

47. Dettori JR, Bullock SH, Sutlive TG, et al. The effects of spinal flexion and extension exercises and their associated postures in patients with acute low back pain. Spine 1995;20:2303-2312.

48. Elnaggar O, Nordin M, Shiekzadeh A, et al. Effects of spinal flexion and extension exercises on low back pain and spinal mobility in chronic mechanical low-back pain patients. Spine 1991;16:967-972.

49. Erhard R, Delitto A, Cibulka M. Relative effectiveness of an extension program and a combined program of manipulation and flexion and extension exercises in patients with acute low back pain syndrome. Physical Therapy 1994;74:1093-1100.

50. Malmivaara A, Hakkinen U, Aro T, et al. The treatment of acute low back pain—bed rest, exercises, or ordinary activity? N Engl J Med 1995;332:351-355.

51. Cook C, Hegedus EJ, Ramey K. Physical therapy exercise intervention based on classification using the patent response method: a systematic review of the literature. J Manual Manip Thera 2005;13:152-162.

52. Slade SC, Keating JL. Unloaded movement facilitation exercise compared to no exercise or alternative therapy on outcomes for people with nonspecific chronic low back pain: a systematic review. J Manipulative Physiol Ther 2007;30:301-311.

53. Miller ER, Schenk RJ, Karnes JL, et al. A comparison of the McKenzie approach to a specific spine stabilization program for chronic low back pain. J Manual Manip Thera 2005;13:103-112.

54. Chorti AG, Chortis AG, Strimpakos N, et al. The prognostic value of symptom responses in the conservative management of spinal pain: a systematic review. Spine 2009;34:2686-2899.

55. George SZ, Bialosky JE, Donald DA. The centralization phenomenon and fear-avoidance beliefs as prognostic factors for acute low back pain: a preliminary investigation involving patients classified for specific exercise. J Orthop Sports Phys Ther 2005;35:580-588.

56. Werneke MW, Hart DL. Centralization: association between repeated end-range pain responses and behavioral signs in patients with acute nonspecific low back pain. J Rehabil Med 2005;37:286-290.

57. May S, Littlewood C, Bishop A. Reliability of procedures used in the physical examination of nonspecific low back pain: a systematic review. Aust J Physiother 2006;52:91-102.

58. Dagenais S, Roffey DM, Wai EK, et al. Can cost utility evaluations inform decision making about interventions for low back pain? Spine J 2009;9:944-957.

59. van der Roer N, Goossens MEJB, Evers SMAA, et al. What is the most cost-effective treatment for patients with low back pain? A systematic review. Best Pract Res Clin Rheumatol 2005;19:671-684.

60. Fritz JM, Delitto A, Erhard RE. Comparison of classification-based physical therapy with therapy based on clinical practice guidelines for patients with acute low back pain: a randomized clinical trial. Spine 2003;28:1363-1371.

61. Manca A, Dumville JC, Torgerson DJ, et al. Randomized trial of two physiotherapy interventions for primary care back and neck pain patients: cost effectiveness analysis. Rheumatology 2007;46:1495-1501.

CHAPTER 11

GERARD A. MALANGA
ERIN T. WOLFF

Common Analgesics

DESCRIPTION

Terminology and Subtypes

Common analgesics is a broad term used to refer to several classes of medications used to manage pain, which in the context of this chapter includes both nonsteroidal anti-inflammatory drugs (NSAIDs), simple analgesics, and muscle relaxants. Although muscle relaxants are not classified as analgesics, they are often used to alleviate symptoms of low back pain (LBP) and therefore also included in this chapter. The term *common analgesics* is also intended to differentiate these medications from opioid analgesics and adjunctive analgesics, which are discussed in Chapters 12 and 13, respectively. The term non-opioid analgesic is also used to describe medications with analgesic properties other than opioids.

Older NSAIDs are sometimes termed *traditional, nonselective,* or *nonspecific* NSAIDs because they inhibit both the cyclooxygenase (COX)-1 and COX-2 enzymes. Newer NSAIDs are commonly known as COX-2 inhibitors (sometimes shortened to coxibs), selective, or specific NSAIDs because they block only the COX-2 isoenzyme.[1,2] *Simple analgesics* is a somewhat vague term of exclusion that typically refers to analgesics that are neither opioid analgesics nor adjunctive analgesics; in this chapter, the term is synonymous with acetaminophen. Muscle relaxants can be categorized as either antispasmodic or antispasticity.[3] *Muscle spasm* refers to an involuntary muscle contraction, whereas *spasticity* refers to persistent muscle contraction.

The two main subtypes of NSAIDs are nonselective and selective (Figure 11-1). Within nonselective NSAIDs, there are salicylates (e.g., aspirin, diflusinal, salsalate), phenylacetics (e.g., diclofenac), indoleacetic acids (e.g., etodolac, indomethacin, sulindac, tolmetin), oxicams (e.g., piroxicam, meloxicam), propionic acids (e.g., ibuprofen, naproxen, ketorolac, oxaprozin), and naphthylkanones (e.g., nabumetone). Within selective NSAIDs, there are only coxibs (e.g., celecoxib, rofecoxib, valdecoxib, and etoricoxib).

Muscle relaxants are a heterogeneous group of medications divided into antispasmodics and antispasticity

medications.[3] Antispasmodic muscle relaxants include two main categories, benzodiazepines and nonbenzodiazepines. Benzodiazepine antispasmodics have many properties and are used as skeletal muscle relaxants, sedatives, hypnotics, anticonvulsants, and anxiolytics; they include medications such as diazepam, fludiazepam, and tetrazepam. Nonbenzodiazepine antispasmodics act at the brain or spinal cord level to decrease muscle spasm associated with LBP and include medications such as cyclobenzaprine and flupirtin. Antispasticity muscle relaxants reduce spasticity associated with upper motor neuron (UMN) disorders and include medications such as dantrolene and baclofen. Simple analgesics include commonly used medications such as acetaminophen.

The World Health Organization generally advocates using a graduated approach to medication use for the management of pain, including chronic LBP (CLBP). This concept is illustrated by the "pain ladder" wherein simple analgesics and NSAIDs occupy the first rung and opioid analgesics occupy higher rungs. The pain ladder should only be climbed if first-line medications prove ineffective for achieving adequate pain management.[3-7]

History and Frequency of Use

Common analgesics have been used to treat LBP for many decades. Predecessor herbal ingredients (e.g., willow bark for aspirin), have been used for hundreds of years for relief of many painful conditions, including LBP.[8]

NSAIDs are the world's most frequently prescribed medications.[9,10] A 2000 US Medical Expenditure Panel Survey[11] found that 44 million prescriptions were written for 25 million patients with LBP, both acute and chronic. Of these, 16% were for nonselective NSAIDs, 10% were for COX-2 inhibitors, and 19% were for muscle relaxants. Most prescription NSAIDs (60%) were ibuprofen and naproxen, and most muscle relaxants (67%) were cyclobenzaprine, carisoprodol, and methocarbamol. A longitudinal study by Cherkin and colleagues[12] found that 69% of patients with LBP in the primary care setting were prescribed NSAIDs,

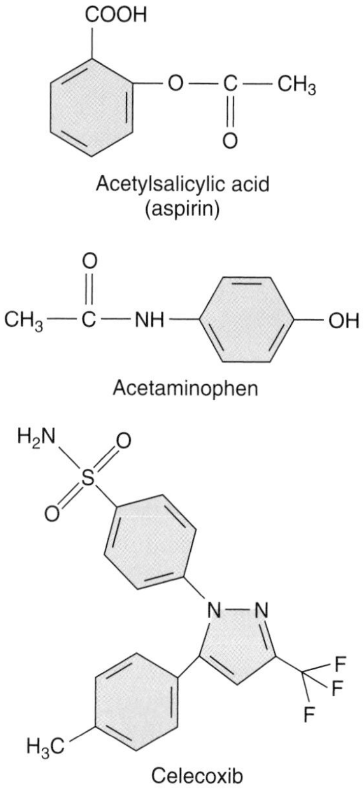

COOH

Acetylsalicylic acid
(aspirin)

Acetaminophen

Celecoxib

Figure 11-1 Molecular structures of several analgesics. (From Wecker L: Brody's human pharmacology, ed. 5. St. Louis, 2010, Mosby.)

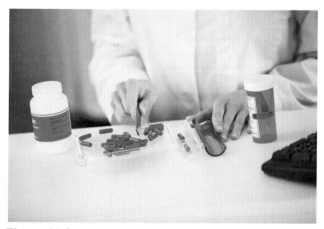

Figure 11-2 Common analgesics may be available as over-the-counter medications or by prescription. (© istockphoto.com/ Sean Locke)

35% received muscle relaxants, 4% received acetaminophen, and only 20% were not prescribed medications. A review of the University of Pittsburgh Healthcare System in 2001 found that 53% of men and 57% of women presenting with LBP were prescribed an NSAID[13]; more severe pain tended to be treated with opioids or muscle relaxants. NSAIDs were prescribed for 27% of patients, opioids and NSAIDs for 26%, opioid and other analgesics for 9%, and COX-2 inhibitors for 3%. A study in Sweden of 302 patients with CLBP reported that patients took an average of two different medications for that condition.[14] The most common class of drug consumed for CLBP was analgesics (59%), followed by NSAIDs (51%), muscle relaxants or anxiolytics (11%), and COX-2 inhibitors (5%). A study of health care use in patients with mechanical LBP enrolled in Kaiser Permanente Colorado indicated that 31% of patients had a claim for NSAIDs.[15]

Practitioner, Setting, and Availability

Any licensed physician may prescribe these classes of drugs, which are available in a variety of settings, including private practices and hospitals. This intervention is widely available in the United States. Many lower doses of NSAIDs, muscle relaxants, and simple analgesics are available as over-the-counter (OTC) medications, although higher doses and some specific medications in these drug classes are only available by prescription.

Procedure

Management of CLBP with common analgesics (as defined above) involves a consultation with a physician who will take a detailed medical and LBP-focused history, and inquire about current medication use. If deemed appropriate, the physician will then prescribe a common analgesic along with instructions about dosage, timing, side effects, and interactions with other medication; this information may also be provided by the dispensing pharmacist (Figure 11-2). A follow-up appointment will likely be scheduled within a few weeks so that the physician can determine whether the common analgesic is achieving the desired effect, adjust the dosage if necessary, change the medication in favor of another common analgesic or different class of medication if required, and provide education about other strategies for managing CLBP.

Regulatory Status

The common analgesics discussed in this chapter are all approved by the US Food and Drug Administration for primary indications related to pain, although not specifically CLBP. These medications are generally available OTC or with a prescription when larger doses are required. However, certain COX-2 inhibitors have been removed from the market following serious safety concerns.

THEORY

Mechanism of Action

Although grouped under the term *common analgesics*, medications classified as NSAIDs, simple analgesics, or muscle relaxants exhibit unique mechanisms of action.

Nonsteroidal Anti-Inflammatory Drugs

NSAIDs function through various degrees of reversible blockade of COX isoenzymes, thus blocking the inflammatory cascade of arachidonic acid to prostaglandins, which mediate inflammation and sensitize peripheral nociceptors.[16]

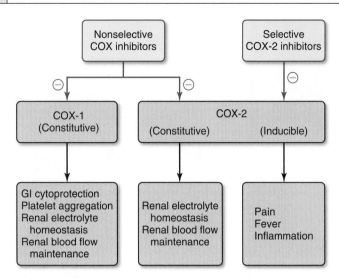

Figure 11-3 Properties of selective (i.e., COX-2) and nonselective (i.e., traditional) nonsteroidal anti-inflammatory drugs. (Modified from Wecker L: Brody's human pharmacology, ed. 5. St. Louis, 2010, Mosby.)

Aspirin is a type of salicylic NSAID with irreversible blockade of both COX isoenzymes, though it binds 170 times more to COX-1 than to COX-2, resulting in inhibition of prostaglandins and platelet aggregation. The exact mechanism of action for non-aspirin salicylates is currently unknown. Another mechanism involved with NSAIDs is inhibition of neutrophil function and phospholipase C activity, which increases intracellular calcium levels and production of arachidonic acid metabolites such as prostaglandins. These mechanisms account for both the anti-inflammatory and analgesic properties of NSAIDs (Figure 11-3).

Simple Analgesics

Acetaminophen possesses both analgesic and antipyretic properties. It is classified as a para-aminophen derivative that weakly inhibits COX isoenzymes, thereby selectively inhibiting prostaglandin synthesis without inhibiting neutrophils. The antipyretic effects of acetaminophen are likely due to its action in the heat regulation center located in the hypothalamus.[16]

Muscle Relaxants

This heterogeneous group of medications generally acts by inhibiting central polysynaptic neuronal events, which indirectly affect skeletal muscle.[17] Antispasticity muscle relaxants act on the central nervous system (CNS) to decrease UMN spasticity pathways. Baclofen is thought to act as a gamma-butyric acid (GABA) analog at GABA-B receptors, thus inhibiting presynaptic calcium influx and excitatory neurotransmitters. Tizanidine acts as an α_2-adrenergic agonist that is thought to inhibit presynaptic motor neurons. The mechanism through which diazepam relaxes skeletal muscle is currently unknown, but is thought to be related to its action on postsynaptic spinal cord GABA transmission. Antispasmodic muscle relaxants act centrally through currently unknown mechanisms. Cyclobenzaprine is thought to act on the brainstem, whereas metaxalone may work by inducing generalized depression of CNS activity.

Indication

Nonsteroidal Anti-Inflammatory Drugs

The primary indications for NSAIDs are generalized muscle aches and pains, soft tissue injuries, and arthritis.[17] NSAIDs can be used for any type of CLBP.

Simple Analgesics

The primary indications for acetaminophen are mild muscular aches, arthritis, and fever.[17] Acetaminophen can be used for any type of CLBP.

Muscle Relaxants

The primary indications for cyclobenzaprine, metaxolone, methocarbamol, and carisoprodol are acute painful musculoskeletal conditions.[16] Baclofen and tizanidine are indicated for spasticity associated with UMN disorders, but are frequently used off-label for painful musculoskeletal conditions. Diazepam is indicated for UMN muscle spasticity and local painful musculoskeletal spasm, as well as anxiety. Because the true mechanism of action on muscle spasm is unknown, the sedating side effects are often used to improve sleep. Muscle relaxants are mostly used for acute LBP or acute exacerbations of CLBP, rather than prolonged CLBP.

Patients with CLBP who are most likely to experience improvements with common analgesics are those without any contraindications or sensitivities to a specific medication, and without risk factors for chronicity such as psychological dysfunction, financial disincentives, or poor social support systems. Given that most of these medications are used only to address symptoms and do not affect any structural changes to the lumbosacral area, they are perhaps best used during acute exacerbations of CLBP rather than on an ongoing basis. The ideal CLBP patient for this type of intervention should also be willing to engage in an active intervention such as therapeutic exercise to address possible physical contributors to their condition.

Assessment

Before receiving common analgesics, patients should first be assessed for LBP using an evidence-based and goal-oriented approach focused on the patient history and neurologic examination, as discussed in Chapter 3. Additional diagnostic imaging or specific diagnostic testing is generally not required before initiating this intervention for CLBP. Prescribing physicians should also inquire about medication history to note prior hypersensitivity, allergy, or adverse events with similar drugs, and evaluate contraindications for these types of drugs. Clinicians may also order a psychological evaluation if they are concerned about the potential for medication misuse or potential for addiction in certain patients.

EFFICACY

Evidence supporting the efficacy of this intervention for CLBP was summarized from recent clinical practice guidelines (CPGs), systematic reviews (SRs), and randomized controlled trials (RCTs). Findings are summarized by study design for each intervention in the following paragraphs.

Clinical Practice Guidelines

Nonsteroidal Anti-Inflammatory Drugs

Five recent national CPGs on the management of CLBP have assessed and summarized the evidence to make specific recommendations about the efficacy of various NSAIDs.

A CPG from Belgium in 2006 found evidence that NSAIDs are not more effective than other conservative approaches including physical therapy, spinal manipulation therapy (SMT), or back school.[18] That CPG found low-quality evidence that NSAIDs are more effective than acetaminophen or placebo. That CPG concluded that there was insufficient evidence to support the efficacy of NSAIDs for CLBP. That CPG also found no evidence to support the efficacy of aspirin for CLBP.[18]

A CPG from the United Kingdom in 2009 found insufficient evidence to support the long-term use of NSAIDs and COX-2 inhibitors for CLBP.[19] That CPG recommended NSAIDs or COX-2 inhibitors as second choice medications only when acetaminophen was not effective for CLBP.[19]

A CPG from Europe in 2004 found strong evidence to support the efficacy of NSAIDs with respect to improvements in pain for up to 3 months in patients with CLBP.[3] That CPG therefore recommended the short-term use of NSAIDs for CLBP.[3]

A CPG from Italy in 2007 found evidence to support the efficacy of NSAIDs with respect to improvements in pain.[20] That CPG also found evidence that different NSAIDs are equally effective.

The CPG from the United States in 2007 found moderate evidence to support the use of NSAIDs for patients with CLBP.[21] That CPG also found insufficient evidence to estimate the efficacy of aspirin for CLBP.[21]

Findings from the above CPGs are summarized in Table 11-1.

Simple Analgesics

Four of the recent national CPGs on the management of CLBP have assessed and summarized the evidence to make specific recommendations about the efficacy of various simple analgesics.

The CPG from the United Kingdom in 2009 recommended acetaminophen as the first choice medication for the management of CLBP.[19]

The CPG from Belgium in 2006 found insufficient evidence to support the use of acetaminophen for CLBP.[18]

The CPG from Italy in 2007 found evidence to support the efficacy of acetaminophen with respect to improvements in pain.[20] That CPG also recommended acetaminophen as the first choice medication for the management of CLBP.

The CPG from the United States in 2007 found moderate-quality evidence to support the efficacy of acetaminophen with respect to improvements in pain.[21]

Findings from the aforementioned CPGs are summarized in Table 11-2.

TABLE 11-1	Clinical Practice Guideline Recommendations on Nonsteroidal Anti-Inflammatory Drugs for Chronic Low Back Pain	
Reference	Country	Conclusion
NSAIDs		
18	Belgium	Insufficient evidence to support use
19	United Kingdom	Recommended for use only if acetaminophen not effective
3	Europe	Recommended for short-term use (up to 3 months)
20	Italy	Evidence to support its use
21	United States	Moderate evidence to support use
COX-2 Inhibitors		
19	United Kingdom	Recommended for use only if acetaminophen not effective
Aspirin		
18	Belgium	No evidence to support use
21	United States	Insufficient evidence to estimate efficacy

TABLE 11-2	Clinical Practice Guideline Recommendations on Simple Analgesics for Chronic Low Back Pain	
Intervention	Country	Conclusion
Acetaminophen		
19	United Kingdom	Recommended
18	Belgium	Insufficient evidence to support use
20	Italy	Recommended
21	United States	Moderate evidence to support use

Muscle Relaxants

Four of the recent national CPGs on the management of CLBP have assessed and summarized the evidence to make specific recommendations about the efficacy of various muscle relaxants.

The CPG from Belgium in 2006 found very low-quality evidence to support the efficacy of muscle relaxants for the management of CLBP and low-quality evidence to support the efficacy of benzodiazepine muscle relaxants for the management of CLBP.[18] That CPG also found no evidence to support the efficacy of diazepam for the management of CLBP and concluded that tetrazepam is effective with respect to short-term improvements in pain. There was conflicting evidence to support the use of nonbenzodiazepine muscle relaxants for CLBP.[18]

The CPG from Europe in 2004 found limited evidence that muscle relaxants are not effective for the relief of muscle spasm.[3] That CPG concluded that muscle relaxants should be considered as one management option for short-term pain relief in patients with CLBP.[3] There was strong evidence to support the efficacy of benzodiazepine muscle relaxants in the pain relief of patients with CLBP and conflicting evidence to support the efficacy of nonbenzodiazepine muscle relaxants for CLBP.[3]

The CPG from Italy in 2007 found evidence to support the efficacy of muscle relaxants with respect to improvements in pain.[20] That CPG concluded that muscle relaxants are an option for the management of CLBP, but should not be used as a first choice medication.

The CPG from the United States in 2007 found insufficient evidence to support the efficacy of muscle relaxants for CLBP.[21] Nevertheless, that CPG concluded that muscle relaxants are one possible option for the management of CLBP. There was also evidence to support a moderate benefit for benzodiazepine muscle relaxants for CLBP.[21]

Findings from the above CPGs are summarized in Table 11-3.

Systematic Reviews

Nonsteroidal Anti-Inflammatory Drugs

Cochrane Collaboration. An SR was conducted in 2008 by the Cochrane Collaboration on NSAIDs for LBP.[9] A total of 65 RCTs were included. Of these studies, 37 included patients with acute or subacute LBP, 7 included patients with CLBP, and 21 included mixed duration LBP populations.[22-85] Meta-analysis showed that NSAIDs were more effective than placebo for acute and chronic LBP without sciatica, but also showed that there were more side effects with NSAID use compared with placebo. This review concluded that NSAIDs provide short-term improvement in pain among patients with acute and chronic LBP without neurologic involvement. The SR also concluded that the different types of NSAIDs are equally effective and that COX-2 inhibitors may exhibit fewer side effects than older NSAIDs, yet recent studies show that COX-2 inhibitors are associated with increased cardiovascular events among certain patients.

American Pain Society and American College of Physicians. An SR was conducted in 2007 by the American Pain Society and the American College of Physicians CPG committee on medication for acute and chronic LBP.[86] That review identified three SRs on NSAIDs (including the Cochrane Collaboration review mentioned earlier).[9,87,88] The second SR evaluated in this review also reached similar conclusions as the Cochrane review.[9,87] The third SR concluded that NSAIDs were not more effective than placebo for LBP with sciatica.[88] Overall, this review concluded that there is good evidence that NSAIDs are effective for short-term pain relief in LBP, and there is little evidence suggesting differences in efficacy between various NSAIDs. However, this review also concluded that there is a paucity of data on serious adverse events related to NSAID use in LBP, which is an important consideration given previous concerns over gastrointestinal (GI) and cardiovascular safety. There were two additional RCTs on CLBP identified in these SRs.[89,90]

Findings from the above SRs are summarized in Table 11-4.

TABLE 11-3	Clinical Practice Guideline Recommendations on Muscle Relaxants for Chronic Low Back Pain	
Intervention	Country	Conclusion
Muscle Relaxants		
18	Belgium	Low-quality evidence to support use
3	Europe	May be considered for short-term use
20	Italy	May be considered but not as first choice
21	United States	Are an option for management of CLBP
Benzodiazepines		
18	Belgium	Low-quality evidence to support efficacy
3	Europe	Strong evidence of efficacy
21	United States	Evidence to support moderate benefit
Diazepam		
18	Belgium	No evidence to support efficacy
Tetrazepam		
18	Belgium	May be considered for short-term use
Non-Benzodiazepines		
18	Belgium	Conflicting evidence supporting use
3	Europe	Conflicting evidence supporting efficacy

CLBP, chronic low back pain.

Simple Analgesics

No recent SRs were identified that reported specifically on the efficacy of simple analgesics as an intervention for LBP.

Muscle Relaxants

Cochrane Collaboration. An SR was conducted in 2003 by the Cochrane Collaboration on muscle relaxants for nonspecific LBP.[91] A total of 30 RCTs were included, of which 77% were found to be of high quality. Of these studies, 23 included patients with acute LBP, 6 included patients with CLBP, and 1 study included mixed duration LBP populations.[27,28,49,55,92-117] The review concluded that there is strong evidence that nonbenzodiazepine muscle relaxants were more effective than placebo in short-term pain relief and overall improvement in acute LBP patients. However, they were associated with significantly more overall adverse events and CNS adverse events than placebo; no differences were found in GI adverse events. The evidence was less clear for the use of benzodiazepines compared with placebo for acute LBP, and muscle relaxants (both benzodiazepines and nonbenzodiazepines) for CLBP. Although pooled analysis of two studies found tetrazepam to be more effective than placebo in short-term pain relief and global improvement in

TABLE 11-4	Systematic Review Findings on Nonsteroidal Anti-Inflammatory Drugs, Simple Analgesics, and Muscle Relaxants for Chronic Low Back Pain			
Reference	# RCTs in SR	# RCTs for CLBP	Conclusion	
9, 141	65	7 chronic 21 mixed populations	NSAIDs more effective than placebo for CLBP without sciatica More side effects with NSAIDs compared to placebo	
86	3 SRs	NR	NSAIDs not more effective than placebo for LBP with sciatica NSAIDs effective for short-term pain relief in LBP	
91	30	6 chronic 1 mixed population	Evidence unclear about use of benzodiazepines compared to muscle relaxants for CLBP No one type of muscle relaxant is more effective than others in treating CLBP Tetrazepam more effective than placebo in short-term pain relief and global improvement in CLBP	
86	4 SRs	NR	Did not summarize findings specifically for CLBP	

CLBP, chronic low back pain; LBP, low back pain; NR, not reported; NSAIDs, nonsteroidal anti-inflammatory drugs; RCT, randomized controlled trial; SR, systematic review.

CLBP, the review did not find that one type of muscle relaxant was more effective than any other.

American Pain Society and American College of Physicians

An SR was conducted in 2007 by the American Pain Society and American College of Physicians CPG committee on medication for acute and chronic LBP.[86] That review identified four SRs on muscle relaxants, including the Cochrane Collaboration review mentioned earlier.[87,88,91,118] Two additional trials not included in the Cochrane review and identified in two additional SRs, also included patients with CLBP.[119,120] Two other SRs reached similar conclusions as the Cochrane review, while a third SR that focused on sciatica[88] found no difference between tizanidine and placebo based on one higher-quality trial.[87,88,91,118] Overall, the SR concluded that there is good evidence that muscle relaxants are effective for short-term pain relief in acute LBP. There is little evidence that there are differences in efficacy between various muscle relaxants. Little evidence was found on the efficacy of the antispasticity medications baclofen and dantrolene for LBP. The review also noted that muscle relaxants are associated with more CNS adverse events than placebo.

Randomized Controlled Trials

Nonsteroidal Anti-Inflammatory Drugs

Eleven RCTs and 12 reports related to those studies were identified.[38,59,60,62-64,73,83,121-124] Their methods are summarized in Table 11-5. Their results are briefly described here.

An RCT conducted by Hickey and colleagues[38] included CLBP patients without neurologic involvement, who had symptoms lasting longer than 6 months. Participants were randomized to either diflunisal (500 mg twice daily) for 4 weeks or paracetamol (1000 mg four times daily) for 4 weeks. At the end of 4 weeks, there was improved pain (0-3 scale) and disability (0-3 scale) in patients from both groups compared with baseline (P values not reported). More patients in the diflunisal group had improved pain and disability than in the paracetamol group (P values not reported). This study was considered of higher quality.

An RCT with a crossover design was conducted by Berry and colleagues[59] on CLBP patients with or without neurologic involvement, who had symptoms for at least 3 months. Participants were each given (1) naproxen (550 mg twice daily), (2) diflunisal twice (550 mg twice daily), or (3) placebo in random sequence, with each treatment lasting for 2 weeks. At the end of the treatment period, there was a significant reduction in pain (visual analog scale [VAS]) in the naproxen group, a significant increase in pain in the placebo group, and no significant change in the diflunisal group. There was a significant difference in pain between the naproxen group and the diflunisal and placebo groups. Disability was not measured in this study. This study was considered of lower quality.

An RCT conducted by Postacchini and colleagues[83] included acute and chronic LBP patients with or without radiating pain. Participants were randomized to (1) diclofenac (10 to 14 days for acute cases, 15 to 20 days for chronic cases; the dose was reported as "full dosage" without providing any further details); (2) chiropractic manipulation; (3) physical therapy; (4) bed rest; (5) back school; or (6) placebo. At the end of 6 months, there was improvement in the mean combined score for pain, disability, and spinal mobility in all groups (P values not reported). The mean combined score in CLBP without radiating pain was highest in the back school group, which was significantly higher than in the other groups. There were no significant differences between any of the treatment groups for acute or chronic LBP with radiating pain, or acute LBP without radiating pain. This study was considered of lower quality.

An RCT conducted by Videman and Osterman[63] included patients with chronic severe LBP with known causes. Participants had CLBP, with or without neurologic involvement, and had symptoms lasting from 1 month to 15 years. Participants were randomized to a 6-week treatment of either piroxicam (50 mg daily) or indomethacin (25 mg three times daily). At the end of the treatment period, there was a statistically significant improvement in pain intensity (VAS) in both groups, but no significant differences between the groups. Disability was not measured in this study. This study was considered of lower quality.

TABLE 11-5   Randomized Controlled Trials of Nonsteroidal Anti-Inflammatory Drugs for Chronic Low Back Pain

Reference	Indication	Intervention	Control (C1)	Control (C2)	Control (C3)	Control (C4)	Control (C5)
38	CLBP without neurologic involvement, symptoms >6 months	Diflunisal 500 mg twice daily × 4 weeks n = 16	Acetaminophen 1000 mg four times daily × 4 weeks n = 14	NA	NA	NA	NA
59*	CLBP with or without neurologic involvement, symptoms >3 months	Naproxen 550 mg twice daily × 2 weeks n = 37	Diflunisal 500 mg twice daily × 2 weeks n = 37	Placebo twice daily × 2 weeks n = 37	NA	NA	NA
83	Acute and CLBP, with or without radiating pain, symptoms <4 weeks (acute), >2 months (chronic)	Diclofenac dose not reported 10-14 days (acute) 15-20 days (chronic) n = 81	Chiropractic manipulation; frequency unknown n = 87	PT; frequency unknown n = 78	Bed rest; frequency unknown n = 29	Back school; frequency unknown n = 50	Placebo n = 73
63	CLBP, with or without neurologic involvement, symptoms >1 month	Indomethacin 25 mg three times daily × 6 weeks n = 14	Piroxicam 20 mg daily × 6 weeks n = 14	NA	NA	NA	NA
64	CLBP, neurologic involvement not reported, symptom duration not reported	Etoricoxib 60 mg daily × 4 weeks n = 224	Diclofenac 50 mg three times daily × 4 weeks n = 222	NA	NA	NA	NA
60	CLBP without neurologic involvement, symptoms >3 months	Etoricoxib 60 mg daily × 12 weeks n = 103	Etoricoxib 90 mg daily × 12 weeks n = 107	Placebo daily × 12 weeks n = 109	NA	NA	NA
62,121	CLBP without neurologic involvement, symptoms >3 months	Rofecoxib 25 mg daily × 4 weeks n = 233	Rofecoxib 50 mg daily × 4 weeks n = 229	Placebo daily × 4 weeks n = 228	NA	NA	NA
73	CLBP with or without neurologic symptoms, symptoms >6 months	Rofecoxib 12.5 mg daily × 6 weeks n = 44	Harpagophytum extract 60 mg daily × 6 weeks n = 44	NA	NA	NA	NA
122	CLBP without neurologic symptoms, symptom duration not reported	Rofecoxib 25 mg daily × 4 weeks n = 126	Rofecoxib 50 mg daily × 4 weeks n = 126	Placebo daily × 4 weeks n = 128			
123	CLBP without neurologic involvement, symptoms >3 months	Etoricoxib 60 mg daily × 12 weeks n = 109	Etoricoxib 90 mg daily × 12 weeks n = 106	Placebo daily × 12 weeks n = 110			
124	CLBP without neurologic involvement, symptoms >3 months	Celecoxib 200 mg twice daily × 6 weeks Study 1: n = 402 Study 2: n = 396	Tramadol HCl 50 mg four times daily × 6 weeks Study 1: n = 389 Study 2: n = 396				

*Crossover design.
CLBP, chronic low back pain; NA, not applicable; NSAIDs, nonsteroidal anti-inflammatory drugs; PT, physical therapy.

An RCT conducted by Zerbini and colleagues[64] included CLBP patients who experienced worsening symptoms ("flare") after prestudy analgesic medication had been discontinued. Participants were randomized to either etoricoxib (60 mg daily) or diclofenac (50 mg three times daily) for 4 weeks. At the end of the treatment period, there was a significant improvement in pain (VAS) and disability (Roland Morris Disability Questionnaire [RMDQ]) in both groups. There was no significant difference in pain or disability between groups. This study was considered of lower quality.

An RCT conducted by Birbara and colleagues[60] included CLBP patients who experienced worsening symptoms ("flare") after prestudy analgesic medication had been discontinued. Participants had symptoms, without neurologic involvement, lasting longer than 3 months. Participants were randomized to (1) etoricoxib (60 mg daily); (2) etoricoxib (90 mg daily); or (3) placebo for 12 weeks. At the end of the treatment period, there was a significant improvement in pain (VAS) and disability (RMDQ) in all three groups. The improvements in pain or disability were significantly greater in both etoricoxib groups compared with the placebo group. There were no significant differences between the 60- and 90-mg etoricoxib dose groups. This study was considered of lower quality.

An RCT conducted by Katz and colleagues[62,121] included CLBP patients who experienced worsening symptoms ("flare") after prestudy analgesic medication had been discontinued. Participants had symptoms, without neurologic involvement, lasting longer than 3 months. Participants were randomized to (1) rofecoxib (25 mg daily); (2) rofecoxib (50 mg daily); or (3) placebo for 4 weeks. At the end of the treatment period, there was a significant improvement in pain (VAS) and disability (RMDQ) in all three groups. The improvements in pain or disability were significantly greater in both rofecoxib groups compared with the placebo group. There were no significant differences between the 25- and 50-mg rofecoxib dose groups. This study was considered of lower quality.

An RCT conducted by Chrubasik and colleagues[73] included CLBP patients with or without leg pain, who had symptoms lasting longer than 6 months. Participants were randomized to either rofecoxib (12.5 mg daily) or *Harpagophytum* extract (60 mg daily) for 6 weeks. At the end of 6 weeks, pain intensity (Arhus LBP index) improved in both groups compared with baseline (*P* values not reported). The difference in pain between the two groups was not statistically significant. Disability was not measured in this study. This study was considered of lower quality.

An RCT conducted by Ju and colleagues[122] included CLBP patients without neurologic involvement who experienced worsening symptoms ("flare") after prestudy analgesic medication had been discontinued. Participants were randomized to (1) rofecoxib (25 mg daily); (2) rofecoxib (50 mg daily); or (3) placebo for 4 weeks. At the end of the treatment period, there were greater improvements in pain (VAS) or disability (RMDQ) in both rofecoxib groups compared with the placebo group. There were no significant differences between the 25- and 50-mg rofecoxib dose groups. Within-group comparisons for pain and disability were not reported. This study was considered of lower quality.

An RCT conducted by Pallay and colleagues[123] included CLBP patients who had symptoms without neurologic involvement, lasting longer than 3 months. Participants were randomized to (1) etoricoxib (60 mg daily); (2) etoricoxib (90 mg daily); or (3) placebo for 12 weeks. At the end of the treatment period, there was a significant improvement in pain (VAS) and disability (RMDQ) in all three groups. The improvements in pain or disability were significantly greater in both etoricoxib groups compared with the placebo group. There were no significant differences between the 60- and 90-mg etoricoxib dose groups. This study was considered of lower quality.

An RCT conducted by O'Donnell and colleagues[124] included CLBP patients without neurologic involvement. Participants were randomized to celecoxib (200 mg twice daily) or tramadol HCl (50 mg four times daily) and examined in two separate studies. At the end of 6 weeks, the percentage of patients experiencing an improvement of greater than 30 on the numerical rating scale for pain among patients randomized to celecoxib was statistically superior to the proportion experiencing improvement in the tramadol group in both studies.

Simple Analgesics
Three RCTs were identified.[38,125,126] Their methods are summarized in Table 11-6, and their results are briefly described here.

An RCT conducted by Hickey[38] included CLBP patients without neurologic involvement, who had symptoms lasting longer than 6 months. Participants were randomized to either diflunisal (500 mg twice daily) or paracetamol (1000 mg four times daily) for 4 weeks. At the end of 4 weeks, there was improved pain (0-3 scale) and disability (0-3 scale) in patients from both groups compared with baseline (*P* values not reported). More patients within the diflunisal group had improved pain and disability than in the paracetamol group (*P* values not reported). This study was considered of higher quality.

Peloso and colleagues[125] performed a 91-day RCT comparing the efficacy and safety of combined tramadol (37.5 mg) and acetaminophen (325 mg) (the combination was termed Ultracet) to placebo in 338 patients with CLBP. Dosing was titrated over 10 days, after which participants took one or two tablets up to four times daily. Participants had pain lasting at least 3 months and did not have neurologic involvement. A total of 147 (43.5%) completed the trial, with 81 and 110 participants withdrawing in the tramadol and placebo groups, respectively. At the end of 91 days, pain scores (VAS) improved in the tramadol group but not in the placebo group compared with baseline (*P* values not reported). There was also a modest improvement in function (RMDQ) in both groups (*P* values not reported). The tramadol plus acetaminophen group had significantly better improvements in pain and function than the placebo group.

Ruoff and colleagues reported a 91-day RCT that compared flexible-dose tramadol (37.5 mg) plus acetaminophen (325 mg) with placebo in patients with CLBP.[126] Dosing was titrated over 10 days, after which participants took a maximum of eight tablets daily. Participants had symptoms lasting at least 3 months and did not have neurologic involvement. At

TABLE 11-6   Randomized Controlled Trials of Simple Analgesics for Chronic Low Back Pain

Reference	Indication	Intervention	Control (C1)
38	CLBP without neurologic involvement, symptoms >6 months	Acetaminophen 1000 mg four times daily × 4 weeks n = 14	Diflunisal 500 mg twice daily × 4 weeks n = 16
125	CLBP without neurologic involvement, symptoms ≥3 months	Combination tramadol 37.5 mg + acetaminophen (325 mg) (1-2 tablets up to four times daily) × 91 days n = 167	Placebo 1-2 tablets up to four times daily × 91 days n = 171
126	CLBP without neurologic involvement, symptoms ≥3 months	Combination tramadol 37.5 mg + acetaminophen (325 mg) (maximum eight tablets daily) × 91 days n = 162	Placebo maximum eight tablets daily × 91 days n = 160

CLBP, chronic low back pain.

TABLE 11-7   Randomized Controlled Trials of Muscle Relaxants for Chronic Low Back Pain

Reference	Indication	Intervention	Control (C1)	Control (C2)
111	Subacute or chronic LBP, neurologic involvement not reported, symptom duration not reported	Tetrazepam 50 mg three times daily × 10 days n = 25	Placebo three times daily × 10 days n = 25	NA
115	CLBP, neurologic involvement not reported, symptom duration not reported	Tetrazepam + PT 50 mg three times daily × 14 days n = 79	Placebo three times daily + PT 14 days n = 73	NA
113	CLBP >20 days, neurologic involvement not reported	Pridinol mesilate 4 mg IM twice daily × 3 days; followed by 2 mg PO BID × 4 days n = 60	Thiocolchicoside 4 mg IM twice daily × 3 days; followed by 2 mg PO BID × 4 days n = 60	NA
112	CLBP, without neurologic involvement, symptom duration not reported	Cyclobenzaprine 10 mg three times daily × 14 days n = 34	Diazepam 5 mg three times daily × 14 days n = 36	Placebo three times daily × 14 days n = 35
114	Muscle spasm associated with spine and proximal joints, symptom duration not reported	Tolperisone; allowed PT 100 mg three times daily × 21 days n = 67	Placebo three times daily; allowed PT 21 days n = 70	NA

CLBP, chronic low back pain; IM, intramuscular; LBP, low back pain; NA, not applicable, PO, orally; PT, physical therapy.

the end of the treatment period, both groups had improved pain (VAS) compared with baseline (*P* values not reported). There was also improvement in disability (RMDQ) compared with baseline (*P* values not reported). The tramadol/acetaminophen group had significantly better pain and disability outcomes compared with the placebo group.

Muscle Relaxants

Five RCTs were identified.[111-115] Their methods are summarized in Table 11-7, and their results are briefly described below.

An RCT by Arbus and colleagues[111] randomized CLBP patients to either tetrazepam (50 mg three times daily) or placebo (three times daily) for 10 days. At 14 days, mean

pain scores improved in both groups compared with baseline (*P* values not reported). The improvement in pain in the tetrazepam group was significantly greater than in the placebo group. Disability was not measured in this study. This study was considered of higher quality.

An RCT by Salzmann and colleagues[115] randomized CLBP patients who did not respond to physical therapy, to either tetrazepam (50 mg three times daily) or placebo (three times daily) for 14 days. At 14 days, the proportion of patients reporting greater than 66.6% reduction of daytime pain increased in both groups compared with baseline. The difference between groups was not statistically significant. Disability was not measured in this study. This study was considered of higher quality.

An RCT by Pipino and colleagues[113] of CLBP patients with muscle spasm randomized participants to either pridinol mesylate or thiocolchicoside. The treatments consisted of 4 mg intramuscular injections twice daily for 3 days followed by 2 mg twice daily taken orally for 4 days. At the end of the treatment period, mean pain intensity (VAS) was reduced in both groups. There was no statistically significant difference between groups. Disability was not measured in this study. This study was considered of lower quality.

An RCT by Basmajian[112] of CLBP patients with muscle spasms for longer than 30 days randomized participants to either (1) cyclobenzaprine (10 mg three times daily); (2) diazepam (5 mg three times daily), or (3) placebo for 14 days. Outcomes were measured after the treatment period, but pain and disability were not measured. This study was considered of lower quality.

An RCT conducted by Pratzel and colleagues[114] included patients with painful reflex muscle spasm associated with diseases of the spinal column or proximal joints. Participants were randomized to tolperisone hydrochloride (300 mg daily) or daily placebo for 21 days. At the end of the treatment period, the change score for the pressure pain threshold increased significantly in both groups compared to baseline. The increase in the tolperisone group was significantly higher than that of placebo. Disability was not measured in this study. This study was considered of higher quality.

SAFETY

Contraindications

Nonsteroidal Anti-Inflammatory Drugs

NSAIDs should not be used in any patient with peptic ulcer disease or congestive heart failure, and should be monitored closely in patients with known renal disease or severe hepatic disease.[13] Naproxen is typical of nonselective NSAIDs and is contraindicated for use in the last 3 months of pregnancy, during the perioperative period for cardiac surgery, in patients with increased risk of bleeding, as well as with asthma, allergic rhinitis, and nasal polyps.[17] Celecoxib, the only remaining COX-2 inhibitor on the US market, is contraindicated in patients with sulfonamide hypersensitivity and, like all NSAIDs, should be used with extra caution in patients with cardiac disease or hypertension.[127]

Simple Analgesics

Acetaminophen should be used with care in the presence of hepatic disease, and should be used with caution in patients who consume alcohol regularly or who are alcoholics. Daily doses of acetaminophen should not exceed 4 grams.[17]

Muscle Relaxants

Because of their sedating effects, muscle relaxants should first be tried when the patient is in a safe situation (e.g., at home) where poor mental clarity would not be detrimental. Benzodiazepines such as diazepam are contraindicated in narrow angle glaucoma.[17] Cyclobenzaprine should not be used within 14 days of monoamine oxidase inhibitors, or in patients with cardiac arrhythmias, coronary artery disease, hyperthyroidism, chronic heart failure, or after an acute myocardial infarction. Metaxalone is not recommended in those with significantly reduced renal or hepatic function, or anemia. Dantrolene is generally contraindicated as a muscle relaxant for CLBP because of potential liver toxicity.

Indications for common analgesics are listed in Table 11-8.

Adverse Events

Nonsteroidal Anti-Inflammatory Drugs

The risk of GI, renal, hepatic, and cardiovascular adverse events in patients taking nonselective NSAIDs is well known.[3,16,17,128] These adverse events are related to the blockade of COX isoenzymes, neutrophil function, and phospholipase activity by NSAIDs. The potential for harms among nonselective NSAIDs may be slightly different. For example, it has been suggested that sulindac may be relatively renal sparing, whereas naproxen may be relatively cardioprotective. A meta-analysis found that ibuprofen and diclofenac had the lowest rates of GI adverse events among nonselective NSAIDs because of the lower doses used in practice.[129]

The advent of COX-2 inhibitors was heralded due to their potential for decreased harms relative to nonselective NSAIDs. However, the literature to date suggests that while associated harms may be different, adverse events associated with COX-2 inhibitors are nevertheless substantial. The Celebrex Long-term Arthritis Safety Study (CLASS) compared celecoxib 400 mg twice daily, ibuprofen 800 mg three times daily, and diclofenac 75 mg twice daily in an observational cohort study with 8059 participants.[128] The incidence of GI adverse events was 0.44% with celecoxib and 1.27% for nonselective NSAIDs. The Vioxx Gastrointestinal Outcomes Research (VIGOR) study similarly compared rofecoxib with naproxen.[130] Although there were fewer GI adverse events with rofecoxib, the risk of myocardial infarction was increased fivefold in the rofecoxib group. Suggestions that these results were attributable to the potential cardioprotective effect of naproxen rather than the harms of rofecoxib were refuted when another study reported similar results in patients taking rofecoxib.[127] Rofecoxib was later withdrawn from the market voluntarily by its manufacturer. Increased cardiovascular adverse events with COX-2 inhibitors are theorized as occurring from a disruption in the normal balance between pro- and anti-thrombotic prostaglandins.[16] Specifically, thromboxane A2 is a platelet activator and aggregator that is mediated by prostaglandin products in the COX-1 isomer pathways, whereas prostaglandin PGI2 vasodilates and inhibits platelet aggregation when the COX-2 isomer is activated. Thrombotic adverse cardiac events may occur when thromboxane A2 dominates prostaglandin PGI2.

A retrospective study of more than 70,000 older patients taking celecoxib, rofecoxib, naproxen, or other NSAIDs found no increased risk of cardiac adverse events when use was less than a year in duration.[131] The CPG from Belgium reported that harms associated with long-term use of nonselective NSAIDs or COX-2 inhibitors in patients with

TABLE 11-8	Approved Indications for Common Analgesics			
Drug Type **Subcategory** **Category**	**Generic Name**	**Trade Name**	**Indication**
Simple analgesic	Acetaminophen	Tylenol (among others)	Fever Pain Muscle aches Minor aches and pains associated with common cold Minor pain of arthritis Menstrual cramps

NSAIDs
  nonselective
  salicylates
	Aspirin	Bufferin (among others)	Pain
			Fever
			Swelling, stiffness and joint pain caused by arthritis

NSAIDs
  nonselective
  phenylacetics
	Diclofenac	Cataflam
		Voltaren
			Rheumatoid arthritis
			Osteoarthritis
			Ankylosing spondylitis

NSAIDs
  nonselective
  indoleacetic acids
	Etodolac	Lodine
		Lodine XL
			Rheumatoid arthritis
			Osteoarthritis

	Indomethacin	Indocin Indocin SR	Acute gouty arthritis Moderate to severe ankylosing spondylitis Osteoarthritis Rheumatoid arthritis
	Sulindac	Clinoril	Osteoarthritis Rheumatoid arthritis Ankylosing spondylitis Acute painful shoulder Acute gouty arthritis
	Tolmetin	Tolectin DS Tolectin 600	Rheumatoid arthritis Osteoarthritis Juvenile rheumatoid arthritis
	Diflunisal	Dolobid	Mild to moderate pain Osteoarthritis Rheumatoid arthritis

NSAIDs
  nonselective
  oxicams
	Meloxicam	Mobic	Rheumatoid arthritis
			Osteoarthritis

	Piroxicam	Feldene	Rheumatoid arthritis Osteoarthritis

NSAIDs
  nonselective
  propionic acids
	Ibuprofen	Advil
		Genpril
		Ibu
		Midol
		Motrin
		Nuprin
			Rheumatoid arthritis
			Osteoarthritis
			Mild to moderate pain
			Dysmenorrheal

	Naproxen	Aleve Anaprox EC-Naprosyn Naprosyn Naprelan	Rheumatoid arthritis Osteoarthritis Ankylosing spondylitis Juvenile rheumatoid arthritis Tendonitis Bursitis Acute gout Pain Dysmenorrhea
	Ketorolac	Toradol	Acute pain in adults
	Oxaprozin	Daypro	Osteoarthritis Rheumatoid arthritis Juvenile rheumatoid arthritis

NSAIDs
  nonselective
  naphthylkanones
	Nabumetone	Relafen	Osteoarthritis
			Rheumatoid arthritis

TABLE 11-8	Approved Indications for Common Analgesics—cont'd		
Drug Type **Subcategory** **Category**	**Generic Name**	**Trade Name**	**Indication**
NSAIDs COX-2 inhibitors	Celecoxib	Celebrex	Osteoarthritis Rheumatoid arthritis Ankylosing spondylitis Pain Dysmenorrhea Reduction of colorectal polyps in familial adenomatous polyposis Juvenile rheumatoid arthritis Unlabeled use—adjunctive therapy in treatment of schizophrenia
	Valdecoxib		Not in the United States
	Rofecoxib	Vioxx	Withdrawn from US market in 2004
	Etoricoxib	Arcoxia	Not in the United States
	Lumiracoxib	Prexige	Not in the United States
	Parecoxib	Dynastat	Not in the United States
Muscle relaxants antispasmodic benzodiazepines	Diazepam	Valium	Management of anxiety disorders Relief of acute symptoms associated with acute alcohol withdrawal Adjunct for relief of skeletal muscle spasm due to reflex spasm to local pathology Spasticity caused by upper motor neuron disorders Athetosis Stiff-man syndrome
	Fludiazepam	Erispan	muscle spasm
	Tetrazepam	Mylostan	muscle spasm
Muscle relaxants antispasmodic nonbenzodiazepines	Cyclobenzaprine	Amrix Fexmid Flexeril	Muscle spasm associated with acute, painful musculoskeletal conditions
	Flupirtin		Muscle spasm
Muscle relaxants antispasticity	Dantrolene	Dantrium Dantrium intravenous	Clinical spasticity resulting from upper motor neuron disorders
	Baclofen	Generic only	Spasticity resulting from multiple sclerosis Concomitant pain Clonus Muscular rigidity

Source: www.drugs.com.
NSAIDs, nonsteroidal anti-inflammatory drugs.

CLBP may be substantial but are likely understudied.[18] A meta-analysis of the VIGOR, CLASS, and two smaller studies reported that use of low-dose aspirin by study participants may have provided cardioprotection.[132] Unfortunately, low-dose aspirin was also associated with an increase in the incidence of GI adverse events from 0.44% to 2.01%.[128] Prolonged use of rofecoxib in patients with CLBP has been associated with a potential increase in cardiovascular risk.[3]

Simple Analgesics
Use of large doses of acetaminophen has been associated with hepatic toxicity. Although the risk of hepatic toxicity was generally thought to be low when exposure to acetaminophen is less than 7.5-10 grams daily, there have been recent concerns about hepatic toxicity due to cumulative acetaminophen dosing from multiple sources and caution is warranted.[17]

Muscle Relaxants
Adverse events related to CNS depression, including dizziness and sedation, have consistently been reported in clinical trials of muscle relaxants.[113,133] There is also a risk of dependency with some muscle relaxants.[3] This is most notable with carisoprodol, which is listed as a controlled substance in some states in the US.[134] Symptoms of withdrawal from some muscle relaxants are also a concern. Sudden discontinued use of long-term benzodiazepines has been associated seizures; its use should be tapered conservatively to avoid symptoms of withdrawal.[17]

COSTS

Fees and Third-Party Reimbursement

In the United States, a recommendation for common analgesics for CLBP can likely be delivered by a clinician in the context of an office or outpatient visit for a new patient using CPT codes 99201 (up to 10 minutes), 99202 (up to 20 minutes), or 99203 (up to 30 minutes). For an established patient, these can likely be provided during an office or outpatient visit using CPT codes 99211 (up to 5 minutes), 99212 (up to 10 minutes), or 99213 (up to 15 minutes). Although time is indicated for the various levels of service and can be a contributing component for selection of the level of office/outpatient visits, the overarching criteria for selection of the level of service should be based on medical necessity and the amount of history, examination, and medical decision-making that is required and documented.

These procedures are widely covered by other third-party payers such as health insurers and worker's compensation insurance. Although some payers continue to base their reimbursements on usual, customary, and reasonable payment methodology, the majority have developed reimbursement tables based on the Resource Based Relative Value Scale used by Medicare. Reimbursements by other third-party payers are generally higher than Medicare.

Typical fees reimbursed by Medicare in New York and California for these services are summarized in Table 11-9.

Common analgesics are typically covered by most third-party payers only if they are prescribed by a physician. Medications available OTC are generally not reimbursed by third-party payers, many of whom now use pharmacy benefits managers (PBMs) to create and maintain formularies of covered medications. PBMs may only include a few medications under each broad class of common analgesics, and may require prior authorization, failure of a cheaper medication, or medical justification for using a more expensive medication within the same class.

The cost of common analgesics varies considerably for each drug class and medication. Older NSAIDs that are now available as generics may cost as little as a few pennies per pill, whereas newer COX-2 inhibitors may cost as much as a few dollars per pill. OTC medications are generally very inexpensive. The average US wholesale cost per tablet in 2005 was $0.03 for aspirin, $0.15 for naproxen, and $2.34

for celecoxib.[135] In Canada in 2003, the daily cost (in Canadian Dollars) of ibuprofen 800 mg three times daily was $0.22, of acetaminophen 1000 mg four times daily was $0.37, of naproxen 500 mg twice daily was $0.42, and of celecoxib 100 mg twice daily was $1.25.[136]

Table 11-10 provides the approximate cost of a 30-day supply of NSAIDs, simple analgesics, and muscle relaxants from a PBM in the United States.

Cost Effectiveness

Evidence supporting the cost effectiveness of this intervention for acute or chronic LBP was summarized based on cost effectiveness analyses (CEAs) and cost utility analyses (CUAs) identified in two recent SRs of interventions for LBP.[137,138] Clinical and economic findings for CEAs and CUAs are summarized below.

An RCT trial in Sweden compared three approaches for patients sick-listed with acute LBP.[139] The manual therapy group received SMT, mobilization, assisted stretching, and exercises. The intensive training group received supervised exercise therapy with a physical therapist, including general and stabilization exercises. The usual care group received various interventions from a general practitioner, including common analgesics and brief education. Clinical outcomes were not reported. Direct medical costs associated with study interventions over 1 year including provider visits, diagnostic testing, and surgery (if needed) were approximately $1054 in the manual therapy group, approximately $1123 in the intensive training group, and approximately $404 in the usual care group. Indirect productivity costs associated with lost work days were approximately $6163 in the manual therapy group, approximately $5557 in the intensive training group, and approximately $7072 in the usual care group. Total costs (direct medical and indirect productivity) over 1 year were therefore approximately $7217 in the manual therapy group, approximately $6680 in the intensive training group, and approximately $7476 in the usual care group. Cost differences between groups were not significant.

Other

A study was conducted to estimate the direct medical costs focusing on analgesic medication used for mechanical LBP as defined by 1 of 66 ICD-9 codes.[13] Data were obtained from utilization records of 255,958 commercial members enrolled in the University of Pittsburgh Medical Center Health System in 2001. Costs were examined from the health plan's perspective. Most costs for analgesics were for opioids (61%), followed by COX-2 inhibitors (23%), NSAIDs (13%), and other medications (2%). Mechanical LBP represented 24% of costs for NSAIDs, and 28% of costs for COX-2 inhibitors.

The costs of adverse events associated with these drugs should also be considered. A Canadian study[140] using the Quebec provincial public health care database found that for each dollar spent on nonselective NSAIDs an extra $0.66 was spent on their side effects. Another Canadian study[136] found that rofecoxib or celecoxib were cost effective in patients with rheumatoid arthritis and osteoarthritis compared with nonspecific NSAIDs plus proton pump inhibitor (PPI).

TABLE 11-9	Medicare Fee Schedule for Related Services	
CPT Code	New York	California
99201	$41	$44
99202	$70	$76
99203	$101	$109
99211	$20	$22
99212	$41	$44
99213	$68	$73

2010 Participating, nonfacility amount.

TABLE 11-10 | **Costs of Common Analgesics from Retail Pharmacy**

Drug Type	Generic Name	Trade Name	Cost (30 day supply)
NSAIDs (nonselective)	Aspirin	Bufferin	OTC
	Diclofenac	Cataflam	100.00 (50 mg tablets)
		Voltaren	$60.00 (50 mg tablets)
	Etodolac	Lodine, Lodine XL	$50.00 (500 mg tablets)
	Indomethacin	Indocin, Indocinn SR	$50.00 (50 mg capsules)
	Sulindac	Clinoril	$50.00 (200 mg tablets)
	Tolmetin	Tolectin DS	$50.00 (400 mg capsules)
		Tolectin 600	$60.00 (600 mg tablets)
	Diflunisal	Dolobid	$50.00 (500 mg tablets)
	Meloxicam	Mobic	$170.00 (15 mg tablets)
	Piroxicam	Feldene	$120.00 (20 mg capsules)
	Ibuprofen	Advil, Genpril, Ibu, Midol, Motrin, Nuprin	OTC
	Naproxen	Aleve	OTC
		Anaprox	$55.00 (275 mg tablets)
		Naprelan	$100.00 (375 mg tablets)
		Naprosyn	$50.00 (375 mg tablets)
	Ketorolac	Toradol	$50.00 (10 mg tablets)
	Oxaprozin	Daypro	$70.00 (600 mg tablets)
	Nabumetone	Relafen	$60.00 (500 mg tablets)
Cox-2 inhibitors	Celecoxib	Celebrex	$110.00 (200 mg capsules)
	Valdecoxib		Not commercially available in US
	Rofecoxib	Vioxx	Withdrawn from US market in 2004
	Etoricoxib	Arcoxia	Not commercially available in United States
	Lumiracoxib	Prexige	Not commercially available in United States
	Parecoxib	Dynastat	Not approved for use in United States
Simple analgesics	Acetaminophen	Tylenol	OTC
	Tramadol	Ultram	$110.00 (100 mg tablets)
	Capsaicin	Zostrix	OTC
Muscle relaxants antispasmodic benzodiazepines	Diazepam	Valium	$80.00 (5 mg tablets)
Muscle relaxants antispasmodic nonbenzodiazepines	Cyclobenzaprine	Amrix	$250.00 (15 mg capsules)
		Fexmid	$100.00 (7.5 mg tablets)
		Flexeril	$50.00 (10 mg tablets)
Muscle relaxants antispasticity	Dantrolene	Dantrium	$50.00 (50 mg capsules)
	Baclofen	Generic only	$20.00 (20 mg tablets)

Source: www.medcohealth.com.
NSAIDs, nonsteroidal anti-inflammatory drugs; OTC, over the counter.

However, this was only the case when patients were over 76 years old (rofecoxib) or 81 years old (celecoxib). When assuming that the risk of GI complications was 50% lower with COX-2 inhibitors, the ages at which the medications became cost effective dropped to 56 and 67 years, respectively. A 2005 study[135] considered GI and cardiovascular events comparing nonselective NSAIDs, NSAIDs plus PPI, and coxibs. For low-risk patients, nonselective NSAIDs were the most cost effective. In patients with high risk, NSAIDs plus PPI seemed to be the most cost effective strategy.

Findings from the above CEAs are summarized in Table 11-11.

SUMMARY

Description

Common analgesics is a term used to refer to several classes of medications that are often used to manage pain, and in this chapter includes NSAIDs, simple analgesics (acetaminophen), and muscle relaxants. Older NSAIDs are sometimes termed traditional, nonselective, or nonspecific NSAIDs because they inhibit both the cyclooxygenase (COX)-1, while COX-2 inhibitors are newer NSAIDs and are sometimes termed selective or specific because they only block the

TABLE 11-11	Cost Effectiveness and Cost Utility Analyses on Nonsteroidal Anti-Inflammatory Drugs, Simple Analgesics, and Muscle Relaxants for Acute or Chronic Low Back Pain				
Ref Country Follow-up	Group	Direct Medical Costs	Indirect Productivity Costs	Total Costs	Conclusion
139 Sweden 1 year	1. Manual therapy 2. Intensive training 3. Usual care (including common analgesics)	1. $1054 2. $1123 3. $404	1. $6163 2. $5557 3. $7072	1. $7217 2. $6680 3. $7476	No significant difference

COX-2 isoenzyme. Antispasmodic muscle relaxants reduce involuntary muscle contraction, whereas antispasticity muscle relaxants reduce persistent muscle contraction. Common analgesics have been used to treat LBP for many decades and NSAIDs are the world's most frequently prescribed medications. Many lower doses of NSAIDs, muscle relaxants, and simple analgesics are available OTC, though higher doses and specific medications in these drug classes are only available by prescription.

Theory

NSAIDs function through various degrees of reversible blockade of COX isoenzymes, thus blocking the inflammatory cascade of arachidonic acid to prostaglandins, which mediate inflammation and sensitize peripheral nociceptors. NSAIDs also inhibit neutrophil function and phospholipase C activity, which increases intracellular calcium levels and production of arachidonic acid metabolites such as prostaglandins. Acetaminophen possesses both analgesic and antipyretic properties. It weakly inhibits COX isoenzymes, thereby selectively inhibiting prostaglandin synthesis without inhibiting neutrophils. Muscle relaxants inhibit central polysynaptic neuronal events, which indirectly act on skeletal muscle. Antispasticity muscle relaxants act on the CNS to decrease UMN spasticity pathways. Antispasmodic muscle relaxants act centrally through unknown mechanisms. NSAIDs and muscle relaxants can be used for any type of LBP, while muscle relaxants are usually reserved for acute exacerbations of CLBP.

Efficacy

Nonsteroidal Anti-Inflammatory Drugs

Recent national CPGs provided recommendations related to NSAIDs for CLBP. Three CPGs found evidence supporting the use of NSAIDs for CLBP, one CPG concluded that there was insufficient evidence supporting the efficacy of NSAIDs for CLBP, and another CPG recommended NSAIDs as second choice medications only if acetaminophen was not effective for CLBP. Recent SRs concluded that NSAIDs are effective for short-term pain relief in LBP, and found little evidence of differences in efficacy between various NSAIDs. At least 12 RCT reports assessed the efficacy of NSAIDs for

CLBP, with 6 observing statistically significant pain relief and 4 reporting statistically significant functional improvement versus other comparators. Two CPGs found no evidence or insufficient evidence supporting aspirin for CLBP.

Simple Analgesics

Recent national CPGs provided recommendations for managing CLBP with simple analgesics. Two CPGs recommended acetaminophen as the first choice medication for the management of CLBP, one CPG found insufficient evidence supporting the use of acetaminophen for CLBP, and another found moderate-quality evidence supporting acetaminophen for CLBP. At least three RCTs assessed the efficacy of acetaminophen for CLBP. One found that NSAIDs were statistically superior for pain relief and two others observed significant improvements in pain and disability for acetaminophen plus tramadol versus placebo.

Muscle Relaxants

Recent national CPGs provided recommendations related to muscle relaxants for CLBP. Three CPGs recommended muscle relaxants as an option for CLBP, while one found very low-quality evidence supporting muscle relaxants for CLBP. One CPG found strong evidence supporting the use of benzodiazepine muscle relaxants for CLBP, another found evidence supporting a moderate benefit, and a third found low-quality evidence supporting its use for CLBP. In addition, two CPGs found conflicting evidence supporting nonbenzodiazepine muscle relaxants for CLBP; one found no evidence supporting diazepam for CLBP and one found that tetrazepam is effective for CLBP. Four SRs concluded that muscle relaxants are effective for short-term pain relief in acute LBP, that the efficacy of various muscle relaxants is equivalent, and that there is a dearth of evidence supporting the use of the antispasticity medications baclofen and dantrolene. Furthermore, the SRs concluded that muscle relaxants and benzodiazepines are associated with more CNS adverse events than placebo. One SR focused on LBP with neurologic involvement found no difference between tizanidine and placebo. At least five RCTs examined the efficacy of muscle relaxants for CLBP, with two finding a statistically significant improvement in pain versus other comparators.

Safety

Nonsteroidal Anti-Inflammatory Drugs

Contraindications for NSAIDs include peptic ulcer disease, congestive heart failure, the last 3 months of pregnancy (naproxen), those at increased risk of bleeding (naproxen), and sulfonamide hypersensitivity selective NSAIDs. Precautions should be taken for those with known renal disease, as well as those with cardiac disease or hypertension (celecoxib). Adverse events associated with NSAID use include GI, renal, hepatic, and cardiovascular-related events. A meta-analysis found that ibuprofen and diclofenac had the lowest rates of GI adverse events among nonselective NSAIDs because of the lower doses used in practice. COX-2 inhibitors have been associated with increased cardiovascular-related adverse events.

Simple Analgesics

Acetaminophen should be used with care in the presence of hepatic disease and should be used with caution in patients who consume alcohol regularly or who are alcoholics; daily dosing should not exceed 4 grams. Use of large doses of acetaminophen has been associated with hepatic toxicity.

Muscle Relaxants

Benzodiazepines such as diazepam are contraindicated in narrow angle glaucoma. Cyclobenzaprine should not be used within 14 days of monoamine oxidase inhibitors, or in patients with cardiac arrhythmias, coronary artery disease, or hyperthyroidism. Metaxalone is not recommended in those with significantly reduced renal or hepatic function. Dantrolene is generally contraindicated as a muscle relaxant for CLBP because of potential liver toxicity. Adverse events related to muscle relaxants include CNS depression (e.g., dizziness, sedation), risk of dependency, and symptoms of withdrawal.

Costs

The Medicare reimbursement for outpatient visits during which a clinician can prescribe common analgesics ranges from $20 to $109 US. The cost of common analgesics varies considerably for each drug class and medication. The costs of side effects associated with these drugs should also be considered. One study found that for each dollar spent on nonselective NSAIDs, an extra $0.66 was spent on their side effects. The cost effectiveness of common analgesics for LBP is unknown.

Comments

Evidence from the CPGs, SRs, and RCTs reviewed suggests that common analgesics and NSAIDs are effective interventions for CLBP. Simple analgesics such as acetaminophen should likely be considered the first choice medication for CLBP, with NSAIDs a close second choice medication if acetaminophen alone fails to improve pain. Inconsistent

evidence was observed regarding the use of muscle relaxants, which were also associated with high rates of adverse events. As such, the use of muscle relaxants in CLBP should likely be reserved for acute exacerbations that are unresponsive to both simple analgesics or NSAIDs.

Evidence is currently not available to clearly distinguish the relative merits of different types of NSAIDs, including COX-2 inhibitors. To select a particular medication, patients should be educated about its expected risks and benefits. A trial dose may then be given for a few days to assess the short-term response. Patients who appear resistant to multiple individual medications may require individualized combinations or other classes of medications such as opioid analgesics or adjunctive analgesics, which are discussed in Chapters 12 and 13.

CHAPTER REVIEW QUESTIONS

Answers are located on page 450.

1. What is the proposed mechanism of action for selective NSAIDs?
   a. inhibition of COX-1 enzymes
   b. promotion of COX-1 enzymes
   c. promotion of COX 2 enzymes
   d. inhibition of COX-2 enzymes
2. Which of the following is not a class of NSAIDs discussed in this chapter?
   a. salicylates
   b. oxicams
   c. procoxibs
   d. propionic acids
3. Which of the following is not a contraindication to one or more common analgesic?
   a. sulfonamide hyposensitivity
   b. reduced renal or hepatic function
   c. narrow angle glaucoma
   d. hyperthyroidism
4. True/false: Both traditional NSAIDs and acetaminophen are thought to act on the COX-1 enzyme.
5. Which rung do common analgesics occupy on the World Health Organization's pain medication ladder?
   a. 1
   b. 2
   c. 3
   d. 4
6. For every dollar spent on NSAIDs, what is the estimated cost of associated adverse events?
   a. $0.16
   b. $2.06
   c. $0.66
   d. $1.06
7. Which common analgesic is associated with the lowest rate of adverse events?
   a. NSAIDs
   b. antispasmodic muscle relaxants
   c. antispasticity muscle relaxants
   d. acetaminophen

REFERENCES

1. Cleary K, Clifford M, Stoianovici D, et al. Technology improvements for image-guided and minimally invasive spine procedures. IEEE Transactions on Information Technology in Biomedicine 2002;6:249-261.

2. Cleland JA, Fritz JM, Brennan GP. Predictive validity of initial fear avoidance beliefs in patients with low back pain receiving physical therapy: is the FABQ a useful screening tool for identifying patients at risk for a poor recovery? Eur Spine J 2008;17:70-79.

3. Airaksinen O, Brox JI, Cedraschi C, et al. European guidelines for the management of chronic nonspecific low back pain. Eur Spine J 2006;15:S192-S300.

4. Arnau JM, Vallano A, Lopez A, et al. A critical review of guidelines for low back pain treatment. Eur Spine J 2006;15:543-553.

5. Bigos S, Bowyer O, Braen G, et al. Acute low back problems in adults. Clinical Practice Guideline Number 14. AHCPR Pub. No. 95-0642. Rockville: U.S. Department of Health and Human Services, Public Health Service, Agency for Health Care Policy and Research; 1994. Report No.: AHCPR Publication no. 95-0642.

6. van Tulder M, Becker A, Bekkering T, et al. European guidelines for the management of acute nonspecific low back pain in primary care. Eur Spine J 2006;15:S169-S191.

7. Institute for Clinical Systems Improvement (ICSI). Adult low back pain. Bloomington, MN: Institute for Clinical Systems Improvement; 2006. p. 1-65.

8. Corcoll J, Orfila J, Tobajas P, et al. Implementation of neuro-reflexotherapy for subacute and chronic neck and back pain within the Spanish public health system: audit results after one year. Health Policy 2006;79:345-357.

9. Roelofs PD, Deyo RA, Koes BW, et al. Non-steroidal anti-inflammatory drugs for low back pain. Cochrane Database Syst Rev 2008;Jan 23;(1):CD000396.

10. Koes BW, Scholten RJ, Mens JM, et al. Efficacy of non-steroidal anti-inflammatory drugs for low back pain: a systematic review of randomised clinical trials. Ann Rheum Dis 1997;56:214-223.

11. Luo X, Pietrobon R, Curtis LH, et al. Prescription of nonsteroidal anti-inflammatory drugs and muscle relaxants for back pain in the United States. Spine 2004;29:E531-E537.

12. Cherkin DC, Wheeler KJ, Barlow W, et al. Medication use for low back pain in primary care. Spine 1998;23:607-614.

13. Vogt MT, Kwoh CK, Cope DK, et al. Analgesic usage for low back pain: impact on health care costs and service use. Spine 2005;30:1075-1081.

14. Ekman M, Jonhagen S, Hunsche E, et al. Burden of illness of chronic low back pain in Sweden: a cross-sectional, retrospective study in primary care setting. Spine 2005;30:1777-1785.

15. Ritzwoller DP, Crounse L, Shetterly S, et al. The association of comorbidities, utilization and costs for patients identified with low back pain. BMC Musculoskeletal Disorders 2006;7:72.

16. Malanga GA, Dennis RL. Use of medications in the treatment of acute low back pain. Clin Occup Environ Med 2006;5:643-653.

17. Physicians' Desk Reference. 58th ed. Montvale, NJ: Thomson PDR; 2006.

18. Nielens H, van Zundert J, Mairiaux P, et al. Chronic low back pain. Good Clinical practice (GCP). Brussels: Belgian Health Care Knowledge Centre (KCE); 2006. KCE reports vol 48C.

19. National Institute for Health and Clinical Excellence (NICE). Low back pain: early management of persistent non-specific low back pain. London: National Institute of Health and Clinical Excellence; 2009. Report No.: NICE clinical guideline 88.

20. Negrini S, Giovannoni S, Minozzi S, et al. Diagnostic therapeutic flow-charts for low back pain patients: the Italian clinical guidelines. Eura Medicophys 2006;42:151-170.

21. Chou R, Qaseem A, Snow V, et al. Diagnosis and treatment of low back pain: a joint clinical practice guideline from the American College of Physicians and the American Pain Society. Ann Intern Med 2007;147:478-491.

22. Aghababian RV, Volturo GA, Heifetz IN. Comparison of diflunisal and naproxen in the management of acute low back strain. Clin Ther 1986;9(Suppl C):47-51.

23. Agrifoglio E, Benvenutti M, Gatto P, et al. Aceclofenac: a new NSAID in the treatment of acute lumbago. Multicentre single blind study vs. diclofenac. Acta Therapeutica 1994;20:33-43.

24. Amlie E, Weber H, Holme I. Treatment of acute low-back pain with piroxicam: results of a double-blind placebo-controlled trial. Spine 1987;12:473-476.

25. Bakshi R, Thumb N, Broll H, et al. Treatment of acute lumbosacral back pain with diclofenac resinate: results of a double-blind comparative trial versus piroxicam. Drug Invest 1994;8:288-293.

26. Basmajian JV. Acute back pain and spasm. A controlled multicenter trial of combined analgesic and antispasm agents. Spine 1989;14:438-439.

27. Berry H, Hutchinson DR. A multicentre placebo-controlled study in general practice to evaluate the efficacy and safety of tizanidine in acute low-back pain. J Int Med Res 1988;16:75-82.

28. Borenstein DG, Lacks S, Wiesel SW. Cyclobenzaprine and naproxen versus naproxen alone in the treatment of acute low back pain and muscle spasm. Clin Ther 1990;12:125-131.

29. Braun H, Huberty R. [Therapy of lumbar sciatica. A comparative clinical study of a corticoid-free monosubstance and a corticoid-containing combination drug.] Med Welt 1982;33:490-491.

30. Brown FL Jr, Bodison S, Dixon J, et al. Comparison of diflunisal and acetaminophen with codeine in the treatment of initial or recurrent acute low back strain. Clin Ther 1986;9(Suppl C):52-58.

31. Bruggemann G, Koehler CO, Koch EM. [Results of a double-blind study of diclofenac + vitamin B1, B6, B12 versus diclofenac in patients with acute pain of the lumbar vertebrae. A multicenter study.] Klin Wochenschr 1990;68:116-120.

32. Colberg K, Hettich M, Sigmund R, et al. The efficacy and tolerability of an 8-day administration of intravenous and oral meloxicam: a comparison with intramuscular and oral diclofenac in patients with acute lumbago. German Meloxicam Ampoule Study Group. Curr Med Res Opin 1996;13:363-377.

33. Evans DP, Burke MS, Newcombe RG. Medicines of choice in low back pain. Curr Med Res Opin 1980;6:540-547.

34. Goldie I. A clinical trial with indomethacin (indomee[R]) in low back pain and sciatica. Acta Orthop Scand 1968;39:117-128.

35. Hingorani K, Biswas AK. Double-blind controlled trial comparing oxyphenbutazone and indomethacin in the treatment of acute low back pain. Br J Clin Pract 1970;24:120-123.

36. Hingorani K, Templeton JS. A comparative trial of azapropazone and ketoprofen in the treatment of acute backache. Curr Med Res Opin 1975;3:407-412.

37. Hosie GAC. The topical NSAID, felbinac, versus oral ibuprofen: a comparison of efficacy in the treatment of acute lower back injury. Br J Clin Res 1993;4:5-17.
38. Hickey RF. Chronic low back pain: a comparison of diflunisal with paracetamol. N Z Med J 1982;95:312-314.
39. Kuhlwein A, Meyer HJ, Koehler CO. [Reduced diclofenac administration by B vitamins: results of a randomized double-blind study with reduced daily doses of diclofenac (75 mg diclofenac versus 75 mg diclofenac plus B vitamins) in acute lumbar vertebral syndromes.] Klin Wochenschr 1990;68: 107-115.
40. Lacey PH, Dodd GD, Shannon DJ. A double blind, placebo controlled study of piroxicam in the management of acute musculoskeletal disorders. Eur J Rheumatol Inflamm 1984;7: 95-104.
41. Metscher B, Kubler U, Jahnel-Kracht H. [Dexketoprofen-trometamol and tramadol in acute lumbago.] Fortschr Med Orig 2001;118:147-151.
42. Muckle DS. Flurbiprofen for the treatment of soft tissue trauma. Am J Med 1986;80:76-80.
43. Nadler SF, Steiner DJ, Erasala GN, et al. Continuous low-level heat wrap therapy provides more efficacy than Ibuprofen and acetaminophen for acute low back pain. Spine 2002;27: 1012-1017.
44. Orava S. Medical treatment of acute low back pain. Diflunisal compared with indomethacin in acute lumbago. Int J Clin Pharmacol Res 1986;6:45-51.
45. Pena M. Etodolac: analgesic effects in musculoskeletal and postoperative pain. Rheumatol Int 1990;10(Suppl):9-16.
46. Pohjolainen T, Jekunen A, Autio L, et al. Treatment of acute low back pain with the COX-2-selective anti-inflammatory drug nimesulide: results of a randomized, double-blind comparative trial versus ibuprofen. Spine 2000;25:1579-1585.
47. Schattenkirchner M, Milachowski KA. A double-blind, multicentre, randomised clinical trial comparing the efficacy and tolerability of aceclofenac with diclofenac resinate in patients with acute low back pain. Clin Rheumatol 2003;22:127-135.
48. Stratz T. [Intramuscular etofenamate in the treatment of acute lumbago. Effectiveness and tolerance in comparison with intramuscular diclofenac-Na.] Fortschr Med 1990;108: 264-266.
49. Sweetman BJ, Baig A, Parsons DL. Mefenamic acid, chlormezanone-paracetamol, ethoheptazine-aspirin-meprobamate: a comparative study in acute low back pain. Br J Clin Pract 1987;41:619-624.
50. Szpalski M, Hayez JP. Objective functional assessment of the efficacy of tenoxicam in the treatment of acute low back pain. A double-blind placebo-controlled study. Br J Rheumatol 1994;33:74-78.
51. Szpalski M, Poty S, Hayez JP, et al. Objective assessment of trunk function in patients with acute low back pain treated with Tenoxicam. A prospective controlled study. Neuro-orthopedics 1990;10:41-47.
52. Vetter G, Bruggemann G, Lettko M, et al. [Shortening diclofenac therapy by B vitamins. Results of a randomized double-blind study, diclofenac 50 mg versus diclofenac 50 mg plus B vitamins, in painful spinal diseases with degenerative changes.] Z Rheumatol 1988;47:351-362.
53. Videman T, Heikkila J, Partanen T. Double-blind parallel study of meptazinol versus diflunisal in the treatment of lumbago. Curr Med Res Opin 1984;9:246-252.
54. Waterworth RF, Hunter IA. An open study of diflunisal, conservative and manipulative therapy in the management of acute mechanical low back pain. N Z Med J 1985;98: 372-375.
55. Weber H. Comparison of the effect of diazepam and levomepromazine on pain in patients with acute lumbago-sciatica. J Oslo City Hosp 1980;30:65-68.
56. Weber H, Holme I, Amlie E. The natural course of acute sciatica with nerve root symptoms in a double-blind placebo-controlled trial evaluating the effect of piroxicam. Spine 1993;18:1433-1438.
57. Ximenes A, Robles M, Sands G, et al. Valdecoxib is as efficacious as diclofenac in the treatment of acute low back pain. Clin J Pain 2007;23:244-250.
58. Yakhno N, Guekht A, Skoromets A, et al. Analgesic efficacy and safety of lornoxicam quick-release formulation compared with diclofenac potassium: randomised, double-blind trial in acute low back pain. Clin Drug Investig 2006;26: 267-277.
59. Berry H, Bloom B, Hamilton EB, et al. Naproxen sodium, diflunisal, and placebo in the treatment of chronic back pain. Ann Rheum Dis 1982;41:129-132.
60. Birbara CA, Puopolo AD, Munoz DR, et al. Treatment of chronic low back pain with etoricoxib, a new cyclo-oxygenase-2 selective inhibitor: improvement in pain and disability—a randomized, placebo-controlled, 3-month trial. J Pain 2003;4:307-315.
61. Coats TL, Borenstein DG, Nangia NK, et al. Effects of valdecoxib in the treatment of chronic low back pain: results of a randomized, placebo-controlled trial. Clin Ther 2004; 26:1249-1260.
62. Katz N, Ju WD, Krupa DA, et al. Efficacy and safety of rofecoxib in patients with chronic low back pain: results from two 4-week, randomized, placebo-controlled, parallel-group, double-blind trials. Spine 2003;28:851-858.
63. Videman T, Osterman K. Double-blind parallel study of piroxicam versus indomethacin in the treatment of low back pain. Ann Clin Res 1984;16:156-160.
64. Zerbini C, Ozturk ZE, Grifka J, et al. Efficacy of etoricoxib 60 mg/day and diclofenac 150 mg/day in reduction of pain and disability in patients with chronic low back pain: results of a 4-week, multinational, randomized, double-blind study. Curr Med Res Opin 2005;21:2037-2049.
65. Aoki T, Kuroki Y, Kageyama T, et al. Multicentre double-blind comparison of piroxicam and indomethacin in the treatment of lumbar diseases. Eur J Rheumatol Inflamm 1983;6: 247-252.
66. Babej-Dolle R, Freytag S, Eckmeyer J, et al. Parenteral dipyrone versus diclofenac and placebo in patients with acute lumbago or sciatic pain: randomized observer-blind multicenter study. Int J Clin Pharmacol Ther 1994;32: 204-209.
67. Ingpen ML. A controlled clinical trial of sustained-action dextropropoxyphene hydrochloride. Br J Clin Pract 1969; 23:113-115.
68. Listrat V, Dougados M, Chevalier X, et al. Comparison of the analgesic effect of tenoxicam after oral or intramuscular administration. Drug Invest 1990;2:51-52.
69. Radin EL, Bryan RS. Phenylbutazone for prolapsed discs? Lancet 1968;2:736.
70. Siegmeth W, Sieberer W. A comparison of the short-term effects of ibuprofen and diclofenac in spondylosis. J Int Med Res 1978;6:369-374.
71. Wiesel SW, Cuckler JM, Deluca F, et al. Acute low-back pain. An objective analysis of conservative therapy. Spine 1980;5: 324-330.
72. Blazek M, Keszthelyi B, Varhelyi M, et al. Comparative study of Biarison and Voltaren in acute lumbar pain and lumbo-ischialgia. Ther Hung 1986;34:163-166.

73. Chrubasik S, Model A, Black A, et al. A randomized double-blind pilot study comparing Doloteffin and Vioxx in the treatment of low back pain. Rheumatology (Oxford) 2003; 42:141-148.

74. Davoli L, Ciotti G, Biondi M, et al. Piroxicam-beta-cyclodextrin in the treatment of low-back pain. Controlled study vs etodolac. Curr Ther Res Clin Exp 1989;46:940-947.

75. Dreiser RL, Le Parc JM, Velicitat P, et al. Oral meloxicam is effective in acute sciatica: two randomised, double-blind trials versus placebo or diclofenac. Inflamm Res 2001;50: S17-S23.

76. Dreiser RL, Marty M, Ionescu E, et al. Relief of acute low back pain with diclofenac-K 12.5 mg tablets: a flexible dose, ibuprofen 200 mg and placebo-controlled clinical trial. Int J Clin Pharmacol Ther 2003;41:375-385.

77. Driessens M, Famaey JP, Orloff S, et al. Efficacy and tolerability of sustained-release ibuprofen in the treatment of patients with chronic back pain. Curr Ther Res Clin Exp 1994;55: 1283-1292.

78. Famaey JP, Bruhwyler J, Geczy J, et al. Open controlled randomized multicenter comparison of nimesulide and diclofenac in the treatment of subacute and chronic low back pain. J Clin Res 1998;1:219-238.

79. Jacobs JH, Grayson MF. Trial of an anti-inflammatory agent (indomethacin) in low back pain with and without radicular involvement. Br Med J 1968;3:158-160.

80. Jaffe G. A double-blind, between-patient comparison of alclofenac ('Prinalgin') and indomethacin in the treatment of low back pain and sciatica. Curr Med Res Opin 1974;2: 424-429.

81. Matsumo S, Kaneda K, Nohara Y. Clinical evaluation of Ketoprofen (Orudis) in lumbago: a double blind comparison with diclofenac sodium. Br J Clin Pract 1991;35:266.

82. Milgrom C, Finestone A, Lev B, et al. Overexertional lumbar and thoracic back pain among recruits: a prospective study of risk factors and treatment regimens. J Spinal Disord 1993;6:187-193.

83. Postacchini F, Facchini M, Palieri P. Efficacy of various forms of conservative treatment in low back pain: a comparative study. Neuro-orthopedics 1988;6:28-35.

84. Waikakul S, Soparat K. Effectiveness and safety of loxoprofen compared with naproxen in nonsurgical low back pain: a parallel study. Clin Drug Investig 1995;10:59-63.

85. Waikakul S, Danputipong P, Soparat K. Topical analgesics, indomethacin plaster and diclofenac emulgel for low back pain: a parallel study. J Med Assoc Thai 1996;79:486-490.

86. Chou R, Huffman LH. Medications for acute and chronic low back pain: a review of the evidence for an American Pain Society/American College of Physicians clinical practice guideline. Ann Intern Med 2007;147:505-514.

87. Schnitzer TJ, Ferraro A, Hunsche E, et al. A comprehensive review of clinical trials on the efficacy and safety of drugs for the treatment of low back pain. J Pain Symptom Manage 2004;28:72-95.

88. Vroomen PC, de Krom MC, Slofstra PD, et al. Conservative treatment of sciatica: a systematic review. J Spinal Disord 2000;13:463-469.

89. De MM, Ooghe R. A double-blind comparison of flurbiprofen and indomethacin suppositories in the treatment of osteoarthrosis and rheumatoid disease. J Int Med Res 1981;9: 495-500.

90. Stevanovic L. Double-blind parallel clinical trial with tenoxicam versus piroxicam in patients suffering from acute lumbalgia and subacute lumboischialgia. Aktuel Rheumatol 1986;11: 196-203.

91. van Tulder MW, Touray T, Furlan AD, et al. Muscle relaxants for nonspecific low back pain: a systematic review within the framework of the Cochrane collaboration. Spine 2003;28: 1978-1992.

92. Baptista R, Brizzi J, Dutra F, Josef H, Keisermann M, de Lucca R. [Terapeutica da lombalgia com a tizanidina (DS 103-282), un novo agente mioespasmolitico. Estudo multicentrico, duplo–cego e comparativo.] Folha Medica 1998; 96:119-123.

93. Baratta RR. A double-blind study of cyclobenzaprine and placebo in the treatment of acute muskuloskeletal conditions of the low back. Curr Ther Res 1982;32:646-652.

94. Berry H, Hutchinson DR. Tizanidine and ibuprofen in acute low-back pain: results of a double-blind multicentre study in general practice. J Int Med Res 1988;16:83-91.

95. Bianchi M. Evaluation of cyclobenzaprine for skeletal muscle spasm of local origin. Clinical Evaluation of Flexeril (Cyclobenzaprine HCL/MSD). Minneapolis: Postgraduate Medicine Communications; 1978. p. 25-29.

96. Boyles W, Glassman J, Soyka J. Management of acute musculoskeletal conditions: thoracolumbar strain or sprain. A double blind evaluation comparing the efficacy and safety of carisoprodol with diazepam. Today's Therapeutic Trends 1983;1:1-16.

97. Bragstad A, Blikra G. Evaluation of a new skeletal muscle relaxant in the treatment of low back pain (a comparison of DS 103-282 with chlorzoxazone). Curr Ther Res 1979;26: 39-43.

98. Casale R. Acute low back pain: symptomatic treatment with a muscle relaxant drug. Clin Jof Pain 1988;4:81-88.

99. Corts Giner JR. [Estudio DS 103–282: relajante muscular en lumbalgia aguda o lumbago (Estudio doble ciego de tizanidina + paracetamol vs. placebo + paracetamol).] Rev Esp de Cir Ost 1989;24:119-124.

100. Dapas F, Hartman SF, Martinez L, et al. Baclofen for the treatment of acute low-back syndrome. A double-blind comparison with placebo. Spine 1985;10:345-349.

101. Gold R. Orphenadrine citrate: sedative or muscle relaxant. Clin Ther 1978;6:451-453.

102. Hennies OL. A new skeletal muscle relaxant (DS 103-282) compared to diazepam in the treatment of muscle spasm of local origin. J Int Med Res 1981;9:62-68.

103. Hindle TH III. Comparison of carisoprodol, butabarbital, and placebo in treatment of the low back syndrome. Calif Med 1972;117:7-11.

104. Hingorani K. Diazepam in backache. A double-blind controlled trial. Ann Phys Med 1966;8:303-306.

105. Hingorani K. Orphenadrin-paracetamol in backache—a double-blind controlled trial. Br J Clin Pract 1971;25: 227-231.

106. Klinger N, Wilson R, Kanniainen C, et al. Intravenous orphenadrine for the treatment of lumbar paravertebral muscle strain. Curr Ther Res 1988;43:247-254.

107. Lepisto P. A comparative trial of dS 103-282 and placebo in the treatment of acute skeletal muscle spasms due to disorders of the back. Ther Res 1979;26:454-459.

108. Moll W. [Therapy of acute lumbovertebral syndromes through optimal muscle relaxation using diazepam. Results of a double-blind study on 68 cases.] Med Welt 1973;24: 1747-1751.

109. Rollings H. Management of acute musculoskeletal conditions—thoracolumbar strain or sprain: a double-blind evaluation comparing the efficacy and safety of carisoprodol with cyclobenzaprine hydrochloride. Curr Ther Res 1983;34: 917-928.

110. Tervo T, Petaja L, Lepisto P. A controlled clinical trial of a muscle relaxant analgesic combination in the treatment of acute lumbago. Br J Clin Pract 1976;30:62-64.

111. Arbus L, Fajadet B, Aubert D, et al. Activity of tetrazepam (Myolastan) in low back pain. A double-blind trial vs placebo. Clin Trials J 1990;27:258-267.

112. Basmajian JV. Cyclobenzaprine hydrochloride effect on skeletal muscle spasm in the lumbar region and neck: two double-blind controlled clinical and laboratory studies. Arch Phys Med Rehabil 1978;59:58-63.

113. Pipino F, Menarini C, Lombardi G, et al. A direct myotonolytic (pridinol mesilate) for the management of chronic low back pain: a multicentre, comparative clinical evaluation. Eur J Clin Res 1991;1:55-70.

114. Pratzel HG, Alken RG, Ramm S. Efficacy and tolerance of repeated oral doses of tolperisone hydrochloride in the treatment of painful reflex muscle spasm: results of a prospective placebo-controlled double-blind trial. Pain 1996;67(2-3): 417-425.

115. Salzmann E, Pforringer W, Paal G, et al. Treatment of chronic low-back syndrome with tetrazepam in a placebo controlled double-blind trial. J Drug Dev 1992;4:219-228.

116. Worz R, Bolten W, Heller B, et al. [Flupirtine in comparison with chlormezanone in chronic musculoskeletal back pain. Results of a multicenter randomized double-blind study]. Fortschr Med 1996;114:500-504.

117. Sirdalud Ternelin Asia-Pacific Study Group. Efficacy and gastroprotective effects of tizanidine plus diclofenac versus placebo plus diclofenac in patients with painful muscle spasms. Curr Ther Res 1998;59:13-22.

118. Browning R, Jackson JL, O'Malley PG. Cyclobenzaprine and back pain: a meta-analysis. Arch Intern Med 2001;161:1613-1620.

119. Brown BR Jr, Womble J. Cyclobenzaprine in intractable pain syndromes with muscle spasm. JAMA 1978;240:1151-1152.

120. Bercel NA. Cyclobenzaprine in the treatment of skeletal muscle spasm in osteoarthritis of the cervical and lumbar spine. Curr Ther Res 1977;22:462-468.

121. Katz N, Rodgers DB, Krupa D, et al. Onset of pain relief with rofecoxib in chronic low back pain: results of two four-week, randomized, placebo-controlled trials. Curr Med Res Opin 2004;20:651-658.

122. Ju WD, Krupa DA, Walters DJ, et al. A placebo-controlled trial of rofecoxib in the treatment of chronic low back pain. Pain Med 2001;2:242-243.

123. Pallay RM, Seger W, Adler JL, et al. Etoricoxib reduced pain and disability and improved quality of life in patients with chronic low back pain: a 3 month, randomized, controlled trial. Scand J Rheumatol 2004;33:257-266.

124. O'Donnell JB, Ekman EF, Spalding WM, et al. The effectiveness of a weak opioid medication versus a cyclo-oxygenase-2 (COX-2) selective non-steroidal anti-inflammatory drug in treating flare-up of chronic low-back pain: results from two randomized, double-blind, 6-week studies. J Int Med Res 2009;37:1789-1802.

125. Peloso PM, Fortin L, Beaulieu A, et al. Analgesic efficacy and safety of tramadol/acetaminophen combination tablets (Ultracet) in treatment of chronic low back pain: a multicenter, outpatient, randomized, double blind, placebo controlled trial. J Rheumatol 2004;31:2454-2463.

126. Ruoff GE, Rosenthal N, Jordan D, et al. Tramadol/acetaminophen combination tablets for the treatment of chronic lower back pain: a multicenter, randomized, double-blind, placebo-controlled outpatient study. Clin Ther 2003;25: 1123-1141.

127. Juni P, Nartey L, Reichenbach S, et al. Risk of cardiovascular events and rofecoxib: cumulative meta-analysis. Lancet 2004;364:2021-2029.

128. Silverstein FE, Faich G, Goldstein JL, et al. Gastrointestinal toxicity with celecoxib vs nonsteroidal anti-inflammatory drugs for osteoarthritis and rheumatoid arthritis: the CLASS study: a randomized controlled trial. Celecoxib Long-Term Arthritis Safety Study. JAMA 2000;284:1247-1255.

129. Henry D, Lim LL, Garcia Rodriguez LA, et al. Variability in risk of gastrointestinal complications with individual nonsteroidal anti-inflammatory drugs: results of a collaborative meta-analysis. BMJ 1996;312:1563-1566.

130. Bombardier C, Laine L, Reicin A, et al. Comparison of upper gastrointestinal toxicity of rofecoxib and naproxen in patients with rheumatoid arthritis. VIGOR Study Group. N Engl J Med 2000;343:1520-1528.

131. Mamdani M, Rochon P, Juurlink DN, et al. Effect of selective cyclooxygenase 2 inhibitors and naproxen on short-term risk of acute myocardial infarction in the elderly. Arch Intern Med 2003;163:481-486.

132. Mukherjee D, Nissen SE, Topol EJ. Risk of cardiovascular events associated with selective COX-2 inhibitors. JAMA 2001;286:954-959.

133. van Tulder MW, Koes B, Malmivaara A. Outcome of non-invasive treatment modalities on back pain: an evidence-based review. Eur Spine J 2006;15:S64-S81.

134. Shen FH, Samartzis D, Andersson GB. Nonsurgical management of acute and chronic low back pain. J Am Acad Orthop Surg 2006;14:477-487.

135. Spiegel BM, Chiou CF, Ofman JJ. Minimizing complications from nonsteroidal antiinflammatory drugs: cost-effectiveness of competing strategies in varying risk groups. Arthritis Rheum 2005;53:185-197.

136. Maetzel A, Krahn M, Naglie G. The cost effectiveness of rofecoxib and celecoxib in patients with osteoarthritis or rheumatoid arthritis. Arthritis Rheum 2003;49:283-292.

137. Dagenais S, Roffey DM, Wai EK, et al. Can cost utility evaluations inform decision making about interventions for low back pain? Spine J 2009;9:944-957.

138. van der Roer N, Goossens MEJB, Evers SMAA, et al. What is the most cost-effective treatment for patients with low back pain? A systematic review. Best Pract Res Clin Rheumatol 2005;19:671-684.

139. Seferlis T, Lindholm L, Nemeth G. Cost-minimisation analysis of three conservative treatment programmes in 180 patients sick-listed for acute low-back pain. Scand J Prim Health Care 2000;18:53-57.

140. Rahme E, Joseph L, Kong SX, et al. Cost of prescribed NSAID-related gastrointestinal adverse events in elderly patients. Br J Clin Pharmacol 2001;52:185-192.

141. Roelofs PD, Deyo RA, Koes BW, et al. Non-steroidal anti-inflammatory drugs for low back pain. Cochrane Database Syst Rev 2008;(1):CD000396.

JEROME SCHOFFERMAN
DANIEL MAZANEC

CHAPTER 12

Opioid Analgesics

DESCRIPTION

Terminology and Subtypes

The term *opioid analgesics* refers to medications that act on opioid receptors and are used for pain relief. Although the term *narcotic* has also been used to describe these medications in the past, opioid analgesic is the preferred term now that the word narcotic has taken on negative connotations.[1] The term *weak (or weaker) opioid analgesics* is sometimes used to refer to compound medications combining simple analgesics such as acetaminophen with low doses of codeine or tramadol. Moderate or strong (or stronger) opioid analgesics, by definition, exclude weak opioid analgesics. The terms mild and major are also occasionally used to differentiate weaker opioids from stronger opioids. Other methods of classifying opioids have been proposed based on their origins (i.e. endogenous, opium alkaloids, semi-synthetic, fully synthetic) or effects on receptors (i.e. full/partial/mixed agonists). Regardless of how they are classified, opioids may also be compared in terms of relative strength by using tables that estimate equivalence doses for different opioids.

Opioid analgesics can be divided into three categories: sustained-release opioids (SROs), immediate-release opioids (IROs), and long-acting opioids (LAOs).[2,3] SROs are also known as continuous release (CR) or extended release (ER), and release medication continuously from the gastrointestinal (GI) tract after ingestion or transdermally via a reservoir; they are therefore used for continuous pain control. SROs include medications such as morphine-ER, oxycodone-CR, oxymorphone-ER, and transdermal fentanyl (TDF). IROs have a rapid onset of analgesia, are short acting, are used for breakthrough pain or acute pain, and include medications such as oxycodone-IR, hydrocodone, and morphine sulfate-IR. LAOs are taken according to a regular dosing schedule to minimize fluctuation in effective concentrations and include medications such as methadone and levorphanol.

Although the terms *addiction* and *dependence* are often used interchangeably, their meanings are very different. Addiction refers to a neurobiologic disease with genetic, psychosocial, and environmental factors characterized by behaviors that include the compulsive use of a psychoactive substance despite the harms endured; it involves loss of control. Dependence is a state of physiologic adaptation induced by the chronic use of any psychoactive substance, and can occur independently of any addiction.[4] Addiction is always a clinical problem, whereas dependence is not.[5,6] The term *pseudoaddiction* is sometimes used to describe a scenario in which patients seek additional medications because their current pain relief is not adequate.[7]

In this context, severe episodes of pain not controlled by usual pain medication are termed *breakthrough pain*. The term *diversion* indicates that medications legitimately prescribed by physicians are appropriated, voluntarily or otherwise, and used by others.

History and Frequency of Use

In patients with severe pain related to cancer, opioid analgesics have been considered the standard of care for pain management for many years, despite the lack of high-quality evidence supporting either efficacy or safety with long-term use. For severe pain not related to cancer, there has long been a bias by many physicians in North America against prescribing opioid analgesics. This perception is likely due to misinformation among physicians about adverse events related to opioid analgesics, regulation and monitoring of certain opioid analgesics, and a lack of understanding about the impact of severe pain on quality of life.[8] This position has slowly been changing in recent decades, perhaps due to legislation in certain states in the US mandating continuing medical education about chronic pain (e.g., California). Studies began to appear approximately 10 years ago that suggested opioid analgesics could be both safe and effective in well-selected patients with chronic low back pain (CLBP).[9,10] Today, many spine centers offer opioid analgesics to patients with moderate or severe CLBP refractory to other medications or interventions (Table 12-1).[9,11,12]

A study was conducted to examine health care utilization in patients with mechanical low back pain (LBP) as defined by one of 66 related ICD-9 codes.[13] Data were obtained from utilization records of Kaiser Permanente Colorado, a health maintenance organization with 410,000 enrollees in the Denver area. Pharmacy records indicated that 29% of patients had a claim for opioids. A study was conducted to estimate the direct medical costs focusing on analgesic medication used for mechanical LBP as defined by one of 66 ICD-9 codes.[13] Data were obtained from utilization records of 255,958 commercial members enrolled in the University of Pittsburgh Medical Center Health System in 2001. Among

TABLE 12-1 | **Opioid Analgesics Commonly Used for Chronic Low Back Pain**

Opioid	Brand Names	Approximate Duration of Analgesia (hours)	Comments
Morphine (ER)	MS-Contin, Oramorph, Kadian, Avinza	8 to 24, depending on product and patient factors	Multiple dose sizes Convenient Gold standard
Fentanyl (transdermal)	Duramorph	up to 72	Five dose sizes Less constipating
Methadone	Dolophine	8	Very inexpensive Initially more complicated to use
Oxycodone	Oxycontin	8 to 12	Multiple dose sizes Convenient Very expensive Higher abuse potential
Levorphanol	Levodromoran	6 to 8	Only 2-mg dose
Oxymorphone	Opana-ER	12	Multiple dose sizes Convenient Newer type of opioid Relatively more data for CLBP
Tramadol	Ultram Ultracet	IR: 6 ER: 24	Very good data Less potent (for moderate pain)

ER, extended release; IR, immediate release.

the 9417 patients (56%) with a pharmacy claim for analgesics related to their LBP, the most frequent analgesic was opioids (33%), followed by opioids and NSAIDs (26%), and opioid and other analgesics (9%). Most opioid use was short-term, with a duration of 1 to 30 days (71%), although a substantial portion had a duration of 31 to 90 days (14%). Smaller proportions of patients used opioids for 90 to 179 days (6%), and more than 180 days (9%). In specialty spine practices, opioids were part of the plan after a single visit for 3% of more than 25,000 patients, 75% of whom had pain for longer than 3 months.[12]

In a university orthopedic spine clinic, opioids were prescribed for 66% of patients and 25% received long-term opioid (LTO) treatment.[11] It has been reported that the proportion of patients receiving opioid analgesics is higher in secondary care settings than in primary care settings and that those with poor physical function and greater distress were more likely to receive them.[14] In a retrospective study of 165,569 employees covered by three large employer-sponsored health plans in the United States, almost half (45%) of the 13,760 patients who had reported LBP had claims for opioid analgesics in the previous year.[15] Factors associated with an increased use of opioid analgesics included comorbidities such as hypertension, arthritis, depression, anxiety, cancer, and prior surgery.

Practitioner, Setting, and Availability

A physician is required to administer this intervention because these medications are only available by prescription. Although any licensed physician can prescribe opioids, pain management specialists are generally more comfortable monitoring patients who require this type of therapy than general practitioners, and they are more experienced at titrating the dose and other medication requirements. Patients may

consult physicians for this therapy in a variety of settings (outpatient pain centers, private pain clinics, private physician offices) and locations. This treatment is widely available across the United States, although specialty spine pain clinics tend to be located in larger cities.

Procedure

Management of CLBP with opioid analgesics involves a consultation with a physician who will take a detailed medical and LBP-focused history, and inquire about current medication use. If deemed appropriate, the physician will then prescribe one or more opioid analgesics along with instructions about dosage, timing, side effects, and interactions with other medication; this information may also be provided by the dispensing pharmacist. A follow-up appointment will likely be scheduled within a few days so that the physician can determine whether the opioid analgesic is achieving the desired effect, adjust the dosage if necessary, change the medication in favor of another opioid analgesic or different class of medication if required, and provide education about other strategies for improving CLBP.

There are two ways to dose opioid analgesics: pain-contingent or time-contingent. Pain-contingent dosing is defined as medication taken when pain occurs (as needed), whereas time-contingent dosing is defined as medication taken on a regular schedule based on the duration of analgesia rather than intensity of symptoms at that time (by the clock). Based on the authors' clinical experience managing patients with CLBP, it appears that time-contingent dosing of opioids generally provides better long-term pain control, fewer side effects, and improved compliance when compared to pain-contingent use. SROs or LAOs are typically taken on a time-contingent basis, whereas IROs are taken on a pain-contingent basis. The duration of action of SROs and LAOs

TABLE 12-2	General Recommendations for the Use of Opioid Analgesics in the Treatment of Chronic Pain
Recommendation	**Components**
A careful evaluation of the patient	History Physical examination Review of imaging Review of medical records
A treatment plan that states the goals of therapy	—
Informed consent (verbal or written)	Potential benefits Potential risks Probable and possible side effects Consequences of abuse, diversion, or illicit use of opioids
Therapeutic trial	If good response with acceptable side effects, continued treatment
Regular follow-up visits for assessment and documentation	Efficacy Side effects Signs of abuse or diversion
Consultation when necessary with specialists	Psychology/psychiatry Chemical dependence
The maintenance of good medical records	—

is somewhat variable, and depends on rates of absorption, distribution, metabolism, and excretion (ADME). Many patients require dosing intervals that are shorter than generic manufacturer recommendations.[16,17] An IRO may be prescribed for breakthrough pain in those taking SROs or LAOs.

An occasional patient may experience better pain control with an IRO administered on a time-contingent basis than with SROs or LAOs. It is not uncommon for the physician to have to try several different opioid analgesics to identify which one is best for a particular patient. An individual patient's response is at least in part based on a genetic predisposition[18]; some CLBP patients may not respond to opioid analgesics at all, despite trying different medications. There is no universally correct dose of opioid analgesics for CLBP; treatment should be initiated at conservative doses until patient response can be assessed. Both the dose and the dosing schedule must be titrated for each patient according to analgesic efficacy and side effects. Most opioids do not have a true ceiling effect and therefore have no maximum dose. However, side effects increase with dose and can interfere with improvements associated with analgesia.

General guidelines for the use of opioid analgesics are summarized in Table 12-2. Specific guidelines for individual medications are summarized here.

Morphine

Morphine, available in both IR and ER formulations, remains the gold standard against which other analgesics are compared. Morphine has been shown to be safe and efficacious

for many patients with CLBP at an average final dose of 105 mg/day (range 6 to 780 mg).[19,20] Sustained-release versions of morphine can provide analgesia for 8 to 24 hours, depending on the formulation and individual patient factors (e.g., ADME). There are many doses of morphine available, which facilitates titration. The dose of morphine can be titrated upward once or twice weekly until a satisfactory level of pain control and side effects is achieved. For breakthrough pain, immediate-release morphine is available in doses of 15 or 30 mg; one every 4 to 6 hours is preferred.

Transdermal Fentanyl

TDF has been shown to be effective in the treatment of CLBP in opioid-naive patients at a mean dose of 57 mg/hr (range 12.5 to 250 mg), though caution is strongly advised when prescribing TDF to opioid-naive patients, and harms should be closely monitored.[16,20,21] TDF can be more convenient than oral formulations because in most patients the patch needs to be changed only every 2 to 3 days. There may also be less constipation with the transdermal route of administration than with oral administration.

Oxycodone

Oxycodone is an effective analgesic for CLBP at an average dose of 60 mg per day, with a wide range.[16,19,22-25] Drawbacks to this otherwise good medication include a relatively high cost, and increased prevalence of abuse and diversion when compared with other opioid analgesics.

Oxymorphone

Oxymorphone is the newest opioid analgesic and perhaps the best studied specifically for CLBP. It is most often administered twice daily, at an average dose of 39 to 79 mg/day.[22,26] Immediate-release oxymorphone is also available for breakthrough pain.

Methadone

Methadone has gained in popularity as an opioid analgesic because it is highly effective, has high biological availability, has no known active metabolites, has no known neurotoxicity, is relatively inexpensive, and may produce less opioid-induced hyperalgesia (OIH) than other opioid analgesics.[27-29] However, methadone can interact with several medications, can cause prolonged QT, should not be used in hepatic failure, and it may be more difficult to initiate this therapy. It is important to note that because of the pharmacokinetics of methadone, its dose should not be increased more frequently than once every 5 to 7 days. Once a steady state is reached, analgesia usually lasts for 8 hours.

Levorphanol

Levorphanol has been shown to be effective in both nociceptive and neuropathic pain.[30] Many patients need 8 to 12 mg every 6 to 8 hours. The 2 mg pill size is therefore inconvenient and has resulted in manufacturer shortages in recent years.

Tramadol

Tramadol is a semisynthetic opioid (analogue of codeine) available alone or combined with acetaminophen (e.g.,

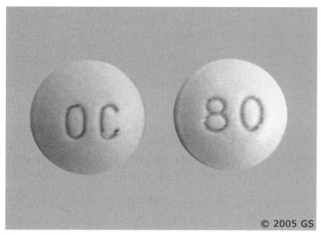

Figure 12-1 Opioid analgesics are only available by prescription. (© Gold Standard, Inc.)

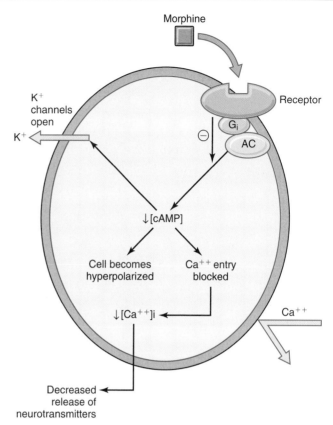

Figure 12-2 Mechanism of action for opioid analgesics (e.g., morphine). (Modified from Wecker L: Brody's human pharmacology, ed. 5. St. Louis, 2010, Mosby.)

Ultracet), and is also available in an extended-release formulation. It has been shown to be effective in patients with CLBP at an average dose of 158 mg/day; the maximum safe daily dose is 400 mg.[19,31-33]

Meperidine

Meperidine (Demerol) should not be used as an LTO because it is poorly absorbed, does not provide reliable analgesia, and its primary metabolite, normeperidine, can accumulate over many days and result in generalized hyperexcitability or seizures.[34]

Regulatory Status

The opioid analgesics discussed in this chapter are all approved by the US Food and Drug Administration for primary indications related to pain, although not specifically CLBP. These medications are only available by prescription, and many are subject to additional monitoring required for controlled substances (Figure 12-1).

THEORY

Mechanism of Action

The analgesic effects of opioids are thought to be related to their ability to bind opioid receptors, which are located primarily in the central nervous system (CNS) and GI system (Figure 12-2). Different medications are thought to exhibit different affinities for specific opioid receptors, including the main μ (mu), κ (kappa), and δ (delta) opioid receptors.[5] Binding to opioid receptors is thought to inhibit transmission of nociceptive input from the peripheral nervous system (PNS), activate descending pathways that modulate and inhibit transmission of nociceptive input along the spinal cord, and also alter brain activity to moderate responses to nociceptive input.[35] As new opioid receptors are discovered and the properties of known opioid receptors are better understood, additional medications may be developed to

selectively act on specific receptors to improve efficacy or decrease side effects (Figure 12-3).

Although tramadol is not chemically related to stronger opioid analgesics, it acts by weakly binding both μ- and δ-opioid receptors in the CNS. Tramadol may also interfere with serotonin and norepinephrine reuptake in descending inhibitory pathways.[13] Tramadol is only partially affected by the opiate antagonist naloxone.[36]

Indication

Short courses of opioid analgesics may be indicated for patients with moderate to severe CLBP who are unable to resume their activities of daily living and have failed to respond to other interventions. The severity of pain reported by patients is subjective, but can nevertheless be measured using simple instruments such as the visual analog scale (VAS) or numerical pain rating scale (NPRS), or more complex instruments such as the McGill pain questionnaire (MPQ) or Brief Pain Inventory (BPI). Repeated administration of these measures in patients with CLBP may be helpful in deciding whether or when opioid analgesics may be warranted if the severity of pain worsens or crosses a particular threshold established by the patient and clinician (Table 12-3).

Additional instruments may also be helpful in identifying those patients with CLBP in whom opioid analgesics may be indicated. From a behavioral and psychological health

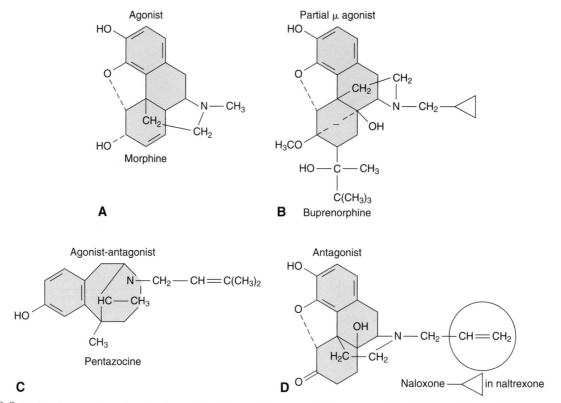

Figure 12-3 Molecular structure of medications with different effects on opioid receptors. (Modified from Wecker L: Brody's human pharmacology, ed. 5. St. Louis, 2010, Mosby.)

TABLE 12-3	Indications for Opioid Analgesics	
Generic Name	Trade Name	Indication
Morphine (ER)	MS-Contin, Oramorph	Moderate to severe pain that requires repeat dosing with potent opioid analgesics for more than a few days
	Kadian, Avinza	Moderate to severe pain that requires a continuous, around-the-clock opioid for an extended period of time
Fentanyl (transdermal)	Duramorph	Pain that is not responsive to non-narcotic analgesics
Methadone	Dolophine	Pain that is not responsive to non-narcotic analgesics, detoxification treatment of opioid addiction, maintenance treatment of opioid addiction
Oxycodone	OxyContin	Moderate to severe pain that requires a continuous, around-the-clock analgesic for an extended period of time
Levorphanol	Levodromoran	Moderate to severe pain where an opioid analgesic is appropriate
Oxymorphone	Opana ER	Moderate to severe pain that requires a continuous, around-the-clock opioid for an extended period of time
Tramadol	Ultram, Ultram ER	Moderate to moderately severe chronic pain in adults who require around-the-clock treatment of their pain for an extended period of time
	Ultracet	Short-term management of acute pain

Source: www.drugs.com.
ER, extended release.

perspective, it has been suggested that patients with chronic pain (including CLBP), can be divided into three categories: (1) adaptive coper, (2) dysfunctional, and (3) interpersonally distressed.[37] A questionnaire has been developed for use by pain management specialists to help make this determination. Of the three categories, only adaptive copers are likely to respond to longer courses of opioid analgesics. Adaptive copers typically demonstrate coherent symptoms, including pain that is consistent with the suspected underlying pathology, function that is concordant with their impairment, and mood that is appropriate to their levels of pain and function. Furthermore, adaptive copers have no history of addictive disease, and reasonable goals and expectations about the proposed intervention.

Patients who are categorized as being dysfunctional or interpersonally distressed should not be prescribed opioid analgesics. As a group, they tend to respond poorly to all biomedical interventions aimed at specific anatomic structures or pathways. Their pain and function often appear out of proportion to the suspected pathology and each other. These patients may also have psychological comorbidities, including depression, character disorder, or a prior history of addiction. Anecdotally, such patients with CLBP may also have a history of consulting with numerous physicians, can appear overly demanding, and request several inappropriate interventions or diagnostic tests.

Assessment

Before receiving opioid analgesics, patients should first be assessed for LBP using an evidence-based and goal-oriented approach focused on the patient history and neurologic examination, as discussed in Chapter 3. Prescribing physicians should also inquire about medication history to note prior hypersensitivity or allergy, or adverse events with similar drugs, and evaluate contraindications for these types of drugs. Clinicians may also wish to order a psychological evaluation if they are concerned about the potential for medication misuse or potential for addiction in certain patients. Diagnostic imaging or other forms of advanced testing is generally not required prior to administering opioid analgesics for CLBP.

EFFICACY

Evidence supporting the efficacy of this intervention for CLBP was summarized from recent clinical practice guidelines (CPGs), systematic reviews (SRs), and randomized controlled trials (RCTs). Observational studies (OBSs) were also summarized where appropriate. Findings are summarized by study design in the following paragraphs.

Clinical Practice Guidelines

Five of the recent national CPGs on the management of CLBP have assessed and summarized the evidence to make specific recommendations about the efficacy of various opioid analgesics.

Weak Opioid Analgesics

The CPG from Belgium in 2006 found moderate-quality evidence to support the efficacy of codeine and tramadol for the management of CLBP.[38] That CPG also found evidence that the efficacy of different weak opioid analgesics was comparable.

The CPG from the United Kingdom in 2009 found insufficient evidence to support either weak opioid analgesics for people who do not obtain adequate pain relief with acetaminophen.[39] That CPG also found limited evidence to support the efficacy of tramadol for CLBP. That CPG concluded that short-term use of weak opioid analgesics could be considered for CLBP, and that the decision to continue should be based on the measured response.

The CPG from Europe in 2004 found strong evidence to support the efficacy of weak opioid analgesics with respect to short-term improvements in pain and function for CLBP.[40] That CPG recommended short-term use of weak opioid analgesics for CLBP.

The CPG from Italy in 2007 found evidence to support the efficacy of tramadol with respect to improvement in pain for CLBP.[41] That CPG also recommended that a combination of acetaminophen and weak opioid analgesics be considered when NSAIDs or acetaminophen do not result in adequate pain relief.

The CPG from the United States in 2007 found moderate evidence to support the efficacy of weak opioid analgesics with respect to improvements in pain.[42] That CPG concluded that weak opioid analgesics could be an option for managing CLBP in patients with severe or disabling pain who do not achieve adequate relief with acetaminophen and NSAIDs.

Strong Opioid Analgesics

The CPG from Belgium in 2006 found very low-quality evidence to support the efficacy of strong opioid analgesics for the management of CLBP.[38]

The CPG from the United Kingdom in 2009 found some evidence to support the short-term use of strong opioid analgesics for people with severe or disabling pain who do not obtain adequate pain relief with acetaminophen or weak opioid analgesics.[39] That CPG also recommended that the decision to continue using strong opioid analgesics should be based on a demonstrated response to treatment. That CPG also reported that patients requiring longer-term use of strong opioid analgesics be referred to pain management specialists who can oversee the use of the medication.

The CPG from the United States in 2007 found moderate evidence to support the efficacy of strong opioid analgesics with respect to improvements in pain.[42] That CPG concluded that strong opioid analgesics could be an option for managing CLBP in patients with severe or disabling pain who do not achieve adequate relief with acetaminophen, NSAIDs, or weak opioid analgesics.

Findings from the above CPGs are summarized in Table 12-4.

Systematic Reviews

Cochrane Collaboration

An SR was conducted in 2006 by the Cochrane Collaboration on opioids for CLBP.[44] A total of four RCTs were included, three comparing tramadol to placebo, and one comparing opioids to naproxen.[24,31-33] Although three of the four trials were deemed to be of higher quality, the authors concluded that there were too few trials to support the use of opioids in CLBP. However, based on the included studies, the authors note that tramadol appears to be more effective than placebo in reducing pain and improving function. A meta-analysis of three RCTs found a standard mean difference (SMD) of 0.71 (95% CI 0.39 to 1.02) for pain relief and an SMD of 0.17 (95% CI 0.04 to 0.30) for improving function. Opioids compared with naproxen were also more effective for pain relief but not for improving function. The authors updated their search in 2007, and identified a further eight potentially relevant studies that are awaiting assessment.[26,45-51]

TABLE 12-4	Clinical Practice Guideline Recommendations on Opioid Analgesics for Chronic Low Back Pain	
Reference	Country	Conclusion
Weak Opioids		
38	Belgium	Moderate evidence to support use
39	United Kingdom	Short-term use could be considered based on measured response
40	Europe	Recommended for short-term use
41	Italy	Recommended when NSAIDs or acetaminophen do not adequately reduce pain
42	United States	Recommended when NSAIDs or acetaminophen do not adequately reduce pain
Strong Opioids		
38	Belgium	Low-quality evidence to support use
39	United Kingdom	Some evidence to support use when acetaminophen or weak opioids do not adequately reduce pain
42	United States	Could be an option when acetaminophen, NSAIDs, or weak opioids do not adequately reduce pain

NSAIDs, nonsteroidal anti-inflammatory drugs.

TABLE 12-5	Systematic Review Findings on Opioid Analgesics for Chronic Low Back Pain		
Reference	# RCTs in SR	# RCTs for CLBP	Conclusion
14	Not specified	NR	Opioid analgesics may be efficacious for short-, but not long-term pain relief (<16 wk)
43	1	1 (not specific to LBP)	Evidence for use of opioids for CLBP is weak
44	4 in original (12 in update)	NR	Role of opioids in CLBP is questionable Tramadol is more effective than placebo in reducing pain and improving function Opioids more effective than naproxen for relieving pain but not improving function
52	14	NR	Fair evidence that tramadol is effective for pain relief

CLBP, chronic low back pain; LBP, low back pain; NR, not reported; RCT, randomized controlled trial; SR, systematic review.

American Pain Society and American College of Physicians

An SR was conducted in 2007 by the American Pain Society and American College of Physicians CPG committee on medications for acute and chronic LBP.[52] This review identified one SR of tramadol for LBP, which included three RCTs, of which two were not included in the Cochrane review above.[53] One of these RCTs included acute LBP patients and the other included CLBP patients.[54,55] The review also identified two additional RCTs on tramadol for LBP and nine other RCTs of opioid therapy.[56,57] Of these nine RCTs, eight not identified in the Cochrane review above.[20,22,23,58-62] The review found that interpreting evidence on the efficacy of opioids for LBP is challenging because there are relatively few trials and results were largely inconclusive. However, the review concluded that there is fair evidence that tramadol is effective for pain relief. They also found that opioids seem to be associated with higher rates of short-term adverse events, particularly constipation and sedation.

Other

A review published in 2007 evaluated opioid analgesics for CLBP.[14] Although this review excluded from its analysis several RCTs that supported the efficacy and safety of opioids

for CLBP, it nevertheless concluded that opioid analgesics may be efficacious for short-term (<16 weeks) but not long-term (>16 weeks) pain relief in patients with CLBP.[20,26,32,33] A meta-analysis of two RCTs reported no significant pain reduction for opioid analgesics when compared with placebo, with an SMD of −0.2 (95% CI −0.49 to 0.11). Authors of this review did not include the study with the longest duration of 13 months and gave less weight to other long-term studies that are lower quality but provided the best available evidence.[9,11,20] Four RCTs included in this review were not included in the Cochrane and American Pain Society reviews described above.[63-66]

A review published in 2002 reported that the evidence supporting the use of opioid analgesics for CLBP was weak, based on only one RCT in which results were not specific to LBP.[43]

Findings from the above SRs are summarized in Table 12-5.

Randomized Controlled Trials

Eleven RCTs describing 12 RCT reports were identified.[19,20,22-24,26,31-33,47,67] Their methods are summarized in Table 12-6. Their results are briefly described below.

TABLE 12-6	Randomized Controlled Trials of Opioid Analgesics for Chronic Low Back Pain			
Reference	Indication	Intervention	Control (C1)	Control (C2)
26	CLBP without neurologic involvement, symptoms ≥3 months	Oxymorphone ER + oxymorphone IR for breakthrough pain ER: Titrated dose every 12 hr × 12 weeks IR: 5 mg every 4-6 hr for 4 days; up to 2 doses/day for rest of 12 weeks n = 105	Placebo + oxymorphone IR for breakthrough pain IR: 5 mg every 4-6 hr for 4 days; up to 2 doses/day for rest of 12 weeks n = 100	NA
47	CLBP without neurologic involvement, symptoms ≥3 months	Oxymorphone ER Titrated dose every 12 hr × 12 weeks to 2 doses/day for rest of 12 weeks n = 70	Placebo Titrated dose every 12 hr × 12 weeks to 2 doses/day for rest of 12 weeks n = 73	NA
22	CLBP with and without neurologic involvement, symptoms ≥2 months	Oxymorphone ER Titrated dose every 12 hr × 18 days n = 80	Oxycodone CR Titrated dose every 12 hr × 18 days n = 75	Placebo Titrated dose every 12 hr × 18 days n = 80
20	CLBP, neurologic involvement NR, symptom duration NR	Transdermal fentanyl Titrated dose every 12 hr × 13 months n = 338	Sustained-release morphine Titrated dose every 12 hr × 13 months n = 342	NA
23*	CLBP, neurologic involvement not reported, symptom duration NR	Oxycodone CR Titrated dose every 12 hr × 4-7 days n = 47	Oxycodone IR Titrated dose (four times daily) × 4-7 days n = 47	NA
24	CLBP, without neurologic involvement, symptoms >6 months	Oxycodone 5 mg (maximum 4 tablets daily) × 16 weeks n = 13	Oxycodone + morphine SR Titrated dose daily × 16 weeks n = 11	NSAID (naproxen) 250 mg (maximum 4 tablets daily) × 16 weeks n = 12
19	CLBP with or without neurologic involvement, duration NR	Sustained-release morphine (daily) × 8 weeks n = 132	Oxycodone ER (twice daily) × 8 weeks n = 134	NA
32	CLBP without neurologic involvement, symptoms ≥3 months	Tramadol 50 mg (maximum 8 tablets daily) × 4 weeks n = 127	Placebo (maximum 8 tablets daily) × 4 weeks n = 127	NA
31	CLBP without neurologic involvement, symptoms ≥3 months	Tramadol 37.5 mg + acetaminophen 325 mg (1-2 tablets up to four times daily) × 91 days n = 167	Placebo 1-2 tablets up to four times daily × 91 days n = 171	NA
33	CLBP without neurologic involvement, symptoms ≥3 months	Tramadol 37.5 mg + acetaminophen 325 mg (maximum 8 tablets daily) × 91 days n = 162	Placebo (maximum 8 tablets daily) × 91 days n = 160	NA
67	CLBP without neurologic involvement, symptoms >3 months	Celecoxib 200 mg (twice daily) × 6 weeks Study 1: n = 402 Study 2: n = 396	Tramadol HCl 50 mg (four times daily) × 6 weeks Study 1: n = 389 Study 2: n = 396	NA

*Crossover design.
CLBP, chronic low back pain; CR, continuous release; ER, extended release; IR, immediate release, NA, not applicable; NR, not reported; NSAID, nonsteroidal anti-inflammatory drug.

Katz and colleagues performed a 12-week RCT to compare pain relief of oxymorphone-ER with placebo in 325 opioid-naive patients with CLBP.[26] Patients had symptoms lasting at least 3 months and their pain did not have neurologic involvement. During the titration period, 120 patients (37%) discontinued treatment because of adverse events, lack of efficacy, or other reasons. In the 205 remaining patients who obtained adequate analgesia and tolerable side effects during titration, pain intensity (VAS) decreased from 69 to 23 mm. These patients were subsequently randomized to continue oxymorphone-ER or changed to placebo. After 12 weeks, pain (VAS) increased in both groups from baseline. Pain increased significantly more in the placebo group compared with the oxymorphone-ER group. Disability related to LBP was not reported.

Hale and colleagues performed a 12-week RCT to compare pain relief of oxymorphone-ER with placebo in 250 opioid-experienced patients with CLBP.[47] Patients had symptoms lasting at least 3 months and their pain did not have neurologic involvement. During the titration period, 108 patients (43%) discontinued treatment because of adverse events, lack of efficacy, or other reasons. In the 143 remaining patients who obtained adequate analgesia and tolerable side effects during titration, there were statistically significant decreases in pain. These patients were subsequently randomized to oxymorphone-ER or placebo. After 12 weeks, pain (VAS) increased in both groups from baseline. Pain increased significantly more in the placebo group compared with the oxymorphone-ER group. Disability related to LBP was not reported.

Peloso and colleagues performed a 91-day RCT comparing the efficacy and safety of flexible-dose tramadol (37.5 mg) plus acetaminophen (325 mg) to placebo in 338 patients with CLBP.[31] Participants had pain lasting at least 3 months and did not have neurologic involvement. A total of 147 (43.5%) completed the trial, with 81 and 110 participants withdrawing in the tramadol and placebo groups, respectively. At the end of 91 days, pain scores (VAS) improved in the tramadol group but not in the placebo group compared to baseline (P values not reported). There was also a modest improvement in function (Roland Morris Disability Questionnaire [RMDQ]) in both groups (P values not reported). The tramadol group had significantly better improvements in pain and function than the placebo group. This study was considered of higher quality.

Schnitzer and colleagues reported a 4-week RCT that compared tramadol (50 mg up to 8 tablets/day) with placebo in 254 patients with CLBP who had had been shown to be tramadol-responders in the open-label phase of the study.[32] Participants had symptoms lasting at least 3 months and did not have neurologic involvement. At the end of 4 weeks, both groups experienced improvements in pain (VAS) and function (RMDQ) compared to study entry (P values not reported); the tramadol group had significantly greater improvements in pain and function compared with the control group. This study was considered of higher quality.

Ruoff and colleagues reported a 91-day RCT that compared flexible dose tramadol 37.5 mg plus acetaminophen 325 mg to placebo in patients with CLBP.[33] Participants had

symptoms lasting at least 3 months and did not have neurologic involvement. At the end of the treatment period, both groups had improved pain (VAS) compared to baseline (P values not reported). There was also improvement in disability (RMDQ) compared to baseline (P values not reported). The tramadol plus acetaminophen group had significantly better pain and disability outcomes compared with the placebo group. This study was considered of higher quality.

Hale and colleagues performed an 18-day multicenter RCT comparing oxymorphone-ER, oxycodone-CR, and placebo in 213 CLBP patients with or without neurologic involvement.[22] Participants had symptoms lasting at least 2 months. After the treatment period, there were significant increases in pain (VAS) in the placebo group compared to baseline, but not in the oxymorphone and oxycodone groups. The mean change in pain intensity was statistically significantly greater in both opioid groups compared with placebo, and there were no differences between opioids. The opioid treatment groups also had significantly better function scores (BPI) than the placebo group. The change in disability related to LBP from baseline was not reported.

Allan and colleagues performed a 13-month unblinded RCT to compare doses of TDF with sustained-release morphine titrated according to patient response in 680 patients with CLBP.[20] At the end of the treatment period, there was a high proportion of participants who reported improved pain (VAS), however, there were no significant differences in pain relief between the groups. There were significant improvements in mean short-form 36 scores for physical functioning in both groups, but no significant differences between the groups.

Hale and colleagues performed a 10-day RCT with a crossover design to compare the efficacy and safety of titrated doses of oxycodone-CR and oxycodone-IR in 47 CLBP patients.[23] Pain intensity decreased from "moderate to severe" at baseline, to "slight" at the end of titration with both oxycodone formulations. At the end of the treatment period, the pain intensity (scale 0-3) was maintained in both groups. There were no significant differences between treatments. Disability related to LBP was not reported.

Jamison and colleagues performed a 16-week RCT to compare naproxen, fixed-dose oxycodone, and a titrated dose of oxycodone plus morphine-ER in 36 patients.[24] Participants had CLBP lasting longer than 6 months, and did not have neurologic involvement. At the end of the treatment period, there was improvement in pain (VAS) in the opioid groups compared to the pre-treatment phase but not in the naproxen group. The difference in pain between groups was statistically significant. Both opioid groups were better than the naproxen group, and the titrated opioid dose group had the lowest mean pain scores. There were no significant differences in activity level (activity diary) between the three groups. This study was considered of lower quality.

Rauck and colleagues performed an 8-week multicenter RCT comparing the effectiveness and safety of a once-a-day morphine sulfate-SR with twice daily oxycodone-CR (mean daily morphine equivalent of at 70 mg and 91 mg, respectively) in 266 patients with moderate to severe CLBP.[19] Both groups had statistically and clinically significant reductions in pain (NPRS). Although there were significantly better outcomes in the morphine group, the authors recognize that the study protocol mandated 12-hour dosing of the oxycodone-CR rather than the 8-hour dosing that is more often necessary, which may have biased the results slightly in favor of the morphine group.

An RCT conducted by O'Donnell and colleagues included CLBP patients without neurologic involvement.[67] Participants were randomized to celecoxib (200 mg twice daily) or tramadol HCl (50 mg four times daily) and examined in two separate studies. At the end of 6 weeks, the percentage of patients experiencing an improvement of greater than 30 on the NPRS among patients randomized to celecoxib was statistically superior to the proportion experiencing improvement in the tramadol group in both studies.

Observational Studies

Simpson and colleagues found a statistically significant improvement in pain in 50 patients who received TDF when compared with their prior regimens of pain-contingent oral opioids for CLBP.[21]

Gammaitoni and colleagues prospectively studied 33 patients with CLBP treated with titrated doses of oxycodone-IR plus acetaminophen three times daily for 4 weeks.[25] Three patients were not able to tolerate the oxycodone and two others withdrew for other reasons. The mean NPRS was reduced from 6.4 to 4.4 and worst NPRS was reduced from 7.7 to 5.6. There were also significant improvements in general activities, mood, walking tolerance, and sleep. Side effects were common, but there were no serious adverse effects. There were no instances of addictive behavior or other abuse in this study.

Schofferman reported a prospective case series of 33 patients with refractory CLBP who were selected by response during the trial titration phase and subsequently treated with opioids for 1 year.[9] Five (15%) patients withdrew because of side effects. In the remaining 28, there were statistically and clinically significant improvements in pain and function at 1 year. The mean NPRS improved from 8.6 to 5.9 and mean Oswestry Disability Index from 64 to 54. There was a biphasic response. In 21 patients, there was an improvement of NPRS from 8.45 to 4.9, whereas 7 others had no change. Overall, of the 33 patients who started the study, opioids were beneficial in 21 (64%).

Mahowald and colleagues retrospectively evaluated opioid use over a period of 3 years in an orthopedic spine clinic.[11] Opioids were prescribed for 152 patients (58 of whom received them long-term), with follow-up data available in 117. Pain was reduced from a mean of 8.3 to 4.5. It is noteworthy that there was no significant dose increase over time and the authors stated that they did not see tolerance in their patients. Side effects were common but well tolerated by most patients. There was a low prevalence of abuse. The authors concluded that there was clinical evidence to support treating CLBP with opioids.

Other

There are multiple studies evaluating the efficacy and safety of opioid analgesics for the treatment of chronic musculoskeletal pain, all of which included, but were not limited to, patients with CLBP. Furlan's meta-analysis of opioids for chronic pain concluded that opioids were more effective than placebo for pain and functional outcomes in patients with nociceptive pain, including CLBP.[68] With respect to side effects, only nausea and constipation were clinically and statistically significantly greater in the opioid groups. Study withdrawal rates averaged 33% in opioid groups and 38% in placebo groups. Markenson and colleagues performed a 90-day RCT comparing oxycodone-CR with placebo in 107 patients with moderate to severe osteoarthritis, 40% to 50% of whom had CLBP.[69] There were statistically significant differences favoring the oxycodone-CR group versus the control group in pain intensity, pain-induced interference with general activity, walking, work, mood, sleep, and enjoyment in life. The improvements in pain were only modest. The discontinuation rate was similar between groups, either related to inadequate pain control or unacceptable side effects.

SAFETY

Contraindications

The only absolute contraindication to an opioid analgesic is an allergy to that specific opioid. Opioid analgesics may be relatively contraindicated in patients with a history of addiction since they are at risk for relapse with exposure to opioids, but some patients can nevertheless be managed successfully by collaborating with an addiction specialist. Greater care is necessary when prescribing opioid analgesics in older adults and in patients with other chronic illnesses that may impact their ability to metabolize these drugs effectively, such as hepatic or renal impairment. The risk of seizure associated with tramadol may be accentuated with the concurrent use of antidepressants, antiepileptics, or opioid analgesics.[70] Tramadol should also be used with caution in those with respiratory illnesses such as obstructive sleep apnea, asthma, or chronic obstructive pulmonary disease.

Adverse Events

The adverse events associated with long-term opioid analgesic use for CLBP are well known and CPGs have generally recommended against their use due to these potential harms (Table 12-7).[38,40] A recent review reported that 59% of patients treated with opioid analgesics for less than 3 months experienced an adverse event.[14] Adverse events were even more common with increased duration of treatment beyond 3 months, occurring in 73% to 90% of patients. Clinical trials have noted that up to one-third of patients discontinued treatment with opioid analgesics due to adverse events. Although adverse events are common with opioid analgesics, they may be partially managed by taking additional medications.[71,72] The main concerns regarding the long-term use of opioid

TABLE 12-7	Adverse Effects Associated with Opioid Analgesics

Symptom	Prevalence (%)
Anorexia	8-11
Constipation	52-65
Dizziness	24-25
Dry mouth	9-18
Headache	6-12
Improper medication-taking behavior	5-24
Myoclonus	2.7-87
Nausea	50-54
Pruritus	15-20
Somnolence	27-30
Substance use disorder	3-43
Sweating	16-26
Urinary retention	9-15
Vomiting	26-29

analgesics include GI problems, CNS depression, serotonin syndrome, metabolite accumulation, endocrine changes, tolerance, addiction, dependence, immune suppression, opioid-induced hyperalgesia (OIH), and fear of disciplinary action by medical licensing boards for the prescribing physicians. Each is briefly discussed in the following paragraphs.

GI side effects are among the most common adverse events associated with opioid analgesics.[73] Constipation occurs as a result of decreased peristaltic propulsive contractions, increased small and large bowel tone, and decreased biliary, pancreatic, and intestinal secretions. Patients beginning opioid analgesics should also initiate a prophylactic bowel regimen including regular use of both a stool softener and a stimulant laxative to preserve normal function. Senna is often useful, and some patients require regular use of polyethylene glycol powder (e.g., Mira-Lax). Nausea and vomiting occur as a result of a central effect of opioid analgesics on the medullary chemoreceptor trigger zone. Nausea may gradually fade after several days, but some patients require an antiemetic. Haloperidol or metoclopramide may be helpful in managing opioid-induced nausea. Organ toxicity resulting from opioid analgesics is rare, and there is no evidence that opioid analgesics are harmful to the liver, kidneys, brain, or other organs.

Sedation and drowsiness are the most common CNS adverse events with opioid analgesics, though a wide range of other neurologic symptoms may also occur, including confusion, hallucinations, nightmares, myoclonus, and dysphoria.[74] Patients typically adjust to the sedating effects within the first week of treatment but in those who continue to feel sedated, daily modafinil may help.[75] There are concerns that important tasks requiring alertness, manual dexterity, and reflex responses might be adversely impacted by the use of opioid analgesics. However, studies suggest that chronic pain itself can impair performance on psychomotor testing, and that patients with chronic pain who receive opioid analgesics actually improved their test results.[76-78] A recent review related to driving impairment in patients treated with opioid analgesics concluded that there was "generally

consistent evidence for no impairment of psychomotor abilities of opioid-maintained patients."[79] Respiratory depression is relatively rare for those taking opioid analgesics, but this risk is increased in persons with significant pulmonary disease, sleep apnea syndrome, or other serious medical conditions.

Because tramadol inhibits both serotonin and norepinephrine reuptake, concomitant administration with selective serotonin reuptake inhibitors may result in "serotonin syndrome."[80] Symptoms of serotonin syndrome include agitation, hyperreflexia, mental status change, myoclonus, tremor, seizures, fever, and may even lead to death. Increased risk of suicide has also been reported with tramadol.

Meperidine is an opioid analgesic with a half-life of approximately 3 hours. Hepatic metabolism of meperidine results in an inactive metabolite, normeperidine, which has a much longer half-life of approximately 20 hours. Repeated, frequent administration of meperidine for analgesic effect may result in toxic accumulation of this long-lived metabolite, particularly in persons with hepatic or renal insufficiency, or older adults.[34,81] Toxic levels of normeperidine have been associated with seizures, tremor, and hallucinations. Meperidine should not be used for long term management of CLBP.

The most common endocrine problem in men taking opioid analgesics is androgen deficiency due to suppression of the gonadotropin-releasing hormone by the hypothalamus. This typically presents clinically as low libido, erectile dysfunction, low energy, fatigue, and depressed mood.[82,83] Women may also experience decreased libido and changes in their menstrual cycle when taking opioid analgesics; concurrent use of testosterone may be effective at reducing these effects.[83] Opioid analgesics may also be associated with osteoporosis and broader hypothalamic pituitary suppression, but the clinical significance of these findings is not yet clear.

Tolerance is the need for progressively higher doses of opioid analgesics to achieve the same degree of pain relief. Tolerance is a biologic process that occurs at the cellular level and differs from addiction. Current evidence suggests that if tolerance occurs with CLBP, it may be related to the progression of the underlying disease.[9,11] Although dose escalations occurred in 29% of patients treated with LTOs for CLBP, 95% of these were related to disease progression, complications of spine surgery, or unrelated medical problems rather than tolerance.[14] Another explanation for dose escalation with opioid analgesics is that the initial relief experienced encourages increased activity, which subsequently produces greater pain. This usually occurs early in the course of opioid analgesic treatment and could perhaps be termed "pseudotolerance" as this implies that the intervention is in fact effective.

The prevalence of addiction in patients treated with opioid analgesics for pain appears to be about the same as it is in the general population (6% to 10%). One of the most common aberrant behaviors in patients treated with opioid analgesics for pain is diversion (e.g., selling the medication to others), which can be confirmed by a urine test that is negative for the prescribed opioid.[84] Other behaviors noted with opioid analgesics include poly-pharmacy or hyperpharmacotherapy (e.g., using multiple opioids simultaneously or combining opioids with other prescription medications), which can be confirmed by a urine test that is positive for opioid analgesics that were not prescribed, or even for other controlled or illegal substances.[84] Patients may also attempt to obtain opioid analgesics from multiple clinicians without informing them of concurrent treatment received elsewhere, or even try forging prescriptions to obtain greater quantities or doses of opioid analgesics.[84]

There has been a great deal of effort to find ways to predict aberrant behavior.[85] It is difficult to predict which patients are at risk for such aberrant behaviors, as neither patient demographics nor the intensity of pain can project their occurrence.[84,86] Other potential predictors for misuse of opioid analgesics include a history of alcohol or other substance abuse, a prior conviction for driving under the influence or possession of drugs, other criminal history, a family history of substance abuse, and significant mental health problems.[84,86,87] Withdrawal syndrome can occur with opioid analgesics if they are suddenly withdrawn or the dose is reduced rapidly.[88]

There is currently evidence from both pre-clinical and clinical studies that opioid analgesics can adversely affect immune function. The mechanism of action for this phenomenon is not fully understood but may be partly mediated by neuroendocrine interactions and direct effects on cells affecting immunity.[89,90] It is not clear whether this effect is clinically important.[90]

Another concern with the use of opioid analgesics is the potential for OIH. Distinct from tolerance, OIH refers to an increased sensitivity to painful stimuli. An SR reported cases of patients who developed allodynia and hyperalgesia, especially with higher doses or rapid dose escalation.[91] In the experimental setting, OIH can occur after using opioid analgesics for as little as one month.[92] This may be detected if a patient who had been doing well with opioid analgesics suddenly develops increased pain in the absence of disease progression with an unexplained expansion and generalization of pain. Such patients may respond to other opioid analgesics or require a complete weaning from opioids.

Fear of disciplinary action by medical boards, specialty societies, or law enforcement agencies is another concern related to prescribing opioid analgesics. The treatment of pain is recognized as a priority by several states and their medical boards have issued statements describing the proper use of opioid analgesics for pain management.[93] It is generally considered appropriate medical practice to prescribe long-term opioid analgesics for chronic pain that cannot otherwise be managed effectively with common or adjunctive analgesics, and physicians who prescribe them for appropriate clinical indications are acting well within the scope of good medical practice. However, it is necessary for physicians to maintain adequate documentation to support their decision to prescribe opioid analgesics. There should be a discussion of efficacy of analgesia, level of function and mood, and an inquiry should be made regarding aberrant drug-related behaviors such as the "four Cs" of addiction: adverse *c*onsequences, impaired *c*ontrol, *c*ompulsive use, and

*c*raving.[84,86,87] With appropriate documentation, fear of regulatory sanction should not constitute a barrier to the use of opioid analgesics in carefully selected appropriate patients with structural spinal pain.

One recent and seemingly promising attempt to predict efficacy, risk, and compliance, rated patients in four domains—diagnosis, intractability, risk, and efficacy.[94] Scores correlated moderately with efficacy and strongly with compliance. As previously noted, patients who are adaptive copers appear most likely to benefit from LTOs whereas those who are dysfunctional or interpersonally distressed appear to do worse in all domains.

COSTS

Fees and Third-Party Reimbursement

In the United States, a recommendation for opioid analgesics for CLBP can likely be delivered by a clinician in the context of an office or outpatient visit for a new patient using CPT codes 99201 (up to 10 minutes), 99202 (up to 20 minutes), or 99203 (up to 30 minutes). For an established patient, these can likely be provided during an office or outpatient visit using CPT codes 99211 (up to 5 minutes), 99212 (up to 10 minutes), or 99213 (up to 15 minutes). Although time is indicated for the various levels of service and can be a contributing component for selection of the level of office/outpatient visits, the overarching criteria for selection of the level of service should be based on medical necessity and the amount of history, examination, and medical decision making that was required and documented.

These procedures are widely covered by other third-party payers such as health insurers and worker's compensation insurance. Although some payers continue to base their reimbursements on usual, customary, and reasonable payment methodology, the majority have developed reimbursement tables based on the Resource-Based Relative Value Scale used by Medicare. Reimbursements by other third-party payers are generally higher than Medicare.

Typical fees reimbursed by Medicare in New York and California for these services are summarized in Table 12-8.

Opioid analgesics are typically covered by most third-party payers, many of whom now use pharmacy benefits managers (PBMs) to create and maintain formularies of

TABLE 12-8	Medicare Fee Schedule for Related Services	
CPT Code	New York	California
99201	$41	$44
99202	$70	$76
99203	$101	$109
99211	$20	$22
99212	$41	$44
99213	$68	$73

2010 Participating, nonfacility amount.

TABLE 12-9	Costs of Opioid Analgesics from a Retail Pharmacy	
Medication	Trade Name	Cost (30 day supply)*
Morphine	MS-Contin	$200.00 (100-mg tablets)
	Oramorph	$200.00 (100-mg tablets)
	Kadian	$400.00 (100-mg capsules)
	Avinza	$330.00 (90-mg capsules)
Fentanyl	Duramorph	$45.00 (1-mg [10 mL] ampule) (assumes 2-mg/day for 30 days at 1 mg/mL)
Methadone	Dolophine	$50.00 (10-mg tablets)
Oxycodone	Oxycontin	$100.00 (20-mg tablets)
Levorphanol	Levodromoran	$50.00 (2-mg tablets)
Oxymorphone	Opana-ER	$170.00 (20-mg tablets)
Tramadol	Ultram, Ultracet	$110.00 (100-mg tablets)

*30-Day supply of brand name drug.
From www.medcohealth.com.

covered medications. PBMs may only include a few medications under each broad class of opioid analgesic, and may require prior authorization, failure of a cheaper medication, or medical justification for using a more expensive medication within the same class. The cost of opioid analgesics varies considerably for each drug class and medication. Generic morphine may cost as little as a few pennies per pill, whereas newer oxycodone may cost as much as a few dollars per pill.

Table 12-9 provides the approximate cost of a 30-day supply of brand name opioid analgesics through a large PBM in the United States.

Cost Effectiveness

The CPG from the United Kingdom in 2009 found that paracetamol, NSAIDs, and weak opioids are generally available as generics and that and treatment costs for these three types of medication are expected to be similar for patients with CLBP (>6 weeks).[39] That CPG also found one study supporting the use of tramadol for patients with CLBP (>6 weeks), but that study also reported that tramadol had higher costs.[39]

The CPG from Europe in 2004 determined that the cost effectiveness of opioids for CLBP (>3 months) was unknown.[40]

Other

As mentioned earlier in this chapter, a study was conducted to estimate the direct medical costs focusing on analgesic medication used for mechanical LBP as defined by 1 of 66 ICD-9 codes.[13] Data were obtained from utilization records of 255,958 commercial members enrolled in the University of Pittsburgh Medical Center Health System in 2001. Costs associated with this intervention were examined from the health plan's perspective. This study reported that the majority of costs for analgesics were for opioids (61%), and that LBP represented 48% of total costs related to opioids. The study also reported that cost of specific opioids prescribed varied considerably, whereas older opioids such as morphine are generally inexpensive, newer opioids can be quite costly.

A study in 2008 reported that the costs associated with opioid analgesics for LBP and neck pain had increased 423% from 1997 to 2004 in the United States.[96]

SUMMARY

Description

The term *opioid analgesics* refers to medications that act on opioid receptors and are used for pain relief. The term *weak opioid analgesics* is often used to refer to compound analgesics combining acetaminophen with low doses of codeine or tramadol. Moderate or strong opioid analgesics can be divided into three categories: sustained-release opioids (SROs, also called continuous-release or extended-release), immediate-release opioids (IROs), and long-acting opioids (LAOs). Although any licensed physician can prescribe opioids, pain management specialists will generally be more comfortable monitoring patients who require this type of therapy than general practitioners, and are more experienced at titrating the dose and managing other medication requirements.

Theory

The analgesic effects of opioids are thought to be related to their ability to bind opioid receptors, which are located primarily in the CNS and GI system. Binding to opioid receptors is thought to inhibit transmission of nociceptive input from the PNS, activate descending pathways that modulate and inhibit transmission of nociceptive input along the spinal cord, and also alter brain activity to moderate responses to nociceptive input. Tramadol is chemically unrelated to opioid analgesics but acts weakly binding both μ- and δ-opioid receptors in the CNS and may also interfere with serotonin and norepinephrine reuptake in descending inhibitory pathways. Short courses of opioid analgesics may be indicated for patients with moderate to severe CLBP who are unable to resume their activities of daily living and have failed to respond to other interventions and medications such as acetaminophen and NSAIDs.

Efficacy

Five CPGs made recommendations related to opioids for CLBP. Two CPGs recommended weak opioids if acetaminophen or NSAIDs do not provide adequate pain relief, while two other CPGs recommended weak opioids only for short-term use. One CPG found moderate-quality evidence supporting the use of weak opioids for CLBP. Two CPGs recommended strong opioids only for severe or disabling pain for which pain relief has not been achieved by other pain medication, while one CPG reported very low-quality evidence supporting strong opioids for CLBP. Two SRs concluded that tramadol is effective for pain relief among patients with CLBP, yet reported that few of the included RCTs were of high quality. One of these SRs concluded that opioids are associated with higher rates of short-term adverse events, particularly constipation and sedation. Another SR concluded that opioids are effective in the short-term for pain relief. At least 12 RCT reports examined the efficacy of opioids, the majority of which reported statistically significant improvement in pain and function versus other comparators.

Safety

Opioids are contraindicated among those with opioid allergies. Patients with a history of addiction should be monitored with caution. The risk of seizure associated with tramadol may be accentuated with the concurrent use of antidepressants, antiepileptics, or opioid analgesics. Long-term use of opioid analgesics has been associated with adverse events, such as GI problems, CNS depression, serotonin syndrome, metabolite accumulation, endocrine changes, tolerance, addiction, dependence, immune suppression, and OIH. Increased suicidal risk has been reported with tramadol. Opioids may also adversely affect immune function.

Costs

A clinician usually prescribes opioid analgesics for CLBP during an outpatient visit; the Medicare reimbursement for this ranges from $22 to $109. The cost of opioid analgesics varies considerably for each drug class and medication. Generic morphine may cost as little as a few pennies per pill, whereas newer oxycodone may cost as much as a few dollars per pill. The cost effectiveness of opioids is unknown.

Comments

Evidence from the CPGs, SRs, and RCTs reviewed suggest that weak opioid analgesics appear effective for short-term pain relief associated with CLBP, while strong opioids appear effective for severe or intolerable pain for which all other types of conservative therapy fail to provide pain relief. There is currently no evidence of superiority for specific medications within the broader classes of weak or strong opioid analgesics. The effectiveness of opioids should be tempered by their potential harms, particularly constipation and sedation. It should be noted that a high proportion of participants withdrew from RCTs of opioid analgesics for LBP due to side effects, indicating the use of opioid analgesics may be limited to a subset of patients with LBP in whom they are well tolerated. Although the potential for addictive behavior or other social problems exists, it appears low when appropriate steps are taken and the therapy is supervised by well trained specialists. Future research in this area would ideally focus on dose titration and opioid rotation to determine the most appropriate treatment for each patient.

CHAPTER REVIEW QUESTIONS

Answers are located on page 450.

1. The gold standard for opioid analgesics is considered to be:
   a. oxycodone
   b. morphine
   c. tramadol
   d. fentanyl
2. Which is the least well-tolerated opioid?
   a. meperidine
   b. levorphanol
   c. methadone
   d. transdermal fentanyl
3. Which of the following is a not an advantage to time-contingent dosing?
   a. lower total dose
   b. eliminated the need for breakthrough medication
   c. less hepatic toxicity
   d. decreased dependence
4. Absolute contraindications to opioid analgesics include:
   a. allergy to prescribed medication
   b. history of opioid addiction
   c. gastrointestinal disorder in older adults
   d. all of the above
5. Which of the following is not a common side effect to opioid analgesics?
   a. constipation
   b. nausea
   c. insomnia
   d. opioid-induced hyperalgesia
6. True or false: Opioid analgesics are more cost effective than common analgesics.
7. True or false: Opioid analgesics act on the gabba receptor in the brain.

REFERENCES

1. Craig DS. Is the word "narcotic" appropriate in patient care? J Pain Palliat Care Pharmacother 2006;20:33-35.
2. Simpson KH. Individual choice of opioids and formulations: strategies to achieve the optimum for the patient. Clin Rheumatol 2002;21:S5-S8.

3. McCarberg BH, Barkin RL. Long-acting opioids for chronic pain: pharmacotherapeutic opportunities to enhance compliance, quality of life, and analgesia. Am J Ther 2001;8: 181-186.

4. Inturrisi CE. Clinical pharmacology of opioids for pain. Clin J Pain 2002 Jul;18:S3-13.

5. Trescot AM, Boswell MV, Atluri SL, et al. Opioid guidelines in the management of chronic non-cancer pain. Pain Physician 2006;9:1-39.

6. Bannwarth B. Risk-benefit assessment of opioids in chronic noncancer pain. Drug Saf 1999;21:283-296.

7. Weissman DE, Haddox JD. Opioid pseudoaddiction—-an iatrogenic syndrome. Pain 1989;36:363-366.

8. Rosenblum A, Marsch LA, Joseph H, et al. Opioids and the treatment of chronic pain: controversies, current status, and future directions. Exp Clin Psychopharmacol 2008;16:405-416.

9. Schofferman J. Long-term opioid analgesic therapy for severe refractory lumbar spine pain. Clin J Pain 1999;15:136-140.

10. Portenoy RK, Foley KM. Chronic use of opioid analgesics in non-malignant pain: report of 38 cases. Pain 1986;25: 171-186.

11. Mahowald ML, Singh JA, Majeski P. Opioid use by patients in an orthopedics spine clinic. Arthritis Rheum 2005; 52:312-321.

12. Fanciullo GJ, Ball PA, Girault G, et al. An observational study on the prevalence and pattern of opioid use in 25,479 patients with spine and radicular pain. Spine 2002;27:201-205.

13. Vogt MT, Kwoh CK, Cope DK, et al. Analgesic usage for low back pain: impact on health care costs and service use. Spine 2005;30:1075-1081.

14. Martell BA, O'Connor PG, Kerns RD, et al. Systematic review: opioid treatment for chronic back pain: prevalence, efficacy, and association with addiction. Ann Intern Med 2007; 146:116-127.

15. Rhee Y, Taitel MS, Walker DR, et al. Narcotic drug use among patients with lower back pain in employer health plans: a retrospective analysis of risk factors and health care services. Clin Ther 2007;29(Suppl):2603-2612.

16. Gallagher RM, Welz-Bosna M, Gammaitoni A. Assessment of dosing frequency of sustained-release opioid preparations in patients with chronic nonmalignant pain. Pain Med 2007;8:71-74.

17. Marcus DA, Glick RM. Sustained-release oxycodone dosing survey of chronic pain patients. Clin J Pain 2004;20:363-366.

18. Lotsch J, Geisslinger G. Current evidence for a genetic modulation of the response to analgesics. Pain 2006;121:1-5.

19. Rauck RL, Bookbinder SA, Bunker TR, et al. The ACTION study: a randomized, open-label, multicenter trial comparing once-a-day extended-release morphine sulfate capsules (AVINZA) to twice-a-day controlled-release oxycodone hydrochloride tablets (OxyContin) for the treatment of chronic, moderate to severe low back pain. J Opioid Manag 2006;2: 155-166.

20. Allan L, Richarz U, Simpson K, Slappendel R. Transdermal fentanyl versus sustained release oral morphine in strong-opioid naive patients with chronic low back pain. Spine 2005;30:2484-2490.

21. Simpson RK Jr, Edmondson EA, Constant CF, et al. Transdermal fentanyl as treatment for chronic low back pain. J Pain Symptom Manage 1997;14:218-224.

22. Hale ME, Dvergsten C, Gimbel J. Efficacy and safety of oxymorphone extended release in chronic low back pain: results of a randomized, double-blind, placebo- and active-controlled phase III study. J Pain 2005;6:21-28.

23. Hale ME, Fleischmann R, Salzman R, et al. Efficacy and safety of controlled-release versus immediate-release oxycodone: randomized, double-blind evaluation in patients with chronic back pain. Clin J Pain 1999;15:179-183.

24. Jamison RN, Raymond SA, Slawsby EA, et al. Opioid therapy for chronic noncancer back pain. A randomized prospective study. Spine 1998;23:2591-2600.

25. Gammaitoni AR, Galer BS, Lacouture P, et al. Effectiveness and safety of new oxycodone/acetaminophen formulations with reduced acetaminophen for the treatment of low back pain. Pain Med 2003;4:21-30.

26. Katz N, Rauck R, Ahdieh H, et al. A 12-week, randomized, placebo-controlled trial assessing the safety and efficacy of oxymorphone extended release for opioid-naive patients with chronic low back pain. Curr Med Res Opin 2007;23: 117-128.

27. Fishman SM, Wilsey B, Mahajan G, et al. Methadone reincarnated: novel clinical applications with related concerns. Pain Med 2002;3:339-348.

28. Sandoval JA, Furlan AD, Mailis-Gagnon A. Oral methadone for chronic noncancer pain: a systematic literature review of reasons for administration, prescription patterns, effectiveness, and side effects. Clin J Pain 2005;21:503-512.

29. Moulin DE, Palma D, Watling C, et al. Methadone in the management of intractable neuropathic noncancer pain. Can J Neurol Sci 2005;32:340-343.

30. Rowbotham MC, Twilling L, Davies PS, et al. Oral opioid therapy for chronic peripheral and central neuropathic pain. N Engl J Med 2003;348:1223-1232.

31. Peloso PM, Fortin L, Beaulieu A, et al. Analgesic efficacy and safety of tramadol/acetaminophen combination tablets (Ultracet) in treatment of chronic low back pain: a multicenter, outpatient, randomized, double blind, placebo controlled trial. J Rheumatol 2004;31:2454-2463.

32. Schnitzer TJ, Gray WL, Paster RZ, et al. Efficacy of tramadol in treatment of chronic low back pain. J Rheumatol 2000 Mar;27:772-778.

33. Ruoff GE, Rosenthal N, Jordan D, Karim R, Kamin M. Tramadol/acetaminophen combination tablets for the treatment of chronic lower back pain: a multicenter, randomized, double-blind, placebo-controlled outpatient study. Clin Ther 2003;25:1123-1141.

34. Armstrong PJ, Bersten A. Normeperidine toxicity. Anesth Analg 1986;65:536-538.

35. Berry P, Covington E, Dahl J, et al. Pain: Current Understanding of Assessment, Management, and Treatments. Washington, DC: National Pharmaceutical Council (NPC); 2001.

36. Mullican WS, Lacy JR. Tramadol/acetaminophen combination tablets and codeine/acetaminophen combination capsules for the management of chronic pain: a comparative trial. Clin Ther 2001;23:1429-1445.

37. Kerns RD, Turk DC, Rudy TE. The West Haven-Yale Multidimensional Pain Inventory (WHYMPI). Pain 1985;23: 345-356.

38. Nielens H, van Zundert J, Mairiaux P, et al. Chronic low back pain. Good Clinical practice (GCP). Brussels: Belgian Health Care Knowledge Centre (KCE); 2006. KCE reports vol 48C.

39. National Institute for Health and Clinical Excellence (NICE). Low back pain: early management of persistent non-specific low back pain. Report No.: NICE clinical guideline 88. London: National Institute of Health and Clinical Excellence; 2009.

40. Airaksinen O, Brox JI, Cedraschi C, et al. European guidelines for the management of chronic nonspecific low back pain. Eur Spine J 2006;15:S192-S300.

41. Negrini S, Giovannoni S, Minozzi S, et al. Diagnostic therapeutic flow-charts for low back pain patients: the Italian clinical guidelines. Eura Medicophys 2006;42:151-170.

42. Chou R, Qaseem A, Snow V, et al. Diagnosis and treatment of low back pain: a joint clinical practice guideline from the American College of Physicians and the American Pain Society. Ann Intern Med 2007;147:478-491.

43. Bartleson JD. Evidence for and against the use of opioid analgesics for chronic nonmalignant low back pain: a review. Pain Med 2002;3:260-271.

44. Deshpande A, Furlan A, Mailis-Gagnon A, et al. Opioids for chronic low-back pain. Cochrane Database Syst Rev 2007;(3): CD004959.

45. Adams EH, Chwiecko P, ce-Wagoner Y, et al. A study of AVINZA (morphine sulfate extended-release capsules) for chronic moderate-to-severe noncancer pain conducted under real-world treatment conditions—-the ACCPT Study. Pain Pract 2006;6:254-264.

46. Gaertner J, Frank M, Bosse B, et al. [Oral controlled-release oxycodone for the treatment of chronic pain. Data from 4196 patients.] Schmerz 2006;20:61-68.

47. Hale ME, Ahdieh H, Ma T, et al. Efficacy and safety of OPANA ER (oxymorphone extended release) for relief of moderate to severe chronic low back pain in opioid-experienced patients: a 12-week, randomized, double-blind, placebo-controlled study. J Pain 2007;8:175-184.

48. Nicholson B, Ross E, Weil A, et al. Treatment of chronic moderate-to-severe non-malignant pain with polymer-coated extended-release morphine sulfate capsules. Curr Med Res Opin 2006;22:539-550.

49. Nicholson B, Ross E, Sasaki J, et al. Randomized trial comparing polymer-coated extended-release morphine sulfate to controlled-release oxycodone HCl in moderate to severe nonmalignant pain. Curr Med Res Opin 2006;22:1503-1514.

50. Portenoy RK, Messina J, Xie F, et al. Fentanyl buccal tablet (FBT) for relief of breakthrough pain in opioid-treated patients with chronic low back pain: a randomized, placebo-controlled study. Curr Med Res Opin 2007;23:223-233.

51. Webster LR, Butera PG, Moran LV, et al. Oxytrex minimizes physical dependence while providing effective analgesia: a randomized controlled trial in low back pain. J Pain 2006;7: 937-946.

52. Chou R, Huffman LH. Medications for acute and chronic low back pain: a review of the evidence for an American Pain Society/American College of Physicians clinical practice guideline. Ann Intern Med 2007;147:505-514.

53. Schnitzer TJ, Ferraro A, Hunsche E, et al. A comprehensive review of clinical trials on the efficacy and safety of drugs for the treatment of low back pain. J Pain Symptom Manage 2004;28:72-95.

54. Metscher B, Kubler U, Jahnel-Kracht H. [Dexketoprofen-trometamol and tramadol in acute lumbago.] Fortschr Med Orig 2001;118:147-151.

55. Muller FO, Odendaal CL, Muller FR, et al. Comparison of the efficacy and tolerability of a paracetamol/codeine fixed-dose combination with tramadol in patients with refractory chronic back pain. Arzneimittelforschung 1998;48:675-679.

56. Raber M, Hofmann S, Junge K, et al. Analgesic efficacy and tolerability of tramadol 100 mg sustained-release capsules in patients with moderate to severe low back pain. Clin Drug Investig 1999;17:415-423.

57. Sorge J, Stadler T. Comparison of the analgesic efficacy and tolerability of tramadol 100 mg sustained-release tablets and tramadol 50 mg capsules for the treatment of chronic low back pain. Clin Drug Investig 1997;14:157-164.

58. Milgrom C, Finestone A, Lev B, et al. Overexertional lumbar and thoracic back pain among recruits: a prospective study of risk factors and treatment regimens. J Spinal Disord 1993;6: 187-193.

59. Baratta RR. A double-blind comparative study of carisoprodol, propoxyphene, and placebo in the management of low back syndrome. Curr Ther Res Clin Exp 1976;20: 233-240.

60. Gostick N, Allen J, Cranfield R, et al. A comparison of the efficacy and adverse effects of controlled release dihydrocodeine and immediate release dihydrocodeine in the treatment of pain in osteoarthritis and chronic back pain. In: Twycross R, editor. The Edinburgh Symposium on Pain Control and Medical Education. London: Royal Society of Medicine; 1989. p. 137-143.

61. Hale M, Speight K, Harsanyi Z, et al. Efficacy of 12 hourly controlled-release codeine compared with as required dosing of acetaminophen plus codeine in patients with chronic low back pain. Pain Res Manag 1997;2:33-38.

62. Salzman RT, Roberts MS, Wild J, et al. Can a controlled-release oral dose form of oxycodone be used as readily as an immediate-release form for the purpose of titrating to stable pain control? J Pain Symptom Manage 1999;18:271-279.

63. Kuntz D, Brossel R. [Analgesic effect and clinical tolerability of the combination of paracetamol 500 mg and caffeine 50 mg versus paracetamol 400 mg and dextropropoxyphene 30 mg in back pain.] Presse Med 1996;25:1171-1174.

64. Tennant F, Moll D, DePaulo V. Topical morphine for peripheral pain. Lancet 1993;342:1047-1048.

65. Richards P, Zhang P, Friedman M, et al. Controlled-release oxycodone relieves moderate to severe pain in a 3-month study of persistent moderate to severe back pain [Abstract]. Pain Med 2002;3:176.

66. Thurel C, Bardin T, Boccard E. Analgesic efficacy of an association of 500-mg paracetamol plus 30-mg codeine versus 400-mg paracetamol plus 30-mg dextropropoxyphene in repeated doses for chronic lower back pain. Curr Ther Res 1991;50:463-473.

67. O'Donnell JB, Ekman EF, Spalding WM, et al. The effectiveness of a weak opioid medication versus a cyclo-oxygenase-2 (COX-2) selective non-steroidal anti-inflammatory drug in treating flare-up of chronic low-back pain: results from two randomized, double blind, 6-week studies. J Int Med Res 2009;37:1789-1802.

68. Furlan AD, Sandoval JA, Mailis-Gagnon A, et al. Opioids for chronic noncancer pain: a meta-analysis of effectiveness and side effects. Can Med Assoc 2006;174:1589-1594.

69. Markenson JA, Croft J, Zhang PG, et al. Treatment of persistent pain associated with osteoarthritis with controlled-release oxycodone tablets in a randomized controlled clinical trial. Clin J Pain 2005;21:524-535.

70. Physicians' Desk Reference. 58th ed. Montvale, NJ: Thomson PDR; 2006.

71. McNicol E, Horowicz-Mehler N, Fisk RA, Bennett K, Gialeli-Goudas M, Chew PW, et al. Management of opioid side effects in cancer-related and chronic noncancer pain: a systematic review. J Pain 2003;4:231-256.

72. Swegle JM, Logemann C. Management of common opioid-induced adverse effects. Am Fam Physician 2006;74:1347-1354.

73. Mehendale SR, Yuan CS. Opioid-induced gastrointestinal dysfunction. Dig Dis 2006;24:105-112.

74. Chapman SL, Byas-Smith MG, Reed BA. Effects of intermediate- and long-term use of opioids on cognition in patients with chronic pain. Clin J Pain 2002;18:S83-S90.

75. Webster L, Andrews M, Stoddard G. Modafinil treatment of opioid-induced sedation. Pain Med 2003;4:135-140.

76. Lorenz J, Beck H, Bromm B. Cognitive performance, mood and experimental pain before and during morphine-induced analgesia in patients with chronic non-malignant pain. Pain 1997;73:369-375.

77. Sjogren P, Thomsen AB, Olsen AK. Impaired neuropsychological performance in chronic nonmalignant pain patients receiving long-term oral opioid therapy. J Pain Symptom Manage 2000;19:100-108.

78. Jamison RN, Schein JR, Vallow S, et al. Neuropsychological effects of long-term opioid use in chronic pain patients. J Pain Symptom Manage 2003;26:913-921.

79. Fishbain DA, Cutler RB, Rosomoff HL, et al. Are opioid-dependent/tolerant patients impaired in driving-related skills? A structured evidence-based review. J Pain Symptom Manage 2003;25:559-577.

80. Ripple MG, Pestaner JP, Levine BS, et al. Lethal combination of tramadol and multiple drugs affecting serotonin. Am J Forensic Med Pathol 2000;21:370-374.

81. Szeto HH, Inturrisi CE, Houde R, et al. Accumulation of normeperidine, an active metabolite of meperidine, in patients with renal failure of cancer. Ann Intern Med 1977;86:738-741.

82. Daniell HW. Hypogonadism in men consuming sustained-action oral opioids. J Pain 2002;3:377-384.

83. Daniell HW. DHEAS deficiency during consumption of sustained-action prescribed opioids: evidence for opioid-induced inhibition of adrenal androgen production. J Pain 2006;7:901-907.

84. Ives TJ, Chelminski PR, Hammett-Stabler CA, et al. Predictors of opioid misuse in patients with chronic pain: a prospective cohort study. BMC Health Serv Res 2006;6:46.

85. Katz NP, Adams EH, Benneyan JC, et al. Foundations of opioid risk management. Clin J Pain 2007;23:103-118.

86. Michna E, Ross EL, Hynes WL, et al. Predicting aberrant drug behavior in patients treated for chronic pain: importance of abuse history. J Pain Symptom Manage 2004;28:250-258.

87. Webster LR, Webster RM. Predicting aberrant behaviors in opioid-treated patients: preliminary validation of the Opioid Risk Tool. Pain Med 2005;6:432-442.

88. Liaison Committee on Pain and Addiction. Definitions Related to the Use of Opioids for the Treatment of Pain. American Academy of Pain Medicine, American Pain Society and American Society of Addiction Medicine; 2001 http://www.ampainsoc.org/advocacy/opioids2.htm.

89. Welters ID. Is immunomodulation by opioid drugs of clinical relevance? Curr Opin Anaesthesiol 2003;16:509-513.

90. Budd K. Pain management: is opioid immunosuppression a clinical problem? Biomed Pharmacother 2006;60:310-317.

91. Angst MS, Clark JD. Opioid-induced hyperalgesia: a qualitative systematic review. Anesthesiology 2006;104:570-587.

92. Chu LF, Clark DJ, Angst MS. Opioid tolerance and hyperalgesia in chronic pain patients after one month of oral morphine therapy: a preliminary prospective study. J Pain 2006;7:43-48.

93. Medical Board of California. Guidelines for Prescribing Controlled Substances for Pain. Sacramento: Medical Board of California; 2002. http://www.medbd.ca.gov/pain_guidelines.html.

94. Belgrade MJ, Schamber CD, Lindgren BR. The DIRE score: predicting outcomes of opioid prescribing for chronic pain. J Pain 2006;7:671-681.

95. Ritzwoller DP, Crounse L, Shetterly S, et al. The association of comorbidities, utilization and costs for patients identified with low back pain. BMC Musculoskeletal Disorders 2006;7:72.

96. Martin BI, Deyo RA, Mirza SK, et al. Expenditures and health status among adults with back and neck problems. JAMA 2008;299:656-664.

VICTOR H. CHANG
PETER G. GONZALEZ
VENU AKUTHOTA

CHAPTER 13

Adjunctive Analgesics

DESCRIPTION

Terminology and Subtypes

Adjunctive analgesics is a term used to describe medications that can be used for pain relief but whose primary indication is not related to pain. This term is also used to differentiate these types of analgesics from the more commonly used drug classes such as simple analgesics, nonsteroidal anti-inflammatory drugs (NSAIDs), and muscle relaxants, which are collectively termed common analgesics in this textbook and discussed in Chapter 11, as well as opioid analgesics, which are discussed in Chapter 12. Adjunctive analgesics are also known as *adjuvant analgesics, nontraditional analgesics,* or *unconventional analgesics.*

Adjunctive analgesics for chronic low back pain (CLBP) discussed in this chapter include the following two main drug classes, each of which contains several subclasses and specific medications: antidepressants (Figure 13-1) and antiepileptics.[1,2]

Numerous other types of medication are occasionally used for symptomatic relief of painful conditions such as CLBP, including corticosteroids, topical anesthetics, cannabinoids, α_2-adrenergic agonists, and N-methyl-D-aspartate (NMDA) receptor antagonists.[1,2] Although these may also be considered adjunctive analgesics, they will not be discussed in this chapter.

Antidepressants

Antidepressants is a generic term used to refer to drug classes such as tricyclic antidepressants (TCAs), selective serotonin reuptake inhibitors (SSRIs), and serotonin-norepinephrine reuptake inhibitors (SNRIs). It should be noted that adrenaline is a synonym for epinephrine and that these two terms are often used interchangeably (e.g., selective noradrenalin reuptake inhibitors). Tetracyclic antidepressants are closely related to TCAs.

Tricyclic Antidepressants. There are different types of TCAs, and their classification has varied over time. Initially, a structural algorithm was used (e.g., tertiary vs. secondary amine TCAs). First-generation TCAs were tertiary amine TCAs, with a balanced inhibition of serotonin and norepinephrine reuptake; these TCAs had adverse effects related to their anticholinergic activity. Subsequently, secondary amine TCAs were discovered, which selectively inhibited

norepinephrine and had less toxicity.[3] Secondary amine TCAs may also be referred to as *noradrenergic TCAs*, while tertiary amine TCAs may be referred to as *balanced reuptake TCAs*.[4] TCAs include amitriptyline, amoxapine, clomipramine, dibenzepin, dosulepin hydrochloride, doxepin, desipramine, imipramine, lofepramine, maprotiline, nortriptyline, protriptyline, and trimipramine. Tetracyclic antidepressants include mirtazapine and maprotiline.

Selective Serotonin Reuptake Inhibitors. SSRIs include citalopram, escitalopram, fluoxetine, fluvoxamine, paroxetine, and sertraline; zimelidine is now available in the United States for the treatment of fibromyalgia.[5]

Serotonin-Norepinephrine Reuptake Inhibitors. SNRIs include venlafaxine, desvenlafaxine, sibutramine, duloxetinel, and milnacipran.

Antiepileptics

Antiepileptics are also known as anticonvulsants. There are three main categories of antiepileptics, named in chronological order of discovery: first generation, second generation, and third generation.[6-8]

First Generation. First-generation antiepileptics include carbamazepine, valproic acid, phenytoin, phenobarbital, primidone, ethotoin, ethosuximide, and methsuximide.

Second Generation. Second-generation antiepileptics include gabapentin, felbamate, tiagabine, levetiracetam, zonisamide, fosphenytoin, vigabatrin, pregabalin, topiramate, lamotrigine, and oxcarbazepine.

Third Generation. Third-generation antiepileptics include acetazolamide, lacosamide, rufinamide, and stiripentol.

Tables 13-1 and 13-2 list specific medications in each of these drug classes, as well as their trade names and indications.

History and Frequency of Use

Several types of medications have been used to manage symptoms of low back pain (LBP), including many that are no longer used (e.g., colchicine).[9] Use of new medications to manage LBP often begins anecdotally, with clinicians observing their effects for other indications and extrapolating those results to how they may impact LBP. This appears to be the case with adjunctive analgesics, which have been used for at least 4 decades to manage LBP but appear to have grown in

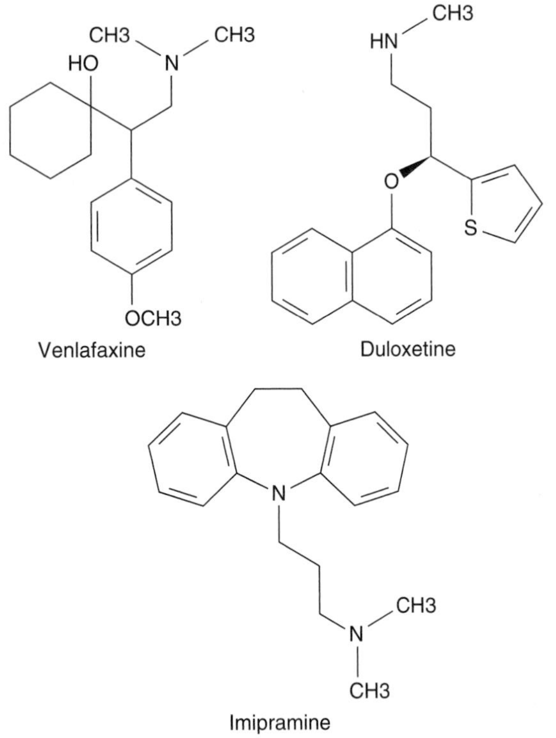

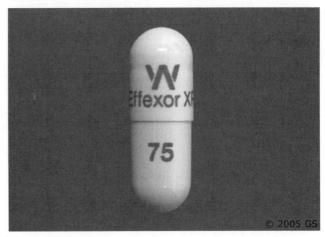

Venlafaxine

Duloxetine

Imipramine

Figure 13-1 Molecular structures for three different adjunctive analgesics.

Figure 13-2 Adjunctive analgesics are only available by prescription. (© Gold Standard, Inc.)

popularity in the past decade.[10] An increasing use of adjunctive analgesics is likely due to a lack of long-term results when using traditional analgesics, prompting clinicians to try other approaches for patients with persistent symptoms. The use of antiepileptic medications as adjunctive analgesics for CLBP likely arose from their US Food and Drug Administration (FDA) approval for neuropathic pain conditions such as postherpetic neuropathy (PHN) and diabetic peripheral neuropathy (DPN).

Medications are the most commonly recommended option for managing LBP and are prescribed to approximately 80% of patients presenting to a primary care provider.[11] There are wide variations in prescribing patterns and little agreement among primary care providers on the optimal medication regimen for LBP; one third of patients with LBP are prescribed more than one medication. It was reported in 1985 that TCAs were prescribed by primary care providers to approximately 2% of patients presenting with LBP.[9] More recently, it was reported that 12% of patients in Belgium with LBP were prescribed antidepressants, and 2% were prescribed antiepileptics.[12] Use of antidepressants and antiepileptics for LBP appears to be higher in older adults; similar figures for adults older than age 60 were 17% and 3%, respectively. A study in Sweden asked 302 patients who presented to 16 physicians at 14 randomly selected outpatient clinics to complete questionnaires on health care resource use in the past 6 months.[13] Antidepressants were the fifth most commonly used class of medication, reported by 8% of patients.

Practitioner, Setting, and Availability

Adjunctive analgesics require a prescription and can be dispensed by any physician with a medical license. This intervention is widely available in a variety of settings throughout the United States, including private medical practices and hospitals. Although they can be used in primary care settings, adjunctive analgesics for CLBP are perhaps best prescribed in secondary care settings. Pain management or other nonsurgical specialists may best be suited to confirm that radicular pain is neuropathic in nature, select amongst the many available adjunctive analgesics, monitor possible interactions between concomitant use of adjunctive and simple or opioid analgesics, assess adverse events commonly reported with adjunctive analgesics, and determine appropriate use of nonmedication interventions that may be required for optimal outcomes.

Procedure

Management of CLBP with adjunctive analgesics involves consultation with a physician who will take a detailed medical and LBP-focused history, and inquire about current medication use. If deemed appropriate, the physician will then prescribe an adjunctive analgesic along with instructions about dosage, timing, side effects, and interactions with other medication; this information may also be provided by the dispensing pharmacist. A follow-up appointment will likely be scheduled within a few weeks so that the physician can determine whether the adjunctive analgesic is achieving the desired effect, adjust the dosage if necessary, change the medication in favor of another adjunctive analgesic or different class of medication if required, and provide education about other strategies for improving CLBP.

Regulatory Status

The adjunctive analgesics discussed in this chapter are all approved by the FDA for other primary indications and are therefore used off-label for CLBP. These medications are only available by prescription (Figure 13-2).

TABLE 13-1	**Medications and Approved Indications by Type of Antiepileptic Adjunctive Analgesic**		
Class Type Medication	Trade Name	Indication	Ref
First-generation carbamazepine	Carbatrol, Epitol, Euetro, Tegretol, Tegretol-XR	Trigeminal neuralgia Partial seizures Generalized tonic-clonic seizures Mixed seizure patterns	5, 27, 85
First-generation valproic acid	Depacon, Depakene, Depakote, Stavzor	Complex partial seizures Simple and complex partial seizures Mania associated with bipolar disorder Migraine prophylaxis	5
First-generation phenytoin	Dilantin, Phenytek	Carries no FDA approval for neuropathic pain, but has reported efficacy for trigeminal neuralgia Tonic-clonic and complex partial seizures Prevention of seizures following head trauma/neurosurgery	5, 72
Second-generation gabapentin	Neurontin	Postherpetic neuralgia Partial seizures Unlabeled uses include: Neuropathic pain, diabetic peripheral neuropathy, fibromyalgia, postoperative pain	5, 81, 86
Second-generation pregabalin	Lyrica	Post-herpetic neuralgia Diabetic peripheral neuropathy Fibromyalgia Partial onset seizure disorder	5, 27, 82
Second-generation topiramate	Topamax	Partial/general tonic-clonic seizures Migraine prophylaxis Seizures associated with Lennox-Gastaut syndrome	5, 27
Second-generation lamotrigine	Lamictal	Partial seizures Primary generalized tonic-clonic seizures Generalized seizures of Lennox-Gestaut syndrome	69, 70
Third-generation lacosamide	Vimpat	Partial-onset seizures Studies have shown efficacy for diabetic neuropathy	5, 29 87, 88

THEORY

Mechanism of Action

The use of adjunctive analgesics for CLBP is based on its presumed etiology, which can broadly be divided into nociceptive or neuropathic pain.[14,15] Nociceptive pain stems from any tissue injury that initiates a nociceptive signal carried by a nerve, and is thought to account for the vast majority of patients with CLBP. Neuropathic pain stems specifically from injury to the nerve itself, which likely contributes to the clinical presentation in only a small fraction of patients with CLBP. Nociceptive CLBP need not be confined to the lumbosacral area and may refer pain along the dermatomal distribution of a spinal nerve root or peripheral nerve. Neuropathic CLBP is radicular in nature and may be felt all along the area of sensory innervation for a spinal or peripheral nerve. The etiology of nociceptive pain is multifaceted and may result from any number of mechanisms of injury to the lumbosacral area, whereas the etiology of neuropathic pain is often due to inflammation secondary to infection, autoimmune, metabolic, or neurologic disorders. The distinction between neuropathic and nociceptive pain is crucial with respect to adjunctive analgesics for CLBP because some medications are intended solely for neuropathic pain and may have no effect in nociceptive pain.[16]

Table 13-3 compares some of the basic characteristics for nociceptive and neuropathic pain.

Various adjunctive analgesics work along different sections of the pain pathway.[17] Pain is activated through a veritable cornucopia of peripheral receptors, often producing a soup of inflammatory mediators that can perpetuate or amplify the nociceptive signal (e.g., bradykinin, leukotrienes, substance P). In patients with chronic pain, it is hypothesized that a windup phenomenon occurs in the dorsal horn, resulting in increased activity of NMDA receptors and activation of voltage-gated calcium channels. If this state endures, central sensitization via modulation of the spinal cord may eventually develop, with descending inhibition of the pain pathway at the spinal cord level. This phenomenon can slowly decrease the threshold required to trigger a nociceptive signal, resulting in greater and more frequent pain.[14,18]

Antidepressants

Tricyclic Antidepressants. TCAs are thought to provide relief for neuropathic pain via the serotonergic and

| TABLE 13-2 | Medications and Approved Indications by Type of Antidepressant Adjunctive Analgesic |

Class Type Medication	Trade Name	Indication	Ref
TCA Amitriptyline	Elavil, Vanatrip, Endep	Relief of symptoms of depression Unlabeled uses include: Analgesic for certain chronic and neuropathic pain	5, 89
TCA Doxepin	Sinequan, Prudoxin, Zonalon	Psychoneurotic patients with depression or anxiety Depression/anxiety related to alcoholism Depression/anxiety related to organic disease Psychotic depressive disorders Depression Moderate pruritus with atopic dermatitis or lichen simplex chronicus (topical) Unlabeled uses include: Analgesic for certain chronic and neuropathic pain	5, 90, 91
TCA Desipramine	Norpramin	Depression Unlabeled uses include: Analgesic adjunct in chronic pain, peripheral neuropathies	5, 90, 92
TCA Imipramine	Tofranil	Depression Nocturnal enuresis in children Unlabeled uses include: Analgesic for certain chronic and neuropathic pain	5, 93
TCA Nortriptyline	Pamelor (US), Aventyl (Canada)	Symptoms of depression Unlabeled uses include: Chronic pain (including neuropathic pain)	5, 94
SNRI Venlafaxine	Effexor	Major depressive disorder Generalized anxiety disorder Social anxiety disorder Panic disorder Unlabeled uses include: Neuropathic pain	5, 89
SNRI Milnacipran	Ixel, Savella	Fibromyalgia	5
SNRI Duloxetine	Cymbalta	Diabetic peripheral neuropathic pain Generalized anxiety disorder Major depressive order Fibromyalgia	5 95
Tetracyclic antidepressant Mirtazapine	Remeron	Major depressive disorder	5
SSRI Paroxetine	Paxil, Pexeva	Major depressive disorder Panic disorder Obsessive-compulsive disorder Social anxiety disorder Generalized anxiety disorder Posttraumatic stress disorder Premenstrual dysphoric disorder Studies have shown efficacy in neuropathic pain	5, 89

Additional source: www.drugs.com.
SNRI, serotonin-norepinephrine reuptake inhibitor; SSRI, selective serotonin reuptake inhibitor; TCA, tricyclic antidepressant; US, United States.

noradrenergic pathways, perhaps due to their stabilization effects on nerve membranes.[19] Although both pathways are involved in TCAs, the ratio of serotonergic to noradrenergic action may differ based on the individual medication. *In vitro*, TCAs demonstrate a mostly balanced inhibition of both serotonin and noradrenalin reuptake; *in vivo*, they are metabolized to secondary amines that primarily affect noradrenalin reuptake.[20] Neuropathic pain relief with TCAs appears to occur independently of any antidepressant effect they may also produce.[21] This is important to note because although the antidepressant effects of TCAs may take several weeks to develop, improvement of pain may occur

TABLE 13-3	Characteristics of Neuropathic and Nociceptive Pain	
Aspect	Neuropathic Pain	Nociceptive Pain
Quality	Numbness, tingling, burning	Dull, achy
Location	Discrete band of pain	Vague pain
Leg involvement	Pain often below knee	Pain often above knee
Neurologic deficit	Occasional	None
Dural tension	Positive	Negative

TABLE 13-4	Mechanisms of Action for Different Antiepileptic Medications
Medication	Mechanism of Action
Carbamazepine	Inhibits voltage-gated Na^{++} channels
Gabapentin	Acts on voltage-gated Ca^{++} channels
Lamotrigine	Acts at Na^{++} and N-type Ca^{++} channels
Oxcarbazepine	Blocks voltage-gated Na^{++} channels May affect C^{++} and K^{++} conductance
Phenytoin	Inhibits voltage-gated Na^{++} channels
Pregabalin	Acts on voltage-gated Ca^{++} channels
Topiramate	Acts on voltage-gated Na^{++} channels Potentiates gamma amino butyric acid transmission Blocks AMPA/glutamate transmission

AMPA, α-amino-3-hydroxy-5-methylisoxazole-4-propionic acid.

substantially sooner. Titration of TCAs to an effective dose with tolerable side effects may take several weeks to achieve and require periodic reevaluation.

Selective Serotonin Reuptake Inhibitors. SSRIs prevent primarily the reuptake of serotonin into the synaptic cleft, thereby increasing available levels of this neurotransmitter. They may also affect other monoamine transporters related to dopamine and norepinephrine, but are not thought to act on their roles in pain pathways.[22] SSRIs are therefore not indicated for neuropathic pain, and any clinical improvement noted in CLBP from their use is likely associated with improvement in secondary emotional disturbances such as depression, anxiety, or insomnia.[21]

Serotonin-Norepinephrine Reuptake Inhibitors. SNRIs affect both serotonergic and noradrenergic pathways. Although mirtazapine has been referred to as a dual-action noradrenergic and specific serotonergic drug, significant serotonergic effects have not been demonstrated in humans.[23] For venlafaxine, the balance between serotonergic and noradrenergic reuptake inhibition relates to dosage. Whereas lower doses of venlaxafine affect primarily serotonin pathways, higher doses affect mainly noradrenalin pathways.[24] In contrast, duloxetine affects both serotonin and noradrenalin pathways in a manner regardless of dosage.[25]

Antiepileptics

First Generation. First-generation antiepileptics such as carbamazepine, valproic acid, and phenytoin are thought to act on the pain pathway through inhibition of voltage-gated sodium channels[26,27]; carbamezepine may also have a stabilizing effect on neuronal membranes.[26] Valproic acid also increases concentrations of gamma-aminobutyric acid (GABA) in the brain.[27] Carbamazepine is typically titrated from 100 to 200 mg to a maximum dose of 1200 mg daily and requires meticulous monitoring of blood levels due to its somewhat narrow therapeutic window.

Second Generation. Until recently, the mechanism of gabapentin was unknown. Gabapentin is classified as a ligand of the voltage-gated calcium channel α_2-Δ subunit, and is structurally related to GABA, although it does not bind directly to GABA receptors and is not converted to GABA. It is thought to act at voltage-gated calcium channels and inhibit

excitatory neurotransmitter release.[27] Pregabalin is also classified as an α_2-Δ ligand and an analog of GABA that similarly does not bind to GABA receptors and is not converted to GABA. It also acts at voltage-gated calcium channels.[26] Topiramate is thought to block voltage-dependent sodium channels, potentiate GABA transmission, and inhibit excitatory neurotransmission. Lamotrigine's proposed antinociceptive effects are attributed to sodium blockade and neural membrane stabilization, as well as to inhibition of the presynaptic release of glutamate.[26]

Gabapentin requires a slow titration, starting at 100 to 300 mg to a maximum dose of 3600 mg daily, typically divided into three or four doses. Pregabalin requires titration from 50 mg three times daily or 75 mg twice daily up to a maximum of 300 mg daily. It does not require as prolonged a titration because of its increased bioavailability and relatively linear pharmacokinetics. At doses of 300 mg/day, topiramate has been reported to alleviate CLBP by reducing pain symptoms and improving mood and quality of life.[28]

Third Generation. Lacosamide is an inhibitor of voltage-gated sodium channels and NMDA receptors.[29]

Table 13-4 provides a summary of the mechanism of action for different generations of antiepileptics.

Indication

Many adjunctive analgesics have been investigated for the treatment of chronic neuropathic pain in general; relatively few studies have focused specifically on CLBP. Most of the literature on this topic relates to the use of adjunctive analgesics for neuropathic pain secondary to conditions such as painful polyneuropathy (PPN), DPN, PHN, central poststroke pain, trigeminal neuralgia, or postmastectomy pain. The use of adjunctive analgesics for CLBP therefore requires extrapolating results from other indications that differ from CLBP in varying degrees. It should be noted that the use of adjunctive analgesics for CLBP is a secondary indication for these medications, which also possess primary indications that may be useful in some patients with CLBP. For example, patients with neuropathic or nociceptive CLBP who also have associated depression may benefit from TCAs, SSRIs, or SNRIs. Similarly, patients with CLBP who report insomnia associated with anxiety about their physical discomfort may benefit from antidepressants with known sleep-inducing properties, such as trazadone or doxepin. Although the indication for prescribing adjunctive analgesics in such cases is not primarily CLBP, symptoms of CLBP may also improve with their use.

Assessment

Before receiving adjunctive analgesics, patients should first be assessed for LBP using an evidence-based and goal-oriented approach focused on the patient history and neurologic examination, as discussed in Chapter 3. Additional diagnostic imaging or specific diagnostic testing is generally not required before initiating these interventions for CLBP. Prescribing physicians should also inquire about medication history to note prior hypersensitivity/allergy or adverse events with similar drugs, and evaluate contraindications for these types of drugs. Clinicians may also wish to order a psychological evaluation if they are concerned about the potential for medication misuse or potential for addiction in certain patients. Diagnostic imaging or other forms of advanced testing is generally not required before administering adjunctive analgesics for CLBP.

EFFICACY

Evidence supporting the efficacy of these interventions for CLBP was summarized from recent clinical practice guidelines (CPGs), systematic reviews (SRs), and randomized controlled trials (RCTs). Observational studies (OBSs) were also summarized where appropriate. Findings are summarized by study design for each intervention.

Clinical Practice Guidelines

Antidepressants

Four recent national CPGs on the management of CLBP assessed and summarized the evidence to make specific recommendations about the efficacy of various antidepressants.

The CPG from Europe in 2004 found that both noradrenergic and noradrenergic-serotonergic antidepressants can be considered as management options for the symptomatic relief of CLBP.[30] That CPG also found moderate evidence that neither noradrenergic nor noradrenergic-serotonergic antidepressants are effective with respect to improvements in function.

The CPG from Belgium in 2006 found conflicting evidence of a moderate effectiveness for both noradrenergic and noradrenergic-serotonergic antidepressants.[12]

The CPG from the United Kingdom in 2009 found that SSRIs should not be used.[31] That CPG also found conflicting evidence concerning the effectiveness of TCAs with respect to improvements in reducing pain and concluded that TCAs

could be considered as one management option for CLBP if other medications do not provide sufficient symptomatic relief.[31]

The CPG from the United States in 2007 found evidence of a small to moderate benefit for antidepressants with CLBP.[32]

Antiepileptics

Three recent national CPGs on the management of CLBP assessed and summarized the evidence to make specific recommendations about the efficacy of various antiepileptics.

The CPG from Europe in 2004 found limited evidence for the efficacy of gabapentin compared with placebo and did not recommend its use.[30]

The CPG from Belgium in 2006 found low-quality evidence supporting the effectiveness of gabapentin.[12]

The CPG from the United States in 2007 found weak evidence to support the efficacy of gabapentin for CLBP with radiculopathy.[32] That CPG also found insufficient evidence to support topiramate for CLBP.

Findings from these CPGs are summarized in Table 13-5.

Systematic Reviews

Antidepressants

Cochrane Collaboration. The Cochrane Collaboration conducted an SR in 2008 on antidepressants for nonspecific LBP.[33] A total of 10 RCTs were included that compared antidepressants with placebo; 9 included patients with CLBP, while 1 did not specify the duration of LBP.[34-43] Overall, the review found inconsistent evidence regarding antidepressants on pain relief in CLBP, with a meta-analysis of six small RCTs giving a standard mean difference (SMD) of −0.04 (95% CI −0.25 to 0.17). The review also concluded that there is no consistent evidence that antidepressants reduce depression in CLBP patients, or that antidepressants improve functional status in LBP patients. Furthermore, there was no difference between two types of antidepressants (TCAs and SSRIs) and placebo in pain relief.

American Pain Society and American College of Physicians. An SR was conducted in 2007 by the American Pain Society and American College of Physicians CPG committee on medication for acute and chronic LBP.[11] That review identified 3 SRs related to antidepressants and LBP, which included 10 unique RCTs.[44-46] Together, these reviews identified three RCTs that were not included in the Cochrane review described above.[47-49] Two of these SRs found antidepressants to be more effective than placebo for pain relief, but found inconsistent evidence for functional improvement.[44,45] One of these SRs performed a meta-analysis of nine trials and estimated an SMD of 0.41 (95% CI 0.22 to 0.61) for pain relief.[45] TCAs were found to be slightly or moderately more effective than placebo for pain relief, but no difference in effect was seen for paroxetine and trazadone. One of these SRs also found that antidepressants were associated with a higher risk of adverse events than placebo, although it also noted that harms were generally not well reported in RCTs.[44] This SR concluded that TCAs are effective for CLBP.

TABLE 13-5	**Clinical Practice Guideline Recommendations on Adjunctive Analgesic Use for Chronic Low Back Pain**

Reference	Country	Conclusion
Antidepressants		
30	Europe	TCAs and SNRIs can be considered as management options for the symptomatic relief of CLBP. Neither is effective with respect to improvements in function
12	Belgium	Conflicting evidence of moderate effectiveness for both TCAs and SNRIs SSRIs were not recommended
31	United Kingdom	SSRIs were not recommended
31	United Kingdom	TCAs can be considered if other medications do not offer relief
32	United States	Evidence of small to moderate benefit
96	Australia	Antidepressants were not recommended
97	Sweden	Antidepressants were not recommended
Antiepileptics		
96	Australia	Antiepileptics were not recommended
30	Europe	Gabapentin was not recommended
12	Belgium	Low-quality evidence supporting the use of gabapentin
32	United States	Weak evidence supporting efficacy for gabapentin
32	United States	Insufficient evidence to support the use of topiramate

CLBP, chronic low back pain; SNRI, serotonin-norepinephrine reuptake inhibitor; SSRI, selective serotonin reuptake inhibitor; TCA, tricyclic antidepressant.

Other. Previous systematic or other reviews have reached different conclusions regarding the efficacy of antidepressants for CLBP or neuropathic conditions.[7,9,10,21,44-46,50,51]

Findings from the aforementioned SRs are summarized in Table 13-6.

Chronic Low Back Pain

A review of six studies published before 1992 concluded that there was insufficient evidence to recommend the use of antidepressants for CLBP.[9]

A review conducted in 1997 included four studies and also failed to find supporting evidence of clinical benefit with antidepressants for CLBP.[50]

A review in 2001, which included nine studies, conducted a meta-analysis and concluded that antidepressants were more effective than placebo for treating CLBP.[44]

A review of SSRIs for CLBP in 2003 concluded, based on a small number of studies, that TCAs and tetracyclic antidepressants produced moderate symptom reductions for patients with CLBP regardless of depression status.[45] However, this review did not distinguish the effectiveness of different classes of antidepressants, and included patients with both neck and low back pain.

A review in 2004 did not distinguish the different antidepressants used and found conflicting evidence as to whether antidepressants improved the functional status of patients with CLBP.[46] That review initially evaluated 22 prior trials of antidepressants for the treatment of back pain, but only 7 met their inclusion criteria; the others lacked a placebo control group, included both neck and low back pain, or used parenteral rather than oral routes. A meta-analysis from that review concluded that antidepressants were more effective than placebo for treating CLBP.[46]

Neuropathic Pain

A review of SSRIs published in 1996 for various neuropathic pain conditions failed to demonstrate their efficacy when used for this purpose.[51] For neuropathic pain conditions, TCAs have been investigated more extensively than SSRIs,

TABLE 13-6	**Systematic Review Findings on Adjunctive Analgesics for Chronic Low Back Pain**

Reference	# RCTs in SR	# RCTs for CLBP	Conclusion
Antidepressants			
98	10	9 (1 of unknown duration)	Inconsistent evidence regarding effect of antidepressants on pain relief, reduction of depression or improved functional status in patients with CLBP
11	10 unique RCTs in 3 SRs	NR	Antidepressants are more effective than placebo for pain relief; inconsistent evidence for functional improvement Associated with higher risk of adverse events compared with placebo Fair evidence that the anticonvulsant gabapentin is effective for pain relief in radiculopathy
Antiepileptics			
52	NR	NR	The reviews did not include RCTs specific to LBP patients

CLBP, chronic low back pain; LBP, low back pain; NR, not reported; RCT, randomized controlled trial; SR, systematic review.

SNRIs, and antiepileptics. In an SR of antidepressants in neuropathic pain conditions, 30% of patients given antidepressants had more than 50% pain relief.

A review published in 2000 estimated that the number needed to treat (NNT), defined as the number of patients needed to treat with a certain drug to obtain one patient with at least 50% pain relief, was 2.6 for TCAs (95% CI 2.2 to 3.3) when comparing several different studies involving several different neuropathic pain conditions.[7]

A more recent review published in 2005 reported substantial variations in NNT values for different TCAs, which may be related to the differences in neuropathic pain diagnoses and the use of drug-level measurements to obtain optimal dosing.[21] When comparing TCAs with balanced reuptake of serotonin and noradrenaline to those TCAs with relatively selective noradrenaline reuptake in patients with PPN, there was a trend toward better effect with the balanced TCAs (NNT 2.1) compared with the noradrenergic TCAs (NNT 2.5). In PHN, a similar trend has been noted (balanced TCA NNT 2.5 vs. noradrenergic TCA NNT 3.1).[21] Although the trend may show favorability toward the balanced TCAs, other issues such as side effects and secondary symptoms (e.g., insomnia) need to be considered. Comparing the individual TCAs among each other is difficult, in that dosages in some trials were titrated to perceived benefits and side effects, whereas other studies targeted optimal plasma drug concentration.

A review of SSRIs in 2005 for various neuropathic pain conditions failed to demonstrate their efficacy when used for this purpose.[10]

Antiepileptics

Cochrane Collaboration. The Cochrane Collaboration conducted SRs in 2005 on anticonvulsants, gabapentin, and carbamazepine for acute and chronic pain.[52-54] Although the reviews found that gabapentin and carbamazepine are effective for pain management, the reviews did not include RCTs specific to LBP.

American Pain Society and American College of Physicians. An SR was conducted in 2007 by the American Pain Society and American College of Physicians CPG committee on medication for acute and chronic LBP, which did not find any SRs on antiepileptics in acute and chronic LBP.[11] The review identified two RCTs of topiramate and gabapentin in LBP.[28,55-57] The authors concluded that there is fair evidence that gabapentin is effective for pain relief in radiculopathy, although improvements were small.

Randomized Controlled Trials

Antidepressants

Nine RCTs were identified.[58-66] Their methods are summarized in Table 13-7. Their results are briefly described here.

An RCT with a crossover design was conducted by Sindrup and colleagues[58] in patients with PPN, who had symptoms lasting longer than 6 months. The etiology of PPN was idiopathic (34.4%), diabetic (46.9%), alcohol-related (6.3%), drug-induced (3.1%), connective tissue disorder (3.1%), and critical illness (3.1%). Participants randomized

to the intervention group received venlafaxine (37.5 mg twice daily in the first week; 75 mg twice daily in the second week; 112.5 mg twice daily in 2 remaining weeks). The control groups received either imipramine (25 mg twice daily in the first week; 50 mg twice daily in the second week; 75 mg twice daily in 2 remaining weeks) or placebo tablets. At the end of 4 weeks, summed pain scores decreased significantly in the venlafaxine and imipramine groups, but not in the placebo group. Improvement in pain was significantly higher in the venlafaxine and imipramine groups compared with the placebo group. There was no significant difference between venlafaxine and imipramine. Disability was not reported in this study.

An RCT conducted by Yucel and colleagues[59] included patients with neuropathic pain. The etiology of the pain was post herpetic neuralgia (13.3%), diabetes (26.7%), traumatic plexus avulsion (5.0%), peripheral nerve injury (8.3%), failed back surgery syndrome (18.3%), phantom pain (15.0%), and poststroke pain (13.3%). Participants were randomized to venlafaxine XR (75 mg daily), venlafaxine XR (150 mg daily), or placebo daily for 8 weeks. At the end of the treatment period, pain intensity (visual analog scale [VAS]) improved significantly for all three groups compared with baseline. Although the improvement was greater in the venlafaxine groups, there were no statistically significant differences between the three groups. There was also a significant increase in the proportion of patients with improved daily activities in all three groups compared with baseline. Again, the difference between groups was not statistically significant.

An RCT with a crossover design was conducted by Tasmuth and colleagues[60] in patients with neuropathic pain who had been treated for breast cancer. Participants experienced pain in the anterior chest wall or axilla and/or median upper arm in an area with sensory disturbances. Participants were randomized to either venlafaxine or placebo for 4 weeks, followed by a 2-week washout period, then 4 weeks of the other treatment. Venlafaxine (18.75 mg once daily) was given in the first week, increasing the dose every subsequent week. At the end of treatment, there were improvements in current pain intensity (VAS, verbal rating scale) in both groups (P values not reported). There were no significant differences between groups. However, the average pain relief (diary) was significantly better for the venlafaxine group compared with placebo group. Disability was not reported in this study.

An RCT was conducted by Rowbotham and colleagues[61] in patients with DPN who had pain symptoms lasting at least 3 months. Participants were randomized to either venlafaxine ER (75 mg once daily), venlafaxine ER (75 mg two or three times daily), or placebo daily for 6 weeks, with dose titration occurring in the first 3 weeks. At the end of 6 weeks, mean pain intensity scores (VAS) improved in all three groups compared with baseline (P values not reported). The largest improvement was seen in the higher dose venlafaxine group and the smallest improvement in the placebo group. The improvement in pain intensity was significantly better in the higher dose venlafaxine group compared with either the placebo or the lower dose venlafaxine group.

TABLE 13-7	Randomized Controlled Trials of Adjunctive Analgesics for Various Neuropathic Pain Conditions				
Reference	Indication	Intervention	Control (C1)	Control (C2)	Control (C3)
58*	Polyneuropathy (34.4% idiopathic; 46.9% diabetic, 6.3% alcohol-related; 3.1% drug-induced; 3.1% connective tissue disorder; 3.1% critical illness), symptoms >6 months	Venlafaxine 37.5 mg twice daily week 1 75 mg twice daily week 2 112.5 mg twice daily weeks 3-4 n = 40	Imipramine 25 mg twice daily week 1 50 mg twice daily week 2 75 mg twice daily weeks 3-4 n = 40	Placebo + paracetamol (500 mg six times daily) if needed n = 40	NA
59	Neuropathic pain (13.3% PHN; 26.7% diabetes; 5.0% traumatic plexus avulsion; 8.3% peripheral nerve injury; 18.3% failed back surgery syndrome; 15.0% phantom pain; 13.3% poststroke pain), symptom duration not reported	Venlafaxine XR 75 mg daily × 8 weeks n = 20	Venlafaxine XR 150 mg daily × 8 weeks n = 20	Placebo 1 tablet daily × 8 weeks n = 20	NA
60*	Neuropathic pain after breast cancer (pain in anterior chest wall and/or axilla and/or median upper arm), symptom duration not reported	Venlafaxine 18.75 mg (1-4 tablets daily) × 4 weeks n = 15	Placebo 1-4 tablets daily × 4 weeks n = 15	NA	NA
61	Diabetic peripheral neuropathic pain, symptoms ≥3 months	Venlafaxine ER 75 mg daily × 6 weeks n = 82	Venlafaxine ER 75 mg two to three times daily × 6 weeks n = 82	Placebo daily × 6 weeks n = 81	NA
62	Major depressive disorder with pain symptoms, symptom duration not reported	Duloxetine 20 mg three times daily × 9 weeks n = 123	Placebo three tablets daily × 9 weeks n = 122	NA	NA
63	Major depressive disorder with pain symptoms, symptom duration not reported	Duloxetine 20 mg three times daily × 9 weeks n = 128	Placebo 3 tablets daily × 9 weeks n = 139	NA	NA
64	Diabetic peripheral neuropathic pain, symptoms >6 months	Duloxetine 20 mg daily × 12 weeks n = 115	Duloxetine 60 mg daily × 12 weeks n = 114	Duloxetine 60 mg twice daily × 12 weeks n = 113	Placebo daily × 12 weeks n = 115
65	Diabetic peripheral neuropathic pain, symptoms >6 months	Duloxetine 60 mg daily × 12 weeks n = 116	Duloxetine 60 mg twice daily × 12 weeks n = 116	Placebo daily × 12 weeks n = 116	NA
66	Diabetic peripheral neuropathic pain, symptoms >6 months	Duloxetine 60 mg daily × 12 weeks n = 114	Duloxetine 60 mg twice daily × 12 weeks n = 112	Placebo daily × 12 weeks n = 108	NA

*Crossover design.
NA, not applicable; PHN, postherpetic neuropathy.

There was no significant difference between the lower dose venlafaxine group and placebo. Disability was not measured in this study.

An RCT was conducted by Detke and colleagues[62] in patients with physical symptoms of pain secondary to major depressive disorder. Participants were randomized to either 60 mg duloxetine or placebo for 9 weeks. At the end of the treatment period, there was an improvement in back pain intensity (VAS) and interference with daily activities (VAS) in the duloxetine group compared with baseline, with little improvement in the placebo group (P values not reported). The improvement in back pain in the duloxetine group was significantly better than that of the placebo group. The difference in interference with daily activities was not statistically significant between the two groups at 9 weeks.

A second RCT was conducted by Detke and colleagues[63] in patients with pain physical symptoms from major depressive disorder. Participants were randomized to either 60 mg duloxetine or placebo for 9 weeks. At the end of the treatment period, improvement in back pain intensity (VAS) was observed in both groups (P values not reported). The difference in back pain was not statistically significant between the two groups at 9 weeks. However, an analysis with the last observation carried forward found that duloxetine produced significantly greater improvement in overall pain from baseline to 9 weeks compared with placebo. Disability was not reported in this study.

An RCT was conducted by Goldstein and colleagues[64] in patients with DPN who had symptoms lasting longer than 6 months. Participants were randomized to (1) 20 mg/day duloxetine, (2) 60 mg/day duloxetine, (3) 120 mg/day duloxetine, or (4) placebo for a duration of 12 weeks. At the end of the treatment period, there was an improvement in pain (24-hour Average Pain Score, 11-point Likert scale) in all groups (P values not reported). The smallest improvement was observed in the placebo group, and greater improvements with increasing doses of duloxetine. There was a significant difference in pain scores between the 60 mg/day and 120 mg/day duloxetine groups compared with the placebo group. There were no significant differences between the 20 mg/day duloxetine group and placebo group, or between the 60 mg/day and 120 mg/day duloxetine groups. Disability was not reported in this study.

An RCT was conducted by Raskin and colleagues[65] in patients with DPN who had symptoms lasting longer than 6 months. Participants were randomized to (1) 60 mg/day duloxetine, (2) 120 mg/day duloxetine, or 3) placebo for a duration of 12 weeks. At the end of the treatment period, there was an improvement in pain (24-hr Average Pain Score, 11-point Likert scale; Brief Pain Inventory [BPI]) and interference with general activity (BPI) in all groups (P values not reported). The improvements were similar in the duloxetine groups and greater than that in the placebo group. There was a significant difference in pain and interference with general activity scores between the 60 mg/day and 120 mg/day duloxetine groups compared to placebo, but no significant difference between the duloxetine groups.

An RCT was conducted by Wernicke and colleagues[66] in patients with DPN who had symptoms lasting longer than 6 months. Participants were randomized to (1) 60 mg/day duloxetine, (2) 120 mg/day duloxetine, or (3) placebo for a duration of 12 weeks. At the end of the treatment period, there was an improvement in pain (24-hr Average Pain Score, 11-point Likert scale; BPI) and interference with general activity (BPI) in all groups (P values not reported). The improvements were similar in the duloxetine groups and greater than that in the placebo group. There was a significant difference in pain between the 60 mg/day and 120 mg/day duloxetine groups compared with the placebo group, but no significant difference between the duloxetine groups. There was also a significant difference in scores for interference with general activity between the 120 mg/day duloxetine group and placebo, but no significant difference between the 60 mg/day duloxetine group and placebo group.

Antiepileptics
No RCTs were identified related to antiepileptics and CLBP.

Observational Studies

Antiepileptics
First Generation. The use of carbamazepine for CLBP or radicular symptoms has not been evaluated in clinical studies. Two case reports have documented its efficacy for the treatment of sciatica.[67]

Third Generation. No studies have been done specifically evaluating pregabalin's role in CLBP. One study was performed evaluating the efficacy of topiramate.[55] The authors' criteria for inclusion were lumbar radiculopathy on clinical presentation and radiographic confirmation of a nerve root compression on magnetic resonance imaging or computed tomography/myelogram. The researchers concluded that topiramate at a mean dose of 200 mg had a small but real analgesic effect. This study is limited by a significant dropout rate (26%) because of intolerable side effects. Another study evaluated topiramate's role in treatment of CLBP.[28] At doses of 300 mg/day, topiramate was found to reduce pain symptoms and improve mood and quality of life. A small, open-label trial treating 14 patients found that at doses of 400 mg/day, lamotrigine reduced pain in patients with intractable sciatica.[68]

Lamotrigine (Lamictal) has no FDA approval for neuropathic pain states, but studies have indicated efficacy in trigeminal neuralgia and DPN.[69,70]

Oxcarbazepine (Trileptal) is not approved by the FDA for any pain states but studies have demonstrated some efficacy in trigeminal neuralgia, PHN, and DPN.[71]

Phenytoin (Dilantin) carries no FDA approval for neuropathic pain, but has reported efficacy for trigeminal neuralgia.[72]

Other antiepileptics such as valproic acid, felbamate, and zonigran lack FDA approval and lack any significant clinical evidence supporting their use for treatment of neuropathic pain.

SAFETY

Contraindications

Contraindications to TCAs include cardiac disease and intolerable adverse events.[58] TCAs should be used with caution in patients with glaucoma, urinary retention, autonomic neuropathy, or advanced age.[73] Caution is recommended when prescribing gabapentin to those with genetic lactose deficiency.[30]

Adverse Events

Antidepressants

Tricyclic Antidepressants. It has been reported that 20% of patients who take antidepressants have experienced an adverse event such as drowsiness, dry mouth, dizziness, or constipation.[30] Other studies have reported that minor adverse events may occur in 30% of patients taking TCAs, whereas 4% had major adverse events.[51] The number needed to harm was 3.7 (95% CI 2.9 to 5.2) for minor adverse events and 22 (95% CI 13.5 to 58) for major adverse events.[51] Given the prevalence of adverse events, there is a delicate balance between benefits and harms when contemplating antidepressants for CLBP.[74] In fact, the main limitation of TCAs for neuropathic pain conditions is adverse events that may worsen as dosage increases (Table 13-8).

Typical adverse events are usually anticholinergic in nature and include blurred vision, cognitive changes, dry mouth, constipation, and sexual dysfunction. Orthostatic hypotension and cardiovascular side effects (conduction defects, arrhythmias, tachycardia, stroke, myocardial infarction) are perhaps the most serious adverse events.[73] Almost 20% of patients treated with nortriptyline after a myocardial infarction may be at risk for cardiac adverse events.[75] In general, adverse events are more common with the older TCAs such as amitriptyline and less common with the newer generation TCAs such as nortriptyline and desipramine.[73] A comparison of nortriptyline to amitriptyline in a study of patients with PHN reported that comparative analgesia was equivalent, with greater tolerability with nortriptyline.[76] In some cases, the adverse events from amitriptyline may be significant enough that elderly patients may opt to remain in pain rather than continue to take the medication.[77] TCAs are sometimes prescribed because some of their side effects may actually be considered beneficial, such as sedation for those patients who have poor sleep at night, appetite stimulation for patients with poor nutrition, or urinary retention for patients with urinary frequency. Some medications may inhibit the effects of TCAs, including CYP2D6 inhibitors, terbinafine, and quinidine.[78]

Serotonin-Norepinephrine Reuptake Inhibitors. Venlafaxine seems to be the least well-tolerated SNRI, combining serotonergic adverse events such as nausea, sexual dysfunction, and withdrawal problems with dose-dependent cardiovascular adverse events, primarily related to hypertension.[79] Although the latter is not typically observed with duloxetine or milnacipran, no direct comparative data are available among the various SNRIs. Adverse events associated with duloxetine include nausea, somnolence, hyperhidrosis, anorexia, vomiting, and constipation.[79] These may be more frequent in the 60 mg twice daily dosage group, as indicated by a higher dropout rate (12%) when compared with the 60 mg daily dosage group (4%).[79] Several studies have also noted the absence of cardiovascular adverse events with duloxetine.[19,62,63,65,80]

Antiepileptics

The clinical usefulness of carbamazepine is limited by significant adverse events including Steven-Johnson syndrome, agranulocytosis, aplastic anemia, and hepatic toxicity. Phenytoin is infrequently used for pain because of adverse events and toxicity. Common adverse events associated with gabapentin include dizziness (23.9%), somnolence (27.4%), peripheral edema (9.7%), ataxia (7.1%), and infection (8.0%).[81] Those related to pregabalin are similar and include dizziness (23.8%), somnolence (11.7%), peripheral edema (11.7%), weight gain (12.8%), and vertigo (8.8%).[82] One study that evaluated the efficacy of topiramate for CLBP reported a dropout rate of 26% because of intolerable side effects.[55] The most common adverse events reported were paresthesia (38%), fatigue/weakness (34%), sedation (34%), and diarrhea (30%). In a small OBS of 14 patients taking lamotrigine 400 mg/day, the most common adverse events encountered were dizziness and diarrhea (Table 13-9).[70]

COSTS

Fees and Third-Party Reimbursement

In the United States, a recommendation for adjunctive analgesics for CLBP can likely be delivered by a clinician in the context of an office or outpatient visit for a new patient using CPT codes 99201 (up to 10 minutes), 99202 (up to 20 minutes), or 99203 (up to 30 minutes). For an established

| TABLE 13-8 | Types of Adverse Events Associated with Specific Tricyclic Antidepressants |

Medication	Sedation	Anticholinergic	Hypotension	Cardiac	Seizures	Weight Gain
Amitriptyline	+++	+++	+++	+++	++	++
Clomipramine	++	+++	++	+++	+++	+
Desipramine	+	+	+	++	+	+
Nortriptyline	+	+	+	++	+	+

+, rare; ++, common; +++, frequent.

TABLE 13-9	Adverse Events Associated with Specific Adjunctive Analgesics		
Ref	Medication	Event	% of Study Population Affected
79	Duloxetine	Nausea, somnolence, hyperhidrosis, anorexia, vomiting, constipation	12% in 60 mg twice daily group 4% in 60 mg once daily group
81	Gabapentin	Dizziness	24
81	Gabapentin	Somnolence	27
81	Gabapentin	Peripheral edema	10
81	Gabapentin	Ataxia	7
81	Gabapentin	Infection	8
82	Pregabalin	Dizziness	24
82	Pregabalin	Somnolence	12
82	Pregabalin	Peripheral edema	12
82	Pregabalin	Weight gain	13
82	Pregabalin	Vertigo	9
55	Topiramate	Paresthesias	38
55	Topiramate	Fatigue/weakness	34
55	Topiramate	Sedation	34
55	Topiramate	Diarrhea	30

TABLE 13-10	Medicare Fee Schedule for Related Services	
CPT Code	New York	California
99201	$41	$44
99202	$70	$76
99203	$101	$109
99211	$20	$22
99212	$41	$44
99213	$68	$73

2010 Participating, nonfacility amount.

TABLE 13-11	Costs of Common Adjunctive Analgesics from Retail Pharmacy	
Medication	Trade Name	Cost (30 day supply)*
Carbamazepine	Tegretol	$50.00 (200 mg tablets)
Gabapentin	Neurontin	$50.00 (100 mg capsules)
Pregabalin	Lyrica	$70.00 (100 mg capsules)
Topiramate	Topamax	$200.00 (100 mg tablets)
Lamotrigine	Lamictal	$150.00 (100 mg tablets)
Oxcarbazepine	Trileptal	$50.00 (150 mg tablets)
Phenytoin	Dilantin	$50.00 (100 mg capsules)
Amitriptyline	Elavil, Vanatrip, Endep	$50.00 (100 mg tablets)
Clomipramine	Anafranil	$300.00 (50 mg capsules)
Doxepin	Sinequan	$50.00 (100 mg capsules)
Desipramine	Norpramin	$150.00 (100 mg tablets)
Nortriptyline	Pamelor, Aventyl	$570.00 (50 mg capsules)
Venlafaxine	Effexor	$75.00 (100 mg tablets)
Milnacipran	Ixel, Savella	$50.00 (100 mg tablets)
Duloxetine	Cymbalta	$125.00 (60 mg capsules)
Mirtazapine	Remeron	$110.00 (100 mg tablets)

*30-day supply of brand name drugs.
From www.medcohealth.com.

patient, these can likely be provided during an office or outpatient visit using CPT codes 99211 (up to 5 minutes), 99212 (up to 10 minutes), or 99213 (up to 15 minutes). Although time is indicated for the various levels of service and can be a contributing component for selection of the level of office/outpatient visits, the overarching criteria for selection of the level of service should be based on medical necessity and the amount of history, examination, and medical decision making that was required and documented.

These procedures are widely covered by other third-party payers such as health insurers and worker's compensation insurance. Although some payers continue to base their reimbursements on usual, customary, and reasonable payment methodology, the majority have developed reimbursement tables based on the Resource Based Relative Value Scale used by Medicare. Reimbursements by other third-party payers are generally higher than Medicare.

Typical fees reimbursed by Medicare in New York and California for these services are summarized in Table 13-10.

Adjunctive analgesics are typically covered by most third-party payers, many of whom now use pharmacy benefits managers (PBMs) to create and maintain formularies of covered medications. PBMs may only include a few medications under each broad class of adjunctive analgesic, and may require prior authorization, failure of a cheaper medication, or medical justification for using a more expensive medication within the same class. The cost of adjunctive analgesics varies considerably for each drug class and medication. Older TCAs that are now available as generics may cost as little as a few pennies per pill, whereas newer SSRIs, SNRIs, and antiepileptics may cost as much as a few dollars per pill.

Table 13-11 provides the approximate cost of a 30-day supply of brand name adjunctive analgesics through a PBM in the United States.

Cost Effectiveness

Evidence supporting the cost effectiveness of these interventions for acute or chronic LBP was summarized based on two recent national CPGs and one OBS.[13,30,31] Findings are summarized here.

The CPG from the United Kingdom in 2009 found that the costs of antidepressants for the treatment of CLBP are expected to be similar to those of acetaminophen.[31]

The CPG from Europe in 2004 found the cost effectiveness of antidepressants for the treatment of CLBP to be unknown.[30]

Other

As described earlier in this chaper, a study in Sweden asked 302 patients who presented to 16 physicians at 14 randomly selected outpatient clinics to complete questionnaires on health care resource use in the past 6 months.[13] Direct costs were calculated based on unit costs from hospital, pharmacy, and national health sources. Annual direct costs per patient for pharmaceuticals were $173 and patients took an average of two medications for CLBP.

SUMMARY

Description

An adjunctive analgesic is a medication that can be used for pain relief but whose primary indication is not related to pain. In this chapter, antidepressants and antiepileptics are considered adjunctive analgesics for CLBP. Antidepressants include drug classes such as TCAs, tetracyclic antidepressants (closely related to TCAs), SSRIs, and SNRIs. There are three main categories of antiepileptics, named in chronological order of discovery: first generation, second generation, and third generation. Adjunctive analgesics have been used for at least 4 decades to manage LBP and their use is increasing, most likely due to anecdotal evidence. Antiepileptics likely gained popularity after the FDA approved their use for neuropathic pain conditions such as PHN and DPN.

Theory

Differentiating between neuropathic and nociceptive pain is central to the mechanism of action of adjunctive analgesics. Neuropathic pain stems specifically from injury to the nerve itself, while nociceptive pain stems from any tissue injury that initiates a nociceptive signal carried by a nerve. TCAs are thought to provide relief for neuropathic pain via the serotonergic and noradrenergic pathways, perhaps due to their stabilization effects on nerve membranes. Neuropathic pain relief with TCAs appears to occur independently of any antidepressant effect they may also produce. Similar to TCAs, SNRIs affect both serotonergic and noradrenergic pathways. SSRIs are not indicated for neuropathic pain and any clinical improvement noted in CLBP from their use is likely associated with improvement in secondary emotional disturbances such as depression, anxiety, or insomnia. First-generation antiepileptics are thought to act on the pain pathway through inhibition of voltage-gated sodium channels. Individual second-generation antiepileptics have their own effects, yet they usually influence GABA receptors and voltage-gated calcium channels. Third-generation antiepileptics inhibit voltage-gated sodium channels and NMDA receptors. The use of adjunctive analgesics for CLBP requires extrapolating results from other indications that differ from CLBP in varying degrees. Adjunctive analgesics may be useful in some patients with CLBP and other comorbidities, such as insomnia, depression or anxiety.

Efficacy

Antidepressants

Four recent national CPGs assessed antidepressants for CLBP. One CPG reported conflicting evidence supporting noradrenergic and noradrenergic-serotonergic antidepressants and another found a small to moderate benefit for antidepressants. One CPG recommended noradrenergic and noradrenergic-serotonergic antidepressants while another recommended TCAs as options for CLBP. An SR concluded that there is inconsistent evidence supporting the use of antidepressants for reducing depression or improving disability in CLBP. Another SR concluded that TCAs are effective for CLBP. At least nine RCTs assessed the efficacy of antidepressants for chronic pain conditions other than LBP, four of which observed statistically significant improvement in pain over placebo or other comparators.

Antiepileptics

Three recent national CPGs assessed antiepileptics for CLBP. One did not recommend gabapentin and two found low-quality or weak evidence supporting gabapentin for CLBP. One CPG found insufficient evidence supporting topiramate for CLBP. SRs concluded that gabapentin and carbamazepine are effective for pain management, yet RCTs specific to LBP were not included. Another SR concluded that gabapentin is effective for pain relief in radiculopathy. Few RCTs have been conducted on antiepileptics for CLBP.

Safety

Contraindications to TCAs include cardiac disease and intolerable adverse events. Adverse events associated with TCAs include blurred vision, cognitive changes, dry mouth, constipation, sexual dysfunction, orthostatic hypotension, and cardiovascular side effects (conduction defects, arrhythmias, tachycardia, stroke, myocardial infarction). Adverse events related to SNRIs include nausea, sexual dysfunction, cardiovascular events (for venlafaxine), somnolence, hyperhidrosis, anorexia, vomiting, and constipation. Carbamazepine is associated with adverse events such as Steven-Johnson syndrome, agranulocytosis, aplastic anemia, and hepatic toxicity. Gabapentin is associated with dizziness, somnolence, peripheral edema, ataxia, and infection. Adverse events related to pregabalin include dizziness, somnolence, peripheral edema, weight gain, and vertigo. Topiramate has been associated with paresthesia, fatigue/weakness, sedation, and diarrhea.

Costs

The Medicare reimbursement for outpatient visits during which a clinician can prescribe adjunctive analgesics ranges from $22 to $109. The cost of adjunctive analgesics varies considerably for each drug class and medication. Older TCAs that are now available as generics may cost as little as a few pennies per pill, whereas newer SSRIs, SNRIs, and antiepileptics may cost as much as a few dollars per pill. One CPG reports that the cost of treatment with older antidepressants is expected to be similar to acetaminophen. Another CPG reports that the cost effectiveness of adjunctive analgesics is unknown.

Comments

Evidence from the CPGs, SRs, and RCTs reviewed show generally conflicting results supporting the use of adjunctive analgesics such as antidepressants or antiepileptics for CLBP. However, this evidence suggests that some specific classes of medications may be helpful in some patients with CLBP. For example, it appears reasonable to consider using low-dose TCAs in mild to moderate CLBP with painful radicular symptoms related to neuropathic pain, after acetaminophen and NSAIDs have been tried and failed. If TCAs do not provide any relief, antiepileptics such as gabapentin can also be considered, though this evidence is derived from indications other than LBP. Furthermore, careful titration of dosing is required for antiepileptics, along with constant vigilance for side effects. If both TCAs and antiepileptics fail to address symptoms associated with CLBP, SNRIs and newer generation antiepileptics might be worth considering. The expense and safety of these medications need to be weighed against their possible efficacy.

CHAPTER REVIEW QUESTIONS

Answers are located on page 451.

1. Which of the following is not a subtype of adjunctive analgesics?
   a. tricyclic antidepressants
   b. selective serotonin reuptake inhibitors
   c. benzodiazepines
   d. serotonin-norepinephrine reuptake inhibitors
2. Which of the following is not a contraindication or precaution to prescribing TCAs?
   a. myopia
   b. urinary retention
   c. autonomic neuropathy
   d. elderly patients with cardiac disease
3. How does a windup phenomenon occur in chronic pain?
   a. decreased activity of NMDA in dorsal horn and activation of voltage-gated calcium channels
   b. increased activity of NMDA in anterior horn and prohibition of voltage-gated calcium channels
   c. increased activity of NMDA in dorsal horn and activation of voltage-gated calcium channels
   d. inhibition activity of NMDA in dorsal horn and activation of voltage-gated potassium channels
4. True or false: Only pain management specialists can prescribe an adjunctive analgesic if the medication is intended for use outside its approved indication.
5. True or false: Pain management specialists are generally more familiar with prescribing adjunctive analgesics for CLBP than primary care physicians.

6. Which of the following is a key difference between nociceptive pain and neuropathic pain?
   a. nociceptive pain stems from the extremities whereas neuropathic pain is in the spine
   b. neuropathic pain can become nociceptive pain if not managed appropriately
   c. nociceptive pain is more common among the elderly and neuropathic pain is more common in the young
   d. neuropathic pain stems from nerve injury while nociceptive pain stems from other tissues
7. Which of the following adjunctive analgesics are FDA-approved for CLBP?
   a. gabapentin
   b. pregabalin
   c. neurontin
   d. none of the above

REFERENCES

1. Torstensen TA, Ljunggren AE, Meen HD, et al. Efficiency and costs of medical exercise therapy, conventional physiotherapy, and self-exercise in patients with chronic low back pain. A pragmatic, randomized, single-blinded, controlled trial with 1-year follow-up. Spine 1998;23:2616-2624.
2. New entry in the DM arena tackles back care issues. Disease Management Advisor 2004;10(5).
3. Baldwin ML, Cote P, Frank JW, et al. Cost-effectiveness studies of medical and chiropractic care for occupational low back pain: a critical review of the literature. Spine J 2001;1: 138-147.
4. Sindrup SH, Jensen TS. Pharmacologic treatment of pain in polyneuropathy. Neurology 2000;55:915-920.
5. McEvoy GK, editor. AHFS Drug Information. Bethesda: American Society of Health System Pharmacists; 2003.
6. Anderson JJ, Ruwe M, Miller DR, et al. Relative costs and effectiveness of specialist and general internist ambulatory care for patients with 2 chronic musculoskeletal conditions. J Rheumatol 2002;29:1488-1495.
7. Simpson KH. Individual choice of opioids and formulations: strategies to achieve the optimum for the patient. Clin Rheumatol 2002;21:S5-S8.
8. Inturrisi CE. Clinical pharmacology of opioids for pain. Clin J Pain 2002;18:3-13.
9. Turner JA, Denny MC. Do antidepressant medications relieve chronic low back pain? J Fam Pract 1993;37: 545-553.
10. Sindrup SH, Otto M, Finnerup NB, et al. Antidepressants in the treatment of neuropathic pain. Basic Clin Pharmacol Toxicol 2005;96:399-409.
11. Chou R, Huffman LH. Medications for acute and chronic low back pain: a review of the evidence for an American Pain Society/American College of Physicians clinical practice guideline. Ann Intern Med 2007;147:505-514.
12. Nielens H, van Zundert J, Mairiaux P, et al. Chronic low back pain. Good Clinical practice (GCP). Brussels: Belgian Health Care Knowledge Centre (KCE); 2006. KCE reports vol 48C.
13. Ekman M, Jonhagen S, Hunsche E, et al. Burden of illness of chronic low back pain in Sweden: a cross-sectional, retrospective study in primary care setting. Spine 2005;30: 1777-1785.

14. Bala MM, Riemsma RP, Nixon J, et al. Systematic review of the (cost-)effectiveness of spinal cord stimulation for people with failed back surgery syndrome. Clin J Pain 2008;24: 741-756.

15. Barber JA, Thompson SG. Analysis of cost data in randomized trials: an application of the non-parametric bootstrap. Statistics Med 2000;19:3219-3236.

16. DM program cuts back pain costs by educating, supporting primary care physicians. Healthcare Demand Dis Management 1999;5:149-153.

17. Gorman DJ, Kam PA, Brisby H, et al. When is spinal pain "neuropathic"? Orthop Clin North Am 2004;35:73-84.

18. Arts MP, Peul WC, Brand R, et al. Cost-effectiveness of micro-endoscopic discectomy versus conventional open discectomy in the treatment of lumbar disc herniation: a prospective randomised controlled trial. BMC Musculoskeletal Disorders 2006;7:42.

19. Goldstein FJ. Adjuncts to opioid therapy. J Am Osteopath Assoc 2002;102:S15-S21.

20. Wong DT, Bymaster FP, Engleman EA. Prozac (fluoxetine, Lilly 110140), the first selective serotonin uptake inhibitor and an antidepressant drug: twenty years since its first publication. Life Sci 1995;57:411-441.

21. Finnerup NB, Otto M, McQuay HJ, et al. Algorithm for neuropathic pain treatment: an evidence-based proposal. Pain 2005;118:289-305.

22. Bastiaenen CHG, de Bie RA, Vlaeyen JWS, et al. Long-term effectiveness and costs of a brief self-management intervention in women with pregnancy-related low back pain after delivery. BMC Pregnancy Childbirth 2008;8:19.

23. Gillman PK. A systematic review of the serotonergic effects of mirtazapine in humans: implications for its dual action status. Hum Psychopharmacol 2006;21:117-125.

24. Harvey AT, Rudolph RL, Preskorn SH. Evidence of the dual mechanisms of action of venlafaxine. Arch Gen Psychiatry 2000;57:503-509.

25. Bymaster FP, Dreshfield-Ahmad LJ, Threlkeld PG, et al. Comparative affinity of duloxetine and venlafaxine for serotonin and norepinephrine transporters in vitro and in vivo, human serotonin receptor subtypes, and other neuronal receptors. Neuropsychopharmacology 2001;25:871-880.

26. McCarberg BH, Barkin RL. Long-acting opioids for chronic pain: pharmacotherapeutic opportunities to enhance compliance, quality of life, and analgesia. Am J Ther 2001;8:181-186.

27. Asche CV, Kirkness CS, McAdam-Marx C, et al. The societal costs of low back pain: data published between 2001 and 2007. J Pain Palliat Care Pharmacother 2007;21:25-33.

28. Muehlbacher M, Nickel MK, Kettler C, et al. Topiramate in treatment of patients with chronic low back pain: a randomized, double-blind, placebo-controlled study. Clin J Pain 2006; 22:526-531.

29. Birkmeyer NJO, Weinstein JN, Tosteson ANA, et al. Design of the Spine Patient outcomes Research Trial (SPORT). Spine 2002;27:1361-1372.

30. Airaksinen O, Brox JI, Cedraschi C, et al. European guidelines for the management of chronic nonspecific low back pain. Eur Spine J 2006;15:S192-S300.

31. National Institute for Health and Clinical Excellence (NICE). Low back pain: early management of persistent non-specific low back pain. London: National Institute of Health and Clinical Excellence; 2009. Report No.: NICE clinical guideline 88.

32. Chou R, Qaseem A, Snow V, et al. Diagnosis and treatment of low back pain: a joint clinical practice guideline from the American College of Physicians and the American Pain Society. Ann Intern Med 2007;147:478-491.

33. Urquhart DM, Hoving JL, Assendelft WW, et al. Antidepressants for non-specific low back pain. Cochrane Database Syst Rev 2008;(1):CD001703.

34. Alcoff J, Jones E, Rust P, et al. Controlled trial of imipramine for chronic low back pain. J Fam Pract 1982;14:841-846.

35. Atkinson JH, Slater MA, Williams RA, et al. A placebo-controlled randomized clinical trial of nortriptyline for chronic low back pain. Pain 1998;76:287-296.

36. Atkinson JH, Slater MA, Wahlgren DR, et al. Effects of noradrenergic and serotonergic antidepressants on chronic low back pain intensity. Pain 1999;83:137-145.

37. Atkinson JH, Slater MA, Capparelli EV, et al. Efficacy of noradrenergic and serotonergic antidepressants in chronic back pain: a preliminary concentration-controlled trial. J Clin Psychopharmacol 2007;27:135-142.

38. Dickens C, Jayson M, Sutton C, et al. The relationship between pain and depression in a trial using paroxetine in sufferers of chronic low back pain. Psychosomatics 2000;41: 490-499.

39. Goodkin K, Gullion CM, Agras WS. A randomized, double-blind, placebo-controlled trial of trazadone hydrochloride in chronic low back pain syndrome. J Clin Psychopharmacol 1990;10:269-278.

40. Katz J, Pennella-Vaughan J, Hetzel RD, et al. A randomized, placebo-controlled trial of bupropion sustained release in chronic low back pain. J Pain 2005;6:656-661.

41. Pheasant H, Bursk A, Goldfarb J, et al. Amitriptyline and chronic low-back pain. A randomized double-blind crossover study. Spine 1983;8:552-557.

42. Treves R, Montaine de la RP, Dumond JJ, et al. [Prospective study of the analgesic action of clomipramine versus placebo in refractory lumbosciatica (68 cases).] Rev Rheum Mal Osteoartic 1991;58:549-552.

43. Jenkins DG, Ebbutt AF, Evans CD. Tofranil in the treatment of low back pain. J Int Med Res 1976;4:28-40.

44. Salerno SM, Browning R, Jackson JL. The effect of antidepressant treatment on chronic back pain: a meta-analysis. Arch Intern Med 2002;162:19-24.

45. Staiger TO, Gaster B, Sullivan MD, et al. Systematic review of antidepressants in the treatment of chronic low back pain. Spine 2003;28:2540-2545.

46. Schnitzer TJ, Ferraro A, Hunsche E, et al. A comprehensive review of clinical trials on the efficacy and safety of drugs for the treatment of low back pain. J Pain Symptom Manage 2004;28:72-95.

47. Ward N, Bokan JA, Phillips M, et al. Antidepressants in concomitant chronic back pain and depression: doxepin and desipramine compared. J Clin Psychiatry 1984;45: 54-59.

48. Hameroff SR, Weiss JL, Lerman JC, et al. Doxepin's effects on chronic pain and depression: a controlled study. J Clin Psychiatry 1984;45:47-53.

49. Schreiber S, Vinokur S, Shavelzon V, et al. A randomized trial of fluoxetine versus amitriptyline in musculo-skeletal pain. Isr J Psychiatry Relat Sci 2001;38:88-94.

50. van Tulder MW, Koes BW, Bouter LM. Conservative treatment of acute and chronic nonspecific low back pain. A systematic review of randomized controlled trials of the most common interventions. Spine 1997;22:2128-2156.

51. McQuay HJ, Tramer M, Nye BA, et al. A systematic review of antidepressants in neuropathic pain. Pain 1996;68: 217-227.

52. Wiffen P, Collins S, McQuay H, et al. Anticonvulsant drugs for acute and chronic pain. Cochrane Database Syst Rev 2005; (3):CD001133.

53. Wiffen PJ, McQuay HJ, Edwards JE, et al. Gabapentin for acute and chronic pain. Cochrane Database Syst Rev 2005;(3): CD005452.

54. Wiffen PJ, McQuay HJ, Moore RA. Carbamazepine for acute and chronic pain. Cochrane Database Syst Rev 2005;(3): CD005451.

55. Khoromi S, Patsalides A, Parada S, et al. Topiramate in chronic lumbar radicular pain. J Pain 2005;6:829-836.

56. McCleane GJ. Does gabapentin have an analgesic effect on background, movement and referred pain? A randomised, double-blind, placebo controlled study. Pain Clin 2001;13: 103-107.

57. Yildirim K, Sisecioglu M, Karatay S, et al. The effectiveness of gabapentin in patients with chronic radiculopathy. Pain Clin 2003;15:213-218.

58. Sindrup SH, Bach FW, Madsen C, et al. Venlafaxine versus imipramine in painful polyneuropathy: a randomized, controlled trial. Neurology 2003;60:1284-1289.

59. Yucel A, Ozyalcin S, Koknel TG, et al. The effect of venlafaxine on ongoing and experimentally induced pain in neuropathic pain patients: a double blind, placebo controlled study. Eur J Pain 2005;9:407-416.

60. Tasmuth T, Hartel B, Kalso E. Venlafaxine in neuropathic pain following treatment of breast cancer. Eur J Pain 2002;6: 17-24.

61. Rowbotham MC, Goli V, Kunz NR, et al. Venlafaxine extended release in the treatment of painful diabetic neuropathy: a double-blind, placebo-controlled study. Pain 2004;110:697-706.

62. Detke MJ, Lu Y, Goldstein DJ, et al. Duloxetine, 60 mg once daily, for major depressive disorder: a randomized double-blind placebo-controlled trial. J Clin Psychiatry 2002;63:308-315.

63. Detke MJ, Lu Y, Goldstein DJ, et al. Duloxetine 60 mg once daily dosing versus placebo in the acute treatment of major depression. J Psychiatr Res 2002;36:383-390.

64. Goldstein DJ, Lu Y, Detke MJ, et al. Iyengar S. Duloxetine vs. placebo in patients with painful diabetic neuropathy. Pain 2005;116:109-118.

65. Raskin J, Pritchett YL, Wang F, et al. A double-blind, randomized multicenter trial comparing duloxetine with placebo in the management of diabetic peripheral neuropathic pain. Pain Med 2005;6:346-356.

66. Wernicke JF, Pritchett YL, D'Souza DN, et al. A randomized controlled trial of duloxetine in diabetic peripheral neuropathic pain. Neurology 2006;67:1411-1420.

67. Lovell J. Carbamazepine and sciatica. Aust Fam Physician 1992;21:784-786.

68. Eisenberg E, Damunni G, Hoffer E, et al. Lamotrigine for intractable sciatica: correlation between dose, plasma concentration and analgesia. Eur J Pain 2003;7:485-491.

69. Zakrzewska JM, Chaudhry Z, Nurmikko TJ, et al. Lamotrigine (lamictal) in refractory trigeminal neuralgia: results from a double-blind placebo controlled crossover trial. Pain 1997; 73:223-230.

70. Eisenberg E, Lurie Y, Braker C, et al. A. Lamotrigine reduces painful diabetic neuropathy: a randomized, controlled study. Neurology 2001;57:505-509.

71. Carrazana E, Mikoshiba I. Rationale and evidence for the use of oxcarbazepine in neuropathic pain. J Pain Symptom Manage 2003;25:S31-S35.

72. McQuay H, Carroll D, Jadad AR, et al. Anticonvulsant drugs for management of pain: a systematic review. BMJ 1995;311: 1047-1052.

73. Dworkin RH, Backonja M, Rowbotham MC, et al. Advances in neuropathic pain: diagnosis, mechanisms, and treatment recommendations. Arch Neurol 2003;60:1524-1534.

74. Hall H, McIntosh G. Low back pain (chronic). Clin Evid (Online) 2008;Oct 1:1116.

75. Roose SP, Laghrissi-Thode F, Kennedy JS, et al. Comparison of paroxetine and nortriptyline in depressed patients with ischemic heart disease. JAMA 1998;279:287-291.

76. Watson CP, Evans RJ, Reed K, et al. Amitriptyline versus placebo in postherpetic neuralgia. Neurology 1982;32: 671-673.

77. Dallocchio C, Buffa C, Mazzarello P, et al. Gabapentin vs. amitriptyline in painful diabetic neuropathy: an open-label pilot study. J Pain Symptom Manage 2000;20:280-285.

78. Verdu B, Decosterd I, Buclin T, et al. Antidepressants for the treatment of chronic pain. Drugs 2008;68:2611-2632.

79. Stahl SM, Grady MM, Moret C, et al. SNRIs: their pharmacology, clinical efficacy, and tolerability in comparison with other classes of antidepressants. CNS Spectr 2005;10:732-747.

80. Goldstein DJ, Lu Y, Detke MJ, et al. Effects of duloxetine on painful physical symptoms associated with depression. Psychosomatics 2004;45:17-28.

81. Rowbotham M, Harden N, Stacey B, et al. Gabapentin for the treatment of postherpetic neuralgia: a randomized controlled trial. JAMA 1998;280:1837-1842.

82. Freynhagen R, Strojek K, Griesing T, et al. Efficacy of pregabalin in neuropathic pain evaluated in a 12-week, randomised, double-blind, multicentre, placebo-controlled trial of flexible- and fixed-dose regimens. Pain 2005;115:254-263.

83. Dagenais S, Roffey DM, Wai EK, et al. Can cost utility evaluations inform decision making about interventions for low back pain? Spine J 2009;9:944-957.

84. van der Roer N, Goossens MEJB, Evers SMAA, et al. What is the most cost-effective treatment for patients with low back pain? A systematic review. Best Pract Res Clin Rheumatol 2005;19:671-684.

85. Brazier J, Roberts J, Tsuchiya A, et al. A comparison of the EQ-5D and SF-6D across seven patient groups. Health Economics 2004;13873-13884.

86. Backonja M, Beydoun A, Edwards KR, et al. Gabapentin for the symptomatic treatment of painful neuropathy in patients with diabetes mellitus: a randomized controlled trial. JAMA 1998;280:1831-1836.

87. Bogefeldt J, Grunnesjo MI, Svardsudd K, et al. Sick leave reductions from a comprehensive manual therapy programme for low back pain: the Gotland Low Back Pain Study. Clin Rehabil 2008;22:529-541.

88. Borkan J, Van Tulder M, Reis S, et al. Advances in the field of low back pain in primary care: a report from the fourth international forum. Spine 2002;27:E128-E132.

89. Boonen A, van den Heuvel R, van Tubergen A, et al. Large differences in cost of illness and wellbeing between patients with fibromyalgia, chronic low back pain, or ankylosing spondylitis. Ann Rheum Dis 2005;64:396-402.

90. Cassidy JD, Carroll L, Cote P, et al. Low back pain after traffic collisions: a population-based cohort study. Spine 2003;28: 1002-1009.

91. Chen CK, Liang HL, Lai PH, et al. Imaging diagnosis of insufficiency fracture of the sacrum. Chung Hua i Hsueh Tsa Chih—Chinese Medical Journal 1999;62:591-597.

92. Cherkin DC, Eisenberg D, Sherman KJ, et al. Randomized trial comparing traditional Chinese medical acupuncture, therapeutic massage, and self-care education for chronic low back pain. Arch Intern Med 2001;161:1081-1088.

93. Chibnall JT, Tait RC, Andresen EM, et al. Race and socioeconomic differences in post-settlement outcomes for African American and Caucasian Workers' Compensation claimants with low back injuries. Pain 2005;114:462-472.

94. Chibnall JT, Tait RC, Merys SC. Disability management of low back injuries by employer-retained physicians: ratings and costs. Am J Industrial Med 2000;38:529-538.

95. Bleichrodt H, Pinto JL, Abellan-Perpinan JM. A consistency test of the time trade-off. J Health Economics 2003;22:1037-1052.

96. Australian Acute Musculoskeletal Pain Guidelines Group. Evidence-based management of acute musculoskeletal pain. Brisbane: Australian Academic Press; 2003.

97. Nachemson A, Jonsson E, Englund L, et al. Neck and back pain: the scientific evidence of causes, diagnosis, and treatment. Philadelphia: Lippincott Williams & Wilkins; 2000.

98. Hayden JA, van Tulder MW, Malmivaara A, et al. Exercise therapy for treatment of non-specific low back pain. Cochrane Database Syst Rev 2005;(3):CD000335.

CHAPTER 14

STEPHANE POITRAS
LUCIE BROSSEAU

Electrotherapeutic Modalities and Physical Agents

DESCRIPTION

Terminology and Subtypes

Physical modalities is a broad term referring to a variety of instruments, machines, and tools traditionally used in physical therapy for musculoskeletal conditions, including chronic low back pain (CLBP). Two important categories of modalities are electrotherapeutic and physical agents.[1,2] Electrotherapeutic modalities involve the use of electricity and include therapies such as transcutaneous electrical nerve stimulation (TENS), electrical muscle stimulation (EMS), and interferential current (IFC).[3] The term *superficial TENS* is also used to differentiate it from TENS administered through a spinal cord stimulator. Electroacupuncture is the application of electrical stimulation, typically with high frequency TENS, through acupuncture needles.

Physical agents are modalities that involve thermal, acoustic (produced by sound waves), or radiant energy, and include interventions such as therapeutic ultrasound (US), superficial heat (hot packs), and cryotherapy (cold packs or ice).[3] US refers to acoustic energy above 20,000 hertz (Hz), and is used for both diagnostic and therapeutic purposes. Therapeutic US uses more energy than diagnostic US, which is also referred to as *sonography.*[4] Phonophoresis is the use of therapeutic US to facilitate the absorption of topical products such as analgesic or anti-inflammatory creams.[5] The term *physical modality* should be distinguished from *physical therapy,* which refers to an allied health profession rather than any specific treatment administered by this profession. This distinction is akin to that between *medication* and *medicine.* The term *passive modalities* is also sometimes used to describe physical modalities in which no active participation is required by the patient, and to distinguish these interventions from active rehabilitation such as supervised exercise therapy, which is also used by physical therapists.

Within electrotherapeutic modalities, common interventions include TENS, EMS, and IFC. TENS delivers an electrical current through superficial electrodes placed on the skin around the area of symptoms and causes a tingling sensation by stimulating sensory nerve fibers. EMS also delivers an electrical current through superficial electrodes placed on the skin, but uses a different type of electrical current than TENS to target motor nerve fibers. IFC is also administered through superficial electrodes and uses a much higher frequency than TENS, which is thought to allow for deeper penetration of the electrical current and is thought to cause less discomfort. There are several types of TENS, EMS, and IFC devices available, including larger units intended for use in clinical settings and smaller, battery-operated units that may be portable and worn under clothing for prolonged use throughout the day (Figure 14-1).

Common physical agents include US, superficial heat, and cryotherapy. US produces sound waves that are transmitted to the affected area through a hand-held, wand-shaped probe using conductive gel. Settings on the US machine may deliver pulsed or continuous waves. Hot packs are typically reusable, moldable bags of gel that are heated and wrapped in moist towels before being placed on the affected area to provide heat (Figure 14-2). Cold packs are typically reusable, moldable bags of gel that are frozen and wrapped in moist towels before being placed on the affected area to provide cold (Figure 14-3). Both hot and cold packs are available as disposable types that create a temporary heating or cooling effect through a chemical reaction initiated by crushing the packs by hand, or as reusable types that need to be placed in the microwave or freezer according to manufacturer recommendations (Figure 14-4). Other types of physical modalities used in the treatment of CLBP and not discussed in this chapter include various types of laser therapy, electromyography/biofeedback, electromagnetic fields, diathermy, and vapocoolant spray.

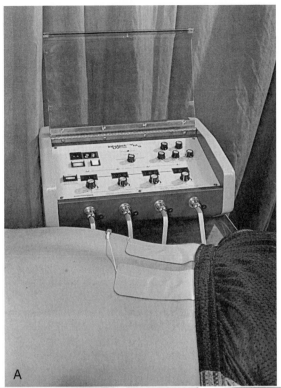

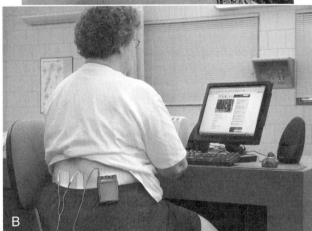

Figure 14-1 Typical stationary (**A**) and portable TENS machines (**B**). (Courtesy of Dewey Neild. In Pagliarulo MA. Introduction to physical therapy, ed 3. St. Louis, Mosby, 2006.)

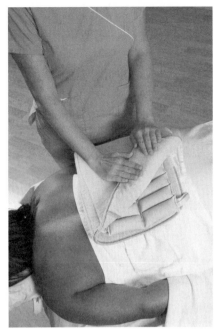

Figure 14-2 Typical moldable and reusable hot pack. (From Salvo S: Massage therapy: principles & practice, ed 3. St. Louis, 2008, Saunders.)

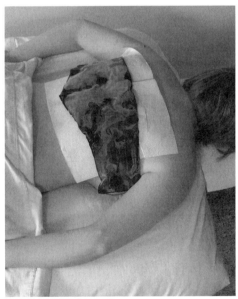

Figure 14-3 Typical moldable and reusable cold pack. (From Salvo S: Massage therapy: principles & practice, ed 3. St. Louis, 2008, Saunders.)

History and Frequency of Use

Electrotherapeutic modalities and physical agents have long been used in the management of musculoskeletal disorders, including CLBP, mostly by physical therapists.[1,2] Heat and cold have likely been used to relieve various types of pain symptoms for millennia. One of the earliest references to using electricity for medical purposes came from the scribe, Largus, who in Rome in 46 AD recommended placing live torpedo fish on painful areas to alleviate symptoms.[6] The use of electrotherapeutic modalities grew following World War I, when injured veterans were treated for musculoskeletal injuries with therapeutic exercise, manual therapy, and

electrical stimulation. IFC was developed in the 1930s, allowing for a more comfortable application of electrical stimulation than its precursors.[6] The first TENS device was approved for use in pain management by the United States Food and Drug Administration (FDA) in the 1970s, and portable units were introduced shortly thereafter.[7] Clinical research comparing various types of electrotherapeutic

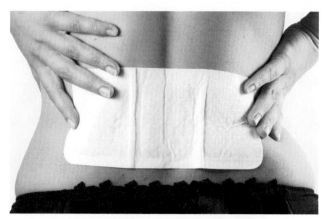

Figure 14-4 Typical disposable adhesive hot pack. (© istockphoto.com/Marlin Allinger)

modalities began to appear in the 1970s. Although modern electrotherapeutic modalities incorporate more sophisticated displays and an increasing number of programmable settings, their internal components are mostly unchanged in recent decades.

Physical modalities, including heat, US, and EMS, are often administered in conjunction with spinal manipulation by chiropractors for the management of low back pain (LBP) where permitted by scope of practice.[8,9]

A prospective study of health care utilization among 1342 patients with LBP who presented to general practitioners in Germany reported that 34% used local heat, 17% used electrotherapy, and 9% used TENS in the subsequent 1 year follow-up.[10] Local heat was the most commonly reported service, electrotherapy was the fourth most common, and TENS was the seventh most common.

Practitioner, Setting, and Availability

Electrotherapeutic modalities and physical agents are typically administered by physical therapists working in various practice settings nationwide, including private practice, rehabilitation centers, specialty spine or sports medicine clinics, and hospitals. Other health professionals involved in the management of CLBP, such as physicians, occupational therapists, chiropractors, and athletic trainers, may also use these types of physical modalities. Additionally, some of these physical modalities can be purchased, borrowed, or rented by patients for use at home following some instruction from the clinician. Portable TENS units, superficial heat, and ice are commonly used in home settings. These interventions are widely available throughout the United States.

Procedure

There are numerous specific treatment protocols for each of the common electrotherapeutic modalities and physical agents, some of which are developed by therapists through anecdotal evidence. For electrotherapeutic modalities such as TENS, EMS, and IFC, the intervention often begins with the provider exposing the patient's skin in the lumbosacral area

and wiping it clean with an alcohol-based solution. Superficial skin electrodes are then placed over areas of pain (TENS, IFC) or on adjacent targeted muscle groups (EMS). To prevent accidental shocks or excessive currents, electrodes are usually placed on the skin while the machines are turned off and then connected to the device. Once the electrodes are in place, the provider will then gradually increase the intensity of the electrical current until a particular goal is achieved. For TENS and IFC, this goal will be a mild to moderate (but not unpleasant) tingling sensation. For EMS, the goal will be the attainment of a mild to moderate muscle contraction that is visible to the provider. The devices are then programmed by the provider to deliver current at constant or varying intensities over a period of 15 to 30 minutes, during which the provider will periodically inquire about the patient's comfort and may increase current intensity to maintain a steady stimulus.

With US, the intervention begins by exposing and cleaning the skin in the lumbosacral area. Conductive gel is then applied to the hand-held US probe and spread over the treatment area. This gel is required to conduct US waves from the probe to the skin since acoustic energy will not travel to the intended target through air. The US device is then activated and a specific intensity of acoustic power (measured in watts/cm^2), frequency (MHz), and cycle (pulsed or continuous) are selected based on target tissue thickness (lower frequency for deeper tissues) and treatment objective (pulsed for nonthermal effects, continuous for thermal effects). The provider then slowly moves the US probe in circular motions over the target area during a specific treatment time, usually 6 to 10 minutes. Unlike TENS, EMS, and IFC, patients may not directly perceive anything at all while the US is being applied using the pulsed setting; a slight warming sensation may be felt by some with the continuous setting. Hot or cold therapy involves the provider applying one or more layers of towels to the targeted area before applying the hot or cold pack. Packs are usually applied either for a specific period of time (e.g., 10-15 minutes) or until a desired effect is achieved (e.g., area feels numb to the touch after applying ice or feels less stiff to move after applying heat).

Regulatory Status

Electrotherapeutic and US equipment is generally regulated by the FDA as class II medical devices. Obtaining this approval mainly requires that the manufacturer submit evidence that the new device is substantially equivalent to a currently approved similar device.

THEORY

Mechanism of Action

Each of these interventions has a general mechanism of action that is summarized in the following paragraphs; it is currently unknown whether these hypotheses also apply specifically to the use of physical modalities for CLBP.

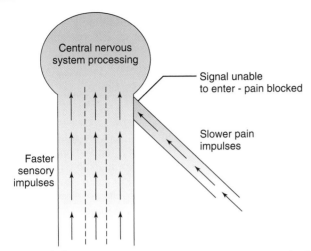

Figure 14-5 Gate control theory of pain. (Modified from Fritz S: Mosby's fundamentals of therapeutic massage, ed. 4. St. Louis, 2009, Mosby.)

Electrotherapeutic Modalities

TENS may use low or high frequencies. At lower frequencies (5-10 Hz), TENS is thought to produce muscle contractions and provide pain reduction for several hours. At higher frequencies (80-100 Hz), TENS is thought to temporarily reduce pain by acting as a counterirritant stimulus.[11] IFC is also thought to temporarily reduce pain by acting as a counterirritant stimulus. EMS provokes muscle contractions in the applied region, which is thought to act as a counterirritant stimulus, reduce muscle spasm, and increase muscle strength and endurance. A counterirritant stimulus is thought to provide pain relief through the gate control theory of pain (Figure 14-5). This theory proposes that input from sensory fibers other than pain (e.g., electrical stimulus) can override input from adjacent nociceptive fibers, thereby inhibiting perception of pain at the spinal cord level. EMS also delivers an electrical current through superficial electrodes placed on the skin, causing one or more adjacent muscles to contract, which is thought to promote blood supply and help strengthen the affected muscle.

Physical Agents

US may be applied in a continuous or pulsed manner. In the continuous setting, US converts nonthermal energy (e.g., acoustic energy) into heat that is thought to increase soft tissue extensibility and act as a counterirritant stimulus, thereby temporarily reducing pain. Pulsed US is thought to promote soft tissue healing by improving blood flow, altering cell membrane activity, and increasing vascular wall permeability in the applied region.[11] US is thought to provide heat that can penetrate soft tissues at a much deeper level (e.g., 5-10 cm) than is possible through superficial heat (e.g., a few millimeters).

Superficial heat is thought to temporarily reduce pain by acting as a counterirritant stimulus, increasing soft tissue extensibility, and reducing muscle tone and spasm; these effects are noted mostly in superficial structures.[11] Superficial heat may also promote muscle and general relaxation through vasodilatation while patients are lying on a treatment table.

Cryotherapy is thought to temporarily reduce pain by acting as a counterirritant stimulus, decreasing nociceptive input and reducing muscle spasm; these effects are noted mostly in superficial structures.[11] It is also thought to promote local vasoconstriction and decrease inflammation.

Indication

Electrotherapeutic modalities and physical agents are generally used for one of the following two main objectives: (1) to reduce pain, swelling, or tissue restriction; and (2) to increase strength, muscle activity, coordination, or rate of healing.[3] These interventions are therefore indicated for nonspecific, mechanical CLBP.

Assessment

Before receiving electrotherapeutic modalities or physical agents, patients should first be assessed for LBP using an evidence-based and goal-oriented approach focused on the patient history and neurologic examination, as discussed in Chapter 3. Additional diagnostic imaging or specific diagnostic testing is generally not required before initiating these interventions for CLBP. The clinician should also inquire about general health to identify potential contraindications to this intervention.

EFFICACY

Evidence supporting the efficacy of these interventions for CLBP was summarized from recent clinical practice guidelines (CPGs), systematic reviews (SRs), and randomized controlled trials (RCTs). Observational studies (OBSs) were also summarized where appropriate. Findings are summarized by study design for each intervention.

Clinical Practice Guidelines

Electrotherapeutic Modalities

Transcutaneous Electrical Nerve Stimulation. Five of the recent national CPGs on the management of CLBP have assessed and summarized the evidence to make specific recommendations about the efficacy of TENS.

The CPG from Belgium in 2006 found low-quality evidence supporting the efficacy of TENS in the management of CLBP.[12]

The CPG from Europe in 2004 found moderate evidence that TENS is not more effective than traction therapy, acupuncture, electroacupuncture, sham TENS, or placebo in the management of CLBP.[13] That CPG did not recommend TENS in the management of CLBP.

The CPG from the United Kingdom in 2009 found weak evidence supporting the efficacy of TENS with respect to improvements in pain.[14] That CPG did not recommend TENS for the management of CLBP.

The CPG from Italy in 2007 did not recommend TENS for the management of CLBP.[15]

The CPG from the United States in 2007 found insufficient evidence to make a recommendation regarding the use of TENS in the management of CLBP.[16]

Interferential Therapy. Three of the recent national CPGs on the management of CLBP have assessed and summarized the evidence to make specific recommendations about the efficacy of IFC.

The CPG from Europe in 2004 found limited evidence that IFC is as effective as traction therapy and massage in the management of CLBP.[13] That CPG also found no evidence that IFC is more effective than sham IFC and did not recommend IFC for CLBP.

The CPG from the United Kingdom in 2009 found insufficient evidence to support the efficacy of IFC for the management of CLBP.[14] That CPG did not recommend IFC for CLBP.

The CPG from the United States in 2007 found insufficient evidence to make a recommendation regarding the use of IFC in the management of CLBP.[16]

Ultrasound. Five of the recent national CPGs on the management of CLBP have assessed and summarized the evidence to make specific recommendations about the efficacy of US.

The CPG from Belgium in 2006 found no evidence to support the efficacy of US in the management of CLBP.[12]

The CPG from Europe in 2004 found limited evidence that US is not effective for the management of CLBP.[13] That CPG also found no evidence that US was more effective than other conservative management options for CLBP. That CPG did not recommend US for CLBP.

The CPG from Italy in 2007 did not recommend US for the management of CLBP.[15]

The CPG from the United Kingdom in 2009 did not recommend US for the management of CLBP.[14]

The CPG from the United States in 2007 found insufficient evidence to make a recommendation regarding the use of US in the management of CLBP.[16]

Electrical Muscle Stimulation

None of the recent national CPGs on the management of CLBP have assessed and summarized the evidence to make specific recommendations about the efficacy of EMS.

Physical Agents

Heat. Three of the recent national CPGs on the management of CLBP have assessed and summarized the evidence to make specific recommendations about the efficacy of heat.

The CPG from Belgium in 2006 found no evidence to support the efficacy of heat in the management of CLBP.[12]

The CPG from Europe in 2004 found no evidence that heat was more effective than other conservative management options for CLPB.[13] That CPG did not recommend the use of heat for CLBP.

The CPG from Italy in 2007 did not recommend heat for the management of CLBP.[15]

Ice. Two of the recent national CPGs on the management of CLBP have assessed and summarized the evidence to make specific recommendations about the efficacy of ice.

TABLE 14-1	Clinical Practice Guideline Recommendation on Electrotherapeutic Modalities and Physical Agents for Chronic Low Back Pain

Reference	Country	Conclusion
TENS		
12	Belgium	Low-quality evidence supporting use
13	Europe	Not recommended
14	United Kingdom	Not recommended
15	Italy	Not recommended
16	United States	Insufficient evidence to make recommendation
Interferential Therapy		
13	Europe	Not recommended
14	United Kingdom	Not recommended
16	United States	Insufficient evidence to make recommendation
Ultrasound		
12	Belgium	No evidence to support efficacy
13	Europe	Not recommended
15	Italy	Not recommended
14	United Kingdom	Not recommended
16	US	Insufficient evidence to make recommendation
Heat		
12	Belgium	No evidence to support efficacy
13	Europe	Not recommended
15	Italy	Not recommended
Ice		
12	Belgium	No evidence to support efficacy
13	Europe	Not recommended

The CPG from Belgium in 2006 found no evidence to support the efficacy of ice in the management of CLBP.[12]

The CPG from Europe in 2004 did not recommend the use of ice for the management of CLBP.[13]

Findings from these CPGs are summarized in Table 14-1.

Systematic Reviews

Electrotherapeutic Modalities

Transcutaneous Electrical Nerve Stimulation

Cochrane Collaboration. An SR was conducted in 2007 by the Cochrane Collaboration on TENS versus placebo for CLBP.[17] A total of four RCTs examining CLBP were identified; two allowed participants with prior back surgery to be included and one allowed patients with LBP with neurologic involvement to be included.[18-21] For pain relief, three RCTs observed statistically significant decreases among those receiving TENS after 2 and 4 weeks of follow-up but only one RCT found clinically meaningful differences.[18,19,21] None of the RCTs observed differences between TENS and placebo on the different types of functional outcomes, except for one RCT that found improved function on the Oswestry Disability Index for TENS but the difference was deemed clinically unimportant.[20,21] Regarding general health status, one RCT observed no statistically significant differences between TENS and placebo, while another RCT found statistically significant benefits for four of eight subsections of the short-form 36 (SF-36) for conventional TENS and the same relationship was observed for two of eight subsections of the SF-36 for acupuncture-like TENS.[19,21] This Cochrane review concluded that there was insufficient evidence supporting the routine use of TENS for CLBP.[17] This SR also concluded that further research on TENS for LBP is warranted and that future RCTs should report baseline information, means and standard deviations for each treatment group, adverse events, and should also monitor use of analgesic medication, and examine long-term follow-up.

American Pain Society and American College of Physicians. An SR was conducted in 2006 by the American Pain Society and American College of Physicians CPG committee on nonpharmacologic therapies for acute and chronic LBP.[22] That review identified one SR related to TENS for CLBP, which was the Cochrane Collaboration review mentioned above.[17] Five SRs that compared other interventions to TENS were also included.[23-28] These SRs included a total of 11 RCTs. No additional RCTs have been identified. In one SR, TENS was not significantly different than acupuncture and conclusions from the other SRs were not reported.[24] One RCT found that TENS was superior to superficial massage for patients with acute and chronic LBP.[29] Other RCTs did not provide sufficient evidence to show a difference between TENS and other interventions (references were not given). This SR concluded that TENS has not been shown to be beneficial for acute, subacute, or chronic LBP.[22]

Interferential Therapy
American Pain Society and American College of Physicians. An SR was conducted in 2006 by the American Pain Society and American College of Physicians CPG committee on nonpharmacologic therapies for acute and chronic LBP.[22] That review did not identify any SRs related to IFC for LBP. However, three RCTs were identified, examining acute LBP, subacute LBP, and subacute and chronic LBP.[30-32] In the RCT examining subacute and chronic LBP, no statistically significant differences were observed between IFC and spinal manipulation or traction.[32] This SR concluded that IFC has not been shown to be beneficial for acute, subacute, or chronic LBP.[22]

Ultrasound
American Pain Society and American College of Physicians. An SR was conducted in 2006 by the American Pain Society and American College of Physicians CPG committee on nonpharmacologic therapies for acute and chronic LBP.[22] That review did not identify any SRs related to US for LBP. However, three RCTs were identified, examining CLBP, LBP of unknown duration, and acute LBP with neurologic involvement.[33-35] One RCT found statistically significant differences between US and sham US, while the other RCT did not find any differences.[33,34] This SR concluded that US has

not been shown to be beneficial for acute, subacute, or chronic LBP.[22]

Electrical Muscle Stimulation
No recent, high-quality SRs were identified that reported specifically on the efficacy of EMS as an intervention for LBP.

Physical Agents
Heat
Cochrane Collaboration. An SR was conducted in 2005 by the Cochrane Collaboration on heat or cold therapy for LBP.[26] A total of nine nonrandomized trials and RCTs were identified. Five examined the effects of heat for acute and subacute LBP, one examined the effects of heat and cold therapy for acute, subacute, and chronic LBP, one examined ice for CLBP, one examined heat for CLBP, and one examined heat and ice for CLBP.[36-39] One nonrandomized trial did not find any differences between heat and ice therapy among acute, subacute, and chronic LBP, while another found that ice massage was statistically significantly better than hot packs for CLBP.[36,39] A third nonrandomized trial compared a wool body belt with a lumbar corset for CLBP but did not report pain results.[38] This Cochrane review concluded that heat wrap reduces pain and disability for acute and subacute LBP and that these effects may be enhanced when combined with exercise.[26] This SR did not make a specific conclusion about CLBP but did conclude that there is conflicting evidence for heat versus cold therapy for LBP.

American Pain Society and American College of Physicians. An SR was conducted in 2006 by the American Pain Society and American College of Physicians CPG committee on nonpharmacologic therapies for acute and chronic LBP.[22] That review identified one SR related to heat therapy for LBP, which was the Cochrane Collaboration review mentioned earlier.[26] No additional RCTs have been identified. This SR concluded that there is good evidence of moderate benefit for heat therapy among acute LBP but did not make a specific conclusion about heat therapy for CLBP.[22]

Ice
Cochrane Collaboration. An SR was conducted in 2005 by the Cochrane Collaboration on heat or cold therapy for LBP.[26] A total of nine nonrandomized trials and RCTs were identified. Five examined the effects of heat for acute and subacute LBP, one examined the effects of heat and cold therapy for acute, subacute, and chronic LBP, one examined ice for CLBP, one examined heat for CLBP, and one examined heat and ice for CLBP.[36-39] One nonrandomized trial did not find any differences between heat and ice therapy among acute, subacute, and chronic LBP, while another found that ice massage was statistically significantly better than hot packs for CLBP.[36,39] A third nonrandomized trial compared ice massage with TENS and did not find any statistical differences in pain relief among patients with CLBP.[37] This Cochrane review concluded that there is insufficient evidence for cold therapy for LBP.[26] This SR also concluded that there is conflicting evidence for heat versus cold therapy for LBP.

Findings from the above SRs are summarized in Table 14-2.

TABLE 14-2	Systematic Review Findings on Electrotherapeutic Modalities and Physical Agents for Chronic Low Back Pain

Reference	# RCTs in SR	# RCTs for CLBP	Conclusion
TENS			
17	4	4 chronic	Insufficient evidence to support routine use of TENS for CLBP
22	6 SRs, 11 RCTs	NR	TENS not beneficial for CLBP
Interferential Therapy			
22	3	1	Not beneficial for CLBP
Ultrasound			
22	3	3	Not beneficial for CLBP
Heat			
26	9	3	Insufficient evidence for CLBP
22	1 SR	—	Insufficient evidence for CLBP
Ice			
26	9	3	Insufficient evidence for CLBP

CLBP, chronic low back pain; NR, not reported; RCT, randomized controlled trial; SR, systematic review; TENS, transcutaneous electrical nerve stimulation.

Randomized Controlled Trials

Electrotherapeutic Modalities

Transcutaneous Electrical Nerve Stimulation. Eight RCTs were identified.[3,18,19,21,40-43] Their methods are summarized in Table 14-3, and their results are briefly described here.

Cheing and Hui-Chan[18] conducted an RCT including patients with CLBP without neurologic involvement. In order to be included, participants had to experience symptoms lasting longer than 6 months. Participants were randomized to either 80-Hz TENS or sham TENS delivered during one 60-minute session. The TENS and sham TENS provider type was not reported. Immediately after treatment, participants in the TENS group experienced statistically significant improvement in pain on one pain score (visual analog scale [VAS] for LBP) compared with baseline but this was not observed for the sham TENS group. Participants in the TENS group had statistically significantly improved pain versus those in the sham TENS group immediately after treatment. No differences were observed immediately after treatment

compared with baseline for either group or between the TENS and sham TENS groups on another pain score (VAS for flexion reflex).

Deyo and colleagues[19] conducted an RCT including patients with CLBP with or without neurologic involvement. In order to be included, participants had to experience symptoms for more than 3 months. Participants were randomized to one of four groups: (1) TENS alone, (2) TENS plus exercise, (3) sham TENS plus exercise, or (4) sham TENS. The TENS group self-administered three daily 45-minute sessions of conventional TENS, 5 days per week over 2 weeks and then self-administered three daily 45-minute sessions of acupuncture-like TENS, 5 days per week over 2 weeks. The sham TENS groups self-administered three daily 45-minute sessions of sham TENS, 5 days per week over 4 weeks. The exercise intervention consisted of three relaxation exercises and nine stretching exercises to be performed at home. After 1 month, only those in the exercise groups experienced statistically significant improvement in pain and function. However, after 2 months, no statistically significant differences were observed between any of the groups regarding pain.

Topuz and colleagues[21] conducted an RCT including patients with CLBP without neurologic involvement. In order to be included, participants had to experience symptoms for more than 3 months. Participants were randomized to one of four groups: (1) conventional TENS, (2) low-frequency TENS, (3) percutaneous neuromodulation therapy (PNT), or (4) placebo TENS. The conventional TENS group received 80 Hz of TENS, the low-frequency TENS group received 4 Hz of TENS, and the PNT group received 4 Hz as well. All groups received treatment administered by a researcher through daily 20-minute sessions 5 days per week over 2 weeks. Immediately after treatment, those in the conventional TENS, low-frequency TENS, and PNT groups experienced statistically significantly improvement in pain and disability compared with baseline values. In addition, statistically significant improvement in pain and disability was observed for conventional TENS, low-frequency TENS, and PNT versus the placebo TENS group immediately after treatment. Individuals in the PNT group experienced statistically significant improvement in pain on one pain outcome compared with the conventional TENS and low-frequency TENS, but this was not the case for another pain outcome or for disability.

Gemignani and colleagues[3] conducted an RCT including patients with ankylosing spondylitis experiencing symptoms for more than 1 month. Neurologic involvement was not reported. Participants were randomized to either TENS (5 Hz) or sham TENS. They received ten 20-minute sessions over 3 weeks. The administrator was not reported. Immediately after treatment, those in the TENS group experienced statistically significant improvement in pain versus baseline scores. The TENS group also experienced statistically significant improvement in pain versus the sham TENS group immediately following the intervention.

Jarzem and colleagues[40] conducted an RCT including patients with CLBP without neurologic involvement. In order to be included, participants had to experience symptoms for

TABLE 14-3	Randomized Controlled Trials of Transcutaneous Electrical Nerve Stimulation for Chronic Low Back Pain				
Reference	Indication	Intervention 1	Intervention 2	Intervention 3	Control
18	CLBP without neurologic involvement, symptoms >6 months	TENS 80 Hz Administrator: NR 1 60-minute session Cointervention: NR n = 15	NA	NA	Sham TENS Administrator: NR 1 60-minute session Cointervention: NR n = 15
19	CLBP with or without neurologic involvement, symptoms >3 months	Conventional TENS 80-100 Hz, acupuncture TENS 2-4 Hz Self-administered 45-minute sessions × 3 sessions/day × 5 days/week × 2 weeks + 45-minute sessions × 3 sessions/day × 5 days/week × 2 weeks acupuncture TENS Cointervention: hot packs, education, analgesic medication n = 36	TENS + exercise 12 sequential exercises: 3 relaxation, 9 stretching Self-administered # exercise sessions NR 45-minute sessions × 3 sessions/day × 5 days/week × 2 weeks conventional + 45-minute sessions × 3 sessions/day × 5 days/week x 2 weeks acupuncture TENS Cointervention: hot packs, education, analgesic medication n = 37	Sham TENS + exercise 12 sequential exercises: 3 relaxation, 9 stretching Self-administered # exercise session NR 45-minute sessions × 3 sessions/day × 5 days/week × 2 weeks conventional + 45-minute sessions × 3 sessions/day × 5 days/week × 2 weeks acupuncture TENS Cointervention: hot packs, education, analgesic medication n = 36	Sham TENS Self-administered 45-minute sessions × 3 sessions/day × 5 days/week × 2 weeks conventional + 45-minute sessions × 3 sessions/day × 5 days/week × 2 weeks acupuncture TENS Cointervention: hot packs, education, analgesic medication n = 36
21	CLBP without neurologic involvement, symptoms >3 months	Conventional TENS 80 Hz Researcher 20-minute sessions × 5 days/week × 2 weeks Cointervention: analgesic medication n = 15	Low-frequency TENS 4 Hz Researcher 20-minute sessions × 5 days/week × 2 weeks Cointervention: analgesic medication n = 15	Percutaneous neuromodulation therapy 4 Hz Researcher 20-minute sessions × 5 days/week × 2 weeks Cointervention: analgesic medication n = 13	Placebo TENS Researcher 20-minute sessions × 5 days/week × 2 weeks Cointervention: analgesic medication n = 12
3	Ankylosing spondylitis, neurologic involvement NR, symptoms >1 month	TENS 5 Hz Administrator: NR 10 20-minute sessions over 3 weeks Cointervention: NR n = 10	NA	NA	Sham TENS Administrator: NR 10 20-minute sessions over 3 weeks Cointervention: NR n = 10
40	CLBP without neurologic involvement, symptoms >3 months	Conventional TENS Self-administered As many sessions as required Cointervention: analgesic medication n = 84	Acupuncture TENS Self-administered As many sessions as required Cointervention: analgesic medication n = 78	Biphasic TENS Self-administered As many sessions as required Cointervention: analgesic medication n = 79	Sham TENS Self-administered As many sessions as required Cointervention: analgesic medication n = 83

Continued

TABLE 14-3	Randomized Controlled Trials of Transcutaneous Electrical Nerve Stimulation for Chronic Low Back Pain—cont'd				
Reference	Indication	Intervention 1	Intervention 2	Intervention 3	Control
41	CLBP with or without neurologic involvement NR, symptoms >6 months	TENS High frequency (100 Hz) and low frequency (Hz NR) Investigator 30-minute session 2×/week × 10 weeks Cointervention: NR n = 14	NA	NA	(1) Placebo TENS Investigator 30-minute session 2×/week × 10 weeks Cointervention: NR n = 14 (2) Control No treatment Cointervention: NR n = 16
42	CLBP without neurologic involvement, symptoms >6 months	TENS Premixed amplitude-modulated frequency of 122 Hz (beat frequency) generated by two medium frequency sinusoidal waves of 4.0 and 4.122 kHz (feed frequency) Administrator NR 15-minute session 1×/week × 5 weeks Cointervention: none n = 8	Acupuncture Acupuncturist 15-minute session 1×/week × 5 weeks Cointervention: none n = 8	TENS + acupuncture Provider type NR 15-minute session 1×/week × 5 weeks Cointervention: none n = 8	Topical poultice Self-administered As needed Cointervention: none n = 8
43	CLBP without neurologic involvement, symptoms >6 months	TENS 4 Hz frequency Physical therapist 40- to 45-minute sessions 4 weeks Cointervention: NR n = 23	Rhythmic stabilization Physical therapist 20-minute sessions 4 weeks Cointervention: NR n = 23	TENS + rhythmic stabilization Physical therapist 40- to 45-minute sessions TENS + 20 minutes rhythmic stabilization 4 weeks Cointervention: NR n = 21	Placebo stimulation Physical therapist 40- to 45-minute sessions 4 weeks Cointervention: NR n = 21

CLBP, chronic low back pain; NA, not applicable; NR, not reported; TENS, transcutaneous electrical nerve stimulation.

more than 3 months. Participants were randomized to one of four groups: (1) conventional TENS, (2) acupuncture-like TENS, (3) biphasic TENS, or (4) sham TENS. The intervention was self-administered at home as many times as the participant wanted. Although all participants improved over time (statistical significance not reported for posttreatment versus baseline scores), no statistically significant differences were observed between the groups after 3 months.

Marchand and colleagues[41] conducted an RCT including patients with CLBP with or without neurologic involvement. In order to be included, participants had to experience symptoms for more than 6 months. Participants were randomized to one of three groups: (1) TENS, (2) placebo TENS, or (3) a control group who did not receive any treatment and were informed that they would receive the intervention in 6 months. The TENS and placebo TENS were administered by an investigator over 30-minute sessions that occurred twice per week for 10 weeks. After 6 months, participants who received TENS and placebo TENS experienced statistically significant improvement in pain compared with baseline scores. In contrast, individuals in the control group did not experience improvement in pain after 6 months. TENS was not statistically significantly different than placebo TENS after 6 months with respect to pain relief.

Itoh and colleagues[42] conducted an RCT including patients with CLBP without neurologic involvement. In order to be included, participants had to experience symptoms for more than 6 months. Participants were randomized to one of four

TABLE 14-4 | **Randomized Controlled Trial of Interferential Current for Chronic Low Back Pain**

Reference	Indication	Intervention 1	Intervention 2	Control
44	CLBP without neurologic involvement, symptoms >3 months	IFC (200 Hz) Physical therapist 10 minutes × 5 × 2 weeks Cointervention: pain medication, bisphosphonates, exercise program (45-minutes × 5 × 2 weeks) n = 45	Horizontal therapy (100 Hz to 4400-12300 Hz) Physical therapist 40 minutes × 5 × 2 weeks Cointervention: pain medication, bisphosphonates, exercise program (45 minutes × 5 × 2 weeks) n = 45	Sham horizontal therapy Physical therapist 40 minutes × 5 × 2 weeks Cointervention: pain medication, bisphosphonates, exercise program (45 minutes × 5 × 2 weeks) n = 30

CLBP, chronic low back pain; IFC, interferential current.

TABLE 14-5 | **Randomized Controlled Trial of Ultrasound for Chronic Low Back Pain**

Reference	Indication	Intervention 1	Intervention 2
45	CLBP without neurologic involvement, symptoms >3 months	US (1 MHz) Physical therapist 10 sessions 3×/week Cointervention: pain medication n = 5	Sham US Physical therapist 10 sessions 3×/week Cointervention: pain medication n = 5

CLBP, chronic low back pain; US, ultrasound.

groups: (1) TENS at painful areas, (2) acupuncture at selected acupoints for LBP, (3) TENS plus acupuncture, and (4) control group who received topical poultice as necessary. An acupuncturist delivered the acupuncture over 5 weekly 15-minute sessions and it was not reported who delivered the 5 weekly 15-minute sessions of TENS. Ten weeks after the first treatment, no statistically significant differences were observed in pain for all groups versus baseline scores. Between group differences were not reported for the pain outcome. Similar results were reported for improvement in disability with no statistically significant differences observed for all groups versus baseline scores. Furthermore, no statistically significant differences were observed between groups regarding disability improvement.

Kofotolis and colleagues[43] conducted an RCT including patients with CLBP without neurologic involvement. The majority of participants experienced symptoms for more than 6 months. They were randomized to one of four groups: (1) low-frequency TENS (40- to 45-minute sessions over 4 weeks), (2) rhythmic stabilization exercise (20-minute sessions over 4 weeks), (3) TENS plus rhythmic stabilization exercise (40- to 45-minute TENS sessions over 4 weeks and 20-minute rhythmic stabilization sessions over 4 weeks), and (4) placebo stimulation (40- to 45-minute sessions over 4 weeks). A physical therapist delivered all treatments. After 2 months of follow-up, patients in the TENS group experienced statistically significant improvement in pain and disability versus the rhythmic stabilization group. The TENS plus rhythmic stabilization group displayed statistically significant improvement in pain versus placebo and TENS-only groups. Furthermore, the TENS plus rhythmic stabilization group displayed statistically significant improvement in dis-

ability versus placebo, TENS-only, and rhythmic stabilization-only groups.

Interferential Current. One RCT was identified.[44] The methods for this RCT are summarized in Table 14-4. The results are briefly described here.

Zambito and colleagues[44] conducted an RCT including patients with CLBP without neurologic involvement. In order to be included, participants had to experience symptoms for at least 3 months. Participants were randomized to one of three groups: (1) IFC for five 10-minute sessions per week over 2 weeks, (2) horizontal therapy for five 40-minute sessions per week over 2 weeks, or (3) sham horizontal therapy for five 40-minute sessions per week over 2 weeks. A physical therapist administered all of the interventions. All groups also participated in an exercise program consisting of 45-minute sessions that occurred 5 times a week for 2 weeks. After 14 weeks, all groups experienced statistically significant improvement in pain according to the Backhill pain score compared with baseline values. Individuals in the horizontal therapy group also experienced statistically significant improvement in pain on the Backhill score versus the sham horizontal therapy group. After 14 weeks of follow-up, participants in the interferential therapy and horizontal therapy groups experienced statistically significant improvement in pain according to the VAS compared with the sham horizontal therapy group.

Ultrasound. One RCT was identified.[33] The methods for this RCT are summarized in Table 14-5. The results are briefly described here.

Ansari and colleagues[33] conducted an RCT including patients with CLBP without neurologic involvement. In order to be included, participants had to experience symptoms for

TABLE 14-6	Randomized Controlled Trial of Electrical Muscle Stimulation for Chronic Low Back Pain		
Reference	Indication	Intervention	Control
45	CLBP without neurologic involvement, symptoms >3 months	EMS + exercise Administrator: NR 30-minute session EMS 30-minute session exercise 3×/week × 8 weeks Cointervention: NR n = 21	Exercise (abdominal, stretching, strengthening, flexibility, extension) Physiatrist 30-minute session exercise 3×/week × 8 weeks Cointervention: NR n = 20

CLBP, chronic low back pain; EMS, electrical muscle stimulation; NR, not reported.

at least 3 months. Participants were randomized to US or sham US for 3 days per week for a total of 10 sessions. A physical therapist administered the US and sham US treatments. Immediately following treatment, both groups experienced statistically significant improvement in function compared with baseline scores. In addition, participants in the US group experienced statistically significant improvement in function compared with those in the sham US group after the intervention. Pain outcomes were not reported in this RCT.

Electrical Muscle Stimulation. One RCT was identified.[45] The methods for this RCT are summarized in Table 14-6. The results are briefly described here.

Durmus and colleagues[45] conducted an RCT including patients with CLBP without neurologic involvement. The majority of participants experienced LBP symptoms for more than 3 months. They were randomized to three 30-minute sessions per week over 8 weeks of EMS plus exercise or exercise alone. A physiatrist administered the exercise therapy but the EMS administrator was not reported. After 2 months both groups experienced statistically significant improvement in pain and disability compared with baseline scores. Furthermore, those in the EMS plus exercise group experienced statistically significant improvement in pain and disability versus the exercise alone group.

Physical Agents
Heat/Ice. No RCTs were identified.

Other
Meta-Analysis. A subset of six RCTs was combined to conduct a meta-analysis comparing the results of high-frequency and low-frequency TENS for CLBP.[3,18,19,21,40,41] Data were analyzed using Review Manager software.[46] Continuous data were analyzed using the weighted mean differences between the intervention and control groups at the end of the study. Dichotomous data were analyzed using relative risks. Meta-analyses were performed when contradictions were found in study results, where possible (similar population, outcome, intervention, and study design). Heterogeneity between studies was tested using the chi-square statistic. Data heterogeneity among the results of different included studies was tested to make sure that only homogeneous data were pooled together. When heterogeneity was not

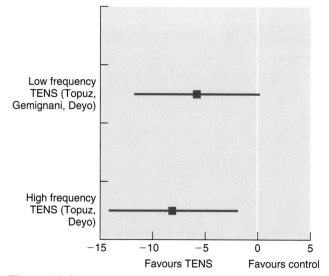

Figure 14-6 High-frequency vs. low-frequency TENS for chronic low back pain: pain intensity outcomes.

significant, fixed-effect models were used. Random effects models were used when heterogeneity was significant. Figures were created using Cochrane Collaboration methodology. The horizontal line represents the standard deviation of the weighted mean difference for a specific outcome of interest (Figures 14-6 and 14-7). If the standard deviation line touches the central vertical line of the graph, the confidence interval is 0 and the difference between the two groups is not statistically significant. Level of significance was set at $P < .05$ for all analyses.

To determine clinical improvement, the absolute benefit and relative difference in the change from baseline were calculated. Absolute benefit was calculated as the improvement in the treatment group less the improvement in the control group, maintaining the original units of measurement. Relative difference was calculated as the absolute benefit divided by the baseline mean (weighted for the intervention and control groups). For dichotomous data, the relative percentage of improvement was calculated as the difference in the percentage of improvement between the intervention and control groups. For meta-analyses, the pooled relative difference was calculated by weighting the relative difference of

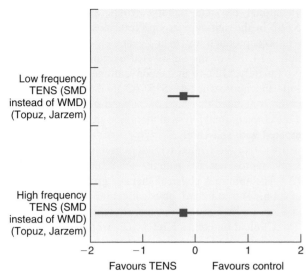

Figure 14-7 High-frequency vs. low-frequency TENS for chronic low back pain: disability outcomes.

each study with its sample size. Outcomes of interest were pain, perceived disability, ability to work, patient satisfaction with treatment, health status, and medication use. Scales demonstrated to be valid and responsive to change were required to support a recommendation.

High-Frequency TENS

A clinically important and statistically significant reduction in pain intensity was obtained in the pooled result of the trials that assessed pain after the TENS protocol (see Figure 14-6).[21] However, there were no clinically or statistically significant differences in the pooled result of perceived disability (see Figure 14-7).[21,40] As for health status, a study found the following results: clinically important and statistically significant improvements in physical role limitations, emotional role limitations, and bodily pain; clinically important improvements without statistical significance in physical function, social function, and general health; no clinical or statistical differences in general mental health and vitality.[21]

Low-Frequency TENS

There was a clinically important improvement without statistical significance in the pooled result of pain intensity.[3,19,21] There were no clinically or statistically significant differences in the pooled result of perceived disability (see Figure 14-7).[21,40] As for health status, a study found the following results: clinically important and statistically significant improvements in emotional role limitations and general mental health; clinically important improvement without statistical significance in physical function, social function, physical role limitations, vitality, bodily pain, and general health.[21] Although not significant, the study that assessed medication found a clinically important reduction in acetaminophen use during the TENS protocol.[3]

SAFETY

Contraindications

Electrotherapeutic physical modalities such as TENS, EMS, and IFC are contraindicated for use over the anterior cervical region, carotid sinuses, heart, transthoracic area, regions with hypoesthesia, and the abdomen of a pregnant woman.[11] Such modalities are also contraindicated in patients with a cardiac pacemaker, implanted defibrillator, or any other implanted electrical device, and venous or arterial thrombosis or thrombophlebitis.[11] Electrotherapeutic modalities should not be used concurrently with diathermy devices.

US is contraindicated for use on lesions due to malignancy, hemorrhage, infection, or ischemia. It should also be avoided over the abdomen of pregnant women, plastic implants, cemented areas of prosthetic joints, regions with hypoesthesia, electronic implants (including neurostimulators), areas that have been exposed to radiotherapy in the past 6 months, fractures, epiphyseal growth plates in skeletally immature patients, thrombotic areas, orbits of the eyes, gonads, and spinal cord after laminectomy.[11]

Superficial heat is contraindicated over regions of acute injury, acute inflammation, hemorrhage, malignancy, impaired sensation, thrombophlebitis, or the abdomen of pregnant women.[11] Applying cold is contraindicated in patients with urticaria, cold intolerance or hypersensitivity, Raynaud's disease or phenomenon, cryoglobulinemia, paroxysmal cold hemoglobinuria, deep open wounds, regenerating peripheral nerves, areas of circulatory compromise or peripheral vascular disease, and areas of impaired somatosensory discrimination.[11]

Adverse Events

CPGs on the management of LBP have reported that the safety of IFC, TENS, superficial heat or ice, and US is currently unknown.[13] Nevertheless, physical modalities are generally regarded as safe interventions. Skin irritation is rare but can occur with the use of electrotherapeutic modalities and physical agents. Even more rarely, skin burns are associated with the inappropriate use of these interventions, such as prolonged continuous use and incorrect placement or settings. Among the RCTs reviewed, minor skin irritations were reported by a minority of subjects in one study.[19]

COSTS

Fees and Third-Party Reimbursement

In the United States, physical modalities that are delivered or supervised by a licensed health practitioner such as a physical therapist can be delivered using CPT codes 97010 (hot or cold packs), 97014 (electrical stimulation), or 97035 (ultrasound). It is often assumed by third-party payers that these modalities are provided in the context of an outpatient visit to a physical therapist, for which a global fee is paid regardless of the number of specific interventions delivered

TABLE 14-7	Medicare Reimbursement for Related Fees	
CPT Code	New York	California
97010	*	*
97014	*	*
97035	$12	$13

*Assumed to be included at no charge in other services provided the same day.

during that visit. Modalities such as heat/ice or TENS may therefore be considered bundled services for which a separate fee cannot be charged.

If delivered in the context of a visit to a physical therapist, these procedures are widely covered by other third-party payers such as health insurers and worker's compensation insurance, with fees that are generally higher than Medicare. Third-party payers will often reimburse a limited number of visits to licensed health providers if they are prescribed by a physician and supported by adequate documentation deeming them medically necessary. Equipment or products required for those interventions are rarely covered by insurers.

Typical fees reimbursed by Medicare in New York and California for these services are summarized in Table 14-7.

Cost Effectiveness

Evidence supporting the cost effectiveness of treatment protocols that compared these interventions, often in combination with one or more cointerventions, with control groups who received one or more other interventions, for either acute or chronic LBP, was identified from two SRs on this topic and is summarized here.[47,48] Although many of these study designs are unable to clearly identify the individual contribution of any intervention, their results provide some insight as to the clinical and economic outcomes associated with these approaches.

An RCT in Norway compared three approaches for patients sick-listed with CLBP.[49] The supervised exercise therapy group received instruction on stabilization and strengthening exercise from a physical therapist. The conventional physical therapy group received one or more interventions including heat, ice, massage, stretching exercises, EMS, or traction. The self-care group received instruction to walk. Participants in all groups received three 1-hour sessions each week for 12 weeks (total 36 sessions). Clinical outcomes after 1 year reported that the supervised exercise therapy and conventional physical therapy groups had greater improvements in pain and function than the self-care group. Direct medical costs associated with the study interventions after 1 year were approximately $375 in the supervised exercise therapy group, approximately $584 in the conventional physical therapy group, and approximately $0 in the self-care group. Indirect productivity costs associated with lost work days after 1 year were approximately $13,816 in the supervised exercise therapy group, approximately $12,062 in the

conventional physical therapy group, and approximately $15,762 in the self-care group. Total costs (direct medical and indirect productivity) over 1 year were therefore approximately $14,191 in the supervised exercise therapy group, approximately $12,646 in the conventional physical therapy group, and approximately $15,762 in the self-care group. Authors concluded that both the supervised exercise therapy and the conventional physical therapy were cost saving when compared with self-care.

An RCT in the United Kingdom compared two physical therapy approaches for patients with subacute or chronic LBP.[50] The minimal physical therapy group received brief education. The standard physical therapy group included education, mobilization, massage, stretching, exercise, heat, or ice. Clinical outcomes after 1 year were similar between the two groups. Direct medical costs for study and nonstudy interventions over 1 year were approximately $376 in the minimal physical therapy group and approximately $486 in the standard physical therapy group. Indirect productivity costs were approximately $1305 in the minimal physical therapy group and approximately $856 in the standard physical therapy group, but these were excluded from the analysis. Because the standard physical therapy group had marginally better clinical outcomes with higher direct medical costs, its incremental cost effectiveness ratio was estimated at approximately $5538 per quality-adjusted life-year, well within the generally accepted threshold for cost utility analyses.

An RCT in Germany compared two approaches for patients with CLBP pain admitted to a 3-week inpatient rehabilitation center.[51] The usual care group included group exercise, EMS, massage, and education. The usual care with cognitive behavioral therapy (CBT) group also included both individual and group CBT sessions. Clinical outcomes after 1 year were mostly similar for improvements in pain and function, though greater improvement was noted in utility gains for the usual care with CBT group. Direct medical costs associated with study and nonstudy interventions over 6 months were approximately $2702 in the usual care group and approximately $2809 in the usual care with CBT group. Indirect productivity costs associated with lost work days over 6 months were approximately $6626 in the usual care group and approximately $5061 in the usual care with CBT group. Total costs (direct medical and indirect productivity) over 6 months were therefore approximately $9328 in the usual care group and approximately $7870 in the usual care with CBT group. Because the usual care with CBT group had better clinical outcomes with lower overall costs, authors concluded that it was cost saving and dominated usual care alone.

The CPG from Europe in 2004 reported that the cost effectiveness of TENS, IFC, US, and heat for treating CLBP (>3 months) is unknown.[13]

Other

An SR reported on a study that determined that an intervention of conventional physical therapy approach, which included electrotherapeutic modalities, was cost effective in patients aged 20 to 65 years with CLBP sick-listed for more than 8 weeks but less than 52 weeks.[52]

TABLE 14-8	Cost Effectiveness and Cost Utility Analyses of Electrotherapeutic Modalities and Physical Agents for Acute or Chronic Low Back Pain				
Reference Country Follow-Up	Group	Direct Medical Costs	Indirect Productivity Costs	Total Costs	Conclusion
49 Norway 1 year	1. Supervised exercise therapy 2. Conventional PT (including heat, ice, EMS) 3. Self-care	1. $375 2. $584 3. $0	1. $13,816 2. $12,062 3. $15,762	1. $14,191 2. $12,646 3. $15,762	Groups 1 and 2 were cost saving compared to group 3
50 United Kingdom 1 year	1. Minimal PT 2. Standard PT (including heat, ice)	1. $376 2. $486	1. $1305 2. $856 (excluded from analysis)	NR	ICER of 2 over 1: $5538/QALY
51 Germany 6 months	1. Usual care (including EMS) 2. Usual care + CBT	1. $2702 2. $2809	1. $6626 2. $5061	1. $9328 2. $7870	Group 2 cost saving and dominated group 1

CBT, cognitive behavioral therapy; EMS, electrical muscle stimulation; ICER, incremental cost effectiveness ratio; NR, not reported; PT, physical therapy; QALY, quality-adjusted life-year

Findings from the aforementioned cost effectiveness analyses are summarized in Table 14-8.

SUMMARY

Description

Physical modalities are a variety of instruments, machines, and tools traditionally used in physical therapy for musculoskeletal conditions, including CLBP. Two important categories of modalities are electrotherapeutic modalities and physical agents. Electrotherapeutic modalities involve the use of electricity and include therapies such as TENS, EMS, and IFC. Physical agents are modalities that involve thermal, acoustic (produced by sound waves), or radiant energy, and include interventions such as therapeutic US, superficial heat (hot packs), and cryotherapy (cold packs or ice). Electrotherapeutic modalities and physical agents are widely available in the United States and are typically administered by physical therapists working in various practice settings nationwide, including private practice, rehabilitation centers, specialty spine or sports medicine clinics, or hospitals. Physicians, occupational therapists, chiropractors, and athletic trainers may also use physical modalities.

Theory

Each electrotherapeutic modality and physical agent has a general mechanism of action. At lower frequencies (5-10 Hz), TENS is thought to produce muscle contractions and provide pain reduction for several hours. At higher frequencies (80-100 Hz), TENS is thought to temporarily reduce pain by acting as a counterirritant stimulus. IFC is also thought to temporarily reduce pain by acting as a counterirritant

stimulus. EMS provokes muscle contractions in the applied region, which is thought to act as a counterirritant stimulus, reduce muscle spasm, and increase muscle strength and endurance. US is thought to provide heat that can penetrate soft tissues at a much deeper level than is possible through superficial heat. Superficial heat is thought to temporarily reduce pain by increasing soft tissue extensibility and by reducing muscle tone and spasm, which may also promote muscle and general relaxation through vasodilatation while lying on a treatment table. Cryotherapy is thought to temporarily decrease nociceptive input and reduce muscle spasm; it may also promote local vasoconstriction and decrease inflammation. All of these interventions are indicated for nonspecific CLBP. Diagnostic imaging or other forms of advanced testing are generally not required before administering these interventions.

Efficacy

Three CPGs do not recommend TENS for CLBP, one found low-quality evidence supporting the efficacy of TENS, and another found insufficient evidence to make a recommendation. A review conducted by the Cochrane Collaboration concluded that there was insufficient evidence supporting the routine use of TENS for CLBP and another SR concluded that TENS has not been shown to be beneficial for CLBP. At least eight RCTs assessed the efficacy of TENS, half of which did not find any statistically significant differences in pain or disability improvement versus other comparators. However, one RCT found that TENS had a statistically significant improvement in pain and two other RCTs found that TENS was superior to comparators on one pain score but not another. Another RCT found that TENS was superior to rhythmic stabilization regarding pain and disability, yet TENS plus rhythmic stabilization was superior to placebo and TENS only for pain improvement while TENS plus rhythmic stabilization was superior to placebo, TENS-only, and rhythmic stabilization-only for improvement in disability.

Two CPGs do not recommend IFC, while one found insufficient evidence to make a recommendation. An SR concluded that IFC has not been shown to be beneficial for CLBP. One RCT found that IFC was superior to placebo on the VAS but not on another pain score.

Three CPGs do not recommend US for CLBP. One found no evidence supporting the efficacy of US, and another found insufficient evidence to make a recommendation. An SR concluded that US has not been shown to be beneficial for CLBP. One small RCT reported that US was statistically superior to sham US regarding improvement in function.

No CPGs or SRs addressed the use of EMS for CLBP. However, one RCT found that EMS plus exercise was superior to exercise alone regarding pain and disability improvement.

Two CPGs do not recommend heat for CLBP and another found no evidence supporting the efficacy of heat therapy. A review conducted by the Cochrane Collaboration and another SR concluded that heat therapy is beneficial for acute and subacute LBP but do not make a specific conclusion for CLBP. One CPG does not recommend ice for CLBP and another found no evidence supporting the efficacy of ice therapy. A review conducted by the Cochrane Collaboration found insufficient evidence supporting cold therapy for LBP.

Safety

Electrotherapeutic physical modalities such as TENS, EMS, and IFC are contraindicated in pregnant women and patients with a cardiac pacemaker, implanted defibrillator, or any other implanted electrical device, or with venous or arterial thrombosis or thrombophlebitis. US is contraindicated in pregnant women and should be avoided over plastic implants, cemented areas of prosthetic joints, regions with hypoesthesia, electronic implants (including neurostimulators), areas that have been exposed to radiotherapy in the past 6 months, fractures, epiphyseal growth plates in skeletally immature patients, thrombotic areas, orbits of the eyes, gonads, and spinal cord after laminectomy. Superficial heat is contraindicated over regions of acute injury, acute inflammation, hemorrhage, malignancy, impaired sensation, thrombophlebitis, and the abdomen of pregnant women. Applying cold is contraindicated in patients with urticaria, cold intolerance or hypersensitivity, Raynaud's disease or phenomenon, cryoglobulinemia, paroxysmal cold hemoglobinuria, deep open wounds, regenerating peripheral nerves, areas of circulatory compromise or peripheral vascular disease, and areas of impaired somatosensory discrimination. Physical modalities are generally regarded as safe, yet skin irritation and skin burns are potential adverse events.

Costs

These modalities are often provided in the context of an outpatient visit to a physical therapist, for which a global fee is paid regardless of the number of specific interventions delivered during that visit. Modalities such as heat/ice or TENS may therefore be considered bundled services for which a separate fee cannot be charged. The cost of these interventions has been assessed in at least three studies, yet all were components of a multifaceted treatment program so the individual contribution of each modality or physical agent could not be determined.

Comments

Evidence from the CPGs, SRs, and RCTs reviewed was generally unable to support the use of electrotherapeutic modalities and physical agents for CLBP. However, some of these interventions, particularly high-frequency TENS, may be useful for temporary pain relief among a subgroup of patients with CLBP who are currently difficult to define using standardized criteria. These results should be interpreted with caution because the majority of the RCTs included were of relatively poor methodologic quality. TENS does not appear to have an impact on perceived disability or long-term pain. Contradictory postintervention results (two studies reported mostly positive outcomes and two mainly negative ones) could be explained by differences in the outcome assessment periods (e.g., short-term vs. immediate-term vs. long-term).[3,19,21,40]

Other questions that remain on the implications of TENS use in the clinical management of CLBP include the following: (1) Does the addition of TENS improve patient satisfaction with overall treatment? (2) Is TENS effective in reducing pain when taking analgesics? (3) What are the consequences of long-term TENS use? (4) Is TENS effective in reducing pain with long-term users? (5) Does TENS use increase fear-avoidance behaviors in patients by focusing treatment on pain? (6) What is the cost effectiveness of TENS when compared with traditional over-the-counter pain medication? It is also not known whether adding TENS to an evidence-based intervention, such as therapeutic exercise, can further improve outcomes. However, one of the studies did assess the interactions between exercise and TENS and found no synergistic impact, but did not provide any specific data on this.[19] These questions should be the focus of future research on TENS for CLBP.

CHAPTER REVIEW QUESTIONS

Answers are located on page 451.
1. Which of the following are the two important categories of modalities used in CLBP?
   a. electrotherapeutic and physical agents
   b. heat and ice
   c. TENS and traction
   d. ultrasound and massage
2. Which of the following is not a type of electrotherapeutic modality?
   a. TENS
   b. EMS
   c. IFC
   d. MRI

3. Which of the following forms of energy are not involved in physical agents?
   a. thermal energy
   b. magnetic energy
   c. acoustic energy
   d. radiant energy

4. Which of the following is the proposed mechanism of action with low frequency TENS?
   a. muscle spasm and pain reduction for several weeks
   b. muscle contraction and hyperalgesia for several hours
   c. muscle contraction and pain reduction for several hours
   d. muscle relaxation and pain reduction for several days

5. Which of the following theories have been proposed for the pain reduction attributed to high frequency TENS?
   a. opioid receptor activation
   b. anterior horn stimulation
   c. counterirritant stimulus
   d. nociceptive excitability

6. True or false: Advanced imaging is recommended prior to TENS.

7. True or false: Superficial heat can penetrate soft tissues at a deeper level than US.

REFERENCES

1. Poitras S, Blais R, Swaine B, et al. Management of work-related low back pain: a population-based survey of physical therapists. Phys Ther 2005;85:1168-1181.
2. Mikhail C, Korner-Bitensky N, Rossignol M, et al. Physical therapists' use of interventions with high evidence of effectiveness in the management of a hypothetical typical patient with acute low back pain. Phys Ther 2005;85:1151-1167.
3. Gemignani G, Olivieri I, Ruju G, et al. Transcutaneous electrical nerve stimulation in ankylosing spondylitis: a double-blind study. Arthritis Rheum 1991;34:788-789.
4. Leighton TG. What is ultrasound? Prog Biophys Mol Biol 2007;93:3-83.
5. ter Haar, G. Therapeutic applications of ultrasound. Prog Biophys Mol Biol 2007;93:111-129.
6. Sabatowski R, Schafer D, Kasper SM, et al. Pain treatment: a historical overview. Curr Pharm Des 2004;10:701-716.
7. Stamp JM. A review of transcutaneous electrical nerve stimulation (TENS). J Med Engineer Technol 1982;6:99-103.
8. Hurwitz EL, Morgenstern H, Harber P, et al. Second prize—the effectiveness of physical modalities among patients with low back pain randomized to chiropractic care: findings from the UCLA low back pain study. J Manipulative Physiol Ther 2002;25:10-20.
9. Hurwitz EL, Morgenstern H, Yu F. Satisfaction as a predictor of clinical outcomes among chiropractic and medical patients enrolled in the UCLA low back pain study. Spine 2005;30:2121-2128.
10. Chenot JF, Becker A, Leonhardt C, et al. Use of complementary alternative medicine for low back pain consulting in general practice: a cohort study. BMC Complement Altern Med 2007;7:42.
11. Allen RJ. Physical agents used in the management of chronic pain by physical therapists. Phys Med Rehabil Clin North Am 2006;17:315-345.
12. Nielens H, van Zundert J, Mairiaux P, et al. Chronic low back pain. Good Clinical practice (GCP). Brussels: Belgian Health Care Knowledge Centre (KCE); 2006. KCE reports vol 48C.
13. Airaksinen O, Brox JI, Cedraschi C, et al. European guidelines for the management of chronic nonspecific low back pain. Eur Spine J 2006;15:S192-S300.
14. National Institute for Health and Clinical Excellence (NICE). Low back pain: early management of persistent non-specific low back pain. London: National Institute of Health and Clinical Excellence; 2009. Report No.: NICE clinical guideline 88.
15. Negrini S, Giovannoni S, Minozzi S, et al. Diagnostic therapeutic flow-charts for low back pain patients: the Italian clinical guidelines. Eura Medicophys 2006;42:151-170.
16. Chou R, Qaseem A, Snow V, et al. Diagnosis and treatment of low back pain: a joint clinical practice guideline from the American College of Physicians and the American Pain Society. Ann Intern Med 2007;147:478-491.
17. Khadilkar A, Odebiyi DO, Brosseau L, et al. Transcutaneous electrical nerve stimulation (TENS) versus placebo for chronic low-back pain. Cochrane Database Syst Rev 2008;(4):CD003008.
18. Cheing GL, Hui-Chan CW. Transcutaneous electrical nerve stimulation: nonparallel antinociceptive effects on chronic clinical pain and acute experimental pain. Arch Phys Med Rehabil 1999;80:305-312.
19. Deyo RA, Walsh NE, Martin DC, et al. A controlled trial of transcutaneous electrical nerve stimulation (TENS) and exercise for chronic low back pain. N Engl J Med 1990;322:1627-1634.
20. Jarzem P. Transcutaneous Electrical Nerve Stimulation [TENS] for Short-Term Treatment of Low Back Pain-Randomized Double Blind Crossover Study of Sham versus Conventional TENS. Journal of Musculoskeletal Pain 2005;13:11-17.
21. Topuz O, Ozfidan E, Ozgen M, et al. Efficacy of transcutaneous electrical nerve stimulation and percutaneous neuromodulation therapy in chronic low back pain. J Back Musculoskel Rehabil 2004;17:127-133.
22. Chou R, Huffman LH. Nonpharmacologic therapies for acute and chronic low back pain: a review of the evidence for an American Pain Society/American College of Physicians clinical practice guideline. Ann Intern Med 2007;147:492-504.
23. Assendelft WJ, Morton SC, Yu EI, et al. Spinal manipulative therapy for low back pain. Cochrane Database Syst Rev 2004;(1):CD000447.
24. Manheimer E, White A, Berman B, et al. Meta-analysis: acupuncture for low back pain. Ann Intern Med 2005;142:651-663.
25. Furlan AD, Brosseau L, Imamura M, et al. Massage for low back pain. Cochrane Database of Systematic Reviews 2002;(2).
26. French S, Cameron M, Walker B, et al. Superficial heat or cold for low back pain. The Cochrane Database of Systematic Reviews 2006;(1).
27. Clarke JA, van Tulder MW, Blomberg SE, et al. Traction for low-back pain with or without sciatica. Cochrane Database of Systematic Reviews 2007;(2).
28. Assendelft WJ, Morton SC, Yu EI, et al. Spinal manipulative therapy for low back pain. A meta-analysis of effectiveness relative to other therapies. Ann Intern Med 2003;138:871-881.
29. Melzack R, Vetere P, Finch L. Transcutaneous electrical nerve stimulation for low back pain. A comparison of TENS and massage for pain and range of motion. Phys Ther 1983;63:489-493.
30. Hurley DA, McDonough SM, Dempster M, et al. A randomized clinical trial of manipulative therapy and interferential therapy for acute low back pain. Spine 2004;29:2207-2216.

31. Hurley DA, Minder PM, McDonough SM, et al. Interferential therapy electrode placement technique in acute low back pain: a preliminary investigation. Arch Phys Med Rehabil 2001; 82:485-493.

32. Werners R, Pynsent PB, Bulstrode CJ. Randomized trial comparing interferential therapy with motorized lumbar traction and massage in the management of low back pain in a primary care setting. Spine 1999;24:1579-1584.

33. Ansari NN, Ebadi S, Talebian S, et al. A randomized, single blind placebo controlled clinical trial on the effect of continuous ultrasound on low back pain. Electromyogr Clin Neurophysiol 2006;46:329-336.

34. Roman MP. A clinical evaluation of ultrasound by use of a placebo technic. Phys Ther Rev 1960;40:649-652.

35. Nwuga VC. Ultrasound in treatment of back pain resulting from prolapsed intervertebral disc. Arch Phys Med Rehabil 1983;64:88-89.

36. Landen BR. Heat or cold for the relief of low back pain? Phys Ther 1967;47:1126-1128.

37. Melzack R, Jeans ME, Stratford JG, et al. Ice massage and transcutaneous electrical stimulation: comparison of treatment for low-back pain. Pain 1980;9:209-217.

38. St.John Dixon A, Owen-Smith BD, Harrison RA. Cold-sensitive, non-specific, low back pain: a comparative trial of treatment. Clin Trial J 1972;4:16-21.

39. Roberts D, Walls C, Carlile J, et al. Relief of chronic low back pain: heat versus cold. In: Evaluation and treatment of chronic pain. 2nd ed. Baltimore: Urban & Schwarzenberg; 1992. p. 263-266.

40. Jarzem PF, Harvey EJ, Arcaro N, et al. Transcutaneous electrical nerve stimulation (TENS) for chronic low back pain. J Musculoskel Pain 2005;13:3.

41. Marchand S, Charest J, Li J, et al. Is TENS purely a placebo effect? A controlled study on chronic low back pain. Pain 1993;54:99-106.

42. Itoh K, Itoh S, Katsumi Y, et al. A pilot study on using acupuncture and transcutaneous electrical nerve stimulation to treat chronic non-specific low back pain. Complement Ther Clin Pract 2009;15:22-25.

43. Kofotolis ND, Vlachopoulos SP, Kellis E. Sequentially allocated clinical trial of rhythmic stabilization exercises and TENS in women with chronic low back pain. Clin Rehabil 2008; 22:99-111.

44. Zambito A, Bianchini D, Gatti D, et al. Interferential and horizontal therapies in chronic low back pain: a randomized, double blind, clinical study. Clin Exp Rheumatol 2006;24:534-539.

45. Durmus D, Akyol Y, Alayli G, et al. Effects of electrical stimulation program on trunk muscle strength, functional capacity, quality of life, and depression in the patients with low back pain: a randomized controlled trial. Rheumatol Int 2009;29: 947-954.

46. Review Manager (RevMan) [computer program]. Nordic Cochrane Centre, 2006.

47. Dagenais S, Roffey DM, Wai EK, et al. Can cost utility evaluations inform decision making about interventions for low back pain? Spine J 2009;9:944-957.

48. van der Roer N, Goossens MEJB, Evers SMAA, et al. What is the most cost-effective treatment for patients with low back pain? A systematic review. Best Pract Res Clin Rheumatol 2005;19:671-684.

49. Torstensen TA, Ljunggren AE, Meen HD, et al. Efficiency and costs of medical exercise therapy, conventional physiotherapy, and self-exercise in patients with chronic low back pain. A pragmatic, randomized, single-blinded, controlled trial with 1-year follow-up. Spine 1998;23:2616-2624.

50. Rivero-Arias O, Gray A, Frost H, et al. Cost-utility analysis of physiotherapy treatment compared with physiotherapy advice in low back pain. Spine 2006;31:1381-1387.

51. Schweikert B, Jacobi E, Seitz R, et al. Effectiveness and cost-effectiveness of adding a cognitive behavioral treatment to the rehabilitation of chronic low back pain. J Rheumatol 2006;33:2519-2526.

52. van der RN, Goossens ME, Evers SM, et al. What is the most cost-effective treatment for patients with low back pain? A systematic review. Best Pract Res Clin Rheumatol 2005;19: 671-684.

RALPH E. GAY
JEFFREY S. BRAULT

CHAPTER 15

Traction Therapy

DESCRIPTION

Terminology and Subtypes

Numerous therapies that mechanically unload the spine have been used to treat chronic low back pain (CLBP) for many years. These interventions are variably known as spinal traction, mechanical traction, spinal distraction, and nonsurgical decompression. The latter term is used to distinguish these approaches from laminectomy or discectomy, which are forms of surgical decompression. *Traction therapy* is a broad term used to refer to any method of separating the lumbar vertebrae along the inferosuperior axis of the spine by using mechanical force.

The most common types of traction therapy are based on the duration of its application, which may be intermittent (alternating traction and relaxation with cycles of up to a few minutes), sustained (20 to 60 minutes) or continuous (hours to days).[1-5] Traction therapy can also be described according to the direction of its primary force, whether axial or distraction. Axial traction attempts to limit the force applied to the superoinferior (e.g., caudadcephalad) axis of the spine, while distraction allows the provider or patient to orient the direction and amount of force along the three cardinal axes by varying the position of the body. Axial traction using at least 30% to 50% of body weight is considered high-dose axial traction (Table 15-1).

Distraction is further subdivided into distraction manipulation and positional distraction. Perhaps the best known type of distraction manipulation is flexion-distraction, which is sometimes referred to as *Cox technique* after one of its main promoters, chiropractor James Cox. In distraction manipulation, the provider attempts to apply distraction force along specific planes (e.g., flexion, extension, lateral flexion, or rotation) to position the targeted spinal segments to receive spinal mobilization or manipulation based on patient symptoms and manual examination findings.[6] Other forms of distraction manipulation traction include the Leander technique and the Saunders ActiveTrac method. The most common example of positional distraction is autotraction, a technique in which the patient controls the direction and force of traction based on the amount of relief experienced.

History and Frequency of Use

Various forms of traction therapy have been used to treat spinal disorders for almost 4000 years, since at least 1800 BC.[7] Hippocrates (fourth to fifth century BC), was likely the first practitioner to create an apparatus to apply spinal traction.[8] By the nineteenth century, the traction bed was used to treat LBP, scoliosis, rickets, and other spinal deformities; other forms of traction therapy using corsets, chairs, and suspension were also promoted at that time by various practitioners.[9] Traction became a common treatment for CLBP in the early twentieth century, when firmer opinions and theories were formulated regarding how it should be applied, including the ideal amount of force, degree of pull, duration of pull, and timing of force intervals.[1] The British physician Cyriax promoted traction therapy for not only CLBP but also for lumbar disc lesions, theorizing that it could produce negative pressure in the disc, thereby reducing disc herniations.[2] Other practitioners suggested that off-axis movements, such as flexion or extension, also be added to axial traction to preferentially reduce back or leg pain, and created the techniques of autotraction and flexion-distraction, as mentioned above.[3,4]

A prospective study of health care utilization among 1342 patients with low back pain (LBP) who presented to general practitioners in Germany reported that 10% used traction in the subsequent 1 year follow-up.[10] Traction was the sixth most commonly reported modality after local heat (34%), massage (31%), spinal manipulation therapy (SMT) (26%), electrotherapy (17%), and acupuncture (13%). The use of traction was statistically significantly higher among those with CLBP, with an odds ratio of 2.0 (95% CI 1.1 to 3.6).

Practitioner, Setting, and Availability

Traction therapy can be applied by chiropractors, physical therapists, or medical physicians trained in the use of specific traction devices for CLBP. Once the treatment parameters are established by the health provider, a clinical assistant may apply some of these interventions under supervision. Traction therapies are widely available in the United States, although specific devices may be limited to proprietary spine centers.

TABLE 15-1	Categories of Traction Therapies Based on Temporal (Sustained vs Intermittent) and Force (Focused vs Dispersed) Variables	
	Sustained	Intermittent
Focused	Positional distraction Autotraction Positional distraction	Distraction-manipulation Flexion-distraction (Cox) Leander technique
Dispersed	Sustained traction Split-table traction Gravity traction LTX 3000	Intermittent traction VAX-D DRX-9000 Split-table traction

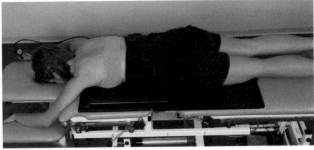

Figure 15-2 Prone lumbar spine traction therapy. (From Olson KA. Manual physical therapy of the spine. St. Louis, 2008, Saunders.)

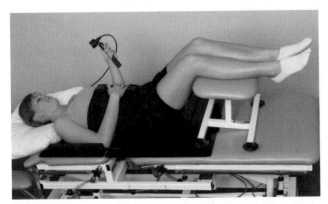

Figure 15-1 Supine lumbar spine traction therapy. (From Olson KA. Manual physical therapy of the spine. St. Louis, 2008, Saunders.)

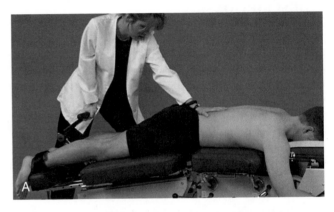

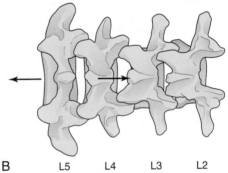

B   L5   L4   L3   L2

Figure 15-3 Flexion-distraction traction therapy. (From Bergmann T, Peterson DH. Chiropractic technique, ed 3. St. Louis, 2011, Mosby.)

Procedure

Traction can be applied in a variety of ways according to the specific device used. With axial traction, patients are most often treated while lying supine on a traction table with their knees and hips partly flexed or over a cushion (Figure 15-1). Typically a harness is applied to both the pelvis and the chest and force is transmitted from the device through the harnesses. Most traction tables are split in the middle; the upper portion remains stationary while the lower portion is mobile, mounted on a track or bearings. The lower portion is slowly pulled away from the upper portion during treatment. This design reduces the force needed to counteract body weight and separate the vertebrae. Although originally applied by manual means or by using weights, axial traction is most often applied with motorized or hydraulic systems today. Modern traction tables can be programmed to gradually increase the amount of force, or cycle through patterns of traction and relaxation as needed.

Patients receiving positional distraction or distraction manipulation are often placed in a prone or side-lying position on a distraction table (Figure 15-2). The lower part of the table can move in several planes, independently of the upper part. The provider can lower or elevate the lower or caudal portions of the table to create distraction (axial traction combined with off-axis motion) in the plane desired. A harness may be used to secure the pelvis or ankles and transmit the distraction forces along the body. Some techniques, for example flexion-distraction, require the provider to use one hand to apply pressure to the spine and the other to operate the table (Figure 15-3). This allows forces to be concentrated in a smaller area as opposed to being dispersed throughout the spine. While some distraction tables are operated manually, others are motorized and can be programmed with varying degrees of movement amplitude, force, and time cycles.

Regulatory Status

Traction therapy equipment is regulated by the US Food and Drug Administration (FDA) as a class II medical device. Obtaining FDA approval usually requires that the manufacturer submits evidence that the new device is substantially equivalent to a currently approved similar device through a 510k marketing application.

THEORY

Mechanism of Action

Several theories have been proposed to explain the possible clinical benefit of traction therapy for CLBP. Axial distraction of the lumbar motion segment is thought to change the position of the nucleus pulposus relative to the posterior annulus fibrosus or change the disc-nerve interface, which could decrease mechanical pressure exerted on the nerve by a displaced disc.[4,5,11,12] These effects are plausible based on studies examining the kinematics of the lumbar spine during traction. In addition to separating the vertebrae, traction has been shown to reduce pressure within the nucleus pulposus and increase the size of the lateral foramen.[13,14] However, it is unlikely that such mechanical changes observed in a prone position would be sustained after a patient resumes an upright, weight-bearing posture. Any lasting clinical response to traction therapy would therefore more likely be related to its biologic effects on the motion segment or neural tissues. Complicating the issue further is that not all traction therapies exert the same force on the spine and animal studies have found the mechanobiology of the disc to be sensitive to the amount, frequency, and duration of loading and unloading.[15]

It is possible that some forms of traction stimulate disc or joint repair, whereas others promote tissue degradation.[16,17] Although these variables have not been systematically examined, even in animal models, what is known regarding disc mechanobiology should alert us to the possibility that not all forms of traction therapy are equal. If distracting the spine can influence disc and joint mechanobiology, different modes of traction may result in different clinical results. Systematic reviews (SRs) of lumbar traction therapy have typically not considered that different effects may exist based on force and time parameters. Clinical studies of traction therapy have most often included patients with a mix of clinical presentations including back-dominant LBP, leg-dominant LBP, or both. However, a patient with predominantly axial LBP and no radiculopathy is likely experiencing pain from a sclerotomal source, such as facet joints or disc, whereas radicular pain, even if caused by disc herniation, may be predominately of neural origin. Although it is reasonable to suspect that traction therapies may affect these conditions differently, there is insufficient evidence to support this hypothesis.

Distraction manipulation and positional distraction are mechanically different than intermittent or sustained axial traction. Rather than allowing forces to be dispersed throughout the lumbar tissues, they attempt to concentrate the forces in a smaller area. Autotraction, for example, allows the patient to concentrate the force by finding the position that most relieves their pain and applying distraction in that position. Distraction manipulation, most often used by chiropractors and physical therapists, is performed on treatment tables that allow the operator to determine the moment-to-moment vector and timing of the distractive force. If manual force is applied to the area of spinal dysfunction while it is in traction, the additional effects of SMT or mobilization (MOB) may also be at play; those interventions are reviewed in Chapter 17.

Although newer forms of traction therapy are frequently proffered and promoted as superior to existing devices, their mechanical effects are based on the same principle of spinal traction or distraction described above, and the clinical results would be expected to be similar.

Indication

The available evidence does not define an ideal patient with CLBP who is most likely to benefit from traction therapy. Traction therapies are most commonly used for CLBP with or without leg pain. There are no examination findings (clinical, imaging, or laboratory) that have been shown to differentiate patients who are likely to benefit from traction. Therefore, the decision to use traction therapy is based on the underlying theory and a lack of benefit from more conservative or less costly treatment options. Because the effects of traction are primarily mechanical, criteria used to identify patients likely to respond to other mechanical treatments such as SMT or MOB might be helpful. In that specific case, patients with CLBP who have not responded to more conservative measures may be suitable candidates for traction therapy.

Assessment

Before receiving traction therapy, patients should first be assessed for LBP using an evidence-based and goal-oriented approach focused on the patient history and neurologic examination, as discussed in Chapter 3. Additional diagnostic imaging or specific diagnostic testing is generally not required. The clinician should also inquire about general health to identify potential contraindications to traction. Radiographs of the lumbar spine may be taken to exclude disease states such as severe osteoporosis or ligamentous instability that might compromise bone or soft-tissue integrity. If signs or symptoms of neurologic compromise are present, appropriate imaging (magnetic resonance imaging or computed tomography) should be obtained to determine the cause.

EFFICACY

Evidence supporting the efficacy of this intervention for CLBP was summarized from recent clinical practice guidelines (CPGs), SRs, and randomized controlled trials (RCTs). Observational studies (OBSs) were also summarized where appropriate. Findings are summarized by study design.

TABLE 15-2	Clinical Practice Guideline Recommendations on Traction Therapy for Chronic Low Back Pain	
Reference	**Country**	**Conclusion**
18	Belgium	Not recommended
19	Europe	Not recommended
20	Italy	Not recommended
21	United Kingdom	Not recommended
22	United States	Fair evidence against use

Clinical Practice Guidelines

Five of the recent national CPGs on the management of CLBP have assessed and summarized the evidence to make specific recommendations about the efficacy of traction therapy.

The CPG from Belgium in 2006 found high-quality evidence against the use of traction for CLBP.[18]

The CPG from Europe in 2004 found no evidence that traction therapy was more effective than other conservative management options or sham traction therapy for CLBP.[19] That CPG did not recommend the use of traction therapy for CLBP.

The CPG from Italy in 2007 did not recommend the use of traction therapy for CLBP.[20]

The CPG from the United Kingdom in 2009 did not recommend the use of traction therapy for CLBP.[21]

The CPG from the United States in 2007 found fair evidence of no benefit for traction therapy in the management of CLBP.[22]

Findings from the above CPGs are summarized in Table 15-2.

Systematic Reviews

Cochrane Collaboration

An SR was conducted in 2006 and updated in 2010 by the Cochrane Collaboration on traction therapy for acute, subacute, and chronic LBP.[23] A total of 25 RCTs were identified: one examined subacute LBP and eight examined chronic LBP.[3,24-29] The remaining RCTs either included patients with a mixed duration of LBP or did not report the duration of LBP.[3,28,30-44] For LBP with or without neurologic involvement, statistically significant differences were not found for (1) traction versus control on any outcome, (2) traction versus interferential treatment for pain and function, (3) static versus intermittent traction, and (4) traction added to physical therapy versus physical therapy alone for pain and function.[25,31,32,34] However, one RCT observed statistically significant global improvement for autotraction versus mechanical traction.[27] For LBP with neurologic involvement, statistically significant differences were not observed for continuous versus intermittent traction.[28,30,35,39,41,42,44]

Furthermore, RCTs of autotraction were inconsistent for LBP with neurologic involvement. One RCT observed short-term improvements in pain after a few weeks but this was not sustained after 3 months of follow-up for traction plus corset versus corset alone.[37] Another RCT found statistically significant improvement for autotraction versus sham traction combined with bed rest and analgesics, yet autotraction was not significantly different from sham traction in another RCT.[38,43] One RCT observed positive results for different types of traction therapy (statistical significance not always reported), yet the rest of the RCTs did not find any statistically significant differences between the different types of traction or for light versus normal force traction.[3,29,35,38]

RCTs of traction versus other interventions (e.g., SMT, exercise, infra-red lamp) usually did not find any statistically significant differences on all outcomes, except for one RCT that observed statistically significant improved pain and disability for traction versus transcutaneous electrical nerve stimulation (TENS) for LBP with neurologic involvement.[3,28,30,33,36,40,42,45]

This review concluded that there is strong evidence that traction is not different from any type of control intervention, moderate evidence that traction is not more effective than other treatments, and limited evidence that there is no difference between traction and physical therapy for LBP with or without neurologic involvement.[23] For LBP with neurologic involvement, it concluded that there was conflicting evidence supporting the different types of traction, moderate evidence for continuous or intermittent traction versus any control intervention, and limited evidence supporting light versus normal force traction. It also concluded that traction therapy research would be improved if LBP symptoms and duration were better described and higher methodological standards were employed.

American Pain Society and American College of Physicians

An SR was conducted in 2006 by the American Pain Society and American College of Physicians CPG committee on nonpharmacologic therapies for acute and chronic LBP.[46] That review identified three SRs related to traction therapy, one of which was the Cochrane Collaboration review mentioned above.[23,47,48] All of the SRs concluded that there was no evidence or insufficient evidence supporting the use of traction for LBP. No additional RCTs have been identified. This SR concluded that traction has not been shown to be beneficial for acute, subacute or chronic LBP.[46]

Findings from the above SRs are summarized in Table 15-3.

Randomized Controlled Trials

Seven RCTs and nine reports related to those studies were identified.[24,26,27,31,32,49-52] Their methods are summarized in Table 15-4. Their results are briefly described here.

Borman and colleagues[24] conducted an RCT including participants with CLBP with or without neurologic involvement. In order to be included, participants had to experience LBP symptoms for more than 6 months. Participants were randomized to physical therapy (hot pack, ultrasound, and active exercises) or physical therapy plus sustained traction (greater than 50% body weight). After 10 treatment sessions

TABLE 15-3	Systematic Review Findings on Traction Therapy for Chronic Low Back Pain		
Reference	# RCTs in SR	# RCTs for CLBP	Conclusion
23	25	8	Conflicting evidence supporting traction Moderate evidence for continuous or intermittent traction versus any control Limited evidence supporting light versus normal force traction
46	3 SRs[23,47,48]	NR	No or insufficient evidence for use of traction for LBP

CLBP, chronic low back pain; LBP, low back pain; NR, not reported; RCT, randomized controlled trial; SR, systematic review.

TABLE 15-4	Randomized Controlled Trials of Traction Therapy for Chronic Low Back Pain				
Reference	Indication	Intervention 1	Intervention 2	Intervention 3	Control
24	CLBP with or without neurologic involvement, symptoms >6 months	Motorized traction + physical therapy program Provider type: NR Program: 5 days/week × 2 weeks, including 20-minute sessions of traction/day Cointervention: hot packs, ultrasound therapy, exercise program n = 21	Physical therapy program Provider type: NR Program: 5 days/week × 2 weeks Cointervention: hot packs, ultrasound therapy, exercise program n = 21	NR	NR
27	Disc herniation, LBP with or without neurologic involvement, symptoms >3 months	Autotraction Provider type: NR 30-60 minute session every 2-3 days (3-10 sessions total) Cointervention: participants could crossover to the other therapy after 4-5 day washout period n = 22	Passive traction Provider type: NR 45-minute daily sessions (5-10 sessions total) Cointervention: participants could crossover to the other therapy after 4-5 day washout period n = 22	NR	NR
31	LBP with or without neurologic involvement, symptom duration NR	Motorized traction + simultaneous massage Orthopedic doctor 6 sessions over 2-3 weeks Cointervention: NR n = 74	Interferential therapy Orthopedist 6 sessions over 2-3 weeks Cointervention: NR n = 72	NR	NR
26	Disc protrusion or herniation, LBP with neurologic involvement, symptoms >3 months	Traction Technician 30-minute sessions 5×/week × 4 weeks + 1×/week × 4 weeks Co-intervention: analgesic medication n = 22	TENS Technician 30-minute sessions 5×/week × 4 weeks + 1×/week × 4 weeks Cointervention: analgesic medication n = 22	NR	NR

Continued

TABLE 15-4	Randomized Controlled Trials of Traction Therapy for Chronic Low Back Pain—cont'd				
Reference	Indication	Intervention 1	Intervention 2	Intervention 3	Control
32, 49, 50	LBP with or without neurologic involvement, symptoms >6 weeks	Motorized traction 35%-50% body weight Physical therapist 20-minute sessions, 12× over 5 weeks Cointervention: education (leaflet), analgesic medication n = 77	Motorized traction 20% body weight Physical therapist 20-minute sessions, 12× over 5 weeks Cointervention: education (leaflet), analgesic medication n = 74	NA	NA
51	LBP with or without neurologic involvement, symptoms 1-3 months	Underwater traction bath Patient's weight + 3 kg Provider type: NR 15-minute sessions, 3×/week × 4 weeks Cointervention: education, analgesic medication n = 35	Balneotherapy Provider type: NR 15-minute sessions, 3×/week × 4 weeks Cointervention: education, analgesic medication n = 44	Underwater massage Provider type: NR 15-minute sessions, 3×/week × 4 weeks Cointervention: education, analgesic medication n = 26	Control Provider type: NA Cointervention: education, analgesic medication n = 53
52	LBP without neurologic involvement, symptoms >4 weeks	Flexion-distraction + trigger point therapy Chiropractor 8 sessions over 3 weeks Cointervention: unclear n = 54	NA	NA	Sham manipulation + effleurage Chiropractor 8 sessions over 3 weeks Cointervention: unclear n = 52

CLBP, chronic low back pain; LBP, low back pain; NA, not applicable; NR, not reported; TENS, transcutaneous electrical nerve stimulation.

over 2 weeks, they found no difference between groups in regard to visual analog scale (VAS), Oswestry Disability Index score, or assessment of global recovery. Likewise, there were no differences 3 months after treatment.

Tesio and Merlo[27] conducted an RCT including participants with disc herniation. In order to be included, participants had to experience LBP for more than 3 months. Participants were randomized to autotraction (3 to 10 sessions of 30 to 60 minutes each) or passive traction (5 to 10 sessions of 45-minutes each). After a 4- to 5-day washout period, participants could cross over to receive the other intervention. After 3 months, participants in the autotraction group experienced statistically significant improvement in pain compared with those in the passive traction group. There was also a statistically significant improvement in disability from baseline among those in the autotraction group.

Werners and colleagues[31] conducted an RCT including participants with LBP with or without neurologic involvement. The duration of symptoms was not reported. Participants were randomized to motorized traction or interferential therapy for a total of six sessions over 2 to 3 weeks. After 3 months, participants in the motorized traction group

experienced statistically significant improvement in pain and disability versus baseline scores. There were no differences between motorized traction and interferential therapy in pain or disability.

Sherry and colleagues[26] conducted an RCT including participants with disc protrusion or herniation. Participants were included if they had LBP with neurologic involvement lasting longer than 3 months. Subjects were randomized to prone traction or TENS delivered by a technician over 30-minute sessions that were preformed 5 times per week for 1 month and once per week for another month. Immediately after treatment, participants in the traction group experienced statistically significant improvement in pain compared to those in the TENS group. After 6 months, participants in the traction group continued to have statistically significant improvement in pain compared with baseline scores.

Beurskens and colleagues[32,49,50] conducted an RCT including participants with LBP with or without neurologic involvement. Participants were included if they had symptoms for more than 6 weeks. Subjects were randomized to motorized traction with 35% to 50% body weight or motorized traction with 20% body weight. Traction was administered to both groups by a physical therapist during twelve 20-minute sessions delivered over 5 weeks. After 5 weeks, no statistically significant differences were observed in either group compared with baseline pain or disability scores. Similarly, no differences were observed between the two groups after 5 weeks for all pain or disability outcomes. These results were also observed after 9 weeks.

Konrad and colleagues[51] conducted an RCT including participants with LBP with or without neurologic involvement. Participants were included if they had symptoms for 1 to 3 months. Subjects were randomized to one of four groups: (1) underwater traction bath, (2) balneotherapy, (3) underwater massage, or (4) control group. The intervention was delivered in the hospital 15 minutes per day, 3 days per week over 4 weeks. After 4 weeks, all of the intervention groups reported statistically significant improvements in pain versus baseline scores, yet this was not sustained at 1 year. Differences between the groups were not reported.

Hawk and colleagues[52] conducted an RCT including participants with LBP without neurologic involvement. Participants were included if they had symptoms for at least 4 weeks. Subjects were randomized to either traction (flexion-distraction) plus trigger point therapy or to sham manipulation plus massage (effleurage). All treatments were delivered by chiropractors in eight sessions over 3 weeks. Immediately after treatment, no statistically significant differences were observed between the two groups regarding pain or disability.

SAFETY

Contraindications

Contraindications to traction therapy are largely based on the mechanical effects of traction on anatomic structures and the physiologic cardiovascular effects of using a harness or putting the patient in an inverted position. Common contraindications to traction therapy include spinal malignancy, spinal cord compression, spinal infection (osteomyelitis, discitis), osteoporosis, inflammatory spondyloarthropathy, acute fracture, aortic or iliac aneurysm, abdominal hernia, pregnancy, severe hemorrhoids, uncontrolled hypertension, and severe cardiovascular or respiratory disease.[5,53]

Adverse Events

There is little information in the literature regarding the adverse events of traction therapy. A few clinical trials have reported some adverse events, the most common being aggravation of the pain syndrome being treated. Of 24 clinical trials summarized in a review, 4 reported no adverse events and 6 reported some, while 14 did not discuss adverse events.[54] One study reported aggravation of neurologic symptoms in 20% of patients with sciatica, which was equal to the rate reported in the placebo group.[35] A case report noted sudden progression of lumbar disc protrusion during VAX-D treatment.[55] No adverse events were observed in an RCT of flexion-distraction for LBP.[56] If continuous traction which restricts patients to bed rest is used, there is potential for adverse events related to prolonged immobilization.[57] Increased intra-abdominal and chest pressure may result in transient cardiopulmonary effects such as shortness of breath or hypertension in susceptible individuals. Gravity traction has been associated with increased blood pressure and there are concerns about possible increased intraocular pressure. CPGs on the management of LBP have reported that traction therapy with forces greater than 50% of body weight could be associated with a potential increase in blood pressure, as well as respiratory constraints, and increased nerve impingement in cases of disc protrusion.[18,19]

Serious adverse events are apparently rare judging by the paucity of reports in the literature. Events such as cauda equina syndrome or fracture are unlikely if appropriate evaluation is performed before starting traction therapy. Nonetheless, the true risk of such adverse events is unknown. Predictors of negative outcome, other than the use of sustained traction, have not been identified in the literature. This may be a function of poor trial quality and the general lack of studies demonstrating efficacy.

COSTS

Fees and Third-Party Reimbursement

In the United States, traction therapy delivered or supervised by a licensed health practitioner such as a physical therapist or chiropractor can be delivered using CPT code 97012 (traction, mechanical). If MOB or SMT is performed concurrently with traction therapy, this can be delivered using CPT codes 98940 (chiropractic manipulation, 1-2 regions), 98925 (osteopathic manipulation, 1-2 regions), or 97140 (manual therapy, each 15 minutes). Although some payers continue to base their reimbursements on usual, customary, and reasonable payment methodology, the majority have developed reimbursement tables based on the Resource Based Relative Value Scale used by Medicare. Reimbursements by other third-party payers are generally higher than Medicare.

Third-party payers will often reimburse a limited number of visits to licensed health providers if they are prescribed by a physician and supported by adequate documentation deeming them medically necessary. Equipment or products required for those interventions are typically considered inclusive in the procedure reported and are not separately reportable. Anecdotally, it has been noted that some providers of traction therapy that use newer, proprietary (and costly) devices may offer a substantial discount to patients who wish to pay out-of-pocket before receiving a fixed number of sessions (e.g., $5000 for 50 sessions).

Typical fees reimbursed by Medicare in New York and California for these services are summarized in Table 15-5.

Cost Effectiveness

Evidence supporting the cost effectiveness of treatment protocols that compared these interventions, often in combination with one or more cointerventions, with control groups who received one or more other interventions, for either acute or chronic LBP, was identified from two SRs on this topic.[58,59] Although many of these study designs are unable to clearly identify the individual contribution of any intervention, their results provide some insight as to the clinical and economic outcomes associated with these approaches.

An RCT in the United States compared two approaches for patients with acute LBP.[60] The first group received care according to the classification of symptoms and examination findings by a physical therapist, including possibly SMT, MOB, traction therapy, and flexion, extension, strengthening, or stabilization exercises. The other group received brief education and general exercise from a physical therapist according to recommendations from CPGs, which were not specified. Clinical outcomes after 1 year favored the therapy according to classification group for improvement in function, though no differences were noted in the SF-36. Direct medical costs associated with the study interventions over 1 year were $604 in the therapy according to classification group and $682 in the CPG recommended care group; direct medical costs for all interventions over 1 year were $883 and $1160, respectively. Indirect productivity costs were not reported, although fewer participants in the therapy according to classification group had missed work due to LBP after 12 months.

An RCT in Norway compared three approaches for patients sick-listed with CLBP.[61] The supervised exercise therapy group received instruction on stabilization and strengthening exercise from a physical therapist. The conventional physical therapy group received one or more interventions including heat, ice, massage, stretching exercises,

electrical muscle stimulation, or traction. The self-care group received instruction to walk. Participants in all groups received three 1-hour sessions each week for 12 weeks (total 36 sessions). Clinical outcomes after 1 year reported that the supervised exercise therapy and conventional physical therapy groups had greater improvements in pain and function than the self-care group. Direct medical costs associated with the study interventions after 1 year were approximately $375 in the supervised exercise therapy group, approximately $584 in the conventional physical therapy group, and approximately $0 in the self-care group. Indirect productivity costs associated with lost work days after 1 year were approximately $13,816 in the supervised exercise therapy group, approximately $12,062 in the conventional physical therapy group, and approximately $15,762 in the self-care group. Total costs (direct medical and indirect productivity) over 1 year were therefore approximately $14,191 in the supervised exercise therapy group, approximately $12,646 in the conventional physical therapy group, and approximately $15,762 in the self-care group. Authors concluded that both the supervised exercise therapy and the conventional physical therapy were cost-saving when compared with self-care.

The CPG from Europe in 2004 determined that the cost effectiveness for traction therapy for CLBP (>3 months) is unknown.[19]

Other

An SR reported on a study which determined that an intervention of conventional physical therapy including traction was cost effective in patients aged 20 to 65 who had CLBP and were sick-listed for more than 8 weeks and less than 52 weeks.[62]

Findings from the aforementioned cost effectiveness analyses are summarized in Table 15-6.

SUMMARY

Description

Traction therapy is a broad term used to refer to several methods of using mechanical force to separate the lumbar

TABLE 15-5	Medicare Fee Schedule for Related Services	
CPT Code	New York	California
97012	$15	$16
98940	$25	$27
98925	$29	$32
97140	$28	$30

2010 Participating, nonfacility amount.

TABLE 15-6	Cost Effectiveness and Cost Utility Analyses on Traction Therapy for Acute or Chronic Low Back Pain				
Reference Country Follow-up	Group	Direct Medical Costs	Indirect Productivity Costs	Total Costs	Conclusion
60 United States 1 year	1. Care according to classification of symptoms (including traction) 2. Brief education + general exercise	1. $883 2. $1160	NR	NR	No conclusion as to cost effectiveness
61 Norway 1 year	1. Supervised exercise therapy 2. Conventional PT (including traction) 3. Self-care	1. $375 2. $584 3. $0	1. $13,816 2. $12,062 3. $15,762	1. $14,191 2. $12,646 3. $15,762	Groups 1 and 2 were cost saving compared to group 3

NR, not reported; PT, physical therapy.

vertebrae along the inferosuperior axis of the spine. Traction can either be intermittent (alternating traction and relaxation with cycles of a few minutes), sustained (maintained for 20 to 60 minutes), or continuous (maintained for hours to days). It can also be described according to the direction of its primary force, whether axial (superoinferior axis of the spine) or distraction (axial force combined with off-axis forces such as flexion or lateral bending). Distraction is further subdivided into distraction manipulation and positional distraction. Various forms of traction therapy have been used to treat spinal disorders for almost 4000 years. Traction is widely available in the United States and can be applied by chiropractors, physical therapists, or medical physicians trained in the use of specific traction devices for CLBP.

Theory

Several theories have been proposed to explain the possible clinical benefit of lumbar traction for CLBP. Axial distraction of the motion segment is thought to change the position of the nucleus pulposus relative to the posterior annulus fibrosus or change the disc-nerve interface, which could decrease mechanical pressure exerted on a nerve by a displaced disc. It is also possible that some forms of traction stimulate disc or joint repair, whereas others promote tissue degradation. Traction is indicated for LBP with or without neurologic involvement. Diagnostic imaging may be required before administering traction therapy for CLBP to exclude disease states such as severe osteoporosis or if signs or symptoms of neurologic compromise are present.

Efficacy

Five CPGs do not recommend traction for CLBP. A review conducted by the Cochrane Collaboration concluded that there is strong evidence that traction is not different from any type of control, moderate evidence that traction is not more effective than other treatments, and limited evidence that there is no difference between traction and physical therapy for LBP with or without neurologic involvement. For LBP with neurologic involvement, this Cochrane review concluded that there was conflicting evidence supporting the different types of traction, moderate evidence for continuous or intermittent traction versus any control, and limited evidence supporting light versus normal force traction. Another high-quality review concluded that traction has not been shown to be beneficial for CLBP. At least seven RCTs assessed the efficacy of traction, the majority of which found no differences between traction and other types of interventions. One RCT found a statistically significant improvement in pain for autotraction versus passive traction.

Safety

Contraindications to traction therapy include spinal malignancy, spinal cord compression, spinal infection (osteomyelitis, discitis), osteoporosis, inflammatory spondyloarthritis,

acute fracture, aortic or iliac aneurysm, abdominal hernia, pregnancy, severe hemorrhoids, uncontrolled hypertension, and severe cardiovascular or respiratory disease. Adverse events associated with traction include aggravation of pain, progression of lumbar disc protrusion, shortness of breath, hypertension, increased blood pressure (gravity traction), cauda equina syndrome, and fracture. Traction therapy with forces greater than 50% of body weight could be associated with a potential increase in blood pressure, as well as respiratory constraints, and increased nerve impingement in cases of disc protrusion.

Costs

The cost per traction session varies from $15 to $32, yet is more expensive if newer, proprietary devices are used (e.g., $5000 for 50 sessions). At least two studies assessed the cost associated with traction for CLBP, yet it was a component of a physical therapy program so the individual contribution of traction to the overall cost effectiveness was unclear.

Comments

Evidence from the CPGs, SRs, and RCTs reviewed suggests that traction therapy may not be effective for patients with CLBP. However, this intervention may be useful for a small subset of patients with CLBP who fail to improve with other conservative interventions. Patients contemplating the use of traction therapy should be advised of associated adverse events, which appear to be relatively minor.

Although "nonsurgical decompression" traction equipment is aggressively promoted in the United States, there is little evidence to suggest that its effect is different than simple intermittent axial traction. It is also unclear if muscle tension plays a major role in modifying vertebral displacement during traction. Furthermore, there is scant data for all categories of traction, including intermittent traction. Because the mechanical input of distraction-manipulation is different than axial traction, the results of RCTs using sustained traction or even intermittent traction should not be generalized to distraction manipulation unless evidence is forthcoming that proves their physiologic and mechanobiologic effects to be the same.

Properly designed RCTs are needed to determine whether there are subgroups of LBP sufferers who benefit from specific traction therapies. Patient variables that might be considered important include age, weight or body mass index, and specific diagnostic category (although controversial). Treatment variables include duration and magnitude of force, direction of off-axis forces, and number of treatments. Additionally, RCTs are needed to specifically evaluate the proprietary forms of traction that are being aggressively marketed to the public. Further studies are needed to conclusively determine whether intermittent traction, positional distraction, or distraction-manipulation is beneficial for CLBP.

CHAPTER REVIEW QUESTIONS

Answers are located on page 451.

1. Which of the following is not a duration-based classification of traction therapy?
   a. continuous
   b. intermittent
   c. sustained
   d. distractional

2. SRs on traction for LBP most often arrive at which of the following conclusions?
   a. traction is safe and effective for both acute and chronic LBP
   b. traction is dangerous and should not be used for LBP
   c. traction is safe but the evidence does not support its use for LBP
   d. traction is effective for acute but not for chronic LBP

3. What is thought to be the most effective force when using axial traction therapy?
   a. 15% to 35% of body weight
   b. 30% to 50% of body weight
   c. 35% to 55% of body weight
   d. 40% to 60% of body weight

4. Which of the following is not a contraindication to traction therapy?
   a. spinal cord compression
   b. pregnancy
   c. LBP with leg pain
   d. osteoporosis

5. What type of traction therapy was popularized by the chiropractor James Cox?
   a. intermittent
   b. continuous
   c. axial
   d. flexion-distraction

6. Which type of diagnostic imaging may occasionally be requested before traction therapy?
   a. magnetic resonance imaging
   b. urinalysis
   c. blood work
   d. discography

REFERENCES

1. Hinterbuchner C. Traction. In: Basmajian JV, editor. Manipulation, traction and massage. Baltimore: Williams & Wilkins; 1985. p. 178.
2. Cyriax J. Conservative treatment of lumbar disc lesions. Physiotherapy 1964;50:300-303.
3. Ljunggren AE, Weber H, Larsen S. Autotraction versus manual traction in patients with prolapsed lumbar intervertebral discs. Scand J Rehabil Med 1984;16:117-124.
4. Cox JM, Feller J, Cox-Cid J. Distraction chiropractic adjusting: clinical application and outcomes of 1,000 cases. Topics Clin Chiropractic 1996;3:45-59.
5. Pellecchia GL. Lumbar traction: a review of the literature. J Orthop Sports Phys Ther 1994;20:262-267.
6. Gay RE, Bronfort G, Evans RL. Distraction manipulation of the lumbar spine: a review of the literature. J Manipulative Physiol Ther 2005;28:266-273.
7. Kumar K. Spinal deformity and axial traction. Spine 1996;21:653-655.
8. Marketos SG, Skiadas P. Hippocrates. The father of spine surgery. Spine 1999;24:1381-1387.
9. Shterenshis MV. The history of modern spinal traction with particular reference to neural disorders. Spinal Cord 1997;35:139-146.
10. Chenot JF, Becker A, Leonhardt C, et al. Use of complementary alternative medicine for low back pain consulting in general practice: a cohort study. BMC Complement Altern Med 2007;7:42.
11. Gudavalli MR. Biomechanics research on flexion-distraction procedure. In: Cox JM, editor. Low back pain: mechanisms, diagnosis and treatment. 6th ed. Philadelphia: Lippincott Williams & Wilkins; 1998. p. 263-268.
12. Knutsson E, Skoglund CR, Natchev E. Changes in voluntary muscle strength, somatosensory transmission and skin temperature concomitant with pain relief during autotraction in patients with lumbar and sacral root lesions. Pain 1988;33:173-179.
13. Ramos G, Martin W. Effects of vertebral axial decompression on intradiscal pressure. J Neurosurg 1994;81:350-353.
14. Gudavalli MR, Cox JM, Baker JA, et al. Intervertebral disc pressure changes during a chiropractic procedure. Adv Bioeng 1997;36:215-216.
15. MacLean JJ, Lee CR, Alini M, et al. The effects of short-term load duration on anabolic and catabolic gene expression in the rat tail intervertebral disc. J Orthop Res 2005;23:1120-1127.
16. Kroeber M, Unglaub F, Guehring T, et al. Effects of controlled dynamic disc distraction on degenerated intervertebral discs: an in vivo study on the rabbit lumbar spine model. Spine 2005;30:181-187.
17. Iatridis JC, MacLean JJ, Ryan DA. Mechanical damage to the intervertebral disc annulus fibrosus subjected to tensile loading. J Biomech 2005;38:557-565.
18. Nielens H, van Zundert J, Mairiaux P, et al. Chronic low back pain. Good Clinical practice (GCP). Brussels: Belgian Health Care Knowledge Centre (KCE); 2006. KCE reports vol 48C.
19. Airaksinen O, Brox JI, Cedraschi C, et al. European guidelines for the management of chronic nonspecific low back pain. Eur Spine J 2006;15:S192-S300.
20. Negrini S, Giovannoni S, Minozzi S, et al. Diagnostic therapeutic flow-charts for low back pain patients: the Italian clinical guidelines. Eura Medicophys 2006;42:151-170.
21. National Institute for Health and Clinical Excellence (NICE). Low back pain: early management of persistent non-specific low back pain. London: National Institute of Health and Clinical Excellence; 2009. Report No.: NICE clinical guideline 88.
22. Chou R, Qaseem A, Snow V, et al. Diagnosis and treatment of low back pain: a joint clinical practice guideline from the American College of Physicians and the American Pain Society. Ann Intern Med 2007;147:478-491.
23. Clarke, Judy A; van Tulder, Maurits W; Blomberg, El Stefan; de Vet, CW Henrica; van der Heijden, Geert J; Bronfort, Gert; Bouter, Lex M. Traction for low-back pain with or without sciatica. Cochrane Database of Systematic Reviews. 5, 2010, Pages 1-75.
24. Borman P, Keskin D, Bodur H. The efficacy of lumbar traction in the management of patients with low back pain. Rheumatol Int 2003;23:82-86.
25. van der Heijden GJ, Beurskens AJ, Koes BW, et al. The efficacy of traction for back and neck pain: a systematic, blinded review of randomized clinical trial methods. Phys Ther 1995;75:93-104.
26. Sherry E, Kitchener P, Smart R. A prospective randomized controlled study of VAX-D and TENS for the treatment of chronic low back pain. Neurol Res 2001;23:780-784.

27. Tesio L, Merlo A. Autotraction versus passive traction: an open controlled study in lumbar disc herniation. Arch Phys Med Rehabil 1993;74:871-876.

28. Weber H, Ljunggren AE, Walker L. Traction therapy in patients with herniated lumbar intervertebral discs. J Oslo City Hosp 1984;34:61-70.

29. Guvenol K, Tuzun C, Peker O, et al. A comparison of inverted spinal traction and conventional traction in the treatment of lumbar disc herniations. Physiother Theory Pract 2000;16: 151-160.

30. Lidstrom A, Zachrisson M. Physical therapy on low back pain and sciatica. An attempt at evaluation. Scand J Rehabil Med 1970;2:37-42.

31. Werners R, Pynsent PB, Bulstrode CJ. Randomized trial comparing interferential therapy with motorized lumbar traction and massage in the management of low back pain in a primary care setting. Spine 1999;24:1579-1584.

32. Beurskens AJ, de Vet HC, Koke AJ, et al. Efficacy of traction for nonspecific low back pain. 12-week and 6-month results of a randomized clinical trial. Spine 1997;22:2756-2762.

33. Coxhead CE, Inskip H, Meade TW, et al. Multicentre trial of physiotherapy in the management of sciatic symptoms. Lancet 1981;1:1065-1068.

34. Letchuman R, Deusinger RH. Comparison of sacrospinalis myoelectric activity and pain levels in patients undergoing static and intermittent lumbar traction. Spine 1993;18: 1361-1365.

35. Reust P, Chantraine A, Vischer TL. [Treatment of lumbar sciatica with or without neurological deficit using mechanical traction. A double-blind study.] Schweiz Med Wochenschr 1988;118:271-274.

36. Bihaug O. [Autotraksjon for ischialgpasienter: en kontollert sammenlikning mellom effekten av Auto–traksjon–B og isometriske ovelser ad modum Hume endall og enkins.] Fysioterapeuten 1978;45:377-379.

37. Larsson U, Choler U, Lidstrom A, et al. Auto-traction for treatment of lumbago-sciatica. A multicentre controlled investigation. Acta Orthop Scand 1980;51:791-798.

38. Lind G. Auto-traction treatment of low back pain and sciatica. An eletromyographic, radiographic and clinical study. Linkoping: University of Linkoping; 1974.

39. Mathews JA, Hickling J. Lumbar traction: a double-blind controlled study for sciatica. Rheumatol Rehabil 1975;14: 222-225.

40. Mathews W, Morkel M, Mathews J. Manipulation and traction for lumbago and sciatica: physiotherapeutic techniques used in two controlled trials. Physiother Pract 1988;4:201-206.

41. Pal B, Mangion P, Hossain MA, et al. A controlled trial of continuous lumbar traction in the treatment of back pain and sciatica. Br J Rheumatol 1986;25:181-183.

42. Sweetman BJ, Heinrich I, Anderson JAD. A randomized controlled trial of exercises, short wave diathermy, and traction for low back pain, with evidence of diagnosis-related response to treatment. J Orthop Rheumatol 1993;6:159-166.

43. Walker L, Svenkerud T, Weber H. [Traksjonbehandling ved lumbago–ischias: en kontrollert undersolske med Spina–trac.] Fysioterapeuten 1982;49:161-163, 177.

44. Weber H. Traction therapy in sciatica due to disc prolapse (does traction treatment have any positive effect on patients suffering from sciatica caused by disc prolapse?). J Oslo City Hosp 1973;23:167-176.

45. Sierpina VS. Progress notes: a review of educational developments in CAM. Altern Ther Health Med 2002;8:104-106.

46. Chou R, Huffman LH. Nonpharmacologic therapies for acute and chronic low back pain: a review of the evidence for an American Pain Society/American College of Physicians clinical practice guideline. Ann Intern Med 2007;147:492-504.

47. Harte AA, Baxter GD, Gracey JH. The efficacy of traction for back pain: a systematic review of randomized controlled trials. Arch Phys Med Rehabil 2003;84:1542-1553.

48. Vroomen PC, de Krom MC, Slofstra PD, et al. Conservative treatment of sciatica: a systematic review. J Spinal Disord 2000;13:463-469.

49. Beurskens AJ, de Vet HC, Koke AJ, et al. Efficacy of traction for non-specific low back pain: a randomised clinical trial. Lancet 1995;346:1596-1600.

50. van der Heijden GJ, Beurskens AJ, Dirx MJ, et al. Efficacy of lumbar traction: a randomised clinical trial. Physiotherapy 1995;81:29-35.

51. Konrad K, Tatrai T, Hunka A, et al. I. Controlled trial of balneotherapy in treatment of low back pain. Ann Rheum Dis 1992;51:820-822.

52. Hawk C, Long CR, Rowell RM, et al. A randomized trial investigating a chiropractic manual placebo: a novel design using standardized forces in the delivery of active and control treatments. J Altern Complement Med 2005;11:109-117.

53. Brault JS, Kappler RE, Grogg BE. Manipulation, traction and massage. In: Braddom RL, editor. Physical medicine and rehabilitation. Philadelphia: Elsevier; 2007. p. 437-457.

54. Clarke J, van Tulder M, Blomberg S, et al. Traction for low back pain with or without sciatica: an updated systematic review within the framework of the Cochrane collaboration. Spine 2006;31:1591-1599.

55. Deen HG Jr, Rizzo TD, Fenton DS. Sudden progression of lumbar disk protrusion during vertebral axial decompression traction therapy. Mayo Clin Proc 2003;78:1554-1556.

56. Gudavalli MR, Cambron JA, McGregor M, et al. A randomized clinical trial and subgroup analysis to compare flexion-distraction with active exercise for chronic low back pain. Eur Spine J 2006;15:1070-1082.

57. Bigos S, Bowyer O, Braen G, et al. Acute low back problems in adults. Clinical Practice Guideline Number 14. AHCPR Pub. No. 95-0642. Rockville: U.S. Department of Health and Human Services, Public Health Service, Agency for Health Care Policy and Research; 1994. Report No.: AHCPR Publication no. 95-0642.

58. Dagenais S, Roffey DM, Wai EK, et al. Can cost utility evaluations inform decision making about interventions for low back pain? Spine J 2009;9:944-957.

59. van der Roer N, Goossens MEJB, Evers SMAA, et al. What is the most cost-effective treatment for patients with low back pain? A systematic review. Best Pract Res Clin Rheumatol 2005;19:671-684.

60. Fritz JM, Delitto A, Erhard RE. Comparison of classification-based physical therapy with therapy based on clinical practice guidelines for patients with acute low back pain: a randomized clinical trial. Spine 2003;28:1363-1371.

61. Torstensen TA, Ljunggren AE, Meen HD, et al. Efficiency and costs of medical exercise therapy, conventional physiotherapy, and self-exercise in patients with chronic low back pain. A pragmatic, randomized, single-blinded, controlled trial with 1-year follow-up. Spine 1998;23:2616-2624.

62. van der Roer N, Goossens ME, Evers SM, et al. What is the most cost-effective treatment for patients with low back pain? A systematic review. Best Pract Res Clin Rheumatol 2005; 19:671-684.

CHAPTER 16

MARTA IMAMURA
ANDREA D. FURLAN
TRISH DRYDEN
EMMA L. IRVIN

Massage Therapy

DESCRIPTION

Terminology and Subtypes

The term *massage*, in this chapter, is defined as soft tissue manipulation using the hands or a mechanical device. Massage includes numerous specific and general techniques that are often used in sequence; some terms for massage techniques are French in origin. *Effleurage* (stroking) refers to light, long, slow, soothing strokes along a broad area of the body using the palms and fingers, and is often used at the beginning of the massage. Deeper effleurage can also be used in an attempt to orient vascular or lymphatic flow in a certain direction (Figure 16-1). *Petrissage* (kneading) uses slightly more force to press and release muscle tissue in circular motions with the stiffened fingers or knuckles, with multiple passes over a small area (Figure 16-2). *Tapotement* (percussion) is rhythmic, somewhat rapid tapping, cupping, or hacking of a broad area using cupped hands, fists, the ulnar border of the hand, or tented fingers (Figure 16-3). *Vibration* is a more rapid technique in which an area is covered with flat hands and fingers and shaken or vibrated lightly.[1] The term *acupressure* is used to describe a type of massage technique in which acupuncture points are stimulated manually using the fingers instead of needles; this technique is also called *massage acupuncture* or *Shiatsu massage*.[2]

On a broad level, what is often referred to as *Swedish massage* (SM) is somewhat homogeneous and involves the application of manual therapy using many of the basic techniques described. However, specific types of massage have also been developed, some of which have defined protocols that differ considerably from one another. Common types of massage include SM, Rolfing, reflexology, myofascial release, and craniosacral therapy.[3] SM is likely the most common type and combines the basic techniques described earlier. Rolfing involves slow, deep friction massage applied to connective tissue throughout the body to break fibrous adhesions and restore mobility to the fascia. Reflexology uses slow and increasing pressure gradually applied with the fingers to specific points along the hands and feet that are

somewhat akin to acupuncture points; reflexology is thought to stimulate specific organs. Deep friction massage involves applying strong, prolonged pressure to a small area of pain (thought to correspond with a trigger point) to temporarily decrease impaired blood flow to that area before releasing the pressure to stimulate reperfusion. Myofascial release involves repeated, slow, deep pressure applied to muscles and connective tissue; a variant of myofascial release in which this pressure is applied while the patient slowly moves the massaged area through its full range of motion is called *active release therapy*.[4] Craniosacral therapy is a gentle form of massage in which light pressure is applied along cranial sutures while deep breathing exercises are performed.[5] Traditional Thai massage (TTM) for low back pain (LBP) is a deep massage with prolonged pressure for usually 5 to 10 seconds per point on low back muscles between L2 and L5.

History and Frequency of Use

Massage may be the earliest and most primitive tool to treat pain.[6] The most ancient references to the use of massage come from China (around 2700 BC), India (around 1500-1200 BC), Babylonia (around 900 BC), Greece (Hippocrates 460-377 BC, Asclepiades, Galen), and Rome (Plato 427-347 BC and Socrates 470-399 BC).[7,8] Massage appears to be gaining popularity in recent years as increasing numbers of people with chronic low back pain (CLBP) are seeking complementary and alternative medicine (CAM). A survey of CAM use among the general adult population in the United States conducted in 1991 reported that massage had been used by 7% of respondents in the past year.[9] Massage was the third most commonly reported CAM therapy after relaxation techniques (13%) and chiropractic (10%). However, only 41% of those who reported using massage had consulted with a health care provider; others presumably received informal massage from family or friends or performed it themselves. The medical conditions for which massage use was highest were back problems and sprains or strains. When this survey was repeated in 1997, the use of massage in the previous 12 months had

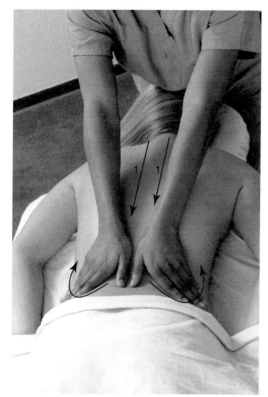

Figure 16-1 Massage therapy technique: effleurage (stroking). (From Salvo S. Massage therapy: principles & practice, ed 3. St. Louis, Saunders, 2008.)

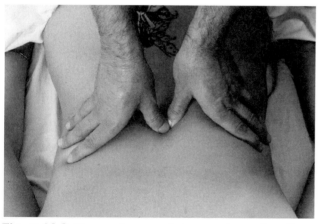

Figure 16-2 Massage therapy technique. petrissage (kneading). (Photo by Yanik Chauvin.)

grown to 11% and was still the third most common CAM therapy, this time after relaxation (16%) and herbal medicine (12%).[10] Among those who reported using massage, the proportion that saw a professional practitioner was increased to 62%. The total number of visits to massage practitioners in 1997 was estimated to exceed 113 million. The medical conditions for which massage use was highest were back problems, neck problems, and fatigue. A prospective study of CAM use among 1342 patients with LBP who presented to general practitioners in Germany

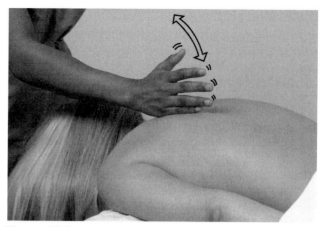

Figure 16-3 Massage therapy technique: tapotement (percussion). (From Salvo S. Massage therapy: principles & practice, ed 3. St. Louis, Saunders, 2008.)

reported that 31% used massage in the subsequent 1 year follow-up.[11] The use of massage was statistically significantly higher among those with CLBP, with an odds ratio of 1.6 (95% CI, 1.1 to 2.3). Massage was the most commonly reported CAM therapy. A survey conducted by the American Massage Therapy Association reported in 2008 that 36% of respondents had received a massage in the last 5 years.[12]

Practitioner, Setting, and Availability

Licensed massage therapists usually deliver massage therapy. This intervention is widely available throughout the United States, where it is regulated as a health profession or controlled health act at the state or even local level, rather than through established national standards. This lack of uniform regulation has resulted in inconsistency regarding the requirements for formal education, clinical training, examinations for licensure, and continuing education for massage therapists. Typical requirements for licensing include as few as 500 hours of education in massage therapy, although some states require double that amount (e.g., Nebraska, New York). The National Certification Board for Therapeutic Massage & Bodywork (NCBTMB) was established to overcome these deficiencies and provide a uniform standard for certification; it is now required by several states. Many massage therapy educational institutions offer training of 1000 hours or more. For example, in several provinces in Canada, educational requirements for licensure is minimally set at 2200 hours, with British Columbia exceeding 3000 hours. The heterogeneity in practitioners can occasionally present challenges for clinicians from other disciplines that wish to refer patients with CLBP for massage therapy but are uncertain about selecting a qualified provider. To a much lesser extent, massage therapy can also be provided by physical therapists or chiropractors as part of an integrated manual therapy approach to CLBP rather than as a standalone intervention.

Procedure

When seeing a massage therapist for the first time, a patient is asked a series of questions related to medical history, prior experiences with massage therapy, preferences for specific massage techniques, and reasons for seeking massage. The goal of these questions is to screen for those patients in whom massage is contraindicated, and to address any concerns or questions patients may have about receiving massage therapy for the first time. Together, the patient and practitioner discuss a treatment plan and the relevant regions of the body to be treated with massage. Prior to discussing the treatment plan, massage therapists may also conduct a physical assessment to determine range of motion and areas of restriction and pain in the soft tissues and joints. At subsequent visits, the provider will ask patients if there have been any changes in their health status since the last visit, as well as how they felt after their last massage. The provider will conduct ongoing physical assessments before and after treatment to assess progress in the treatment plan.

To begin an individual massage therapy treatment, the practitioner will leave the treatment room (if the patient does not need help getting on or off the massage table), and will ask the patient to prepare for the massage by removing clothing as required for optimal treatment (and as is comfortable for the patient). They will then lie or sit on the massage table or chair, as requested, and be covered by a sheet or blanket (Figure 16-4). Only the parts of the body that the patient has consented to have treated are uncovered to respect the patient's modesty. A competent provider will adapt to the patient's preferences and treatment needs for positioning and draping. Massage for LBP is often conducted with the patient in the prone position, but this can (and should) be modified if the patient is unable to remain in this position comfortably or to help the therapist access areas to be treated.

When addressing a focused condition such as LBP, massage may still be applied beyond the area of complaint and include surrounding areas, or even the whole body if general relaxation or other goals are desired. Massage typically uses a combination of the techniques described earlier, progressing from lightest to deepest, repeating the cycle on different regions of the body. Depending on the practitioner or setting, massage may constitute the primary intervention or may be considered an adjunct to prepare the patient for exercise or other interventions. In physical therapy or chiropractic, for example, a short massage may be administered before other manual therapies such as mobilization (MOB) or spinal manipulation therapy (SMT).

Regulatory Status

Not applicable.

THEORY

Mechanism of Action

At its most basic, massage therapy can be viewed as a simple way to aid in relaxation, promote a sense of well-being, and

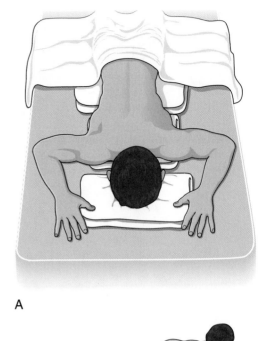

A

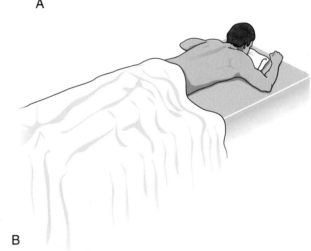

B

Figure 16-4 Massage therapy for low back pain: patient partially disrobed on a massage table.

ease feelings of muscular tension, all of which may ultimately lead to decreased pain and improved physical function. The mechanism of action for massage therapy is not fully understood. It is thought to achieve its results through a complex interplay of both physical and mental modes of action. Massage therapy delivered to soft and connective tissues may induce local biochemical changes that modulate local blood flow and regulate oxygenation.[13] These local effects may subsequently influence neural activity at the spinal cord segmental level, thereby modulating the activities of subcortical nuclei that influence both mood and pain perception.[14]

Massage therapy may also increase the pain threshold at the central nervous system (CNS) level by stimulating the release of neurotransmitters such as endorphins and serotonin. It may also act through the gate-control theory of pain, which proposes that local stimulus (e.g., massage therapy or other interventions) to an affected area stimulates large-diameter nerve fibers, which inhibit T-cells in the spinal cord that project into the CNS, then followed by pain relief.[15] Massage therapy has also been proposed to increase local blood circulation, improve muscle flexibility, intensify the movement of lymph, and loosen adherent connective tissue.[6] These actions may alternately improve reuptake of local nociceptive and inflammatory mediators, increase pain-free range of motion, and improve muscle function.

Indication

Massage is indicated for a wide variety of conditions, including CLBP, in which pain relief, reduction of swelling, or mobilization of adhesive tissues is desired.[6] It is uncertain which patient characteristics are associated with improved outcomes for massage therapy in CLBP. The general profile of patients included in randomized controlled trials (RCTs) reporting positive outcomes for benefit of massage was adults (18 years and older) with nonspecific CLBP and without infection, neoplasm, metastasis, osteoporosis, rheumatoid arthritis, fracture, inflammatory process, or radicular syndrome. Prior studies have reported that gender, race, work status, and family income did not influence the outcomes obtained with massage therapy.[16]

Assessment

Before receiving massage therapy, patients should first be assessed for LBP using an evidence-based and goal-oriented approach focused on the patient history and neurologic examination, as discussed in Chapter 3. The massage therapist should also inquire about general health to identify potential contraindications to this intervention. Diagnostic imaging or other forms of advanced testing is generally not required before administering massage therapy for CLBP.

EFFICACY

Evidence supporting the efficacy of these interventions for CLBP was summarized from recent clinical practice guidelines (CPGs), systematic reviews (SRs), and RCTs. Observational studies (OBSs) were also summarized where appropriate. Findings are summarized by study design.

Clinical Practice Guidelines

Five of the recent national CPGs on the management of CLBP have assessed and summarized the evidence to make specific recommendations about the efficacy of massage therapy.

The CPG from Belgium in 2006 found low-quality evidence to support the efficacy of massage therapy in the management of CLBP.[17]

The CPG from Europe in 2004 found limited evidence that massage, when combined with exercise and brief

TABLE 16-1	Clinical Practice Guideline Recommendations on Massage Therapy for Chronic Low Back Pain	
Reference	Country	Conclusion
17	Belgium	Low-quality evidence to support use
18	Europe	Not recommended
19	Italy	Not recommended
20	United Kingdom	Limited evidence to support use
21	United States	Moderate evidence to support efficacy

education, is more effective than massage alone, exercise alone, or sham laser therapy, with respect to short-term improvements in pain and function.[18] That CPG also found limited evidence that massage is more effective than exercise, brief education, acupuncture, relaxation training, or sham massage with respect to short-term improvements in pain and function. There was limited evidence that massage is as effective as SMT, transcutaneous electrical nerve stimulation (TENS), or a corset, with respect to improvements in pain. That CPG also found limited evidence that massage is less effective than TENS with respect to improvements in pain. There was limited evidence that massage is less effective than SMT with respect to improvements in function. That CPG did not recommended massage for the management of CLBP.

The CPG from Italy in 2007 did not recommend massage for CLBP.[19]

The CPG from the United Kingdom in 2009 found limited evidence to support the efficacy of massage with respect to short-term improvements in pain and function.[20]

The CPG from the United States in 2007 found moderate-quality evidence to support the efficacy of massage for patients who do not obtain adequate pain relief with self-care alone.[21]

Findings from the above CPGs are summarized in Table 16-1.

Systematic Reviews

Cochrane Collaboration

In 2008 the Cochrane Collaboration conducted an SR on massage for nonspecific LBP.[22,23] A total of 13 RCTs were identified, including 1 RCT on acute LBP, 3 trials of subacute and chronic LBP, 6 trials for CLBP, and 3 trials of mixed LBP duration.[16,24-35] The review concluded that massage might be beneficial for patients with subacute and chronic nonspecific LBP, especially if combined with exercise and delivered by a licensed therapist. Massage was shown to be efficacious in the long term (at least 1 year). One study showed that acupuncture massage was better than SM, and another trial showed that Thai massage is similar to SM, but these findings were not confirmed.[28,29]

TABLE 16-2		Systematic Review Findings on Massage Therapy for Chronic Low Back Pain	
Reference	# RCTs in SR	# RCTs for CLBP	Conclusion
22, 23	13	6 chronic 3 subacute and chronic 3 mixed population	Massage might be beneficial for patients with subacute and chronic nonspecific LBP, especially if combined with exercise Massage is efficacious in long term (>1 year)
36	2 SRs (22, 37)	NR	Fair evidence that massage is similarly effective as other noninvasive interventions for CLBP

CLBP, chronic low back pain; LBP, low back pain; NR, not reported; RCT, randomized controlled trial; SR, systematic review.

American Pain Society and American College of Physicians

An SR was conducted in 2007 by the American Pain Society and American College of Physicians CPG committee on non-pharmacologic therapies for acute and chronic LBP.[36] That review identified two SRs related to massage therapy and LBP, including the Cochrane Collaboration review mentioned previously.[22,23,37] The review found consistent conclusions between the two SRs. They found that there was not enough evidence to evaluate the efficacy of massage in acute LBP and that there was fair evidence that massage is similarly effective as other noninvasive interventions for CLBP. This review did not identify any additional RCTs.

Findings from the above SRs are summarized in Table 16-2.

Randomized Controlled Trials

Ten RCTs and 11 reports were identified.[16,24-28,30,31,38-40] Their methods are summarized in Table 16-3. Their results are briefly described here.

Preyde[27] conducted an RCT including patients with LBP without neurologic involvement. In order to be included, participants had to experience symptoms for 1 week to 8 months. Participants were randomized to one of four groups: (1) comprehensive massage therapy, including soft tissue manipulation, exercise, and posture education; (2) soft tissue manipulation only; (3) remedial exercise, including stretching and posture education; or (4) sham laser therapy. Massage therapists administered the comprehensive massage therapy and soft tissue manipulation for six 30- to 35-minute sessions

over 1 month, while a personal trainer and massage therapist delivered the remedial exercise and sham laser therapy for six 15- to 20-minute sessions over 1 month and six 20-minute sessions over 1 month, respectively. After 1 month of follow-up, participants in the comprehensive massage therapy group experienced statistically significant improvement in pain and function compared with those in the sham laser group and remedial exercise group. The soft tissue manipulation group was not different than the remedial exercise group, yet these groups both displayed statistically significant improvement in function over the sham laser therapy group.

Hsieh and colleagues[25,26] conducted an RCT including patients with CLBP whose symptoms lasted more than 4 months. Neurologic involvement was not reported. Participants were randomized to either acupressure delivered by an acupressure therapist or a program delivered by a physical therapist consisting of traction, SMT, thermotherapy, infrared light therapy, electrical stimulation, and exercise. The intervention was delivered via six sessions over 4 weeks. After 6 months of follow-up, participants in the acupressure group experienced statistically significant improvement in pain and disability versus those in the physical therapist program.

Cherkin and colleagues[16] performed an RCT including patients with CLBP without neurologic involvement. To be included, participants had to experience symptoms lasting longer than 6 weeks. Participants were randomized to one of three groups: (1) traditional Chinese medical acupuncture, (2) massage, or (3) self-care consisting of education through a book and videos. A licensed acupuncturist delivered acupuncture and a licensed massage therapist administered massage during 10 sessions over 10 weeks. After 1 year of follow-up, participants in the massage group experienced statistically significant improvement in pain and function versus the acupuncture group. However, no statistically significant differences were observed between the massage and self-care groups regarding pain and function after 1 year.

Geisser and colleagues[30] conducted an RCT including patients with CLBP without neurologic involvement. In order to be included, participants had to experience symptoms for more than 3 months. Participants were randomized to one of four groups: (1) manual therapy plus specific exercise (self-correction and stretching twice per day, strengthening 3 times per week), (2) sham manual therapy plus specific exercise (self-correction and stretching twice per day, strengthening 3 times per week), (3) manual therapy plus nonspecific exercise (stretching twice per day, 20 minutes of aerobics 3 times per week), or (4) sham manual therapy plus nonspecific exercise (stretching twice per day, 20 minutes of aerobics 3 times per week). A physical therapist delivered manual therapy or sham manual therapy to the groups once per week for 6 weeks, and administered all other interventions. Immediately after treatment, participants in the manual therapy plus specific exercise group experienced statistically significant improvement in pain versus baseline scores. However, this group also experienced a statistically significant increase in disability compared with baseline scores. For the other groups, no differences were observed in pain or disability for post-treatment versus baseline scores. Differences between groups were not reported.

TABLE 16-3	Randomized Controlled Trials of Massage Therapy for Chronic Low Back Pain				
Reference	Indication	Intervention 1	Intervention 2	Intervention 3	Control
27	LBP without neurologic involvement, symptoms 1 week to 8 months	Comprehensive massage therapy (including soft tissue manipulation, exercise, posture education) Massage therapist 30-35 minutes/ session × 6 sessions over 1 month Cointervention: analgesic medication n = 25	Soft tissue manipulation (same soft tissue manipulation as those in the massage therapy group) Massage therapist 30-35 minutes/session × 6 sessions over 1 month Cointervention: analgesic medication n = 25	Remedial exercise (stretching trunk, hips, and thighs, posture education) Personal trainer and massage therapist 15-20 minutes/ session × 6 sessions over 1 month n = 22	Sham laser therapy Personal trainer and massage therapist 20 minutes/session × 6 sessions over 1 month n = 26
26	CLBP, neurologic involvement NR, symptoms >4 months	Acupressure Acupressure therapist 6 sessions over 4 weeks Cointervention: NR n = 64	Physical therapy program (pelvic manual traction, spinal manipulation, thermotherapy, infrared light therapy, electrical stimulation, exercise therapy) Physical therapist 6 sessions over 4 weeks Cointervention: NR n = 65	NA	NA
16	LBP without neurologic involvement, symptoms >6 weeks	Traditional Chinese medical acupuncture Acupuncturist 10 sessions over 10 weeks Cointervention: analgesic medication n = 94	Massage Massage therapist 10 sessions over 10 weeks Cointervention: analgesic medication, exercise n = 78	NA	Self-care, education (book, videos), exercise video Cointervention: analgesic medication n = 90
30	CLBP without neurologic involvement, symptoms >3 months	Manual therapy + specific exercise (self-correction, stretching, strengthening) Physical therapist 1 session/week × 6 weeks manual therapy + self-correction and stretches 2×/day, strengthening 3×/week × 6 weeks Cointervention: analgesic medication, education n = 21	Sham manual therapy + specific exercise (self-correction, stretching, strengthening) Physical therapist 1 session/week × 6 weeks sham manual therapy + self-correction and stretches 2×/day, strengthening 3×/week × 6 weeks Cointervention: analgesic medication, education n = 18	Manual therapy + nonspecific exercise (stretching, aerobics) Physical therapist 1 session/week × 6 weeks manual therapy + stretches 2×/day, aerobics 20 minutes × 3×/week × 6 weeks Cointervention: analgesic medication, education n = 15	Sham manual therapy + non-specific exercise (stretching, aerobics) Physical therapist 1 session/week × 6 weeks sham manual therapy + stretches 2×/day, aerobics 20 minutes × 3×/week × 6 weeks Cointervention: analgesic medication, education n = 18

Continued

TABLE 16-3	Randomized Controlled Trials of Massage Therapy for Chronic Low Back Pain—cont'd

Reference	Indication	Intervention 1	Intervention 2	Intervention 3	Control
31	CLBP without neurologic involvement, symptoms >6 months	Massage therapy Massage therapist 30-minute session × 2×/week × 5 weeks Cointervention: NR n = 12	Progressive relaxation 30-minute session × 2×/week × 5 weeks at home Cointervention: weekly compliance calls n = 12	NA	NA
25	LBP, neurologic involvement NR, symptoms >1 month and <10 years	Acupressure Acupressure therapist 6 sessions over 4 weeks Cointervention: NR n = 69	Physical therapy program (pelvic manual traction, spinal manipulation, thermotherapy, infrared light therapy, electrical stimulation, exercise therapy) Physical therapist 6 sessions over 4 weeks Cointervention: NR n = 77	NA	NA

CLBP, chronic low back pain; LBP, low back pain; NA, not applicable; NR, not reported.

Hernandez-Reif and colleagues[31] conducted an RCT including patients with CLBP without neurologic involvement. In order to be included, participants had to experience symptoms for more than 6 months. One group received massage administered by massage therapists for 30 minutes twice per week for 5 weeks. The second group performed progressive relaxation exercise at home for 30 minutes twice per week for 5 weeks. Immediately after treatment, participants in the massage therapy group experienced statistically significant improvement in pain versus baseline scores. There were no differences between baseline and post-treatment scores for participants in the progressive relaxation group. Differences between groups were not reported.

Chatchawan and colleagues[28] conducted an RCT including patients with LBP due to myofascial trigger points. In order to be included, participants had to experience symptoms for more than 4 weeks. Exclusion based on neurologic involvement was not reported. Participants were randomized to either TTM or SM. The intervention was delivered by massage therapists via six 30-minute sessions of massage plus 10 minutes of stretching over 3 to 4 weeks. After 1 month of follow-up, participants in both groups experienced statistically significant improvement in pain and disability compared with baseline scores. However, no differences were observed between the two groups regarding pain or disability after 1 month.

Yip and Tse[24] conducted an RCT including patients with subacute or chronic LBP with or without neurologic involvement. In order to be included, participants had to experience symptoms on most days over the past 4 weeks. Participants were randomized to acupoint stimulation followed by acupressure with lavender oil for eight sessions over 3 weeks or to usual care. One week after the end of treatment, participants in the intervention group experienced statistically significant improvement in pain and disability compared to those in the usual care group.

Little and colleagues[38] conducted a factorial design RCT in the United Kingdom in patients with CLBP recruited from primary care settings. The interventions were (1) normal care, (2) massage, and (3) 6 or (4) 24 lessons in the Alexander technique. Half of each group was also randomized to a prescription for exercise from a doctor plus behavioral counseling from a nurse. The outcomes measured were improvement in pain intensity, disability (Roland-Morris Disability Questionnaire [RMDQ]), and quality of life (short form [SF-36]). The authors demonstrated significant reductions in the disability scores and days in pain at 3 months in all intervention groups. No significant difference was observed between the massage and the normal care groups. At 1 year, the group who had exercise followed by lessons in the Alexander technique was better than massage, both in terms of the number of days without pain and in the disability scores. The authors do not clearly describe the massage technique that was employed nor the amount of training and experience of the massage therapists.

Quinn and colleagues[40] conducted a randomized controlled pilot study comparing the effectiveness of weekly sessions of reflexology delivered for 40 minutes per week for 6 consecutive weeks compared with sham reflexology in patients with chronic nonspecific LBP. The group of patients receiving pressure over the inner part of both plantar areas of the feet demonstrated higher decrease of pain intensity on

VAS (2.5 points) than patients in the sham group of regular foot massage (0.2 points).

Zaproudina and colleagues[39] conducted an RCT to evaluate the effectiveness of a popular and traditional manual therapy used in Finland named *traditional bone setting* for chronic nonspecific LBP. This therapy uses a gentle, painless whole-body manual mobilization. Compared with conventional physical therapy that includes massage, therapeutic stretching, exercise therapy, home training, and ergonomic instructions, there were no significant differences in the short- or long-term.

SAFETY

Contraindications

Contraindications to massage may include acute inflammation, skin infection, recent fracture, burns, deep vein thrombosis, or active tumor in the area to be treated.[41] Precautions should be taken when providing massage to patients using anticoagulant therapy and in those diagnosed with hemophilia or myositis ossificans.[42]

Adverse Events

Massage is generally recognized as a safe intervention, with minimal risk of adverse events. No serious adverse events were reported by any of the patients in the studies reviewed. Some specific techniques of massage such as deep friction, compression, or ischemic compression, might result in greater soreness or ecchymosis.[16,43] In one high-quality study with 180 participants, 11% to 12% reported temporary (10 to 15 minutes) soreness after receiving massage.[28] In another high-quality study with 78 participants, 13% reported significant discomfort or pain during or shortly after treatment.[16] When massage oil was applied, hypersensitivity reactions such as rashes or pimples occurred in 6% of participants.[28]

COSTS

Fees and Third-Party Reimbursement

In the United States, treatment with massage that is delivered by a licensed health care practitioner a such as a massage therapist, physical therapist, or chiropractor in an outpatient setting can be delivered using CPT codes 97124 (therapeutic massage, each 15 minutes) or 97140 (manual therapy, each 15 minutes).

These procedures are often covered by other third-party payers such as health insurers and worker's compensation insurance. Although some payers continue to base their reimbursements on usual, customary, and reasonable payment methodology, the majority have developed reimbursement tables based on the Resource Based Relative Value Scale used by Medicare. Reimbursements by other third-party payers are generally higher than Medicare. Third-party payers often reimburse a limited number of visits to licensed

TABLE 16-4	Medicare Fee Schedule for Related Services	
CPT Code	New York	California
97124	$24	$26
97140	$28	$30

2010 Participating, nonfacility amount.

health care providers if they are prescribed by a physician and supported by adequate documentation deeming them medically necessary.

Typical fees reimbursed by Medicare in New York and California for these services are summarized in Table 16-4.

Cost Effectiveness

Evidence supporting the cost effectiveness of treatment protocols that compared these interventions, often in combination with one or more cointerventions, with control groups who received one or more other interventions, for either acute or chronic LBP, was identified from two SRs on this topic and is summarized here.[44,45] Although many of these study designs are unable to clearly identify the individual contribution of any intervention, their results provide some insight as to the clinical and economic outcomes associated with these approaches.

Critchley and colleagues[46] conducted an RCT in the United Kingdom comparing three approaches for patients with CLBP. The individual physical therapy approach included a maximum of 12 sessions with SMT, MOB, massage, home exercises, and brief education. The spinal stabilization approach included a maximum of eight sessions with abdominal and multifidus exercises. The pain management approach included a maximum of eight sessions with education, exercises, cognitive behavioral therapy (CBT), and fear avoidance training. Clinical outcomes after 18 months were similar for all groups, with improvements noted in pain, function, and utility. Direct medical costs for study and nonstudy interventions paid by the National Health Service over 18 months were approximately $872 for individual physical therapy, approximately $698 for spinal stabilization, and approximately $304 for pain management. Indirect productivity costs were not reported. Over 18 months, the three groups experienced gains in quality-adjusted life-years (QALYs) of 0.99, 0.90, and 1.00, respectively. By virtue of having lower direct medical costs and greater gains in utility, the pain management approach was reported to dominate over both individual physical therapy and spinal stabilization.

Cherkin and colleagues[16] conducted an RCT in the United States comparing three approaches for patients with CLBP. The traditional Chinese medicine (TCM) group received needle acupuncture with electrical or manual stimulation of needles, and possibly moxibustion; manual therapy was not permitted. The massage group received a variety of techniques, although acupressure was not permitted. The brief education group received education about LBP from a book and videos. Clinical outcomes after 12 months favored the massage group over the TCM group for improvement in both pain and function; medication use was also lowest in the massage group. Direct medical costs associated with study interventions over 12 months were $352 in the TCM group, $377 in the massage group, and $50 in the brief education group. Direct medical costs associated with nonstudy interventions including provider visits, medication use, and diagnostic imaging over 12 months were $252 in the TCM group, $139 in the massage group, and $200 in the brief education group. Total direct medical costs for both study and nonstudy interventions over 12 months were therefore $604 in the TCM group, $516 in the massage group, and $250 in the brief education group. Indirect productivity costs were not reported. Authors concluded that although cost differences between groups were not significant, massage appeared to be more effective than TCM.

Torstensen and colleagues[47] conducted an RCT in Norway comparing three approaches for patients sick-listed with CLBP. The supervised exercise therapy group received instruction on stabilization and strengthening exercise from a physical therapist. The conventional physical therapy group received one or more interventions including heat, ice, massage, stretching exercises, electrical muscle stimulation (EMS), or traction. The self-care group received instruction to walk. Participants in all groups received three 1-hour sessions each week for 12 weeks (total 36 sessions). Clinical outcomes after 1 year reported that the supervised exercise therapy and conventional physical therapy groups had greater improvements in pain and function than the self-care group. Direct medical costs associated with the study interventions after 1 year were approximately $375 in the supervised exercise therapy group, approximately $584 in the conventional physical therapy group, and approximately $0 in the self-care group. Indirect costs associated with lost workdays after 1 year were approximately $13,816 in the supervised exercise therapy group, approximately $12,062 in the conventional physical therapy group, and approximately $15,762 in the self-care group. Total costs (direct medical and indirect productivity) over 1 year were therefore approximately $14,191 in the supervised exercise therapy group, approximately $12,646 in the conventional physical therapy group, and approximately $15,762 in the self-care group. Authors concluded that both the supervised exercise therapy and the conventional physical therapy were cost saving when compared with self-care.

Rivero-Arias and colleagues[48] conducted an RCT in the United Kingdom comparing two physical therapy approaches for patients with subacute or chronic LBP. The minimal physical therapy group received brief education. The standard physical therapy group included education, MOB, massage, stretching, exercise, heat, or ice. Clinical outcomes after 1 year were similar between the two groups. Direct medical costs for study and nonstudy interventions over 1 year were approximately $376 in the minimal physical therapy group and approximately $486 in the standard physical therapy group. Indirect productivity costs were approximately $1305 in the minimal physical therapy group and approximately $856 in the standard physical therapy group, but these were excluded from the analysis. Since the standard physical therapy group had marginally better clinical outcomes with higher direct costs, its incremental cost-effectiveness ratio (ICER) was estimated at approximately $5538 per QALY, well within the generally accepted threshold for cost utility analyses.

Whitehurst and colleagues[49] conducted an RCT in the United Kingdom comparing two approaches for patients with acute LBP. The brief pain management group included education, general exercise, and CBT. The physical therapy group included MOB, SMT, massage, back exercise, and brief education. Clinical outcomes after 1 year were similar between the two groups. Direct medical costs for study and nonstudy interventions over 1 year were approximately $254 in the brief pain management group and approximately $354 in the physical therapy group. Indirect productivity costs were not considered. Because the physical therapy group had marginally better clinical outcomes with higher direct costs, its ICER was estimated at approximately $4710 per QALY, well within the generally accepted threshold for cost utility analyses.

Schweikert and colleagues[50] conducted an RCT in Germany comparing two approaches for patients with CLBP pain admitted to a 3-week inpatient rehabilitation center. The usual care group included group exercise, EMS, massage, and education. The usual care with CBT group also included both individual and group CBT sessions. Clinical outcomes after 1 year were mostly similar for improvements in pain and function, although greater improvement was noted in utility gains for the usual care with CBT group. Direct medical costs associated with study and nonstudy interventions over 6 months were approximately $2702 in the usual care group and approximately $2809 in the usual care with CBT group. Indirect productivity costs associated with lost workdays over 6 months were approximately $6626 in the usual care group and approximately $5061 in the usual care with CBT group. Total costs (direct medical and indirect productivity) over 6 months were therefore approximately $9328 in the usual care group and approximately $7870 in the usual care with CBT group. Since the usual care with CBT group had better clinical outcomes with lower overall costs, authors concluded that it was cost saving and dominated usual care alone.

The European Guidelines for the management of chronic nonspecific LBP published in 2004 reported that the cost effectiveness of massage in the treatment of CLBP (>3 months) is unknown.[18]

In the RCT by Preyde, the cost (in Canadian dollars) of six sessions of massage combined with exercise and education was $300, whereas massage alone cost $240, and exercise alone or sham laser cost $90 each.[27] In this study, massage combined with exercise and education had the most positive outcomes but also cost more.

Other

Hollinghurst and colleagues[51] conducted a factorial design RCT in the United Kingdom in 579 patients with CLBP recruited from primary care settings. The interventions were (1) normal care (control group), (2) massage, and (3) 6 or (4) 24 lessons in the Alexander technique. Half of each group

TABLE 16-5	Cost Effectiveness and Cost Utility Analyses of Massage Therapy for Acute or Chronic Low Back Pain				
Ref **Country** **Follow-up**	**Group**	**Direct Medical Costs**	**Indirect Productivity Costs**	**Total Costs**	**Conclusion**
46 United Kingdom 18 months	1. Individual PT (including massage) 2. Spinal stabilization 3. Pain management	1. $872 2. $698 3. $304	NR	NR	Gains in QALY: 1. 0.99 2. 0.90 3. 1.00 Group 3 reported to dominate other interventions
16 United States 1 year	1. TCM 2. Massage 3. Brief education	1. $604 2. $516 3. $250	NR	NR	No significant difference
47 Norway 1 year	1. Supervised exercise therapy 2. Conventional PT (including massage) 3. Self-care	1. $375 2. $584 3. $0	1. $13,816 2. $12,062 3. $15,762	1. $14,191 2. $12,646 3. $15,762	Groups 1 and 2 were cost saving compared with group 3
48 United Kingdom 1 year	1. Minimal PT 2. Standard PT (including massage)	1. $376 2. $486	1. $1305 2. $856 (excluded from analysis)	NR	ICER of 2 over 1: $5538/QALY
49 United Kingdom 1 year	1. Brief pain management 2. PT (including massage)	1. $254 2. $354	NR	NR	ICER of 1 over 2: $4710/QALY
50 Germany 6 months	1. Usual care (including massage) 2. Usual care	1. $2702 2. $2809	1. $6626 2. $5061	1. $9328 2. $7870	Group 2 cost saving and dominated group 1

ICER, incremental cost-effectiveness ratio; NR, not reported; PT, physical therapy; QALY, quality-adjusted life-year; TCM, traditional Chinese medicine.

was also randomized to a prescription for exercise from a doctor plus behavioral counseling from a nurse. The outcomes measured included costs to the National Health Service and to participants, comparison of costs with RMDQ score, days in pain, QALYs, and comparison of National Health Service costs with QALY gains. Of the three "single" interventions (massage, six lessons in Alexander technique, and exercise), exercise provided the best value on all three outcomes. Adding an extra therapy provides greater benefit at extra cost in all cases, with six lessons in the Alexander technique plus exercise looking to be best value. In conclusion, this study found that an exercise prescription and six lessons in Alexander technique were both more than 85% likely to be cost effective at values above a proposed threshold of $30,000 per QALY.

Lind and colleagues[52] examined the costs of health care for individuals with back pain (related ICD-9 codes). Utilization data were obtained from two large insurers in the state of Washington for the year 2002. Of the 497,597 eligible insured, 104,358 (22%) made 652,593 visits related to LBP that represented 15% of all outpatient visits. A total of 13% of visits were made to massage therapists. The largest group of insured (45%) sought care from only conventional providers and had mean costs of $506, whereas those who sought care from only CAM providers (43%) had mean costs of $342, and a third group of insured who saw both conventional and CAM providers (12%) had mean costs of $1079. The average cost allowed per visit was $128 for conventional providers and $50 for CAM providers.[53]

Findings from cost effectiveness analyses are summarized in Table 16-5.

SUMMARY

Description

Massage can be defined as soft tissue manipulation using the hands or a mechanical device. Massage includes numerous specific and general techniques that are often used in sequence, such as effleurage (stroking), petrissage (kneading), and tapotement (percussion). Common types of massage include SM, Rolfing, reflexology, myofascial release, and craniosacral therapy. Massage may be the earliest and most primitive tool to treat pain and the most commonly reported CAM therapy in a recent nationwide survey conducted in the United States. It is usually delivered by licensed massage therapists, yet can also be administered by physical therapists or chiropractors, on a limited basis.

Theory

The mechanism of action for massage therapy is not fully understood. Massage therapy may induce local biochemical changes that modulate local blood flow and regulate oxygenation in muscles, subsequently influencing neural activity at the spinal cord segmental level, thereby modulating the activities of subcortical nuclei that influence both mood and pain perception. It may also increase the pain threshold at the CNS level by stimulating the release of neurotransmitters such as endorphins and serotonin. It may inhibit T-cells in the spinal cord that project into the CNS, leading to pain relief, increased local blood circulation, improved muscle flexibility, intensified movement of lymph, and loosened adherent connective tissue. Massage therapy is indicated for CLBP to provide pain relief, reduction of swelling or mobilization of adhesive tissues. Diagnostic imaging or other forms of advanced testing is generally not required prior to administering massage therapy for CLBP.

Efficacy

Five of the recent national CPGs on the management of CLBP have assessed and summarized the evidence to make specific recommendations about the efficacy of massage therapy. One CPG found low-quality evidence supporting massage therapy for CLBP, two CPGs did not recommend massage for CLBP, another reported limited evidence, and the fifth reported moderate-quality evidence supporting massage for CLBP. A review conducted by the Cochrane Collaboration concluded that massage might be beneficial for patients with nonspecific CLBP, especially if combined with exercise and delivered by a licensed therapist. Another high-quality review concluded that there was fair evidence that massage is similarly effective as other noninvasive interventions for CLBP. At least ten RCTs assessed the efficacy of massage for CLBP, many of which reported statistically significant improvement in pain and/or disability when compared to baseline or other comparators.

Safety

Contraindications to massage include acute inflammation, skin infection, recent fracture, burns, deep vein thrombosis, or active tumor in the area to be treated. Precautions should be taken in patients with hemophilia, myositis ossificans, or concurrent use of anticoagulants. Massage is generally recognized as a safe intervention, with minimal risk of adverse events. Minor adverse events include soreness, ecchymosis, and hypersensitivity reactions to massage oil.

Costs

Massage generally costs $24 to $30 for 15 minutes of therapy. The cost effectiveness of massage for CLBP has been examined by at least six studies, yet all were components of a multi-faceted treatment program so the individual contribution of massage could not be determined.

Comments

Evidence from the CPGs, SRs, and RCTs reviewed shows somewhat mixed results when evaluating the efficacy of massage therapy for CLBP. However, results suggest that massage therapy may be effective for a subset of patients with CLBP, especially when combined with exercise and patient education. There is still uncertainty about the precise mechanisms of action for massage therapy, which makes it challenging to design appropriate clinical studies. More research is needed to determine the type of massage that is indicated for different presentations, such as patients with higher baseline pain scores, muscle spasm, sleep disturbances, stress, and anxiety symptoms. It is important to assess whether a patient's beliefs and expectations play a role in the response to massage therapy.

Future trials should also investigate the synergic effect of massage and other therapies such as exercise, acupuncture, SMT, or medications. There is some evidence suggesting that the training and experience of the massage therapist might influence outcomes, and this needs to be confirmed in further high-quality trials. There is uncertainty about the most appropriate duration and number of sessions of massage therapy; therefore, future studies are encouraged to assess the effectiveness of different regimens of massage therapy. There is a paucity of high-quality studies that assess the cost effectiveness of massage therapy. Lastly, researchers should pay attention to the introduction of bias when measuring subjective outcomes (e.g., pain) on patients who are unblinded to the intervention they received. Future studies using an inert control group should also control for the possible effects of interpersonal contact and support provided during massage therapy.

CHAPTER REVIEW QUESTIONS

Answers are located on page 451.

1. Which of the following is not a type of massage?
   a. Shiatsu
   b. Rolfing
   c. Danish
   d. reflexology
   e. myofascial release
2. Which of the following is not involved in the proposed mechanism of action for massage?
   a. small-diameter nerve fibers
   b. decreased T-cell activity
   c. increased blood circulation
   d. loosened adherent connective tissue
   e. increased lymphatic circulation
3. Which of the following is considered a potential contraindication to massage?
   a. hemophilia
   b. nonconsolidated fracture
   c. deep vein thrombosis
   d. skin infection
   e. all of the above

4. When was the use of massage to relieve pain first reported?
   a. 80 years ago
   b. 350 years ago
   c. 1200 years ago
   d. 1800 years ago
   e. 2700 years ago
5. Which type of advanced imaging should be used prior to massage therapy for common LBP?
   a. x-rays
   b. MRI
   c. CT
   d. discography
   e. none of the above
6. True or false: National CPGs consistently recommend massage for CLBP.
7. Which of the following is not a technique used in massage therapy?
   a. effleurage
   b. kneading
   c. patisserie
   d. tapotement
8. True or false: Massage therapy originated in Thailand.

Acknowledgement to Victoria Pennick for English proofing the chapter.

REFERENCES

1. Goats GC. Massage—the scientific basis of an ancient art: Part 1. The techniques. Br J Sports Med 1994;28:149-152.
2. World Health Organization. Acupuncture: review and analysis of reports on controlled clinical trial. Geneva: World Health Organization; 2002.
3. Sherman KJ, Dixon MW, Thompson D, et al. Development of a taxonomy to describe massage treatments for musculoskeletal pain. BMC Complement Altern Med 2006;6:24.
4. Barnes MF. The basic science of myofascial release: morphologic change in connective tissue. J Bodywork Movement Ther 1997;1:231-238.
5. Green C, Martin CW, Bassett K, et al. A systematic review of craniosacral therapy: biological plausibility, assessment reliability and clinical effectiveness. Complement Ther Med 1999;7:201-207.
6. Lee MHM, Itoh K, Yang G-FW. Physical therapy and rehabilitation medicine: massage. In: Bonica JJ, editor. The management of pain. Philadelphia: Lea & Febiger; 1990. p. 1777-1778.
7. Kanemetz HL. History of massage. In: Basmajian JV, editor. Manipulation, traction and massage. Baltimore: Williams & Wilkins; 1985. p. 211-255.
8. Atchison JW, Stoll ST, Cotter AC. Manipulation, traction, and massage: massage. In: Braddom RL, editor. Physical medicine and rehabilitation, 2nd ed. Philadelphia: WB Saunders; 2007. p. 1413-1439.
9. Eisenberg DM, Kessler RC, Foster C, et al. Unconventional medicine in the United States. Prevalence, costs, and patterns of use. N Engl J Med 1993;328:246-252.
10. Eisenberg DM, Davis RB, Ettner SL, et al. Trends in alternative medicine use in the United States, 1990-1997: results of a follow-up national survey. JAMA 1998;280:1569-1575.
11. Chenot JF, Becker A, Leonhardt C, et al. Use of complementary alternative medicine for low back pain consulting in general practice: a cohort study. BMC Complement Altern Med 2007;7:42.
12. American Massage Therapy Association. 2008 Massage Therapy Consumer Survey Fact Sheet. American Massage Therapy Association 2009 [cited 2009 Sep 14]; Available from: URL: http://www.amtamassage.org/media/consumersurvey_factsheet-2008.html.
13. Goats GC. Massage–the scientific basis of an ancient art: Part 2. Physiological and therapeutic effects. Br J Sports Med 1994;28:153-156.
14. Sagar S, Dryden T, Wong K. Massage therapy for cancer patients: a reciprocal relationship between body and mind. Curr Oncol 2007;14:45-56.
15. Melzack R, Wall PD. The challenge of pain. 2nd ed. London: Penguin Books; 1996.
16. Cherkin DC, Eisenberg D, Sherman KJ, et al. Randomized trial comparing traditional Chinese medical acupuncture, therapeutic massage, and self-care education for chronic low back pain. Arch Intern Med 2001;161:1081-1088.
17. Nielens H, van Zundert J, Mairiaux P, et al. Chronic low back pain. Good Clinical practice (GCP) Brussels: Belgian Health Care Knowledge Centre (KCE); 2006. KCE reports vol 48C.
18. Airaksinen O, Brox JI, Cedraschi C, et al. European guidelines for the management of chronic nonspecific low back pain. Eur Spine J 2006;15:S192-S300.
19. Negrini S, Giovannoni S, Minozzi S, et al. Diagnostic therapeutic flow-charts for low back pain patients: the Italian clinical guidelines. Eura Medicophys 2006;42:151-170.
20. National Institute for Health and Clinical Excellence (NICE). Low back pain: early management of persistent non-specific low back pain. London, 2009, National Institute of Health and Clinical Excellence. Report No.: NICE clinical guideline 88.
21. Chou R, Qaseem A, Snow V, et al. Diagnosis and treatment of low back pain: a joint clinical practice guideline from the American College of Physicians and the American Pain Society. Ann Intern Med 2007;147:478-491.
22. Furlan AD, Brosseau L, Imamura M, et al. Massage for low-back pain: a systematic review within the framework of the Cochrane Collaboration Back Review Group. Spine 2002;27:1896-1910.
23. Furlan AD, Imamura M, Dryden T, et al. Massage for low-back pain. Cochrane Database Syst Rev 2008;(4):CD001929.
24. Yip YB, Tse SH. The effectiveness of relaxation acupoint stimulation and acupressure with aromatic lavender essential oil for non-specific low back pain in Hong Kong: a randomised controlled trial. Complement Ther Med 2004;12:28-37.
25. Hsieh LL, Kuo CH, Yen MF, et al. A randomized controlled clinical trial for low back pain treated by acupressure and physical therapy. Prev Med 2004;39:168-176.
26. Hsieh LL, Kuo CH, Lee LH, et al. Treatment of low back pain by acupressure and physical therapy: randomised controlled trial. BMJ 2006;332:696-700.
27. Preyde M. Effectiveness of massage therapy for subacute low-back pain: a randomized controlled trial. CMAJ 2000;162:1815-1820.
28. Chatchawan U, Thinkhamrop B, Kharmwan S. Effectiveness of traditional Thai massage versus Swedish massage among patients with back pain associated with myofascial trigger points. J Bodywork Movement Ther 2005;9:298-309.

29. Franke A, Gebauer S, Franke K, et al. [Acupuncture massage vs Swedish massage and individual exercise vs group exercise in low back pain sufferers—a randomized controlled clinical trial in a 2 × 2 factorial design.] Forsch Komplementarmed Klass Naturheilkd 2000;7:286-293.

30. Geisser ME, Wiggert EA, Haig AJ, et al. A randomized, controlled trial of manual therapy and specific adjuvant exercise for chronic low back pain. Clin J Pain 2005;21:463-470.

31. Hernandez-Reif M, Field T, Krasnegor J, et al. Lower back pain is reduced and range of motion increased after massage therapy. Int J Neurosci 2001;106:131-145.

32. Field T, Hernandez-Reif M, Diego M, et al. Lower back pain and sleep disturbance are reduced following massage therapy. J Bodywork Movement Ther 2007;11:141-145.

33. Mackawan S, Eungpinichpong W, Pantumethakul R, et al. Effects of traditional Thai massage versus joint mobilization on substance P and pain perception in patients with non-specific low back pain. J Bodywork Movement Ther 2007;11:9-16.

34. Poole H, Glenn S, Murphy P. A randomised controlled study of reflexology for the management of chronic low back pain. Eur J Pain 2007;11:878-887.

35. Farasyn A, Meeusen R, Nijs J. A pilot randomized placebo-controlled trial of roptrotherapy in patients with subacute non-specific low back pain. J Back Musculoskel Rehabil 2006;19:111-117.

36. Chou R, Huffman LH. Nonpharmacologic therapies for acute and chronic low back pain: a review of the evidence for an American Pain Society/American College of Physicians clinical practice guideline. Ann Intern Med 2007;147:492-504.

37. Cherkin DC, Sherman KJ, Deyo RA, et al. A review of the evidence for the effectiveness, safety, and cost of acupuncture, massage therapy, and spinal manipulation for back pain. Ann Intern Med 2003;138:898-906.

38. Little P, Lewith G, Webley F, et al. Randomised controlled trial of Alexander technique lessons, exercise, and massage (ATEAM) for chronic and recurrent back pain. BMJ 2008;337:a884.

39. Zaproudina N, Hietikko T, Hanninen OO, et al. Effectiveness of traditional bone setting in treating chronic low back pain: a randomised pilot trial. Complement Ther Med 2009;17:23-28.

40. Quinn F, Hughes CM, Baxter GD. Reflexology in the management of low back pain: a pilot randomised controlled trial. Complement Ther Med 2008;16:3-8.

41. Vickers A, Zollman C. ABC of complementary medicine. Massage therapies. BMJ 1999;319:1254-1257.

42. Rachlin I. Physical therapy treatment approaches for myofascial pain syndromes and fibromyalgia; therapeutic massage in the treatment of myofascial pain syndromes and fibromyalgia. In: Rachlin ES, Rachlin I, editors. Myofascial pain and fibromyalgia. Trigger point management. St. Louis: Mosby; 2002. p. 467-487.

43. Simons DG, Travell JG, Simons LS. Apropos of all muscles: trigger point release. In: Simons DG, editor. Travell & Simons' myofascial pain and dysfunction: the trigger point manual. Upper half of body, 2nd ed. Baltimore: Williams & Wilkins; 1999. p. 94-177.

44. Dagenais S, Roffey DM, Wai EK, et al. Can cost utility evaluations inform decision making about interventions for low back pain? Spine J 2009;9:944-957.

45. van der Roer N, Goossens MEJB, Evers SMAA, et al. What is the most cost-effective treatment for patients with low back pain? A systematic review. Best Pract Res Clin Rheumatol 2005;19:671-684.

46. Critchley DJ, Ratcliffe J, Noonan S, et al. Effectiveness and cost-effectiveness of three types of physiotherapy used to reduce chronic low back pain disability: a pragmatic randomized trial with economic evaluation. Spine 2007;32:1474-1481.

47. Torstensen TA, Ljunggren AE, Meen HD, et al. Efficiency and costs of medical exercise therapy, conventional physiotherapy, and self-exercise in patients with chronic low back pain. A pragmatic, randomized, single-blinded, controlled trial with 1-year follow-up. Spine 1998;23:2616-2624.

48. Rivero-Arias O, Gray A, Frost H, et al. Cost-utility analysis of physiotherapy treatment compared with physiotherapy advice in low back pain. Spine 2006;31:1381-1387.

49. Whitehurst DGT, Lewis M, Yao GL, et al. A brief pain management program compared with physical therapy for low back pain: results from an economic analysis alongside a randomized clinical trial. Arthrit Rheum 2007;57:466-473.

50. Schweikert B, Jacobi E, Seitz R, et al. Effectiveness and cost-effectiveness of adding a cognitive behavioral treatment to the rehabilitation of chronic low back pain. J Rheumatol 2006;33:2519-2526.

51. Hollinghurst S, Sharp D, Ballard K, Barnett J, et al. Randomised controlled trial of Alexander technique lessons, exercise, and massage (ATEAM) for chronic and recurrent back pain: economic evaluation. BMJ 2008;337:a2656.

52. Lind BK, Lafferty WE, Tyree PT, et al. The role of alternative medical providers for the outpatient treatment of insured patients with back pain. Spine 2005;30:1454-1459.

53. Dagenais S, Caro J, Haldeman S. A systematic review of low back pain cost of illness studies in the United States and internationally. Spine J 2008;8:8-20.

GERT BRONFORT
MITCHELL HAAS
RONI EVANS
GREGORY KAWCHUK
SIMON DAGENAIS

CHAPTER 17

Spinal Manipulation and Mobilization

DESCRIPTION

Terminology and Subtypes

For the purpose of this chapter, *spinal manipulation therapy* (SMT) is defined as the application of high-velocity, low-amplitude (HVLA) manual thrusts to the spinal joints slightly beyond the passive range of joint motion.[1] *Spinal mobilization* (MOB) is defined as the application of manual force to the spinal joints within the passive range of joint motion that does not involve a thrust.

There are many subtypes of SMT currently in use, including several named technique that propose specific methods of combining patient assessment and management. The most common type of SMT technique has been termed *diversified* because it incorporates many of the aspects taught in these different systems. It consists of the application of HVLA thrusts to the spine with the practitioner's hand to distract spinal zygapophyseal joints slightly beyond their passive range of joint motion into the paraphysiologic space (Figure 17-1).[1] There are many specific HVLA techniques available to practitioners of SMT, which can also be modified according to patient need. This type of SMT has also been termed short-lever SMT, because the thrust is applied directly to the spine (Figure 17-2). It is distinguished from long-lever SMT, originally from the osteopathic tradition, in which force is not provided to the spine directly, but from rotation of the patient's thigh and leg (Figure 17-3). MOB is the application of manual force to the spinal joints within the passive range of joint motion; it does not involve a thrust and may include traction through the use of specialized treatment tables. There are other types of SMT that are not covered by this review, including instrument-assisted procedures and low-force manual procedures.

History and Frequency of Use

Although the practice of spinal manipulation is now frequently associated with chiropractic, which began as a profession in 1895, it predates any modern health profession and dates back thousands of years. It is believed that SMT was practiced in China as far back as 2700 BC.[2] In India, SMT was historically practiced as an act of hygiene and related techniques were considered a component of surgery.[2] Hippocrates, in his book *On Joints*, was the first to give a formal definition to the technique of manipulation; his belief in the spine as the epicenter of holistic bodily health is well known (Figure 17-4).[2] As a testament to its long history of use, there are now more randomized controlled trials (RCTs) examining SMT for low back pain (LBP) than those for any other intervention.[3]

The use of SMT appears to be gaining popularity in recent years as increasing numbers of people with chronic low back pain (CLBP) seek complementary or alternative medicine (CAM). A survey of CAM use among the general adult population in the United States conducted in 1991 reported that chiropractic (as a proxy for SMT) had been used by 10% of respondents in the past year.[4] Chiropractic was the second most commonly reported CAM therapy after relaxation techniques (13%). However, only 70% of those who reported using chiropractic had consulted with a professional health care provider; others presumably received informal chiropractic from family or friends or did not accurately report their utilization. The medical conditions for which chiropractic use was highest were back problems, arthritis, and headache. When this survey was repeated in 1997, the use of chiropractic in the previous 12 months had grown to 11% and was the fourth most common CAM therapy after relaxation (16%), herbal medicine (12%), and massage (11%).[4] Among those who reported using chiropractic, the proportion who saw a professional practitioner increased to 90%. The total number of visits to chiropractic practitioners in 1997 was estimated at 192 million. The medical conditions for which chiropractic use was highest were back problems, neck problems, arthritis, headaches, and sprains or strains. A prospective study of CAM use among 1342 patients with LBP who presented to general practitioners (GP) in Germany reported that 26% received SMT in the subsequent 1 year follow-up.[5] The use of SMT was statistically significantly higher among those whose GP offered SMT, with an odds ratio of 5.8 (95% CI, 3.1 to 10.0). SMT was the second most commonly reported CAM therapy after massage (31%).

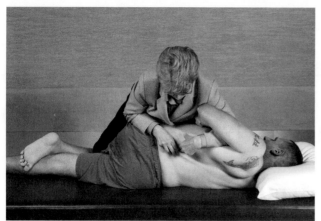

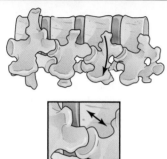

Figure 17-1 Spinal manipulation therapy with distraction of zygapophyseal joints. (Drawing from Bergmann T, Peterson DH. Chiropractic technique, ed 3. St. Louis, Mosby, 2011.)

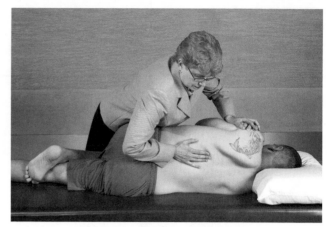

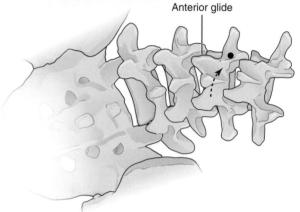

Figure 17-2 Spinal manipulation therapy: short-lever technique with manual thrust applied by hand to the spine. (Drawing from Bergmann T, Peterson DH. Chiropractic technique, ed 3. St. Louis, Mosby, 2011.)

Practitioner, Setting, and Availability

In most jurisdictions, SMT is considered a controlled health act and must be delivered by a licensed health care practitioner. The vast majority of SMT (previously estimated at 94%) in North America is provided by doctors of chiropractic (DCs), who receive extensive training in manual examination and manual therapies during their 4 years of education and clinical internship; licensing requirements differ considerably outside the United States.[6] Some SMT is provided by doctors of osteopathy and physical therapists, who receive additional training in SMT where permitted by state licensure, and also by naturopathic doctors where permitted. SMT is most often administered in the private practice of DCs. In rare cases, SMT may occasionally be performed in conjunction with anesthesia or injections, which would require that it be performed in an outpatient surgical center. Medicine-assisted manipulation, including manipulation under anesthesia, is discussed in Chapter 18. SMT is widely available throughout the United States, with an estimated 60,000 licensed DCs practicing across the country.

Procedure

Before performing SMT, the practitioner must conduct a thorough physical examination that includes manual palpation of the lumbar and sacral areas to assess local tenderness and inflammation, and identify areas of segmental dysfunction/hypomobility to which SMT will be applied. SMT for LBP is typically performed with the patient in a side-lying position on a cushioned treatment table. The practitioner then positions the patient's torso, hips, arms, and legs according to the desired type of SMT, places the "stabilizing" hand on the patient's arms, and contacts the legs using the practitioner's thigh or leg. The practitioner places the thrusting "treatment" hand over either the superior or inferior vertebra of the target spinal motion segment to which SMT will be applied. The practitioner introduces a slow force to preload the target spinal joints, and then administers an HVLA thrust with the direction, velocity, and amplitude determined by the examination and desired joint movement (Figure 17-5). The manual thrust can be assisted by a "body drop" produced when the practitioner contracts his or her abdominal and leg muscles.[7] This thrust is often accompanied by an audible cracking or popping sound, which represents the formation and dissolution of small gas bubbles within the joint cavity resulting from pressure changes as the articular surfaces momentarily separate in response to the HVLA thrust.[8,9]

Regulatory Status

Not applicable.

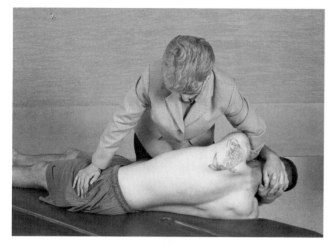

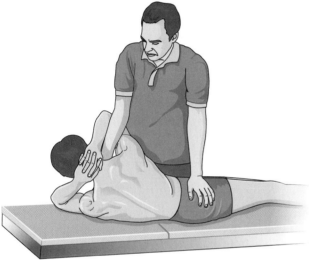

Figure 17-3 Spinal manipulation therapy: long-lever technique with rotation of the pelvis (two examples).

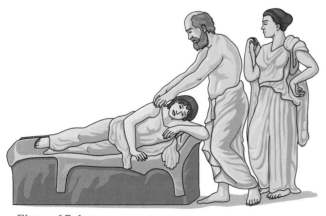

Figure 17-4 Early example of spinal manipulation therapy.

THEORY

Mechanism of Action

The precise mechanism of action for many manual therapies, including SMT and MOB, is not fully understood.[10] Many

hypotheses have focused on singular aspects of these interventions, such as the immediate biomechanical consequences of applying an external force to the tissues of the spine. It is generally thought that if the target tissues that receive this force are relatively rigid (e.g., bone), they may displace, whereas if the target tissue are relatively pliable, they may deform. Several studies related to SMT and MOB have examined the immediate biomechanical effects of tissue displacement or deformation, including altering orientation or position of anatomic structures, unbuckling of structures, release of entrapped structures, and disruption of adhesions.[11,12] Other hypotheses regarding the mechanism of action for SMT and MOB have focused on the downstream consequences of target tissue displacement or deformation, including neurologic and cellular responses.[10] Evidence suggests that SMT may impact primary afferent neurons in paraspinal tissues, the motor control system, and central pain processing.[13] It should be noted that such reductionistic approaches may not be appropriate to fully comprehend all the effects of a multifaceted clinical encounter that may also involve aspects such as the nonspecific effects of therapeutic touch, and potential healing effects of empathy shown by a practitioner spending time with their patient.[12]

Indication

Various countries and organizations have published clinical practice guidelines (CPGs) for the treatment of LBP based on systematic reviews (SRs) of evidence. In general, the recommended indication for SMT or MOB is nonspecific mechanical CLBP. Little research has been performed to evaluate which CLBP patients are best suited for SMT or MOB. Generally, SMT or MOB may be recommended for CLBP patients who do not have any contraindications. In addition, SMT or MOB may not be the best choice for patients who cannot increase activity/workplace duties, are physically deconditioned, or have psychosocial barriers to recovery.[14] Recent work on acute LBP has begun to suggest characteristics to identify which patients who may respond favorably to SMT, including duration of LBP less than 16 days, symptoms that remain proximal to the knee, Fear-Avoidance Belief Questionnaire (FABQ) scores less than 19, hypomobility of the lumbar spine, and hip rotation greater than 35 degrees.[15] In a study with a 6-month follow-up, when three of these five markers were present, subjects were observed to experience significantly greater benefits from SMT. More studies are needed to identify which CLBP patients are likely to benefit from SMT or MOB.

Assessment

Prior to receiving SMT or MOB, patients should first be assessed for LBP using an evidence-based and goal-oriented approach focused on the patient history and neurologic examination, as discussed in Chapter 3. Additional diagnostic imaging or specific diagnostic testing is generally not required prior to initiating these interventions for CLBP. The clinician should also inquire about general health to identify potential contraindications to these interventions.

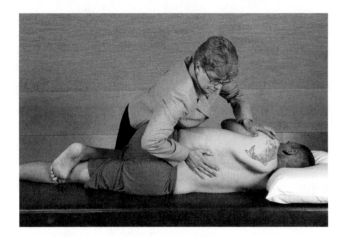

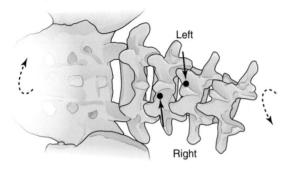

Figure 17-5 Spinal manipulation therapy with specific thrust direction, velocity, and amplitude. (Drawing from Bergmann T, Peterson DH. Chiropractic technique, ed 3. St. Louis, Mosby, 2011.)

TABLE 17-1	Clinical Practice Guideline Recommendations on Spinal Manipulation Therapy or Mobilization for Chronic Low Back Pain	
Reference	**Country**	**Conclusion**
16	Belgium	Moderate evidence to support short-term efficacy
17	Europe	Recommended for short-term improvements in pain
18	Italy	Recommended spinal manipulation therapy after patient screened for potential risks
19	United Kingdom	Recommended maximum of 9 sessions over 12 weeks
20	United States	Moderate evidence to support efficacy
24	Switzerland	Unclear evidence
112	Denmark	Recommended
113	Germany	Unclear evidence
114	Sweden	Recommended
25	Finland	Unclear evidence

EFFICACY

Evidence supporting the efficacy of these interventions for CLBP was summarized from recent CPGs, SRs, and RCTs. Observational studies (OBSs) were also summarized where appropriate. Findings are summarized by study design.

Clinical Practice Guidelines

Five of the recent national CPGs on the management of CLBP have assessed and summarized the evidence to make specific recommendations about the efficacy of SMT.

The CPG from Belgium in 2006 found moderate-quality evidence to support the efficacy of SMT when compared to no treatment with respect to short-term improvements in pain.[16] That CPG also found moderate-quality evidence that SMT is not more effective than other conservative interventions including nonsteroidal anti-inflammatory drugs (NSAIDs), usual care from a GP, physical therapy (PT), exercise, or back school for CLBP.

The CPG from Europe in 2004 recommended that SMT be considered as one option for short-term improvements in pain for the management of CLBP.[17]

The CPG from Italy in 2007 suggested that SMT be performed only by trained clinicians after screening patients for potential risk factors such as serious spinal pathology.[18]

The CPG from the United Kingdom in 2009 recommended SMT as one option for the management of CLBP.[19]

That CPG also recommended offering a maximum of 9 sessions of SMT over a period of up to 12 weeks.

The CPG from the United States in 2007 found moderate-quality evidence to support the efficacy of SMT for the management of CLBP.[20]

Five other CPGs have also assessed and summarized the evidence to make specific recommendations about the efficacy of SMT.

Findings from the above CPGs are summarized in Table 17-1.

Systematic Reviews

Cochrane Collaboration

The Cochrane Collaboration conducted an SR in 2004 on SMT for LBP.[21] A total of 28 RCTs were identified, 2 of which included patients with CLBP and 26 of which included both acute and chronic LBP patients or patients with back pain of an unspecified duration.[22-49] Using meta-regression, the review found that compared with sham therapy, spinal manipulation gave clinical short-term improvements in pain and function for acute LBP. There was also statistically significant short-term pain improvement and clinically significant short-term improvement in function for acute LBP when SMT was compared with therapies judged to be ineffective or possibly even harmful (i.e., traction, corset, bed rest, home care, topical gel, no treatment, diathermy, minimal massage). However, there were no differences in efficacy between SMT and conventional therapies (i.e., analgesics, PT, exercises, back school) for acute LBP. There were similar findings for CLBP. This Cochrane review concluded that SMT is not

TABLE 17-2	Systematic Review Findings on Spinal Manipulation Therapy or Mobilization for Chronic Low Back Pain		
Reference	# RCTs in SR	# RCTs for CLBP	Conclusion
21	28	2 chronic 26 acute and chronic or LBP of unspecified duration	SMT gave short-term improvements when compared with sham therapy No differences in efficacy between spinal manipulation and conventional therapies
50	12 SRs	NR	AEs in SMT are very rare SMT more effective than other effective interventions

AE, adverse events; CLBP, chronic low back pain; LBP, low back pain; NR, not reported; RCT, randomized controlled trial; SMT, spinal manipulation therapy; SR, systematic review.

superior to other standard treatments for patients with acute or chronic LBP.

American Pain Society and American College of Physicians

An SR was conducted in 2007 by the American Pain Society and American College of Physicians CPG committee on non-pharmacologic therapies for acute and chronic LBP.[50] That review identified 12 SRs on SMT, including the Cochrane review described earlier and four other SRs on harms associated with SMT.[3,21,51-66] The review found that five higher-quality SRs reached consistent conclusions as the Cochrane review.[53,55,56,59,60] Two lower-quality SRs based on sparse data found that SMT was more effective than other effective interventions.[3,58] The review also concluded that serious adverse events in SMT are very rare, based on consistent results from five SRs.[59,64-67] Two other RCTs were identified by this review, which also had similar conclusions as the Cochrane review.[68,69] A third other RCT was identified that evaluated a decision tool to identify patients who may benefit from spinal manipulation.[15] This SR concluded that there is moderate efficacy of SMT for subacute and chronic LBP.

Findings from the aforementioned SRs are summarized in Table 17-2.

Other

A recent narrative review of SRs of RCTs on SMT by Ernst and Canter concluded that SMT is not an effective intervention given the possibility of adverse events, and suggested that SMT is not a recommended treatment.[70] That review was severely limited in its approach because of an incomplete quality assessment of RCTs, lack of prespecified rules to evaluate the evidence, and several erroneous assumptions.[71] For example, Ernst concluded that bias exists when SRs of SMT are performed by chiropractors (including some of the authors of this chapter). This unfounded claim was refuted and addressed by using transparency in our review, including *a priori* defined standards, and acceptable methods for conducting SRs.[71-73] Clinicians should exercise caution when generalizing the findings of SRs to their practice. Disparate patient populations are likely to be included in SRs and potentially important distinguishing characteristics, such as condition severity, are not always carefully defined. In addition, diverse SMT and MOB therapeutic approaches are applied by providers with different backgrounds and training, which may affect outcomes.

TABLE 17-3	Summary Conclusions From Other Systematic Reviews on Spinal Manipulation Therapy for Chronic Low Back Pain	
Reference	Author, Year	Conclusion
70	Ernst, 2006	Evidence against efficacy of SMT for CLBP
55	Ferreira, 2002	Inconclusive evidence about efficacy of SMT for CLBP
74	van Tulder, 1997	Evidence supporting efficacy of SMT for CLBP
75	van Tulder, 2006	Evidence supporting efficacy of SMT for CLBP
3	Bronfort, 2004	Evidence supporting efficacy of SMT for CLBP

The conclusions from several recent SRs that have been conducted on the efficacy of SMT for LBP are summarized in Table 17-3.

Randomized Controlled Trials

Twenty RCTs and 25 reports related to those studies were identified.[23,26,28,31,33-34,37,39,46-47,69,76-89] Their methods are summarized in Table 17-4. Their results are briefly described here.

Koes and colleagues[37,76] conducted an RCT including patients with LBP or neck pain lasting longer than 6 weeks. It should be noted that our group was able to obtain data from these study investigators in which outcomes were reported separately for LBP and neck pain; our conclusions for between group differences are based on these data rather than those in published reports. Inclusion based on neurologic involvement was not reported. Participants were randomized to one of four groups: (1) SMT, (2) PT (e.g., massage, exercise, heat, ultrasound), (3) PT modalities (e.g., detuned short-wave diathermy, ultrasound), or (4) usual care (e.g., analgesic medication, rest, exercise, posture education). Physical therapists delivered SMT, PT, and PT modalities, while a clinician delivered usual care. Participants in the SMT group received an average of 5.4 sessions over 3 months, while those in the PT and PT modalities groups received an average of 14.7 and 11.1 sessions, respectively, over 3 months. The usual care group received one session only. After 12 months, those in

Text continued on page 238

TABLE 17-4	Randomized Controlled Trials of Spinal Manipulation Therapy or Mobilization for Chronic Low Back Pain					
Reference	Indication	Intervention 1	Intervention 2	Intervention 3	Intervention 4	Control
39, 77	LBP with or without neurologic involvement, duration of symptoms NR	SMT Chiropractor 10 sessions Cointervention: traction, corset, exercise n = 384	Hospital management # sessions NR Cointervention: manipulation, traction, corset, exercise n = 357	NA	NA	NA
33, 78	LBP or mid-back pain, neurologic involvement NR, symptoms >7 weeks	MOB Traditional bonesetter Max 10 1-hour sessions over 6 weeks (mean 8.1 sessions) n = 45	PT (heat, cold, ultrasound, shortwave diathermy, TENS, massage) Physical therapist Max 10 1-hour sessions over 6 weeks (mean 9.9 sessions) Cointervention: stretching exercise n = 35	Exercise (mostly at home: stretching, strengthening) Physical therapist Max 10 1-hour sessions over 6 weeks (mean 4.5 sessions) n = 34	NA	NA
37, 76	LBP and neck pain, neurologic involvement NR, symptoms >6 weeks	SMT Physical therapist Mean 5.4 sessions over 3 months Cointervention: PT, surgery, injection n = 36	PT (massage, exercise, heat, electrotherapy, ultrasound, shortwave diathermy) Physical therapist Mean 14.7 sessions over 3 months Cointervention: manual therapy, massage n = 36	PT modalities (shortwave diathermy, ultrasound) Physical therapist 20-minute sessions 2×/ week × 6 weeks (mean 11.1 sessions over 3 months) Cointervention: manual therapy, surgery n = 40	NA	Usual care (e.g., analgesic medication, rest, exercise, posture education) Clinician 1 session Cointervention: PT, manual therapy, massage, surgery n = 32
28*	Sciatica (with or without LBP), average duration of symptoms 14.3 weeks	SMT Physical therapist 5-10 sessions Cointervention: back school, diathermy n = 228	Traction Physical therapist 5-10 sessions Cointervention: back school, diathermy n = 228	Exercise Physical therapist 5-10 sessions Cointervention: back school, diathermy n = 228	Corset Physical therapist 5-10 sessions Cointervention: back school, diathermy n = 228	NA
31	LBP without neurologic involvement, symptoms >4 weeks but <1 year	SMT Osteopath (nonmedical practitioner) 1×/week × 4 weeks Cointervention: analgesic medication n = 41	Active diathermy Physical therapist 3×/week × 4 weeks Cointervention: analgesic medication n = 34	NA	NA	Detuned diathermy Physical therapist 3×/week × 4 weeks Cointervention: analgesic medication n = 34

TABLE 17-4	Randomized Controlled Trials of Spinal Manipulation Therapy or Mobilization for Chronic Low Back Pain—cont'd					
Reference	Indication	Intervention 1	Intervention 2	Intervention 3	Intervention 4	Control
46	LBP with or without neurologic involvement, symptoms >50 days	SMT Chiropractor Mean 10.5 sessions Cointervention: NR n = 70	Back education Clinician Mean 10.5 sessions Cointervention: NR n = 69		NA	Sham SMT Chiropractor Mean 10.5 sessions Cointervention: NR n = 70
34	Sacroiliac disorder, LBP without neurologic involvement, symptoms >4 weeks	SMT Chiropractor 3 sessions/week (10 sessions max) Cointervention: NR n = 19	Back school Physical therapist 3 sessions/week (10 sessions max) Cointervention: NR n = 18	NA	NA	NA
26	LBP without neurologic involvement, symptoms >6 weeks	SMT Chiropractor 10 sessions over 5 weeks Cointervention: strengthening exercise, analgesic medication n = 71	SMT Chiropractor 10 sessions over 5 weeks Cointervention: stretching exercise, analgesic medication n = 51	NSAIDs Naproxen (500 mg twice daily) × 5 weeks Cointervention: strengthening exercise n = 52	NA	NA
47	LBP without neurologic involvement, symptoms >3 weeks	SMT Chiropractor 2-3 sessions/ week × 2 weeks Cointervention: NR n = 11	NA	NA	NA	Sham SMT Chiropractor 2-3 sessions/ week × 2 weeks Cointervention: soft tissue massage n = 18
69	LBP without neurologic involvement, symptoms >4 weeks	SMT Chiropractor, osteopath Max 8 20-minute sessions over 12 weeks Cointervention: NR n = 353	SMT + exercise Chiropractor, osteopath, physical therapist Max 8 20-minute sessions over 6 weeks + max 8 60-minute sessions over 6 weeks Cointervention: NR n = 333	Exercise Physical therapist Max 8 60-minute sessions over 4-8 weeks Cointervention: NR n = 353 n = 310	NA	Usual care Clinician Cointervention: NR n = 353 n = 338
79, 80	CLBP without neurologic involvement, symptoms >13 weeks	SMT Chiropractor 20-minute session × 2×/ week over 9 weeks Cointervention: NR n = 35	Acupuncture Acupuncturist 20-minute session × 2×/week over 9 weeks Cointervention: NR n = 34	NSAIDs and paracetamol Sports physician 20-minute session × 2×/ week over 9 weeks Cointervention: NR n = 40	NA	NA

Continued

TABLE 17-4	Randomized Controlled Trials of Spinal Manipulation Therapy or Mobilization for Chronic Low Back Pain—cont'd					
Reference	Indication	Intervention 1	Intervention 2	Intervention 3	Intervention 4	Control
81	CLBP without neurologic involvement, symptoms >13 weeks	SMT Chiropractor 6 20-minute sessions over 3-4 weeks Cointervention: NR n = 36	Acupuncture Acupuncturist 6 20-minute sessions over 3-4 weeks Cointervention: NR n = 20	Analgesic medication not specified Clinician 20-minute session × 2×/ week over 9 weeks Cointervention: NR n = 21	NA	NA
23	CLBP without neurologic involvement, symptoms >6 months	Strengthening exercise (lumbar extension, and lumbar flexion, lateral flexion, and rotation machines, isotonic and isokinetic, seated and standing; latissimus pull down + bike for 10 minutes) Physical therapist 10 rep/set, 1 set, 3/week, 8 weeks, PRE-increase load n = 50	Stabilization exercise (McKenzie-type extension exercises + home exercise with same movements) Physical therapist 10 rep/set, 2-3 sets, 3×/week, 8 weeks + home exercise daily n = 50	SMT Physical therapist 3×/week, 8 weeks n = 50	Passive therapies (heat, TENS, ultrasound) Physical therapist 3×/week, 8 weeks n = 50	Control: No treatment n = 50
84, 90	CLBP with or without neurologic involvement, symptoms >3 months	MOB Chiropractors 2-4 sessions/ week × 4 weeks Cointervention: n = 123	PT (exercise: strengthening, flexibility, cardiovascular; ultrasound, cold) Physical therapist 2-4 sessions/week × 4 weeks n = 112	NA	NA	NA
82*	CLBP without neurologic involvement, symptoms >3 months	SMT or SMT plus physical modalities (heat/ice, ultrasound, electrotherapy, massage) Chiropractor 1 visit/week × 3 weeks Cointervention: NR n = 18	SMT or SMT plus physical modalities (heat/ice, ultrasound, electrotherapy, massage) Chiropractor 2 visits/week × 3 weeks Cointervention: NR n = 18	SMT or SMT plus physical modalities (heat/ice, ultrasound, electrotherapy, massage) Chiropractor 3 visits/week × 3 weeks Cointervention: NR n = 18	SMT or SMT plus physical modalities (heat/ice, ultrasound, electrotherapy, massage) Chiropractor 4 visits/week × 3 weeks Cointervention: NR n = 18	NA

TABLE 17-4	Randomized Controlled Trials of Spinal Manipulation Therapy or Mobilization for Chronic Low Back Pain—cont'd				
Reference	Indication	Intervention 1	Intervention 2	Intervention 3	Intervention 4	Control
86	LBP without neurologic involvement, symptoms >6 weeks	MOB Physical therapist 45-minute session 1×/week × 6 weeks Cointervention: analgesic medication n = 23	Stabilization exercise Physical therapist 45-minute session 1×/week × 6 weeks Cointervention: analgesic medication n = 24	NA	NA	NA
87	CLBP with or without neurologic involvement, symptoms >50% days in the past year	MOB Traditional bonesetter 5 sessions over 2 weeks Cointervention: analgesic medication n = 35	PT (massage + exercise: stretching, stabilization) Fitness center specialist Average of 5 treatments over 2 weeks Cointervention: analgesic medication n = 35	NA	NA	NA
89	LBP with or without neurologic involvement, symptom duration NR	SMT + exercise (strengthening, flexibility) + education Chiropractor # sessions NR over 4 weeks Cointervention: electrical muscle stimulation, ultrasound n = 169	SMT + exercise (strengthening, flexibility) + education + physical modalities (heat/cold, ultrasound, electrical muscle stimulation) Chiropractor # sessions NR over 4 weeks Cointervention: NR n = 172	NA	NA	NA
88	Neck pain and LBP without neurologic involvement, mixed symptom duration	SMT Chiropractor Average 4.9 sessions Cointervention: exercise, traction n = 138	PT Physical therapist Average 6.4 sessions Cointervention: SMT, traction, exercise, ultrasound, TENS, acupuncture n = 115	NA	NA	NA
85	Lumbar disc herniation, LBP with neurologic involvement, average symptoms 31 weeks	SMT Osteopath Average 11 15-minute sessions over 12 weeks Cointervention: education n = 20	Chemonucleolysis Orthopedic surgeon 1 treatment Cointervention: NR n = 2	NA	NA	NA

*This RCT used a factorial design so all combinations of treatments were employed.
CLBP, chronic low back pain; LBP, low back pain; MOB, mobilization; NSAIDs, nonsteroidal anti-inflammatory drugs; PT, physical therapy; NA, not applicable; NR, not reported; SMT, spinal manipulation therapy; TENS, transcutaneous electrical nerve stimulation.

the SMT and PT groups experienced statistically significant improvement in pain and function versus baseline scores.

Meade and colleagues[39,77] conducted an RCT including patients with LBP with or without neurologic involvement; duration of symptoms was not reported. Participants were randomized to either SMT performed by a chiropractor or hospital care (including SMT, along with other interventions). The SMT group received a maximum of 10 sessions, while the number of sessions for the hospital care group was not reported. After 3 years, those in the SMT group experienced statistically significant improvement in pain and function versus those in the hospital care group.

Coxhead and colleagues[28] conducted an RCT including patients with sciatic pain (with or without LBP). They did not specify a minimum symptom duration but participants had LBP for an average of 14.3 weeks before entering the trial. Participants were randomized to 1 of 4 groups: (1) SMT, (2) traction, (3) exercise, or (4) corset. All groups were also given diathermy and participated in back school. Physical therapists delivered the intervention over 5 to 10 sessions. After 4 weeks, those receiving SMT experienced statistically significant improvement in pain versus those receiving the other interventions.

Gibson and colleagues[31] conducted an RCT including patients with LBP without neurologic involvement. In order to be included, participants had to experience LBP for more than 4 weeks but less than 1 year. Participants were randomized to one of three groups: (1) SMT, (2) active diathermy, or (3) detuned diathermy. The SMT group received one session per week over 4 weeks, which was administered by an osteopath who was a nonmedical practitioner. The active and detuned diathermy groups received three sessions per week over 4 weeks, which was administered by a physical therapist. After 4 weeks of follow-up, all groups experienced statistically significant improvement in pain versus baseline scores. Between-group comparisons were not conducted because the authors reported these were not possible.

Hemmilä and colleagues[33,78] conducted an RCT including patients with LBP or mid-back pain lasting longer than 7 weeks. Inclusion based on neurologic involvement was not reported. Participants were randomized to one of three groups: (1) MOB performed by a traditional bonesetter, (2) PT (including heat, cold, ultrasound, shortwave diathermy, transcutaneous electrical nerve stimulation [TENS], massage), or (3) exercise (stretching and strengthening usually performed at home). The MOB group received the intervention from practitioners with no formal medical training, while the PT and exercise groups received the intervention from physical therapists. The mean number of sessions per group over the 6-week intervention was 8.1 for the MOB, 9.9 for the PT, and 4.5 for the exercise groups. After 1 year of follow-up, those in the MOB group experienced statistically significant improvement in disability versus those in the exercise group.

Triano and colleagues[46] conducted an RCT including patients with LBP with or without neurologic involvement. In order to be included, participants had to experience LBP for at least 50 days. Participants were randomized to one of three groups: (1) SMT, (2) back education, or (3) sham SMT. All groups received an average of 10.5 sessions. SMT and sham SMT were administered by a chiropractor and a

clinician administered back education. After 4 weeks of follow-up, no statistically significant differences were observed between groups.

Herzog and colleagues[34] conducted an RCT including patients with sacroiliac disorder. In order to be included, participants had to have LBP without neurologic involvement and symptoms lasting longer than 4 weeks. Participants were randomized to SMT with a chiropractor or back school with a physical therapist. The intervention was administered three times per week for a maximum of 10 sessions. After 4 weeks of follow-up, no statistically significant differences were observed between groups for pain or disability.

Bronfort and colleagues[26] conducted an RCT including patients with LBP without neurologic involvement. In order to be included, participants had to experience symptoms for more than 6 weeks. Participants were randomized to one of three groups: (1) SMT plus strengthening exercise, (2) SMT plus stretching exercise, or (3) NSAIDs (naproxen 500 mg twice daily) plus strengthening exercise. A chiropractor delivered 10 sessions of SMT over 5 weeks, while those in the NSAID group received treatment over 5 weeks. After 1 year of follow-up, no statistically significant differences were observed between groups for pain or disability.

Waagen and colleagues[47] conducted an RCT including patients with LBP without neurologic involvement. In order to be included, participants had to experience symptoms for more than 3 weeks. Participants were randomized to either SMT or sham SMT. A chiropractor administered SMT or sham SMT to the groups for two to three sessions per week over 2 weeks. After 2 weeks of follow-up, the SMT group experienced statistically significant improvement in pain compared with baseline scores. This was not observed for the sham SMT group. Differences between the groups were not reported.

The UK BEAM trial team[69] conducted an RCT including patients with LBP without neurologic involvement. In order to be included, participants had to experience symptoms for more than 4 weeks. Participants were randomized to one of four groups: (1) SMT (maximum of eight 20-minute sessions over 12 weeks), (2) SMT plus exercise (maximum of eight 20-minute sessions of SMT over 6 weeks plus a maximum of eight 60-minute sessions of exercise over 6 weeks), (3) exercise (a maximum of eight 60-minute sessions over 4 to 8 weeks), or (4) usual care. Chiropractors or osteopaths administered SMT and physical therapists administered the exercise program. After 1 year of follow-up, the exercise group experienced statistically significant improvement in pain and disability compared with baseline scores. In addition, those in the SMT group and SMT plus exercise group experienced statistically significant improvement in pain and disability compared with baseline scores after 1 year of follow-up. No significant differences were reported in pain or disability after 1 year between the SMT group and exercise group. No differences were observed between the exercise group and usual care group after 1 year regarding pain or disability.

Giles and Müller[79,80] conducted an RCT including patients with chronic spinal pain (including CLBP) lasting longer than 13 weeks; outcomes were reported separately for LBP and neck pain. In order to be included, participants could not have neurologic involvement. Participants were randomized to one of three groups: (1) SMT, (2) acupuncture, or (3) analgesic medication (NSAIDs, paracetamol). SMT was delivered by a chiropractor and an acupuncturist delivered acupuncture during 20-minute sessions that occurred twice per week for 9 weeks; a sports physician prescribed analgesic medication. Immediately after treatment, those in the SMT group experienced statistically significant improvement in pain and disability when compared to baseline scores, though no differences were reported between groups.

Giles and Müller[81] conducted an RCT including patients with chronic spinal pain (including CLBP) lasting longer than 13 weeks; outcomes were reported separately for LBP and neck pain. In order to be included, participants could not have neurologic involvement. Participants were randomized to one of three groups: (1) SMT, (2) acupuncture, or (3) unspecified analgesic medication. SMT was delivered by a chiropractor and an acupuncturist delivered acupuncture during six 20-minute sessions that occurred over 3 to 4 weeks; a clinician prescribed analgesic medication. Immediately after treatment, those in the SMT group experienced statistically significant improvement in pain and disability versus baseline scores. None of the other two groups experienced significant differences in pain or disability compared with baseline scores. Differences between the three groups were not reported.

Haas and colleagues[82] conducted an RCT including patients with CLBP without neurologic involvement. In order to be included, participants had to experience LBP for at least 3 months. Participants were randomized to one of four groups using a factorial design: (1) SMT or SMT plus physical modalities for one visit per week, (2) SMT or SMT plus physical modalities for two visits per week, (3) SMT or SMT plus physical modalities for three visits per week, or (4) SMT or SMT plus physical modalities for four visits per week. The intervention was delivered over 3 weeks by a chiropractor. After 12 weeks of follow-up, a dose-response relationship was noted whereby participants who received a higher number of SMT sessions reported greater improvement in pain, but not disability.

Cambron and colleagues[84,90] conducted an RCT including patients with CLBP with or without neurologic involvement. In order to be included, participants had to experience LBP for at least 3 months. Participants were randomized to MOB or PT consisting of exercise, ultrasound, and cold therapy. MOB was administered by a chiropractor, while physical therapists delivered PT. The intervention was administered for two to four sessions over 4 weeks. After 53 weeks of follow-up, all groups experienced statistically significant improvement in pain and disability versus baseline scores; there were no significant differences between groups.

Burton and colleagues[85] conducted an RCT including patients with lumbar disc herniation. In order to be included, participants had to have LBP with neurologic involvement. Participants had an average of 31 weeks of symptom duration. They were randomized to either SMT administered by an osteopath or chemonucleolysis administered by an orthopedic surgeon. The SMT group received an average of eleven 15-minute sessions over 12 weeks while the chemonucleolysis group received one treatment. After 12 months

of follow-up, no differences in pain or disability were observed between the two groups.

In an RCT by Timm,[23] individuals with CLBP without neurologic involvement, who had symptoms lasting longer than 6 months and had one-level L5 laminectomy were randomly assigned to one of five groups: (1) lumbar strengthening exercise; (2) lumbar stabilization and extension range of motion exercise; (3) SMT; (4) passive modalities including hot packs, TENS, and ultrasound; or (5) no treatment. The lumbar strengthening exercise group performed lumbar extensor progressive resistance exercises (PREs) on isokinetic and isotonic machines. Cointerventions for the strengthening exercise group included lumbar flexion and rotation, latissimus dorsi PREs on machines, and bike exercise. Treatments were administered three times a week for 8 weeks. At 8 weeks, improvements in disability (Oswestry Disability Index) were observed in all groups, with the largest improvements in the lumbar extensor and stabilization exercise groups. The improvements in disability for the lumbar extensor exercise and stabilization exercise groups were significantly greater than the SMT, passive modalities, and control groups.

Rasmussen-Barr and colleagues[86] conducted an RCT including patients with LBP without neurologic involvement. In order to be included, participants had to experience LBP for at least 6 weeks. Participants were randomized to either MOB or stabilization exercise. A physical therapist performed all interventions via weekly 45-minute sessions over 6 weeks. After 12 months of follow-up, the stabilization group experienced statistically significant improvement in pain and disability compared with baseline scores. No differences in pain or disability were observed among the MOB group after 12 months of follow-up. In addition, no statistically significant differences in pain or disability were observed between groups after 1 year of follow-up.

Ritvanen and colleagues[87] conducted an RCT including patients with LBP with or without neurologic involvement. In order to be included, participants had to experience LBP for at least half of the days in the past year. Participants were randomized to either MOB administered by traditional bonesetters or PT including massage and exercise administered by a fitness center specialist. Both groups received approximately five treatments over 2 weeks. Immediately after treatment, both groups experienced statistically significant improvement in pain and disability compared with baseline scores. However, no differences in pain or disability were observed between the two groups immediately after treatment.

Skargren and colleagues[88] conducted an RCT including patients with neck pain or LBP without neurologic involvement. Participants had a mixed duration of symptoms. They were randomized to either SMT with a chiropractor (average of 4.9 sessions) or PT with a physical therapist (average of 6.4 sessions) over the intervention period. After 1 year of follow-up, no differences were observed between the two groups in pain or disability.

Hurwitz and colleagues[89] conducted an RCT including patients with LBP with or without neurologic involvement. Participants had a mixed duration of symptoms and were randomized to one of four groups, half of whom were primarily managed by a chiropractor (n = 341), and half of whom were primarily managed by a medical physician (n = 340). This study only reported on the two groups who received chiropractic care, half of whom (n = 172) were randomized to also receive physical modalities, consisting of heat/cold, ultrasound, and electrical muscle stimulation. Both groups whose results were reported in this study also received instruction on exercises (strengthening and flexibility) and back care education. The number of treatment sessions was not reported but the intervention was administered over 4 weeks. After 6 months of follow-up, no differences in pain or disability were observed between the groups who received chiropractic care alone when compared to chiropractic care and physical modalities; both groups improved over baseline.

SAFETY

Contraindications

Contraindications to SMT include all of the red flags associated with LBP due to potentially serious spinal pathology, such as fever, unrelenting night pain or pain at rest, pain with below-knee numbness or weakness, leg weakness, loss of bowel or bladder control, progressive neurologic deficit, direct trauma, unexplained weight loss, and history of cancer.[91] Other contraindications include fracture, severe osteoporosis, or trauma causing tissue disruption to the treated area.

As with all forms of conservative interventions for CLBP, the likelihood of obtaining positive outcomes with SMT is decreased in patients who have severe comorbidities or psychosocial risk factors associated with chronicity. Instruments such as the Yellow Flags Questionnaire have defined several factors to identify patients with LBP who are at higher risk for developing chronicity and a worsened prognosis.[92] These factors are not specific to SMT and include beliefs about appropriateness of working with current pain levels, perceived chance of recovery in 6 months, light work, stress, and previous number of sick days.[92] Low patient expectations and low satisfaction with the care received have also been associated with poor outcomes for SMT and LBP, suggesting that patients who do not expect to improve with SMT and respond poorly to an initial trial of care may fare better with other interventions.[93,94] Other factors associated with poor outcomes for SMT and LBP include pain radiating below the knee, baseline levels of pain or disability, income, and smoking.[95,96]

Adverse Events

SMT can be associated with relatively benign temporary adverse events (AEs) including mild localized soreness or pain, which typically does not interfere with activities of daily living.[97] A large, prospective observational study of 1058 patients who received 4712 sessions of SMT from 102 DCs in Norway reported the following common AEs: local discomfort (53%), headache (12%), tiredness (11%), radiating discomfort (10%), and dizziness (5%).[98] Most of these AEs occurred within 4 hours of SMT (64%), were of mild-to-moderate severity (85%), and disappeared the same day

(74%).[98] It should be noted that this study included AEs from SMT applied to the cervical, thoracic, or lumbar areas. The risk of AEs for SMT applied uniquely to the lumbosacral region for CLBP is therefore likely to be lower.

Rare AEs that have been reported following SMT in the lumbar region include lumbar disc herniation (LDH) and cauda equina syndrome (CES).[97] Because of the low incidence of severe AEs, the risk attributable to SMT cannot be evaluated in RCTs. An SR on the safety of SMT for LBP uncovered four studies, which reported the following estimates of risk: 1 CES per 128 million SMT, 1 CES per 100 million SMT, less than 1 CES or LDH per 1 million SMT, 1 LDH per 8 million SMT, and 1 CES per 4 million SMT.[65] On the basis of these estimates and other reports of AEs, the review authors estimated the risk of LDH or CES following SMT at one event per 3.72 million SMT.[65]

Discrepancies in the estimates of risk reported in the four studies discussed here are likely attributable to heterogeneous methodology and retrospective data sources, in addition to the imprecise nature of combining data from case reports and legal malpractice claims to estimate the numerator with utilization data to estimate the denominator. It should be noted that some of the cases of CES or LDH included in these estimates of risk occurred during manipulation under anesthesia, which has been associated with a greater risk of disc injury than SMT. Although underreporting of rare AEs associated with SMT may lead to underestimating the true risk, other reports have wrongly attributed AEs to SMT.[99] Thus the existing estimates are associated with substantial uncertainty and will only improve when more data become available from well-designed prospective studies.[100]

COSTS

Fees and Third-Party Reimbursement

In the United States, treatment with SMT that is delivered by licensed health care practitioner such as a chiropractor or physician can be delivered using CPT codes 98940 (chiropractic manipulation, 1-2 regions), 98925 (osteopathic manipulation, 1-2 regions), or 97140 (manual therapy, each 15 minutes).

Third-party payers will often reimburse a limited number of visits if they are supported by adequate documentation deeming them medically necessary. Although some payers continue to base their reimbursements on usual, customary, and reasonable payment methodology, the majority have developed reimbursement tables based on the Resource Based Relative Value Scale used by Medicare. Reimbursements by other third-party payers are generally higher than Medicare.

Typical fees reimbursed by Medicare in New York and California for these services are summarized in Table 17-5.

Cost Effectiveness

Evidence supporting the cost effectiveness of treatment protocols that compared these interventions, often in

TABLE 17-5	Medicare Fee Schedule for Related Services	
CPT Code	New York	California
98940	$25	$27
98925	$29	$32
97140	$28	$30

2010 Participating, nonfacility amount.

combination with one or more cointerventions, with control groups who received one or more other interventions, for either acute or chronic LBP, was identified from two SRs on this topic and is summarized here.[101,102] Although many of these study designs are unable to clearly identify the individual contribution of any intervention, their results provide some insight as to the clinical and economic outcomes associated with these approaches.

An RCT in the United States compared three approaches for patients with acute LBP presenting to a health maintenance organization (HMO).[27] The PT group received nine visits centered on the McKenzie method. The chiropractic group received nine visits of SMT. The brief education group received only an educational booklet. Clinical outcomes after 3 months reported greater improvement in pain for the PT and chiropractic groups. Direct medical costs associated with study and nonstudy interventions provided by the HMO over 2 years were $437 in the PT group, $429 in the chiropractic group, and $153 in the brief education group. Indirect productivity costs were not reported.

An RCT in Finland compared two approaches for patients with CLBP in the rehabilitation unit of an orthopedic hospital.[101] One group received brief education by a physician and an educational booklet. The other group received MOB, stretching, and stabilization exercises from a manual therapist, as well as an educational booklet. Clinical outcomes after 12 months were mostly similar between the two groups, though slightly greater improvements were noted in pain and function in the manual therapist group. Direct medical costs associated with study and nonstudy interventions over 12 months were $431 in the brief education group and $470 in the manual therapist group. Indirect productivity costs from lost workdays over 12 months were $2450 in the brief education group and $1848 in the manual therapist group. Total costs (direct medical and indirect productivity) over 12 months were $2681 in the brief education group and $2318 in the manual therapist group. Total costs decreased in both groups when compared with historical health utilization and lost workdays before having enrolled in the study, but cost differences between the groups were not significant.

An RCT in the United Kingdom compared three approaches for patients with CLBP.[104] The individual PT approach included a maximum of 12 sessions with SMT, MOB, massage, home exercises, and brief education. The spinal stabilization approach included a maximum of eight sessions with abdominal and multifidus exercises. The pain management approach included a maximum of eight sessions with education, exercises, cognitive behavioral therapy (CBT), and fear avoidance training. Clinical outcomes after

18 months were similar for all groups, with improvements noted in pain, function, and utility. Direct medical costs for study and nonstudy interventions paid by the National Health Service over 18 months were approximately $872 for individual PT, approximately $698 for spinal stabilization, and approximately $304 for pain management. Indirect productivity costs were not reported. Over 18 months, the three groups experienced gains in quality-adjusted life-years (QALYs) of 0.99, 0.90, and 1.00, respectively. By virtue of having lower direct medical costs and greater gains in utility, the pain management approach was reported to dominate over both individual PT and spinal stabilization.

An RCT in the United States compared two approaches for patients with acute LBP.[105] The first group received care according to the classification of symptoms and examination findings by a physical therapist, including possibly SMT, MOB, traction therapy, and flexion, extension, strengthening, or stabilization exercises. The other group received brief education and general exercise from a physical therapist according to recommendations from CPGs, which were not specified. Clinical outcomes after 1 year favored the therapy according to classification group for improvement in function, though no differences were noted in the SF-36. Direct medical costs associated with the study interventions over 1 year were $604 in the therapy according to classification group and $682 in the CPG recommended care group; direct costs for all interventions over 1 year were $883 and $1160, respectively. Indirect productivity costs associated with lost productivity were not reported, although fewer participants in the therapy according to classification group had missed work due to LBP after 12 months.

An RCT from Canada compared two approaches for patients who had been injured at work and subsequently suffered from CLBP.[106] The functional restoration group included CBT, fear avoidance training, education, biofeedback, and group counseling, as well as strengthening and stretching exercises. The usual care group could receive a variety of interventions, including PT, acupuncture, back school, SMT, medication, or supervised exercise therapy. Clinical outcomes were not reported. Direct medical costs associated with the study intervention were $2507 higher in the functional restoration group. Indirect productivity costs associated with lost workdays were $3172 lower in the functional restoration group. Total costs for interventions, lost workdays, and disability pensions were $7068 lower in the functional restoration group. These differences were not statistically significant.

An RCT in Sweden compared three approaches for patients sick-listed with acute LBP.[107] The manual therapy group received SMT, MOB, assisted stretching, and exercises. The intensive training group received supervised exercise therapy with a physical therapist, including general and stabilization exercises. The usual care group received various interventions from a GP, including common analgesics and brief education. Clinical outcomes were not reported. Direct medical costs associated with study interventions over 1 year including provider visits, diagnostic testing, and surgery (if needed) were approximately $1054 in the manual therapy group, approximately $1123 in the intensive training group, and approximately $404 in the usual care group. Indirect productivity costs associated with lost workdays were approximately $6163 in the manual therapy group, approximately $5557 in the intensive training group, and approximately $7072 in the usual care group. Total costs (direct medical and indirect productivity) over 1 year were therefore approximately $7217 in the manual therapy group, approximately $6680 in the intensive training group, and approximately $7476 in the usual care group. Cost differences between groups were not significantly different.

An RCT in the United Kingdom compared two PT approaches for patients with subacute or chronic LBP.[108] The minimal PT group received brief education. The standard PT group included education, MOB, massage, stretching, exercise, heat, or ice. Clinical outcomes after 1 year were similar between the two groups. Direct medical costs for study and nonstudy interventions over 1 year were approximately $376 in the minimal PT group and approximately $486 in the standard PT group. Indirect productivity costs were approximately $1305 in the minimal PT group and approximately $856 in the standard PT group, but these were excluded from the analysis. Since the standard PT group had marginally better clinical outcomes with higher direct medical costs, its incremental cost-effectiveness ratio (ICER) was estimated at approximately $5538 per QALY, well within the generally accepted threshold for cost utility analyses.

An RCT in the United Kingdom compared two approaches for patients with acute LBP.[109] The brief pain management group included education, general exercise, and CBT. The PT group included MOB, SMT, massage, back exercise, and brief education. Clinical outcomes after 1 year were similar between the two groups. Direct medical costs for study and nonstudy interventions over 1 year were approximately $254 in the brief pain management group and approximately $354 in the PT group. Indirect productivity costs were not considered. Since the PT group had marginally better clinical outcomes with higher direct medical costs, its ICER was estimated at approximately $4710 per QALY, well within the generally accepted threshold for cost utility analyses.

An RCT in the United Kingdom compared four approaches for patients with subacute or chronic LBP.[110] The usual care from a GP group included various unspecified interventions, brief education, and advice to remain active. The usual care from a GP with exercise group included various unspecific interventions, plus individual and group supervised exercise therapy classes. The usual care from a GP with SMT group included various unspecified interventions and SMT. The usual care from a GP with SMT and exercise group included various unspecified interventions, brief education, advice to remain active, group and individual supervised exercise therapy classes, and SMT. Clinical outcomes after 1 year were mostly similar, with improvement in pain, function, and utility, though greater improvement was reported for utility gains in the usual care with SMT and usual care with SMT and exercise groups. Direct medical costs associated with study and nonstudy interventions over 1 year were approximately $503 in the usual care group, approximately $707 in the usual care with exercise group, approximately $787 in the usual care with SMT group, and approximately $685 in the usual care with SMT and exercise group. Indirect

productivity costs were not reported. Since the usual care with SMT and exercise group had lower direct medical costs and greater gains in QALYs than usual care with exercise or usual care with SMT, authors concluded that it was cost saving and dominated those two other choices; its ICER when compared to usual care was estimated at approximately $5509 per QALY, well within the generally accepted threshold for cost utility analyses.

Other

A survey reported that the mean annual expenses among those with LBP or neck pain related to receiving care from a chiropractor (presumably for SMT/MOB), increased from $94 (95% CI, $68 to $120) to $157 (95% CI, $127 to $187) from 1997 to 2005.[111]

Findings from these cost-effectiveness analyses are summarized in Table 17-6.

SUMMARY

Description

SMT can be defined as the application of HVLA manual thrusts to the spinal joints slightly beyond the passive range of joint motion, while MOB can be defined as the application of manual force to the spinal joints within the passive range of joint motion that does not involve a thrust. The most common type of SMT technique is termed *diversified* because it incorporates many different SMT techniques. SMT is believed to date as far back as 2700 BC and is widely available throughout the United States. Doctors of chiropractic usually deliver SMT but some doctors of osteopathy and physical therapists may also do so.

Theory

The precise mechanism of action for SMT and MOB is not fully understood. Many hypotheses have focused on singular aspects of these interventions, such as the immediate biomechanical consequences of applying an external force to the tissues of the spine. Other hypotheses regarding the mechanism of action for SMT and MOB have focused on the downstream consequences of target tissue displacement or deformation, including neurologic and cellular responses. It should be noted that such reductionist approaches might not fully take all effects of a multifaceted clinical encounter into account. In general, the recommended indication for SMT or MOB is nonspecific mechanical CLBP. Diagnostic imaging or other forms of advanced testing is generally not required prior to administering SMT or MOB for CLBP.

Efficacy

Five recent national CPGs made recommendations about the efficacy of SMT for CLBP. Two CPGs reported moderate-quality evidence supporting SMT for CLBP, two CPGs reported that SMT is an option for managing CLBP, and one CPG reported that SMT can be used for patients who have

TABLE 17-6 | **Cost Effectiveness and Cost Utility Analyses of Massage Therapy for Acute or Chronic Low Back Pain**

Ref Country Follow-up	Group	Direct Medical Costs	Indirect Productivity Costs	Total Costs	Conclusion
27 United States 2 years	1. PT 2. Chiropractic 3. Brief education	1. $437 2. $429 3. $153	NR	NR	No conclusion as to cost effectiveness
103 Finland 1 year	1. Brief education by physician 2. Treatment by manual therapist (including MOB)	1. $431 2. $470	1. $2450 2. $1848	1. $2881 2. $2318	No significant difference
104 UK 18 months	1. Individual PT (including SMT and MOB) 2. Spinal stabilization 3. Pain management (including fear avoidance training)	1. $872 2. $698 3. $304	NR	NR	Gains in QALY: 1. 0.99 2. 0.90 3. 1.00 Group 3 reported to dominate other interventions
105 United States 1 year	1. Care according to classification of symptoms (including SMT and MOB) 2. Brief education + general exercise	1. $883 2. $1160	NR	NR	No conclusion as to cost effectiveness
106 Canada NR	1. Functional restoration (including back school) 2. Usual care (including SMT)	1. $2507 higher than group 2 2. NR	1. $3172 lower than group 2 for lost work days 2. NR	1. $7068 lower than group 2 (lost work days + disability pensions) 2.	No significant difference
107 Sweden 1 year	1. Manual therapy (including SMT and MOB) 2. Intensive training 3. Usual care (including brief education)	1. $1054 2. $1123 3. 404	1. $6163 2. $5557 3. $7072	1. $7217 2. $6680 3. $7476	No significant difference
108 UK 1 year	1. Minimal PT 2. Standard PT (including MOB)	1. $376 2. $486	1. $1305 2. $856 (excluded from analysis)	NR	ICER of 2 over 1: $5538/QALY
109 UK 1 year	1. Brief pain management 2. PT (including SMT and MOB)	1. $254 2. $354	NR	NR	ICER of 1 over 2: $4710/QALY
110 UK 1 year	1. Usual care 2. Usual care + exercise 3. Usual care + SMT 4. Usual care + exercise + SMT	1. $503 2. $707 3. $787 4. $685	NR	NR	ICER of 4 over 1: $5509/QALY

ICER, incremental cost effectiveness ratio; MOB, mobilization; NR, not reported; PT, physical therapy; QALY, quality-adjusted life-year; SMT, spinal manipulation therapy.

been screened for potential risk factors. Five SRs have concluded that SMT is superior to interventions deemed ineffective or possibly even harmful but not necessarily superior to conventional therapies (i.e., analgesics, PT, exercises, back school) for CLBP. Five SRs concluded that serious adverse events with SMT are very rare. Another SR concluded that SMT is not a recommended treatment, yet this SR was methodologically challenged because of incomplete quality assessment, lack of prespecified rules to evaluate the evidence, and several erroneous assumptions. At least 20 RCTs examined the efficacy of SMT or MOB, many of which reported statistically significant improvement in pain or disability when compared to other methods of conservative care or baseline scores.

Safety

Contraindications to SMT include red flags such as fever, unrelenting night pain or pain at rest, pain with below-knee numbness or weakness, leg weakness, loss of bowel or bladder control, progressive neurologic deficit, direct trauma, unexplained weight loss, and history of cancer. Other contraindications include fracture, severe osteoporosis, or trauma causing tissue disruption to the treated area. SMT is associated with relatively benign temporary adverse events including local discomfort, headache, tiredness, radiating discomfort, and dizziness. Rare adverse events may include LDH.

Costs

The Medicare reimbursement for SMT or MOB varies from $25 to $32. Additional fees may also apply if adjunct therapies are administered, such as heat, ice, electrical muscle stimulation, assisted stretching, myofascial release, massage, or supervised exercise. At least nine studies examined the costs associated with SMT or MOB for CLBP. One RCT concluded that usual care with SMT and exercise was cost saving and superior to usual care with exercise or usual care with SMT. The other RCTs examined SMT or MOB as components of multifaceted treatment programs so their individual contributions to the overall cost effectiveness could not be determined.

Comments

Evidence from the CPGs, SRs, and RCTs reviewed suggests that SMT and MOB are effective in the management of CLBP. Results from methodologically sound, well reported SRs suggest that SMT and MOB are at least as effective as other efficacious and commonly used interventions, such as exercise and NSAIDs, and may be more effective for short-term relief of pain than other interventions, such as acupuncture. Evidence also suggests that serious adverse events associated with SMT are very rare, though minor and self-limiting adverse events appear common. Future trials should attempt to define subgroups of patients with CLBP in whom this intervention is most likely to achieve clinically meaningful improvement. This should be done by using validated and reliable diagnostic classification criteria, establishing the optimal number of treatment visits, and evaluating the cost effectiveness of care using appropriate scientific methodology.

CHAPTER REVIEW QUESTIONS

Answers are located on page 451.

1. Which of the following is the correct definition of spinal manipulation therapy?
   a. low-velocity, low-amplitude manual thrusts within passive range of motion
   b. high-velocity, low-amplitude manual thrusts beyond passive range of motion
   c. low-velocity, high-amplitude manual thrusts beyond passive range of motion
   d. high-velocity, high-amplitude manual thrusts beyond anatomic range of motion
2. How is mobilization defined in this chapter?
   a. application of manual thrust to a joint outside passive range of motion
   b. application of manual force to a muscle within active range of motion
   c. application of manual force to a joint within passive range of motion
   d. application of electrical force to a joint within passive range of motion
3. Which of the following is not a potential contraindication to SMT?
   a. pain below knee
   b. loss of bowel or bladder control
   c. progressive neurologic deficit
   d. saddle area numbness
4. Which of the following does not help predict a favorable response to SMT?
   a. patients with duration of LBP less than 16 days
   b. patients with FABQ scores lower than 19
   c. hypomobility of the lumbar spine
   d. patients with symptoms that remain distal to the knee
5. True or false: SMT originated in Africa 2700 years ago.
6. True or false: x-rays, MRI, or CT must be performed prior to SMT.
7. Which of the following health care providers typically does not deliver SMT?
   a. massage therapists
   b. physical therapists
   c. chiropractors
   d. osteopaths
8. Which of the following is not a proposed theory for the mechanism of action of SMT?
   a. energy release from HVLA
   b. biomechanical response
   c. cellular responses
   d. neurophysiologic response attenuation

REFERENCES

1. Haldeman S, Phillips RB. Spinal manipulative therapy in the management of low back pain. In: Frymoyer JW, Ducker TB, Hadler NM, et al, editors. The adult spine: principles and practice. New York: Raven Press; 1991. p. 1581-1605.
2. Wiese G, Callender A. History of spinal manipulation. In: Haldeman S, Dagenais S, Budgell B, editors. Principles and practice of chiropractic, 3rd ed. New York: McGraw-Hill; 2005.
3. Bronfort G, Haas M, Evans RL, et al. Efficacy of spinal manipulation and mobilization for low back pain and neck pain: a systematic review and best evidence synthesis. Spine J 2004;4:335-356.
4. Eisenberg DM, Davis RB, Ettner SL, et al. Trends in alternative medicine use in the United States, 1990-1997: results of a follow-up national survey. JAMA 1998;280:1569-1575.

5. Chenot JF, Becker A, Leonhardt C, et al. Use of complementary alternative medicine for low back pain consulting in general practice: a cohort study. BMC Complement Altern Med 2007;7:42.

6. Shekelle PG, Adams AH, Chassin MR, et al. Spinal manipulation for low-back pain. Ann Intern Med 1992;117:590-598.

7. Peterson DH, Bergmann TF. Chiropractic technique. 2nd ed. St. Louis: Mosby; 2002.

8. Unsworth A, Dowson D, Wright V. "Cracking joints." A bioengineering study of cavitation in the metacarpophalangeal joint. Ann Rheum Dis 1971;30:348-358.

9. Watson P, Kernohan WG, Mollan RA. A study of the cracking sounds from the metacarpophalangeal joint. Proc Inst Mech Eng [H] 1989;203:109-118.

10. Khalsa PS, Eberhart A, Cotler A, et al. The 2005 conference on the biology of manual therapies. J Manipulative Physiol Ther 2006;29:341-346.

11. Shekelle PG. Spinal manipulation. Spine 1994;19:858-861.

12. Evans DW. Mechanisms and effects of spinal high-velocity, low-amplitude thrust manipulation: previous theories. J Manipulative Physiol Ther 2002;25:251-262.

13. Pickar JG. Neurophysiological effects of spinal manipulation. Spine J 2002;2:357-371.

14. Institute for Clinical Systems Improvement (ICSI). Adult low back pain. Institute for Clinical Systems Improvement 2006:1-65. Available at: http://www.guideline.gov/summary/summary.aspx?doc_id=9863&nbr=005287&string=adult+AND+low+AND+back+AND+pain.

15. Childs JD, Fritz JM, Flynn TW, et al. A clinical prediction rule to identify patients with low back pain most likely to benefit from spinal manipulation: a validation study. Ann Intern Med 2004;141:920-928.

16. Nielens H, van Zundert J, Mairiaux P, et al. Chronic low back pain. Good Clinical practice (GCP) Brussels: Belgian Health Care Knowledge Centre (KCE); 2006. KCE reports vol 48C.

17. Airaksinen O, Brox JI, Cedraschi C, et al. European guidelines for the management of chronic nonspecific low back pain. Eur Spine J 2006;15:S192-S300.

18. Negrini S, Giovannoni S, Minozzi S, et al. Diagnostic therapeutic flow-charts for low back pain patients: the Italian clinical guidelines. Eura Medicophys 2006;42:151-170.

19. National Institute for Health and Clinical Excellence (NICE). Low back pain: early management of persistent non-specific low back pain. London, 2009, National Institute of Health and Clinical Excellence. Report No.: NICE clinical guideline 88.

20. Chou R, Qaseem A, Snow V, et al. Diagnosis and treatment of low back pain: a joint clinical practice guideline from the American College of Physicians and the American Pain Society. Ann Intern Med 2007;147:478-491.

21. Assendelft WJ, Morton SC, Yu EI, et al. Spinal manipulative therapy for low back pain. Cochrane Database Syst Rev 2004;(1):CD000447.

22. Ongley MJ, Klein RG, Dorman TA, et al. A new approach to the treatment of chronic low back pain. Lancet 1987;2:143-146.

23. Timm KE. A randomized-control study of active and passive treatments for chronic low back pain following L5 laminectomy. J Orthop Sports Phys Ther 1994;20:276-286.

24. Andersson GB, Lucente T, Davis AM, et al. A comparison of osteopathic spinal manipulation with standard care for patients with low back pain. N Engl J Med 1999;341:1426-1431.

25. Bronfort G. Chiropractic versus general medical treatment of low back pain: a small scale controlled clinical trial. Am J Chiropract Med 1989;2:145-150.

26. Bronfort G, Goldsmith CH, Nelson CF, et al. Trunk exercise combined with spinal manipulative or NSAID therapy for chronic low back pain: a randomized, observer-blinded clinical trial. J Manipulative Physiol Ther 1996;19:570-582.

27. Cherkin DC, Deyo RA, Battie M, et al. A comparison of physical therapy, chiropractic manipulation, and provision of an educational booklet for the treatment of patients with low back pain. N Engl J Med 1998;339:1021-1029.

28. Coxhead CE, Inskip H, Meade TW, et al. Multicentre trial of physiotherapy in the management of sciatic symptoms. Lancet 1981;1:1065-1068.

29. Doran DM, Newell DJ. Manipulation in treatment of low back pain: a multicentre study. BMJ 1975;2:161-164.

30. Evans DP, Burke MS, Lloyd KN, et al. Lumbar spinal manipulation on trial. Part I: clinical assessment. Rheumatol Rehabil 1978;17:46-53.

31. Gibson T, Grahame R, Harkness J, et al. Controlled comparison of short-wave diathermy treatment with osteopathic treatment in non-specific low back pain. Lancet 1985;1:1258-1261.

32. Glover JR. Arthrography of the joints of the lumbar vertebral arches. Orthop Clin North Am 1977;8:37-42.

33. Hemmilä HM, Keinanen-Kiukaanniemi SM, Levoska S, et al. Does folk medicine work? A randomized clinical trial on patients with prolonged back pain. Arch Phys Med Rehabil 1997;78:571-577.

34. Herzog W, Conway PJ, Willcox BJ. Effects of different treatment modalities on gait symmetry and clinical measures for sacroiliac joint patients. J Manipulative Physiol Ther 1991;14:104-109.

35. Hoehler FK, Tobis JS, Buerger AA. Spinal manipulation for low back pain. JAMA 1981;245:1835-1838.

36. Kinalski R, Kuwik W, Pietrzak D. The comparison of the results of manual therapy versus physiotherapy methods used in treatment of patients with low back pain syndromes. J Manual Med 1989;4:44-46.

37. Koes BW, Bouter LM, van Mameren H, et al. Randomised clinical trial of manipulative therapy and physiotherapy for persistent back and neck complaints: results of one year follow-up. BMJ 1992;304:601-605.

38. MacDonald RS, Bell CM. An open controlled assessment of osteopathic manipulation in nonspecific low-back pain. Spine 1990;15:364-370.

39. Meade TW, Dyer S, Browne W, et al. Randomised comparison of chiropractic and hospital outpatient management for low back pain: results from extended follow up. BMJ 1995;311:349-351.

40. Pope MH, Phillips RB, Haugh LD, et al. A prospective randomized three-week trial of spinal manipulation, transcutaneous muscle stimulation, massage and corset in the treatment of subacute low back pain. Spine 1994;19:2571-2577.

41. Postacchini F, Facchini M, Palieri P. Efficacy of various forms of conservative treatment in low back pain: a comparative study. Neuro-orthopedics 1988;6:28-35.

42. Rupert RL, Wagnon R, Thompson P, et al. Chiropractic adjustments: results of a controlled clinical trial in Egypt. ICA Int Rev Chiro 1985;58-60.

43. Sims-Williams H, Jayson MI, Young SM, et al. Controlled trial of mobilisation and manipulation for patients with low back pain in general practice. BMJ 1978;2:1338-1340.

44. Sims-Williams H, Jayson MI, Young SM, et al. Controlled trial of mobilisation and manipulation for low back pain: hospital patients. BMJ 1979;2:1318-1320.

45. Skargren EI, Carlsson PG, Oberg BE. One-year follow-up comparison of the cost and effectiveness of chiropractic and physiotherapy as primary management for back pain. Sub-group analysis, recurrence, and additional health care utilization. Spine 1998;23:1875-1884.

46. Triano JJ, McGregor M, Hondras MA, et al. Manipulative therapy versus education programs in chronic low back pain. Spine 1995;20:948-955.

47. Waagen GN, Haldeman S, Cook G, et al. Short term trial of chiropractic adjustments for the relief of chronic low back pain. Manual Med 1986;2:63-67.

48. Wreje U, Nordgren B, Aberg H. Treatment of pelvic joint dysfunction in primary care—a controlled study. Scand J Prim Health Care 1992;10:310-315.

49. Zylbergold RS, Piper MC. Lumbar disc disease: comparative analysis of physical therapy treatments. Arch Phys Med Rehabil 1981;62:176-179.

50. Chou R, Huffman LH. Nonpharmacologic therapies for acute and chronic low back pain: a review of the evidence for an American Pain Society/American College of Physicians clinical practice guideline. Ann Intern Med 2007;147: 492-504.

51. Assendelft WJ, Morton SC, Yu EI, et al. Spinal manipulative therapy for low back pain. A meta-analysis of effectiveness relative to other therapies. Ann Intern Med 2003;138: 871-881.

52. Avery S, O'Driscoll ML. Randomised controlled trials on the efficacy of spinal manipulation therapy in the treatment of low back pain. Physical Therapy Reviews 2004;9: 146-152.

53. Brown A, Angus A, Chen S, et al. Costs and outcomes of chiropractic treatment for low back pain. Ottawa: Canadian Coordinating Office for Health Technology, 2005. Report No.: 56.

54. Ernst E, Canter P. Chiropractic spinal manipulation treatment for back pain? A systematic review of randomised clinical trials. Physical Therapy Reviews 2003;8:85-91.

55. Ferreira ML, Ferreira PH, Latimer J, et al. Does spinal manipulative therapy help people with chronic low back pain? Aust J Physiother 2002;48:277-284.

56. Ferreira ML, Ferreira PH, Latimer J, et al. Efficacy of spinal manipulative therapy for low back pain of less than three months' duration. J Manipulative Physiol Ther 2003;26: 593-601.

57. Gay RE, Bronfort G, Evans RL. Distraction manipulation of the lumbar spine: a review of the literature. J Manipulative Physiol Ther 2005;28:266-273.

58. Woodhead T, Clough A. A systematic review of the evidence for manipulation in the treatment of low back pain. J Orthop Med 2005;27:99-120.

59. Cherkin DC, Sherman KJ, Deyo RA, et al. A review of the evidence for the effectiveness, safety, and cost of acupuncture, massage therapy, and spinal manipulation for back pain. Ann Intern Med 2003;138:898-906.

60. Vroomen PC, de Krom MC, Slofstra PD, et al. Conservative treatment of sciatica: a systematic review. J Spinal Disord 2000;13:463-469.

61. Ernst E, White A. Life-threatening adverse reactions after acupuncture? A systematic review. Pain 1997;71:123-126.

62. Jadad AR, Moore RA, Carroll D, et al. Assessing the quality of reports of randomized clinical trials: is blinding necessary? Control Clin Trials 1996;17:1-12.

63. Mendelson G, Selwood TS, Kranz H, et al. Acupuncture treatment of chronic back pain. A double-blind placebo-controlled trial. Am J Med 1983;74:49-55.

64. Ernst E. Prospective investigations into the safety of spinal manipulation. J Pain Symptom Manage 2001;21: 238-242.

65. Oliphant D. Safety of spinal manipulation in the treatment of lumbar disk herniations: a systematic review and risk assessment. J Manipulative Physiol Ther 2004;27:197-210.

66. Stevinson C, Ernst E. Risks associated with spinal manipulation. Am J Med 2002;112:566-571.

67. Meeker WC, Haldeman S. Chiropractic: a profession at the crossroads of mainstream and alternative medicine. Ann Intern Med 2002;136:216-227.

68. Hurwitz EL, Morgenstern H, Harber P, et al. A randomized trial of medical care with and without physical therapy and chiropractic care with and without physical modalities for patients with low back pain: 6-month follow-up outcomes from the UCLA low back pain study. Spine 2002;27: 2193-2204.

69. UK BEAM Trial Team. United Kingdom back pain exercise and manipulation (UK BEAM) randomised trial: effectiveness of physical treatments for back pain in primary care. BMJ 2004;329:1377-1381.

70. Ernst E, Canter PH. A systematic review of systematic reviews of spinal manipulation. J R Soc Med 2006;99:189-193.

71. Bronfort G, Haas M, Moher D, et al. Review conclusions by Ernst and Canter regarding spinal manipulation refuted. Chiropr Osteopat 2006;14:14.

72. Oxman AD, Cook DJ, Guyatt GH. Users' guides to the medical literature. VI. How to use an overview. JAMA 1994;272: 1367-1371.

73. Kaptchuk TJ. Effect of interpretive bias on research evidence. BMJ 2003;326:1453-1455.

74. van Tulder MW, Koes BW, Bouter LM. Conservative treatment of acute and chronic nonspecific low back pain: a systematic review of randomized controlled trials of the most common interventions. Spine 1997;22:2128-2156.

75. van Tulder MW, Koes B, Malmivaara A. Outcome of noninvasive treatment modalities on back pain: an evidence-based review. Eur Spine J 2006;15:S64-S81.

76. Koes BW, Bouter LM, van Mameren H, et al. The effectiveness of manual therapy, physiotherapy, and treatment by the general practitioner for nonspecific back and neck complaints. A randomized clinical trial. Spine 1992;17:28-35.

77. Meade TW, Dyer S, Browne W, et al. Low back pain of mechanical origin: randomised comparison of chiropractic and hospital outpatient treatment. BMJ 1990;300:1431-1437.

78. Hemmilä HM, Keinänen-Kiukaanniemi S, Levoska S, et al. Long-term effectiveness of bone-setting, light exercise therapy, and physiotherapy for prolonged back pain: a randomized controlled trial. J Manipulative Physiol Ther 2002;25:99-104.

79. Giles LG, Müller R. Chronic spinal pain: a randomized clinical trial comparing medication, acupuncture, and spinal manipulation. Spine 2003;28:1490-1502.

80. Müller R, Giles LG. Long-term follow-up of a randomized clinical trial assessing the efficacy of medication, acupuncture, and spinal manipulation for chronic mechanical spinal pain syndromes. J Manipulative Physiol Ther 2005;28:3-11.

81. Giles LGF, Müller R. Chronic spinal pain syndromes: a clinical pilot trial comparing acupuncture, a nonsteroidal anti-inflammatory drug, and spinal manipulation. J Manipulative Physiol Ther 1999;22:376-381.

82. Haas M, Groupp E, Kraemer DF. Dose-response for chiropractic care of chronic low back pain. Spine J 2004;4: 574-583.

83. Tesio L, Merlo A. Autotraction versus passive traction: an open controlled study in lumbar disc herniation. Arch Phys Med Rehabil 1993;74:871-876.

84. Cambron JA, Gudavalli MR, Hedeker D, et al. One-year follow-up of a randomized clinical trial comparing flexion distraction with an exercise program for chronic low-back pain. J Altern Complement Med 2006;12:659-668.

85. Burton AK, Tillotson KM, Cleary J. Single-blind randomised controlled trial of chemonucleolysis and manipulation in the treatment of symptomatic lumbar disc herniation. Eur Spine J 2000;9:202-207.

86. Rasmussen-Barr E, Nilsson-Wikmar L, Arvidsson I. Stabilizing training compared with manual treatment in sub-acute and chronic low-back pain. Man Ther 2003;8:233-241.

87. Ritvanen T, Zaproudina N, Nissen M, et al. Dynamic surface electromyographic responses in chronic low back pain treated by traditional bone setting and conventional physical therapy. J Manipulative Physiol Ther 2007;30:31-37.

88. Skargren EI, Oberg BE, Carlsson PG, et al. Cost and effectiveness analysis of chiropractic and physiotherapy treatment for low back and neck pain. Six-month follow-up. Spine 1997;22:2167-2177.

89. Hurwitz EL, Morgenstern H, Harber P, et al. Second prize—the effectiveness of physical modalities among patients with low back pain randomized to chiropractic care: findings from the UCLA low back pain study. J Manipulative Physiol Ther 2002;25:10-20.

90. Gudavalli MR, Cambron JA, McGregor M, et al. A randomized clinical trial and subgroup analysis to compare flexion-distraction with active exercise for chronic low back pain. Eur Spine J 2006;15:1070-1082.

91. Bigos S, Bowyer O, Braen G, et al. Acute low back problems in adults. Clinical Practice Guideline Number 14. AHCPR Pub. No. 95-0642. Rockville: U.S. Department of Health and Human Services, Public Health Service, Agency for Health Care Policy and Research; 1994. Report No.: AHCPR Publication no. 95-0642.

92. Linton SJ, Hallden K. Can we screen for problematic back pain? A screening questionnaire for predicting outcome in acute and subacute back pain. Clin J Pain 1998;14:209-215.

93. Goldstein MS, Morgenstern H, Hurwitz EL, et al. The impact of treatment confidence on pain and related disability among patients with low-back pain: results from the University of California, Los Angeles, low-back pain study. Spine J 2002;2:391-399.

94. Hurwitz EL, Morgenstern H, Yu F. Satisfaction as a predictor of clinical outcomes among chiropractic and medical patients enrolled in the UCLA low back pain study. Spine 2005;30:2121-2128.

95. Nyiendo J, Haas M, Goldberg B, et al. Pain, disability, and satisfaction outcomes and predictors of outcomes: a practice-based study of chronic low back pain patients attending primary care and chiropractic physicians. J Manipulative Physiol Ther 2001;24:433-439.

96. Haas M, Goldberg B, Aickin M, et al. A practice-based study of patients with acute and chronic low back pain attending primary care and chiropractic physicians: two-week to 48-month follow-up. J Manipulative Physiol Ther 2004;27:160-169.

97. Dvorak J, Kranzlin P, Muhleman D, et al. Musculoskeletal complications. In: Haldeman S, editor. Principles and practice of chiropractic. Norwalk: Appleton & Lange; 1992; p. 549-577.

98. Senstad O, Leboeuf-Yde C, Borchgrevink C. Frequency and characteristics of side effects of spinal manipulative therapy. Spine 1997;22:435-441.

99. Powell FC, Hanigan WC, Olivero WC. A risk/benefit analysis of spinal manipulation therapy for relief of lumbar or cervical pain. Neurosurgery 1993;33:73-78.

100. Assendelft WJ, Bouter LM, Knipschild PG. Complications of spinal manipulation: a comprehensive review of the literature. J Fam Pract 1996;42:475-480.

101. Dagenais S, Roffey DM, Wai EK, et al. Can cost utility evaluations inform decision making about interventions for low back pain? Spine J 2009;9:944-957.

102. van der Roer N, Goossens MEJB, Evers SMAA, et al. What is the most cost-effective treatment for patients with low back pain? A systematic review. Best Pract Res Clin Rheumatol 2005;19:671-684.

103. Niemisto L, Lahtinen-Suopanki T, Rissanen P, et al. A randomized trial of combined manipulation, stabilizing exercises, and physician consultation compared to physician consultation alone for chronic low back pain. Spine 2003;28:2185-2191.

104. Critchley DJ, Ratcliffe J, Noonan S, et al. Effectiveness and cost-effectiveness of three types of physiotherapy used to reduce chronic low back pain disability: a pragmatic randomized trial with economic evaluation. Spine 2007;32:1474-1481.

105. Fritz JM, Delitto A, Erhard RE. Comparison of classification-based physical therapy with therapy based on clinical practice guidelines for patients with acute low back pain: a randomized clinical trial. Spine 2003;28:1363-1371.

106. Mitchell RI, Carmen GM. The functional restoration approach to the treatment of chronic pain in patients with soft tissue and back injuries. Spine 1994;19:633-642.

107. Seferlis T, Lindholm L, Nemeth G. Cost-minimisation analysis of three conservative treatment programmes in 180 patients sick-listed for acute low-back pain. Scand J Prim Health Care 2000;18:53-57.

108. Rivero-Arias O, Gray A, Frost H, et al. Cost-utility analysis of physiotherapy treatment compared with physiotherapy advice in low back pain. Spine 2006;31:1381-1387.

109. Whitehurst DGT, Lewis M, Yao GL, et al. A brief pain management program compared with physical therapy for low back pain: results from an economic analysis alongside a randomized clinical trial. Arthrit Rheum 2007;57:466-473.

110. UK Beam Trial Team. United Kingdom back pain exercise and manipulation (UK BEAM) randomised trial: cost effectiveness of physical treatments for back pain in primary care. BMJ 2004;329:1381.

111. Martin BI, Deyo RA, Mirza SK, et al. Expenditures and health status among adults with back and neck problems. JAMA 2008;299:656-664.

112. Arkuszewski Z. The efficacy of manual treatment in low back pain: a clinical trial. Manual Med 1986;2:68-71.

113. Aure OF, Nilsen JH, Vasseljen O. Manual therapy and exercise therapy in patients with chronic low back pain: a randomized, controlled trial with 1-year follow-up. Spine 2003;28:525-532.

114. Beyerman KL, Palmerino MB, Zohn LE, et al. Efficacy of treating low back pain and dysfunction secondary to osteoarthritis: chiropractic care compared with moist heat alone. J Manipulative Physiol Ther 2006;29:107-114.

CHAPTER 18

SIMON DAGENAIS
JOHN MAYER
SCOTT HALDEMAN

Medicine-Assisted Manipulation Therapy

DESCRIPTION

Terminology and Subtypes

Medicine-assisted manipulation (MAM) is a broad term used to define manipulation of the spine after any type of anesthesia or analgesia, whether facilitated by injections or oral medications. It is often used interchangeably with the term *manipulation under anesthesia* (MUA), which is the oldest and perhaps most commonly used form of MAM.

The various types of MAM discussed in this chapter include MUA, manipulation under joint anesthesia (MUJA), and manipulation under epidural steroid injections (MUESIs). MUA refers to manipulation of the spine while the patient is under general anesthesia or conscious sedation (Figure 18-1). MUJA refers to manipulation of the spine after fluoroscopically guided intra-articular injections of anesthetic or corticosteroid agents. MUESI refers to manipulation of the spine after epidural steroid administration (Figure 18-2).

History and Frequency of Use

Various forms of MAM have been used since the 1930s and several studies were published on MUA in the 1940s and 1950s when it was practiced by some orthopedic surgeons and osteopathic physicians.[1] Early methods for MUA were very different than the modern practice of MAM. Complications from general anesthesia and forceful, long-lever, high-amplitude nonspecific manipulation procedures led to decreased use of early MUA procedures in favor of surgery or other pain management therapies.[1,2] Once it had been largely abandoned by orthopedic surgeons in the 1960s, MUA was modified and revived in the 1990s by chiropractors and, to a lesser extent, osteopathic physicians. The resurgence of MAM was likely the result of increased interest in spinal manipulation therapy (SMT) and the advent of safer, shorter-acting anesthesia agents used for conscious sedation.[1]

Although SMT is commonly used for low back pain (LBP), the use of MAM is relatively rare; no reliable estimates are available on frequency of utilization.

Practitioner, Setting, and Availability

The physician administering the conscious sedation for MUA should be an anesthesiologist, whereas the physician administering the epidural for MUESI or joint injection for MUJA can be an anesthesiologist, pain management physician, physiatrist, or orthopedist. The manual therapist should be extensively trained and licensed to provide SMT without anesthesia, and receive MUA certification from accredited continuing medical education or continuing chiropractic education courses. Certification typically consists of 8 to 12 hours of classroom instruction, an equal amount of practical instruction, and completion of a number of procedures proctored by an experienced MUA therapist. Specific requirements for MUA certification vary by state. For example, Missouri requires 25 hours of instruction and 6 proctored procedures, Wisconsin requires completion of a continuing chiropractic education course and 15 proctored procedures, and Texas requires 24 hours of instruction and 5 proctored procedures.[3] The secondary manual therapist who assists the primary manual therapist should also be certified in MUA.

MUA is typically performed in an outpatient surgical center.[2] MUJA requires a fluoroscopy suite and is typically performed in an outpatient surgical/imaging center.[4] MUESI can be performed in a private practice or outpatient surgical center. The availability of MAM is largely determined by the presence of trained manual therapists working in multidisciplinary settings with medical specialists to administer the anesthesia. The availability of this therapy is therefore difficult to generalize. For instance, there are reports that physicians and chiropractors in the smaller town of Tyler, TX, treated 1000 patients with MUJA over a 7-year period.[4] There is one report that MUA has been performed in more than 20,000 patients based on a literature review and clinician interviews in the United States and United Kingdom.[5]

Procedure

Manipulation under Anesthesia

The treatment procedures for MUA as practiced today are very different than those practiced by orthopedic surgeons in the 1940s and 1950s.[1,2] Performing MUA requires a

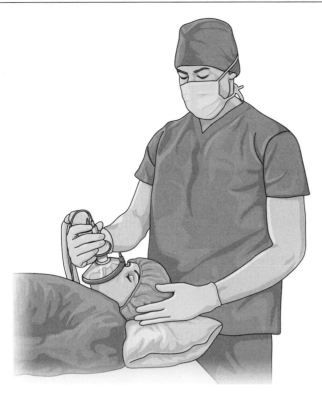

Figure 18-1 Manipulation under anesthesia may involve general anesthesia or conscious sedation.

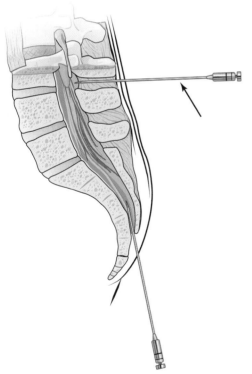

Figure 18-2 Manipulation under epidural anesthesia may involve a caudal, transforaminal, or interlaminar epidural steroid injection. (From Kirkaldy-Willis WH, Bernard TH: Managing low back pain, ed. 4. Philadelphia, 1999, Churchill Livingstone.)

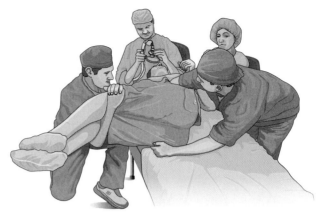

Figure 18-3 Manipulation under anesthesia requires a multidisciplinary team that may include an anesthesiologist, a primary manual therapist, an assistant manual therapist, and a nurse.

multidisciplinary team that may include an anesthesiologist, a trained primary manual therapist (e.g., chiropractor, osteopath), a trained secondary manual therapist, a physical therapist, and a nurse (Figure 18-3).[6] Communication and respect between team members is considered a crucial factor to success with MUA.[7] The MUA procedure generally consists of four stages: sedation, mobilization/stretching/traction, manipulation, and post-MUA care.[2]

The procedure begins with an anesthesiologist who induces deep conscious sedation with intravenous propofol or midazolam and monitors the patient with a cardiac monitor, blood pressure cuff, and oximeter.[1] This form of conscious sedation is considered safer than general anesthesia. The manual therapist then performs a series of mobilization, stretching, and traction procedures to the spine and lower extremities. Less force is applied during these procedures than when the patient is fully awake and use of conscious sedation preserves joint end feel, which helps the therapist determine the amount of force needed.[5]

The procedure may start by passive stretching of the gluteal and hamstring muscles by repeating a motion similar to a single straight leg raise test, progressively increasing the upper range of motion (Figure 18-4). Other stretching procedures might include progressive knee to chest, followed by hip capsule stretching and mobilization in all planes of motion (e.g., Fabere's procedure). Lumbosacral traction may then be applied by repeatedly bringing both knees to the chest while stabilizing the sacrum and manually applying caudal axial distraction. The lateral abdominal and paraspinal muscles may then be stretched by bringing both knees down from the chest to each side of the body while stabilizing the upper body. Other stretching or mobilization procedures may also be applied as needed.

After the stretching and traction procedures, the patient is typically placed in a side-lying position to receive SMT with a high-velocity, short-amplitude thrust applied to a spinous process by hand, while both manual therapists stabilize the upper torso and lower extremities (Figure 18-5). In addition to the lumbosacral area, SMT may also be applied to the

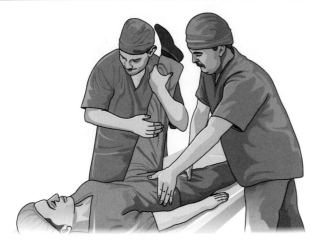

Figure 18-4 Manipulation under anesthesia may include passive stretching of the gluteal and hamstring muscles, progressively increasing the upper range of motion.

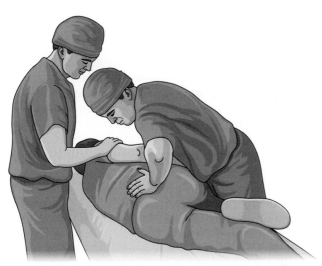

Figure 18-5 Manipulation under anesthesia may require a less forceful thrust by avoiding muscle guarding.

thoracolumbar or cervical area if necessary to address the chronic low back pain (CLBP). These procedures generally take 15 to 20 minutes.

Immediate post-MUA care includes observation by a nurse until the patient recovers from the anesthesia, after which the patient is discharged with instructions to remain active and use heat or ice for short-term analgesic control. Post-MUA care may include 4 to 8 weeks of active rehabilitation and additional manual therapy such as myofascial release techniques, mobilization, SMT, stretching, traction, and therapeutic modalities.

Some proponents of MUA recommend performing the same procedure on 3 consecutive days to achieve optimal results, but there is little scientific evidence to support this practice. The rationale for performing MUA on 3 consecutive days is that each procedure can be gentler because the therapist is not attempting to release all fibrous adhesions in

only one session, which may require greater force. Other practitioners—based on opinion and personal experience—prefer to administer serial MUA only if the patient responds positively to the first procedure but symptoms remain that could perhaps be addressed with one to two more sessions.

Manipulation under Epidural Steroid Injection

MUESI begins with an epidural injection of a corticosteroid and local anesthetic (e.g., 80 mg Depo-Medrol and 3 mL lidocaine 1%) and then proceeds similarly to the MUA procedure described, with fewer general stretching/ mobilization/ traction maneuvers because muscle guarding may still be present.[8]

Manipulation under Joint Anesthesia

MUJA begins with fluoroscopically guided intra-articular injection into zygapophyseal joints with local anesthetic.[7] If greater than 50% improvement in pain is noted, the injection is sometimes repeated with a corticosteroid. The patient may then receive SMT and stretching/mobilization procedures to the lumbosacral area. It has been proposed that 6 to 8 sessions of SMT may be performed over 10 to 14 days after MUJA while the analgesic properties of the injection remain.[4]

Regulatory Status

Not applicable.

THEORY

Mechanism of Action

The use of MAM grew from mostly clinical observation that the combined effects of anesthesia or analgesia obtained through medication as well as SMT were greater when administered simultaneously.[1] Several theories have been offered by practitioners to explain this phenomenon. A commonly proposed mechanism of action for MAM is that the anesthesia or analgesia provided by the medication helps to temporarily decrease local pain and muscle guarding that could interfere with the effective delivery of manual therapies such as SMT, mobilization, traction, and stretching. The general and local relaxation brought about by medication is thought to allow the manual therapist to more effectively break up joint and soft tissue adhesions that would otherwise be impossible if the patient was guarding against these motions. The use of anesthesia or analgesia may also allow SMT to be performed in patients who cannot otherwise tolerate the procedure when fully awake because of excessive guarding or pain.[2]

This enhanced state of readiness may allow practitioners to use less force than would otherwise be required to overcome patient resistance or apprehension.[5] It has also been suggested that MAM can eliminate deeper adhesions that may be present in ligaments, tendons, muscles, or joints, thereby increasing pain-free range of motion.[5] This may occur by manually disrupting abnormal cross-linking in collagen fibers that form after incomplete healing from injury, without precipitating the acute inflammation cascade that may result in scar tissue formation.[6] With MUESI and MUJA, the use of corticosteroid may help address the inflammatory component of CLBP while manual therapy addresses its mechanical component, creating a synergistic treatment effect.[8] However, there is no experimental research specifically on MUA, MUESI, or MUJA to confirm or refute these theories.

Indication

The general indication for MAM proposed by practitioners is nonspecific mechanical CLBP that has failed to respond to more conservative treatment options. There is general agreement among guidelines and training materials for MUA that patients should first try 4 to 8 weeks of SMT and other conservative care before considering MUA, unless SMT cannot be attempted because of severe pain or muscle spasm.[1,2,4,6-9] The specific indication for MUA is fairly consistent in the clinical literature and consists of CLBP with a hypomobility or soft tissue component. Some practitioners also consider patients with failed back surgery, nerve entrapment, chronic myositis, chronic fibrositis, motion restriction after trauma, or chronic muscle contracture reasonable candidates for MUA or other forms of MAM.[3] It has been estimated that 3% to 10% of chiropractic patients may be appropriate candidates for MUA.[2] These purported indications are based solely on the clinical opinion and experience of MUA therapists and have not been confirmed by controlled scientific studies.

Anecdotal experience suggests that the ideal patient who is most likely to respond to MAM is someone with nonspecific mechanical CLBP resulting from suspected hypomobility from articular or myofascial adhesions who responds positively to manual therapies but experiences only short-term improvement.[2] This patient should be otherwise healthy, have no contraindications to anesthesia/analgesia, and have no red flags or psychosocial yellow flags associated with a poor prognosis for LBP.[10]

Assessment

Before receiving MAM, patients should first be assessed for LBP using an evidence-based and goal-oriented approach focused on the patient history and neurologic examination, as discussed in Chapter 3. Additional diagnostic imaging or specific diagnostic testing is generally not required before initiating this intervention for CLBP. The physician should also inquire about medication history to note prior hypersensitivity/allergy or adverse events with similar drugs, and evaluate contraindications for the types of drugs used during MAM. Although it has been suggested that anteroposterior, lateral, oblique, flexion/extension, and lateral bending lumbar spine x-rays can help identify specific vertebral levels that may be corrected during the procedure and contrast magnetic resonance imaging can help distinguish disc herniation from fibrosis, there is no scientific evidence to confirm that these imaging studies impact the outcomes of treatment.[2,6,11] Preanesthesia clearance must also be obtained by the anesthesiologist before MUA.

EFFICACY

Evidence supporting the efficacy of these interventions for CLBP was summarized from recent clinical practice guidelines (CPGs), systematic reviews (SRs), and randomized controlled trials (RCTs). Observational studies (OBSs) were also summarized where appropriate. Findings are summarized by study design.

Clinical Practice Guidelines

None of the recent national CPGs on the management of CLBP have assessed and summarized the evidence to make specific recommendations about the efficacy of MAM.

One other CPG related only to chiropractic interventions gave MUA an equivocal rating because of insufficient evidence to support or refute its value.[12]

Systematic Reviews

No recent, high-quality SRs by the Cochrane Collaboration were identified that reported specifically on the efficacy of MAM as an intervention for LBP.

Other

An independent health technology assessment group recently conducted an SR of MUA for LBP.[3] To uncover relevant evidence, multiple databases were searched including MEDLINE, EMBASE, CINAHL, Cochrane Library, Allied and Alternative Medicine, CHID, ECRI, Mantis, Rehab-DATA, and the US National Guideline Clearinghouse. The computerized database search was complemented by hand-searching related journals and searching gray literature. Study eligibility criteria were as follows: more than 10 patients, published after 1970, and related to MUA for LBP. That assessment uncovered five studies related to MUA for LBP including one RCT, a prospective cohort study, and three retrospective case series.[9,13-16] The three retrospective case series were excluded because of poor study quality. In the other studies, the length of LBP for participants was not reported and it was therefore not possible to determine whether it constituted CLBP. The SR concluded that the evidence evaluated on MUA for LBP was small, of poor quality, and could not support drawing any evidence-based conclusions.[3]

A review of MAM was published earlier in *The Spine Journal* by members of our research group.[1] The literature was searched using PubMed and the review included all studies related to MUA, MUJA, and MUESI for acute or chronic spinal disorders. The review uncovered 10 case series related to MUA for LBP, sciatica, or lumbar disc herniations, although it was unclear whether participants had acute or chronic LBP. The majority (80%) of those studies had been published in the 1930s (n = 1), 1950s (n = 3), 1960s (n = 2), or 1970s (n = 2) when the procedure was mostly performed by orthopedic surgeons or osteopathic physicians and differed considerably from MUA as currently taught and practiced. Nevertheless, almost all (90%) of those case series reported generally positive findings that ranged from

TABLE 18-1	Systematic Review Findings of Medicine-Assisted Manipulation for Chronic Low Back Pain		
Reference	# RCTs in SR	# RCTs for CLBP	Conclusion
3	1	0	Small and poor-quality evidence could not support drawing evidence-based conclusions for MUA
1	10 case series	0	All of the case series reported generally positive results but studies had poor methodologic quality and 8/10 were published more than 30 years ago

CLBP, chronic low back pain; MUA, manipulation under anesthesia; RCT, randomized controlled trial; SR, systematic review.

short-term improvements in pain to long-term changes in function. The review also uncovered evidence related to other forms of MAM including four case series on MUESI for CLBP, one case series on SMT with caudal anesthesia for LBP (duration unknown), and one case series on MUJA for CLBP. All of the case series reported generally positive results. The review noted that although findings reported in most case series for MUA, MUESI, and MUJA were positive, they had poor methodologic quality, lacked control groups, and had an incomplete understanding of the purported benefits of combining SMT with anesthesia/analgesia.

Findings from the SRs are summarized in Table 18-1.

Randomized Controlled Trials

No RCTs were identified evaluating MAM as an intervention for CLBP.

Observational Studies

Six observational studies were identified and are summarized here (Tables 18-2 and 18-3).

An observational study examined a prospective cohort of patients with CLBP who received 4 to 6 weeks of chiropractic care with SMT, manual therapy, and exercise.[17] Participants were eligible if they had CLBP for more than 3 months, reduced lumbopelvic flexibility as measured by failure to bring fingertips to floor, and were 18 to 60 years old; exclusion criteria were fracture, infection, tumor, nonmechanical cause of LBP, active rheumatoid disease, tobacco use, coagulation disorder, contraindications to anesthesia, severe coexisting disease, and worker's compensation or litigation related to the current episode of LBP. Those who failed to achieve substantial improvements in pain, function, or flexibility after 4 to 6 weeks were given the option of receiving one to three sessions of MUA with conscious sedation and

internal traction of the sacrococcygeal region. Of the 68 participants recruited into the study, 42 (62%) received MUA and 26 (38%) continued to receive chiropractic care and acted as a control group. Outcomes were measured at baseline, 6 weeks, 3 months, 6 months, and 12 months using the North American Spine Society composite questionnaire that included pain, disability, quality of life, patient expectations of treatment outcomes, and comorbidities. Baseline differences were noted between groups in pain and disability and participants who eventually received MUA presented with significantly worse symptoms upon entering the study and failed to improve as much as the control groups after 4 to 6 weeks of chiropractic care. After receiving MUA, however, their improvement increased considerably and they overtook the control group behind which they had lagged after 3 months. There were no differences in outcomes between groups in subsequent follow-up at 6 or 12 months. Authors concluded that participants with CLBP presenting with greater symptoms were more likely to receive a recommendation for MUA, which appeared to offer them increased improvements over chiropractic care without MUA.

A study was conducted examining a prospective cohort of patients with CLBP presenting for care to chiropractors affiliated with surgical centers offering MUA.[14] Participants were included if they were older than 18 years, had CLBP for more than 6 months, had clinical eligibility for MUA as established by the National Association for Manipulation Under Anesthesia Practitioners, and had received at least 4 weeks of SMT before enrolling in the study. Although all participants received a recommendation for MUA, not all were approved for the procedure by their insurance companies. Those who did (n = 38) and did not (n = 49) receive insurance approval were compared after one to four daily MUA procedures (mean, 2.7) and 4 weeks of chiropractic care (MUA group) or continued chiropractic care only (chiropractic group). MUA consisted of conscious sedation with propofol, stretching, mobilization, and SMT. Outcomes were assessed with the Numerical Pain Rating Scale (NPRS) and Roland Morris Disability Questionnaire (RMDQ) at baseline, after their last MUA procedure, and 4 weeks later. NPRS scores at baseline, post-MUA, and 4 weeks later were 7.3, 4.4, and 3.7 for the MUA group and 6.8, 5.9, and 5.0 for the chiropractic group. RMDQ scores at baseline, post-MUA, and 4 weeks later were 10.9, 7.8, and 5.3 for the MUA group and 6.9, 5.6, and 4.3 for the chiropractic group. Although both groups improved, there were greater changes from baseline in both outcomes in the MUA group; it was unclear whether these differences were statistically significant.

An observational cohort study reported on patients presenting for care to chiropractors with a variety of spinal complaints.[9] Eligibility criteria included consideration for MUA based on a diagnostic/treatment algorithm (e.g., 2 to 6 weeks of failed conservative care) and absence of contraindications or severe coexisting disease. Of the 200 potentially eligible participants, 177 were enrolled and 168 (95%) completed follow-up visits. Participants presented with cervicocranial, cervical, thoracic, lumbar, or pelvic complaints. Although the areas of complaint were dichotomized into cervical or lumbar for study purposes, the number of

TABLE 18-2	Designs of Observational Studies of Medicine Assisted Manipulation for Chronic Low Back Pain			
Reference	Study Design	Indication	Intervention	Control
17	Prospective cohort	LBP with or without neurologic involvement, symptoms >3 months	MAM: 4-6 wk SMT followed by 1-3 treatments of modified MUA with internal traction and mobilization of the sacrococcygeal region n = 42	4-6 weeks SMT followed by 4-12 weeks of additional SMT n = 26
14	Prospective cohort	LBP with or without neurologic involvement, symptoms >6 months	MAM: 1-4 MUA procedures over consecutive days followed by specific MUA rehabilitation lasting 4-6 weeks n = 38	SMT, passive modalities, HEP, 3×/week, 4 weeks n = 49
9	Prospective cohort without an unexposed group	LBP, neurologic involvement NR, symptoms >2-6 weeks	MAM: 3 MUA procedures followed by SMT, passive modalities, HEP for several weeks n = 177	NA
18	Case series	CLBP with or without neurologic involvement, symptoms >3 months	MUESI: 1 ESI and SMT n = 10	NA
8	Retrospective case series	Cervical back pain or LBP with neurologic involvement, symptoms >4-6 weeks	MUESI: ESI, flexion-distraction mobilization n = 60	SMT, 1-3 sessions
7	Case reports	LBP with or without neurologic involvement, symptoms >4 weeks	MUJA: 1 intra-articular injection of anesthetic and corticosteroid followed by SMT for several times over 2 weeks n = 4	NA

CLBP, chronic low back pain; ESI, epidural steroid injection; HEP, home exercise program; LBP, low back pain; MAM, medicine-assisted manipulation; MUA, manipulation under anesthesia; MUESI, manipulation under epidural steroid injection; MUJA, manipulation under joint anesthesia; NA, not applicable; NR, not reported; SMT, spinal manipulation therapy.

participants in each category was not reported. Outcomes were assessed by visual analog scale (VAS) and range of motion before and after MUA and at 6 months post-MUA. Lumbar range of motion increased an average of 83%, and lumbar VAS improved from 7.3 at baseline to 4.9 post-MUA and to 3.0 after 6 months. Return to work and analgesic consumption also improved, although results were not presented separately for the cervical and lumbar patients.

A case series was presented in which 10 participants with mechanical CLBP who had failed to achieve greater than 50% improvement with conservative care such as medication, epidural steroid injections, physical therapy, and a minimum of six sessions of SMT received MUESI.[18] Participants were excluded if they had any contraindications to SMT or severe coexisting disease. The MUESI procedure included 10 mg oral diazepam and injection of 10 mL containing lidocaine, saline, and 15 mg betamethasone into the epidural space under fluoroscopic guidance, followed by

SMT within 30 to 60 minutes of the injection. Outcomes were assessed upon completing conservative care and 30 days after the MUESI using a self-reported global improvement scale (0%-100%). The mean self-reported improvement after MUESI was 25% and represented a statistically significant change from baseline ($P = .0015$).

A retrospective case series reported on 60 patients with mechanical LBP and radiculopathy who had failed to respond to prior conservative care with mobilization, SMT, exercise, and nonsteroidal anti-inflammatory drugs and were treated with MUESI.[8] Participants were excluded if they had cauda equina syndrome or other severe coexisting disease. The epidural steroid injection was performed using 80 mg Depo-Medrol and 3 mL of 1% lidocaine, after which flexion-distraction mobilization and SMT were applied. Outcomes were assessed according to the following three categories of improvement: (1) significant (resolution of pain, no further care), (2) temporary (reduction of pain but further

TABLE 18-3 | **Outcomes of Observational Studies of Medicine-Assisted Manipulation for Chronic Low Back Pain**

Reference	Outcomes and Follow-Up Period	Intervention	Control	Results
17	Pain/disability (101-point scale based on NASS composite instrument) Improvement—3 months/12 months	Improvement: 39%	Improvement: 13%	Mean difference between groups: 4.4 (NS)
17	HRQOL (SF-36)—Improvement 3 months/12 months	33%	14%	Mean difference between groups: 0.3 (NS)
14	Pain (NPRS)—4 weeks after last MUA	50%	26%	P value NR
14	Disability (RMDQ)—4 weeks after last MUA	Disability: 51%	Disability: 38%	P value NR
9	Pain (VAS)—6 months after last MUA	Pain: 59%		P value NR
9	ROM—6 months after last MUA	NR	NR	P value NR
8	Improvement (symptoms and need for care)—12 months	20/60 (33%) significant 27/60 (45%) temporary 13/60 (22%) no change		
7	Pain relief (unspecified)—4 months—6 months	Nearly complete relief (n = 1) 3 pain-free (n = 3)		
18	Global improvement (self-reported scale)—1 month	25%		$P = .002$

CON, control; HRQOL, health-related quality of life; MAM, medicine-assisted manipulation; MUA, manipulation under anesthesia; NASS, North American Spine Society; NPRS, Numerical Pain Rating Scale; NR, not reported; NS, not significant; RMDQ, Roland Morris Disability Questionnaire; ROM, range of motion; VAS, visual analog scale.

Follow-up: Time from onset of intervention, unless otherwise noted.

Results: Mean change (improvement) scores from treatment initiation, unless otherwise noted.

nonsurgical care needed), and (3) no change (required subsequent surgery). After 12-month follow-up, 20 of 60 (33%) had significant improvement, 27 of 60 (45%) had temporary improvement, and 13 of 60 (22%) had no change.

Four cases were presented in which patients with CLBP who obtained partial, short-term relief with conservative or manual therapy but failed to improve completely received MUJA.[7] Upon successfully locating the source of their pain through challenge injections to the zygapophyseal joints or sacroiliac joints under fluoroscopy, patients underwent SMT to that area several times for 2 weeks after the injection. Outcomes were assessed subjectively before and after MUJA. Results were considered encouraging in that one patient had nearly complete pain relief after 4 months and three remained pain-free at 6 months.

SAFETY

Contraindications

There are no specific contraindications to MUA beyond those of its individual components (e.g., anesthesia and SMT).[1] In general, these contraindications include spinal malignancy, hypermobility, instability, acute inflammation, infection, fracture, progressive neurologic deficits, large aortic aneurysms, bleeding disorders, severe osteoporosis, acute gout, spinal cord compression, severe canal stenosis, sequestered nucleus pulposus, or cardiopulmonary conditions precluding anesthesia.[3]

It has also been suggested that procedures such as MUA are not appropriate for patients who could improve with a simpler, more cost effective therapy that does not involve anesthesia.[19] Judging from participant exclusion criteria used in previous studies on MAM, it would appear that patients with nonmechanical CLBP, active rheumatoid disease, tobacco use, severe coexisting disease, severe obesity, and involvement in worker's compensation or litigation are less likely to respond favorably to MUA, MUJA, or MUESI.[1]

Adverse Events

Older forms of MUA as practiced many decades ago using more forceful long-lever techniques were associated with adverse events (AEs) such as cauda equina syndrome, paralysis, and fracture.[1] However, more recent studies evaluating newer, presumably gentler techniques of MUA have not reported any serious AEs.[1] Temporary flare-ups in lumbosacral pain have been reported and are attributed to the stretching of adhesions and mobilization of inflamed joints achieved by MUA; such flare-ups are easily treated with appropriate post-MUA care (e.g., stretching, analgesics, heat/ice).[5]

A review of the MAM literature reported a total of 11 AEs in 17 studies with a total of 1525 participants (prevalence <1%).[1] These AEs included eight cases of increased lumbosacral pain, one case of myelographic evidence of herniated intervertebral disc, and two cases of respiratory distress that resolved with Valium.[1] Most observational studies have reported no AEs from MUA.[1,7,9,14,18] An additional review of MUA reported no AEs in any of the published studies, indicating they are likely rare.[3]

One cohort study on both cervical and lumbar MUESI reported two wet taps and one vagal response, although it was unclear whether those were related to cervical or lumbar procedures.[8] If malpractice insurance premiums may be used as a proxy for the perceived harms associated with a procedure, it should be noted that two large chiropractic malpractice insurers provide MUA coverage at no additional charge to their members.[2]

COSTS

Fees and Third-Party Reimbursement

In the United States, treatment with MUA that is delivered by a licensed health care practitioner such as a chiropractor or physician in an outpatient setting can be delivered using a variety of CPT codes. Some of these CPT codes may include 22505 (manipulation of the spine under anesthesia), 98940 (chiropractic manipulation, 1-2 regions), 98925 (osteopathic manipulation, 1-2 regions), 97140 (manual therapy, each 15 minutes), 97124 (massage, each 15 minutes), or 97112 (neuromuscular re-education, each 15 minutes). Because a second manual therapist is usually present to assist with this procedure, two providers may charge these fees, with slightly reduced fees for the MUA assistant. Although there are no specific codes for the manual therapy component of MUJA or MUESI, it has been suggested that the SMT component of those procedures should not cost any more than traditional SMT.[4]

Additional professional fees will also be charged by the physician administering the anesthesia, joint anesthesia, or epidural steroid injection for MAM. The outpatient surgical center in which the procedure takes place also charges facility fees for use of their operating room, recovery room, disposable medical equipment, nurses, radiology, and other services. Fees may also be charged for traveling to the outpatient facility and preparing reports. Because of these ancillary fees, the total cost of an MUA procedure can reach $5000 or more, although there is wide variation in fees.

Reimbursement policies regarding MUA vary widely from state to state. It was reported in 2003 that MUA was generally covered by the Texas Worker's Compensation board, Texas Board of Insurance, and HSG administrators of Pennsylvania.[3] The same report also noted that MUA was

TABLE 18-4	Medicare Fee Schedule for Related Services	
CPT Code	New York	California
22505	$114	$121
98940	$25	$27
98925	$29	$32
97140	$28	$30
97124	$24	$26
97112	$31	$33

2010 Participating, nonfacility amount.

generally not covered by BlueCross/BlueShield of Tennessee and North Carolina, nor was it covered by Aetna; it was also stated at the time that there was no Medicare coverage policy on MUA.[3] MUA was covered intermittently in California by the Worker's Compensation Board and various private insurers when preapproval was obtained, but recent changes in legislation have cast serious doubts on the future of MUA in California (Table 18-4).[20]

Insurance carriers may argue that MUA is experimental or investigational. However, denials for such reasons can be appealed. CPT code 22505 is considered a category 1 CPT code, which the CPT Advisory Committee and the CPT Editorial Panel have stated do not represent experimental or emerging technology. In order for a procedure to be listed as a category 1 CPT code, it must have gone through clinical trials and a review process by a panel of practitioners who have made recommendations to classify the procedure as a category 1 code for specific indications.[20]

Cost Effectiveness

No cost effectiveness analyses were identified which evaluated the cost effectiveness of MAM as an intervention for LBP.

SUMMARY

Description

Medicine-assisted manipulation is a broad term used to define manipulation of the spine after any type of anesthesia or analgesia, whether facilitated by injections or oral medications. There are various types of MAM, including MUA, MUJA, and MUESIs. Although various forms of MAM have been used since the 1930s, the use of MAM for LBP is quite rare, and reliable estimates of frequency of utilization are not available. An anesthesiologist should administer the conscious sedation for MUA, whereas nonsurgical or surgical spine specialists should administer the epidural steroidal injection or joint injection for MUESI and MUJA, respectively. These procedures are typically performed in secondary care settings, such as specialty spine clinics and pain management clinics. MUJA requires that the center be able to perform fluoroscopy.

Theory

The use of MAM grew from mostly clinical observation that the combined effects of anesthesia or analgesia obtained through medication as well as SMT were greater when administered simultaneously. A commonly supported mechanism of action for MAM is that the anesthesia or analgesia provided by the medication helps to temporarily decrease local pain and allows the therapist to more effectively break up joint and soft tissue adhesions that would not be possible if the patient was guarding against these motions. The use of anesthesia or analgesia may also allow SMT to be performed in patients who cannot tolerate the procedure when fully awake because of excessive guarding or pain. The indication for MAM is nonspecific mechanical CLBP that has failed to respond to more conservative treatment options. Diagnostic imaging or other forms of advanced testing is generally not required before administering MAM for CLBP.

Efficacy

None of the recent national CPGs make specific recommendations about the efficacy of MAM for LBP, yet a chiropractic CPG reported insufficient evidence supporting MUA. An SR conducted by an independent health technology assessment group concluded that the evidence evaluated on MUA for LBP was small, of poor quality, and could not support drawing any evidence-based conclusions. Another SR reported that although findings reported in most case series for MUA, MUESI, and MUJA were positive, they had poor methodologic quality, lacked control groups, and had an incomplete understanding of the purported benefits of combining SMT with anesthesia/analgesia. No eligible RCTs were uncovered related to MUA, MUJA, or MUESI.

Safety

There are no specific contraindications to MUA beyond those of its individual components (e.g., anesthesia and SMT). In general, these contraindications include spinal malignancy, hypermobility, instability, acute inflammation, infection, fracture, progressive neurologic deficits, large aortic aneurysms, bleeding disorders, severe osteoporosis, acute gout, spinal cord compression, severe canal stenosis, sequestered nucleus pulposus, or cardiopulmonary conditions precluding anesthesia. Older forms of MUA as practiced many decades ago using more forceful long-lever techniques were associated with adverse events such as cauda equina syndrome, paralysis, and fracture. However, more recent studies evaluating newer, gentler techniques of MUA only report minor adverse events, such as increased lumbosacral pain, herniated intervertebral disc, respiratory distress, wet taps, and vagal response.

Costs

The total cost of an MUA procedure can reach $5000 or more, although there is wide variation in fees. The cost effectiveness of MUA, MUJA, and MUESI has not been evaluated.

Comments

Evidence from the CPGs, SRs, and OBSs reviewed was conflicting regarding the use of MAM for CLBP. As noted in previous studies, generalizing prior MUA literature is very challenging because of participant heterogeneity and differences between treatment procedures used several decades ago and those used today.[1,14] Overall, the methodologic quality of the studies uncovered related to MUA, MUESI, and MUJA is weak, and evidence consists mainly of OBSs. However, most studies on these procedures have reported generally positive results, indicating that patients who undergo their procedures have a reasonable short-term prognosis. There is currently insufficient evidence to make any definitive conclusions concerning the efficacy of MUA, MUJA, or MUESI for CLBP.

As with other manual therapies, it is challenging to conduct quality research in MAM. Eligibility for MUA often includes a requirement for prior failed SMT, making SMT alone a poor control group because those proceeding to MUA would have already been identified as not responding to SMT.[3] However, a study in which participants at baseline are deemed eligible for MUA, MUJA, and MUESI, and randomly allocated to the procedure or an alternative treatment approach would provide information as to the relative outcome after two treatment approaches even if there was no blinding of participants or clinicians. An independent observer, however, is essential. The recent examples from studies comparing outcomes in patients who had lumbar surgery with those who did not have surgery could serve as templates for clinical trials to determine the efficacy of MUA. There is a strong need for comparative clinical trials, large cohort studies, and experimental studies to support the theories on which these treatment approaches are based.

Despite being used for more than 80 years, there is currently insufficient research to help clinicians, policy makers, and especially patients make a decision about whether to consider MAM for CLBP. At present, MAM can be considered one of the multiple treatment approaches that have been proposed for the management of CLBP whose primary justification is the mostly positive experience of clinicians, a few OBSs, and some presumably satisfied patients. These procedures deserve the same consideration that is given to other treatment approaches with similarly weak supporting evidence, and further research is required.

CHAPTER REVIEW QUESTIONS

Answers are located on page 451.
1. Which of the following is not a variant of manipulation under anesthesia?
   a. manipulation under epidural steroid injection
   b. manipulation under conscious sedation
   c. manipulation under joint anesthesia
   d. manipulation under open discectomy
2. True or false: MAM is a cost effective procedure.
3. True or false: Many national CPGs have assessed MAM.

4. True or false: All forms of MAM require fluoroscopy.

5. True or false: MAM is widely performed across the United States.

6. Which historical milestones revived the practice of MAM?

   a. increased interest in trigger point injections

   b. advent of shorter-acting anesthetics

   c. advent of anesthetics for epidural steroid injections

   d. invention of new manipulation techniques

7. Which of the following diagnostic imaging tests must be performed prior to MAM?

   a. CT

   b. MRI

   c. x-rays

   d. none of the above

8. Which of the following is generally an indication for MAM?

   a. spondylolisthesis

   b. spinal stenosis

   c. spinal hypomobility due to suspected soft tissue adhesions

   d. degenerative disc disorder

REFERENCES

1. Kohlbeck FJ, Haldeman S. Medication-assisted spinal manipulation. Spine J 2002;2:288-302.

2. Cremata E, Collins S, Clauson W, et al. Manipulation under anesthesia: a report of four cases. J Manipulative Physiol Ther 2005;28:526-533.

3. ECRI Health Technology Assessment Group. Manipulation under anesthesia for treatment of low back pain: an evidence-based assessment. Plymouth, PA: ECRI; 2003.

4. Michaelsen MR. Manipulation under joint anesthesia/analgesia: a proposed interdisciplinary treatment approach for recalcitrant spinal axis pain of synovial joint origin. J Manipulative Physiol Ther 2000;23:127-129.

5. Gordon RC. An evaluation of the experimental and investigational status and clinical validity of manipulation of patients under anesthesia: a contemporary opinion. J Manipulative Physiol Ther 2001;24:603-611.

6. Davis CG, Fernando CA, da Motta MA. Manipulation of the low back under general anesthesia: case studies and discussion. J Neuromusculoskel Syst 1993;1:126-134.

7. Dreyfuss P, Michaelsen M, Horne M. MUJA: manipulation under joint anesthesia/analgesia: a treatment approach for recalcitrant low back pain of synovial joint origin. J Manipulative Physiol Ther 1995;18:537-546.

8. Dougherty P, Bajwa S, Burke J, et al. Spinal manipulation postepidural injection for lumbar and cervical radiculopathy: a retrospective case series. J Manipulative Physiol Ther 2004;27:449-456.

9. West DT, Mathews RS, Miller MR, et al. Effective management of spinal pain in one hundred seventy-seven patients evaluated for manipulation under anesthesia. J Manipulative Physiol Ther 1999;22:299-308.

10. Krismer M, van TM. Strategies for prevention and management of musculoskeletal conditions. Low back pain (non-specific). Best Pract Res Clin Rheumatol 2007;21:77-91.

11. Greenman PE. Manipulation with the patient under anesthesia. J Am Osteopath Assoc 1992;92:1159-1170.

12. The World Chiropractic Alliance. The Guidelines for Chiropractic Quality Assurance and Practice Parameters (Mercy Guidelines). The World Chiropractic Alliance 1993. Available at: http://www.worldchiropracticalliance.org/positions/mercy.htm.

13. Siehl D, Olson DR, Ross HE, et al. Manipulation of the lumbar spine with the patient under general anesthesia: evaluation by electromyography and clinical-neurologic examination of its use for lumbar nerve root compression syndrome. J Am Osteopath Assoc 1971;70:433-440.

14. Palmieri NF, Smoyak S. Chronic low back pain: a study of the effects of manipulation under anesthesia. J Manipulative Physiol Ther 2002;25:E8-E17.

15. Morey LW Jr. Osteopathic manipulation under general anesthesia. J Am Osteopath Assoc 1973;73:116-127.

16. Burn JM. Treatment of chronic lumbosciatic pain. Proc R Soc Med 1973;66:544.

17. Kohlbeck FJ, Haldeman S, Hurwitz EL, et al. Supplemental care with medication-assisted manipulation versus spinal manipulation therapy alone for patients with chronic low back pain. J Manipulative Physiol Ther 2005;28:245-252.

18. Nelson L, Aspegren D, Bova C. The use of epidural steroid injection and manipulation on patients with chronic low back pain. J Manipulative Physiol Ther 1997;20:263-266.

19. Kolsi I, Delecrin J, Berthelot JM, et al. Efficacy of nerve root versus interspinous injections of glucocorticoids in the treatment of disk-related sciatica. A pilot, prospective, randomized, double-blind study. Joint Bone Spine 2000;67:113-118.

20. California Academy for Manipulation Under Anesthesia. California Academy for Manipulation Under Anesthesia guidelines. Cornerstone Professional Education Inc 2001. Available at http://www.backpainaway.info.

CHAPTER 19

JOEL J. GAGNIER

Nutritional, Herbal, and Homeopathic Supplements

DESCRIPTION

Terminology and Subtypes

The United States Dietary Supplement Health and Education Act of 1994 defines a nutritional supplement as "a product (other than tobacco) that is intended to supplement the diet that bears or contains one or more of the following dietary ingredients: a vitamin, a mineral, an herb or other botanical, an amino acid, a dietary substance for use by man to supplement the diet by increasing the total daily intake, or a concentrate, metabolite, constituent, extract, or combinations of these ingredients" (Figure 19-1).[1] The equivalent legislation in Canada is the Natural Health Products (NHPs) Regulations, which defines an NHP as a natural source "substance that is manufactured, sold, or represented for use in: (1) the diagnosis, treatment, mitigation, or prevention of a disease, disorder or abnormal physical state or its symptoms in humans; (2) restoring or correcting organic functions in humans; or (3) modifying organic functions in humans, such as modifying those functions in a manner that maintains or promotes health."[2]

Nutritional supplements are often associated with complementary and alternative medicine (CAM), which encompasses a group of diverse medical and health care systems, practices, and products that are not considered part of conventional medicine.[3] The main types of nutritional supplements that will be discussed in this chapter are herbal medicines, vitamins, minerals, and homeopathic remedies. The use of other supplements, such as accessory nutrients (e.g., coenzyme Q10), macronutrients (e.g., fatty acids, amino acids), and other macromolecules (e.g., glucosamine, bee pollen) are not reviewed in the chapter. Nutritional supplements are also termed *dietary supplements* or *supplements*.

Herbal Medicines

Herbal medicines, also called herbal medicinal products, are a diverse group of heterogeneous substances and products that can be delivered in a number of ways, including as whole herbs, herbal materials, herbal preparations, and finished herbal products that contain, as active ingredients, plants or plant materials. The term *herbal medicine* excludes single compounds that are derived and purified from plants or synthesized in laboratory settings.[4] By definition, herbal medicines are used for medicinal purposes and may be taken by oral ingestion, injection, or applied topically. Oral herbal medicines include raw plant material (dried or fresh), liquid extracts (with alcohol, aqueous, or glycerin solvents), and solid extracts (e.g., lyophilized or freeze dried) (Figures 19-2 and 19-3). Some forms of herbal medicine are given via intramuscular (IM) or intravenous routes. Topical forms include creams, gels, ointments, oils, plasters, and poultices.

Vitamins and Minerals

Vitamins are a group of substances essential for normal metabolism, growth, development, and regulation of cell function. They work together with enzymes, cofactors (substances that assist enzymes), and other substances necessary for normal bodily functions. The two main types of vitamins are fat-soluble (e.g., vitamins A, D, E, K) and water-soluble (e.g., vitamins B and C). Minerals are similarly defined as a group of substances essential for normal metabolism, growth, development, body structure, cell function regulation, and electrolyte balance. The two main types of minerals are macrominerals (e.g., calcium, phosphorus, sodium) and trace minerals (e.g., zinc, selenium, manganese).[5] There are many forms of vitamins and minerals as well as many routes of administration. For example, vitamin C can be manufactured

Supplement Facts

Serving Size 1 Capsule

Amount Per Capsule	% Daily Value
Calories 20	
Calories from Fat 20	
Total Fat 2 g	3%*
Saturated Fat 0.5 g	3%*
Polyunsaturated Fat 1 g	†
Monounsaturated Fat 0.5 g	†
Vitamin A 4250 IU	85%
Vitamin D 425 IU	106%
Omega-3 fatty acids 0.5 g	†

* Percent Daily Values are based on a 2,000 calorie diet.
† Daily Value not established.

Ingredients: Cod liver oil, gelatin, water, and glycerin.

Figure 19-1 A nutritional supplement contains a vitamin, mineral, herb, botanical, amino acid, dietary substance, or a concentrate, metabolite, constituent, extract, or combination thereof. (Courtesy US Food and Drug Administration.)

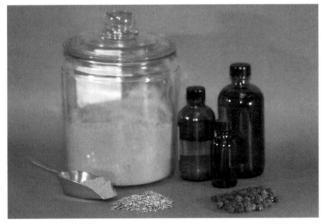

Figure 19-2 Herbal supplements as dried plant materials and liquid plant extracts. (Photo by Martin Wall Photography.)

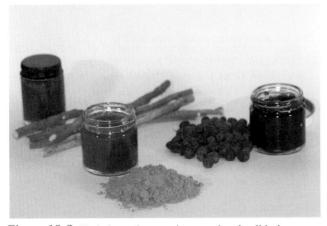

Figure 19-3 Herbal supplements in natural and solid plant extract states. (Photo by Martin Wall Photography.)

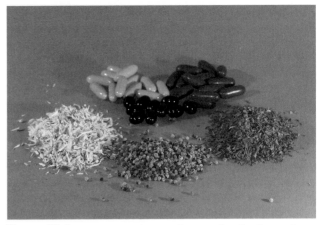

Figure 19-4 Vitamin supplements in natural and gel capsule forms. (Photo by Martin Wall Photography.)

as ascorbic acid or ascorbate, and calcium is available as calcium carbonate, calcium citrate, or calcium lactate. Vitamin and mineral supplements are frequently mixed with other vitamins, minerals, or herbal medicines that are thought to enhance their action. Different types of vitamins and minerals can be compounded in a variety of ways, including as capsules, tablets, liquids, gels, or creams (Figure 19-4).

Homeopathic Remedies

Homeopathy is a system of healing established by Samuel Hahnemann two centuries ago that is founded on the "law of similars" *(similia similibus curentur)*. This principle states that if a substance is capable of inducing a series of symptoms in a healthy living system, microscopically low doses of the same substance can also be used to cure those same symptoms under certain circumstances.[6] Homeopathic supplements are generally termed *remedies* and can be made from virtually any naturally occurring substance (e.g., herbal, animal, mineral). Thousands of homeopathic remedies are in existence, each of which may come in different potencies. In this context, *potency* refers to the relative strength of homeopathic remedies. Unlike conventional chemical potency, homeopathic potency is thought to be greatest when it has gone through a higher number of serial dilutions. The number of serial dilutions is indicated by a digit and a letter, where X = 1/10 dilution, C = 1/100 dilution, M = 1/1000 dilution, and LM = 1/50,000 dilution (e.g., 5X = 5 serial 1/10 dilutions, or 1/100,000).[7] Homeopathic remedies can be delivered as liquids, tablets, creams, gels, or sprays and can be made up of single or multiple ingredients (Figure 19-5).

History and Frequency of Use

Herbal Medicines

Herbal medicines have been used throughout written history, and probably even longer. Archaeological evidence suggests the use of herbal medicines for various conditions as early as 60,000 years ago.[8] More recently, the use of specific extracts of herbal medicines was popular in the United States and Canada from the nineteenth century until the 1930s before slowly falling out of favor with the advent of modern

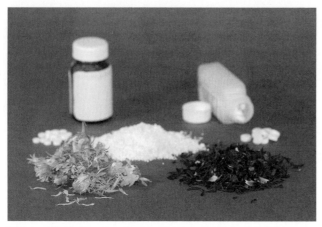

Figure 19-5 Homeopathic supplements in natural and dried pellet forms. (Photo by Martin Wall Photography.)

pharmaceuticals. Resurgence was noted in the 1970s when studies from several European countries (most notably Germany) began applying scientific principles to testing the use of herbal medicines in clinical settings. Preclinical and clinical research on this topic has been increasing at a staggering rate in recent years.

Vitamins and Minerals

Early theories on the cause of beriberi—a condition caused by severe vitamin B_1 (thiamine) deficiency—implicated the formation of toxins following improper cooking, preservation, or storage of food. However, experiments using standardized food suggested the existence of accessory factors that were essential for metabolic processes and could not be synthesized by an organism. In 1912, Cashmir Funk named these accessory factors "vitamines" because they were considered vital amines (thiamine from rice husks contained nitrogen, almost called *amine* at the time). The term was later changed to *vitamin* when scientists from 1912 to 1948 identified, purified, and synthesized all of the vitamins and noted that they did not all contain amines.[9] The importance of minerals to cell structure and function can be traced back to experiments that measured the specific mineral contents of tissues and fluids.[10] Once minerals were identified and measured, research was undertaken to explore their specific functions and utility in the prevention and treatment of various clinical conditions.

Homeopathic Remedies

Homeopathy was founded by Samuel Hahnemann, a German physician, in 1796 when he first published a work describing the "law of similars" built upon observations made after administering various substances to healthy individuals.[6] Such studies are known as *provings* in homeopathy and involve carefully recording all symptoms experienced after ingesting large quantities of herbal, animal, or mineral substances. Once raw materials are identified that can produce specific symptoms, they are serially diluted and administered to patients complaining of those same symptoms. There has been a large amount of research to improve the incomplete scientific understanding of homeopathic remedies.[6]

Use of Supplements. The use of nutritional supplements appears to be gaining popularity in recent years as increasing numbers of people with chronic low back pain (CLBP) seek CAM. A survey of CAM use among the general adult population of the United States conducted in 1991, reported that herbal medicine had been used by 3% of respondents in the past year, megavitamin therapy by 2%, and homeopathy by 1%.[11] However, only 10% of those who reported using herbal medicine had consulted with a health care provider; similar figures were 12% and 32% for megavitamin therapy and homeopathy, respectively. When this survey was repeated in 1997, the use of herbal medicine in the previous 12 months had grown dramatically to 12%, whereas megavitamin use was 6%, and homeopathy use was 3%.[11] Herbal medicine was the second most common CAM therapy after relaxation (16%). The proportion of users who saw a professional practitioner increased to 15% for herbal medicine, 24% for megavitamin therapy, and 17% for homeopathy. The total number of visits to practitioners for these interventions in 1997 was estimated at 10 million, 22 million, and 2 million, respectively. The medical conditions for which herbal medicine use was highest included allergies and insomnia; megavitamin use was highest for high blood pressure.

A prospective study of CAM use among 1342 patients with low back pain (LBP) who presented to general practitioners in Germany reported that 3% received homeopathy, less than 2% saw a naturopathic healer, and less than 1% used herbal medicine in the subsequent 1 year follow-up.[12] The use of homeopathy was statistically significantly higher among females, with an odds ratio of 2.8 (95% confidence interval, 1.3 to 6.1). The Baseline Natural Health Products Survey conducted in 2005 found that 71% of Canadians had used an NHP at least once in the past year.[13] LBP is one of the most commonly reported indications for CAM use. A survey in Canada reported that 37% of those with LBP visited a CAM practitioner, compared with only 17% in the general population.[14] The number of randomized controlled trials (RCTs) related to CAM has been doubling every 5 years; the Cochrane Collaboration Complementary Medicine field contains more than 6500 studies.[15] In addition, principles of CAM are now incorporated into some undergraduate medical education programs.[16]

Practitioner, Setting, and Availability

Herbs, vitamins, minerals, and homeopathic supplements can be purchased from a number of sources, including retail stores such as pharmacies, health food stores, or grocery stores. Nutritional supplements can also be obtained directly from the health care providers who prescribe their use, including naturopaths, doctors of Chinese medicine, homeopaths, chiropractors, and physicians. These products are widely available throughout the United States.

Procedure

In their simplest forms, these interventions consist of patients using self-prescribed supplements purchased in health food stores, pharmacies, or grocery stores based on the advice of friends, family, or advertisements. Patients who consult with health care providers who do not specialize in these interventions (e.g., most primary care providers) may receive generic advice to follow manufacturer recommendations and avoid known drug interactions. Alternatively, patients may consult with health care providers who specialize in CAM interventions and supplements, including naturopaths, homeopaths, and some chiropractors, or physicians who undergo additional training. Before prescribing specific products, these providers will typically conduct a history and physical examination to arrive at a diagnosis that will inform their choice of specific supplements, doses, and instructions for use. Follow-up visits may be required to monitor response to care and adjust the type, frequency, or dose of recommended supplements. Although many individuals use supplements without any guidance, the number of visits to CAM providers has been rapidly increasing in North America.[17]

TABLE 19-1	Herbal Medicines Commonly Used for Chronic Low Back Pain
English Name	**Latin Name**
Myrrh	Commiphora molmol
Cayenne	Capsicum frutescens
White willow	Salix alba
Tea tree	Melaleuca alternifolia
Dong quai	Angelica sinensis
Aloe	Aloe vera
Thyme	Thymus officinalis
Peppermint	Menthe piperita
Wolf's bane	Arnica montana
Curcumin	Curcuma longa
Feverfew	Tanacetum parthenium
Devil's claw	Harpagophytum procumbens
Ginger	Zingiber officinale

Regulatory Status

Nutritional supplements are regulated by the US Food and Drug Administration (FDA) under the Dietary Supplement Health and Education Act of 1994 (DSHEA). Broadly speaking, this legislation places the responsibility on the manufacturer to ensure that a dietary supplement is safe before it is marketed; no evidence is required to support its efficacy, as is currently the case with over-the-counter and prescription medications.[18] Manufacturers of dietary supplements are generally not required to register their products with the FDA before marketing. Once sold to the public, the FDA is responsible for taking action against manufacturers if their products are unsafe or make false claims in advertising (e.g., that they can be used to treat a specific medical condition).

THEORY

Mechanism of Action

The mechanism of action for many nutritional supplements is currently unknown. Every particular product within the broader categories of herbal medicines, vitamins and minerals, and homeopathic remedies may have a unique mechanism of action. Each category is briefly described here.

Herbal Medicines

Several herbal medicines have been used for pain relief, including *Commiphora molmol, Capsicum frutescens, Salix alba, Melaleuca alternifolia, Angelica sinensis, Aloe vera, Thymus officinalis, Menthe piperita, Arnica montana, Curcuma longa, Tanacetum parthenium, Harpagophytum procumbens,* and *Zingiber officinale,* among others.[19] Many

of these herbal medicines have been the subject of extensive biochemical research in recent decades to understand their biochemical and pharmacologic properties.[20] When studied, herbal medicines are often found to contain a variety of active compounds that exhibit different properties. This may help explain why some herbs have been used for so many different indications.

For example, *Z. officinale* has traditionally been used not only for musculoskeletal conditions such as arthritis, soft tissue injuries, and LBP, but also for gastrointestinal indications such as constipation, indigestion, and vomiting, as well as infection, hypertension, and dementia.[21] Isolated components of *Z. officinale* were reported to have anti-inflammatory, antiemetic, antilipidemic, antioxidant, and immune modulation properties. One or more of these effects may be related to its use for CLBP; the same observation likely holds true of other herbal medicines (Table 19-1).

Vitamins and Minerals

Various vitamins and minerals have been proposed as beneficial for musculoskeletal conditions such as CLBP. These include vitamins B_1, B_6, B_{12}, and C, as well as the minerals zinc and manganese, among others. These substances are known to regulate various biochemical reactions in the body and their specific mechanisms of action on musculoskeletal tissues have been elucidated for many of these substances. In some cases vitamin and mineral supplements may be beneficial because they rectify insufficient levels obtained from a normal diet and they may also produce pharmacologic effects when ingested in quantities beyond normal daily allowances. For example, several vitamins and minerals, at normal daily intakes, play a role in the development and repair of connective and muscle tissue, including vitamin C, zinc, manganese, and biotin.[22] Also, some of the B vitamins, when taken in larger than daily intakes, are thought to have antinociceptive and anti-inflammatory properties.

Homeopathic Remedies

The mechanism of action of homeopathy is currently unknown and somewhat controversial. There is little agreement in the scientific community as to how a remedy, when diluted beyond any measurable level, can credibly exert any measurable physiologic effects.

Indication

Nutritional supplements are indicated for nonspecific mechanical CLBP when other medications are contraindicated or have failed, or based on patient preference. It is not currently known which subset of patients with CLBP may benefit most from this intervention.

Assessment

Before receiving nutritional, herbal, or homeopathic supplements, patients should first be assessed for LBP using an evidence-based and goal-oriented approach focused on the patient history and neurologic examination, as discussed in Chapter 3. Additional diagnostic imaging or specific diagnostic testing is generally not required prior to initiating these interventions for CLBP. Prescribing clinicians should also inquire about medication history to note prior hypersensitivity/ allergy or adverse events with similar products, and evaluate contraindications for these types of products. A nutritional evaluation may also be appropriate to estimate levels of vitamins and herbals that are already being provided through dietary sources.

EFFICACY

Evidence supporting the efficacy of these interventions for CLBP was summarized from recent clinical practice guidelines (CPGs), systematic reviews (SRs), and RCTs. Observational studies (OBSs) were also summarized where appropriate. Findings are summarized by study design for each intervention.

Clinical Practice Guidelines

Three of the recent national CPGs on the management of CLBP have assessed and summarized the evidence to make specific recommendations about the efficacy of nutritional, herbal, and homeopathic supplements.

The CPG from Belgium in 2006 found low-quality evidence to support the efficacy of herbal supplements in the management of CLBP.[23]

The CPG from Europe in 2004 found strong evidence that topical capsicum plasters are more effective than placebo with respect to short-term improvements in pain.[24] That CPG reported that topical capsicum plasters could be considered as one of the management options for CLBP.

The CPG from the United States in 2007 found evidence to support small to moderate benefits for capsicum, *H. procumbens*, or *S. alba* for acute exacerbations of CLBP.[25]

Findings from the above CPGs are summarized in Table 19-2.

TABLE 19-2	Clinical Practice Guideline Recommendations on Nutritional, Herbal, and Homeopathic Supplements for Chronic Low Back Pain		
Reference	Country	Conclusion	
Herbal Supplements			
23	Belgium	Low-quality evidence to support efficacy	
25	United States	Evidence of small to moderate benefit with *Capsicum, H. procumbens*, or *S. alba*	
Topical Capsicum Plasters			
24	Europe	Recommended	

Systematic Reviews

Herbal Medicines

Cochrane Collaboration. An SR was conducted in 2005 by the Cochrane Collaboration on herbal therapy for acute, subacute, and chronic LBP.[26] A total of 10 RCTs were included, 2 of which examined acute or subacute LBP and 8 of which examined chronic LBP.[27-34] Two RCTs (n = 325) compared *Harpagophytum procumbens* (devil's claw) versus placebo. Both RCTs included participants suffering from acute exacerbations of CLBP (greater than 6 months) and found strong evidence that a daily dose of 50 mg harpagoside (the purported active constituent of *H. procumbens*) aqueous extract reduced pain more than placebo in the short-term.[27,31] In addition, 100 mg harpagoside reduced pain more than placebo for at least 5 days in the fourth week of treatment.[31]

Two RCTs compared *Salix daphnoides* and *Salix purpurea*. Both RCTs included participants suffering from acute exacerbations of CLBP.[30,34] One trial did not report clinically relevant outcomes; the other RCT (n = 210) found that an extract of willow bark, containing *S. daphnoides* and *S. purpurea* yielding the equivalent of 120 mg salicin per day led to more pain free patients in the short-term than placebo and that a dose yielding the equivalent of 240 mg of salicin per day reduced pain to a greater extent than placebo or 120 mg salicin.[30,34]

One RCT (n = 154) found that a plaster of *C. frutescens* with 11 mg capsaicinoids reduced pain and improved function more than placebo for the treatment of acute episodes of nonspecific CLBP in the short term.[33] One RCT (n = 88) compared *Harpagophytum procumbens* with rofecoxib (a cyclooxygenase-2 inhibitor) and observed no differences in pain and function between 60 mg daily harpagoside aqueous extract of *H. procumbens* and 12.5 mg daily rofecoxib in the treatment of acute episodes of CLBP in the short term.[28] One RCT (n = 228) compared *Salix alba* versus rofecoxib and observed no differences in pain and function between daily 240 mg salicin extract of *S. alba* and daily 12.5 mg rofecoxib in treatment of acute episodes of CLBP in the short term.[34] This SR concluded that *Harpagophytum procumbens, Salix alba,* and *Capsicum frutescens* are treatment options for acute exacerbations of CLBP.

Other. A review conducted in 2006 examined the effects of *Salix* (white willow bark) preparations for musculoskeletal pain.[35] This review included seven studies, two of which were included in the Cochrane Review previously mentioned. The other studies were not RCTs or were not focused on LBP. This review concluded that there is moderate evidence that ethanolic willow bark extract is effective for LBP.

A review conducted in 2007 examined the effects of anti-inflammatory drugs for osteoarthritis and CLBP.[36] The review included 13 SRs but did not specify which reviews pertained specifically to CLBP. One of these was the Cochrane Collaboration SR mentioned previously. This review concluded that strong evidence supports avocado soybean fraction and *Harpagophytum* preparations (>50 mg harpagoside daily), moderate evidence supports ginger and rose hip and seed powder, insufficient evidence exists for *Boswellia serrata* gum resin, and inconsistent evidence exists for willow bark extract. However, the conclusions did not specify which interventions were related to LBP and which were related to osteoarthritis.

A review on topical treatment for CLBP evaluated the efficacy of capsaicin plasters.[37] This review included 1 RCT with 154 participants and 1 RCT with 301 participants.[32,33] The first RCT found significant improvement in nonspecific CLBP with a 60.8% positive response rate to capsaicin plasters over three weeks. Similar results were reported in the second RCT, which had a 67% positive response rate to capsaicin plasters, compared with 49% positive response rate to placebo plasters.

Vitamins and Minerals

No recent, high-quality SRs were identified that reported specifically on the efficacy of vitamins and minerals as an intervention for LBP.

Homeopathic Remedies

No recent, high-quality SRs were identified that reported specifically on the efficacy of homeopathic supplements as an intervention for LBP.

Findings from the above SRs are summarized in Table 19-3.

Randomized Controlled Trials

Herbal Medicines

Capsaicin Plaster. Two RCTs were identified.[32,33] Their methods are summarized in Table 19-4. Their results are briefly described below.

An RCT conducted by Keitel and colleagues[33] included CLBP patients with no neurologic involvement and symptoms lasting longer than 3 months. Participants were randomized to either daily capsaicin plaster or daily placebo for 3 weeks. At the end of the treatment period, both groups had a reduction of mean combined pain scores (Arhus low back rating scale) compared with baseline. The capsaicin group had significantly better improvements in pain than the placebo group. Improvements in disability (Arhus low back rating scale) were achieved, with no significant differences between groups.

TABLE 19-3	Systematic Review Findings on Nutritional, Herbal, and Homeopathic Supplements for Chronic Low Back Pain		
Reference	# RCTs in SR	# RCTs for CLBP	Conclusion
26	10	8	*H. procumbens, S. alba,* and *C. frutescens* seem to reduce pain more than placebo
35	7	NR	Moderate evidence that ethanolic willow bark extract is effective for LBP
36	13 SRs (did not specify which pertained to CLBP)	NR	
37	2	2	Capsaicin has moderate to poor efficacy in treating LBP

CLBP, chronic low back pain; LBP, low back pain; NR, not reported; RCT, randomized controlled trial; SR, systematic review.

An RCT conducted by Frerick and colleagues[32] included CLBP patients with no neurologic involvement and symptoms lasting longer than 3 months. Participants were randomized to either daily capsaicin plaster or daily placebo for 3 weeks. At the end of the treatment period, the mean combined pain score (Arhus low back rating scale) decreased significantly in the capsaicin group compared with baseline, but no significant change was observed in the placebo group. The improvement in pain in the capsaicin group was significantly higher than that in the placebo group. An improvement in disability (Arhus low back rating scale) was achieved in both groups (*P* values not reported). The improvement in disability in the capsaicin group was significantly greater than that of the placebo group.

Lavender Oil One RCT included 61 participants with subacute or chronic LBP.[38] The active group received acupoint stimulation followed by acupressure with lavender oil for eight sessions over 3 weeks. One week after the end of treatment, the active group had a 39% greater reduction in pain (visual analog scale [VAS]) than the usual care group (*P* < .001), as well as improved walking time and greater lateral spine flexion. Because it is impossible to assess the individual contribution of each intervention in this trial, there is limited evidence for lavender oil in the treatment of CLBP.

TABLE 19-4	Randomized Controlled Trials of Nutritional, Herbal, and Homeopathic Supplements for Chronic Low Back Pain		
Reference	Indication	Intervention	Control
33	CLBP without neurologic involvement, symptoms ≥3 months	Capsaicin plaster Daily × 3 weeks n = 77	Placebo Daily × 3 weeks n = 77
32	CLBP without neurologic involvement, symptoms ≥3 months	Capsaicin plaster Daily × 3 weeks n = 159	Placebo Daily × 3 weeks n = 160
38	Subacute and chronic LBP with or without neurologic involvement, symptoms most days in past 4 weeks	Acupoint stimulation + acupressure with lavender oil 35-40 minutes × 8 sessions over 3 weeks Cointervention: NR n = 32	Usual care Cointervention: NR n = 29
22	CLBP with or without neurologic involvement, symptoms >6 months	Once daily 1000 mg B_{12} (intramuscularly) 2-week period Cointervention: paracetamol n = 30	Placebo (2-mL ampoules, intramuscularly) 2-week period Cointervention: paracetamol n = 30

CLBP, chronic low back pain; LBP, low back pain; NR, not reported.

Vitamins and Minerals

Intramuscular Vitamin B_{12}. An RCT tested the efficacy and safety of IM vitamin B_{12} injections (IM B_{12}; Tricortin 1000 mg) in 60 participants with CLBP or sciatic neuritis of mechanical origin not requiring surgery and without signs of B_{12} deficiency.[22] Injections of placebo or B_{12} were given once per day for 2 weeks. Both groups experienced decreased pain, with the active treatment group having a greater decrease ($P < .0001$). In the active treatment group, the VAS score changed from 75.5 to 9.5 ($P < .0001$) and in the placebo group from 70.6 to 36.8 ($P < .0001$). The disability index was decreased in both groups, with the active treatment group having a significantly greater decrease ($P < .0002$). Mean consumption of paracetamol rescue medication was also significantly lower in the active treatment group ($P < .0001$). There is moderate evidence that IM B_{12} is effective when compared with placebo for CLBP.

Homeopathic Remedies

No RCTs were identified.

SAFETY

Contraindications

In general, caution should be exercised when recommending nutritional supplements to patients with CLBP who are concurrently taking over-the-counter or prescription medications, to minimize the risk of harmful interactions. Specific nutritional supplements may also have other contraindications related to renal or hepatic impairment, or other medical conditions that could impact metabolism and excretion.

Adverse Events

Herbal Medicines

Capsicum can cause upper abdominal discomfort including fullness, gas, bloating, nausea, epigastric pain and burning, diarrhea, and belching when taken by mouth.[5] Sweating and flushing of the head and neck, lacrimation, headache, faintness, and rhinorrhea have also been reported with capsicum. Excessive amounts can potentially lead to gastroenteritis or hepatic necrosis. There are also reports of dermatitis in breast-fed infants whose mothers' food is heavily spiced with capsicum from food sources rather than nutritional supplements. Topically, capsicum can cause burning, stinging, and erythema. Although these effects tend to diminish over time, approximately 10% of patients discontinue treatment because of these effects. When taken intranasally, capsicum can cause nasal burning and pain, lacrimation, sneezing, and excessive nasal secretion; these effects appear to diminish with repeated applications. Patients may be pretreated with intranasal lidocaine to decrease the pain of intranasal capsaicin treatment. Inhalation of capsicum can cause coughing, dyspnea, nasal congestion, eye irritation, and allergic alveolitis. Capsicum can be extremely irritating to the eyes and mucous membranes (its concentrated oily extract is used in pepper self-defense sprays). Anecdotal evidence suggests that fair-skinned individuals may react more violently to topical capsicum formulas. *Harpagophytum procumbens* (devil's claw) may increase stomach acid, decrease blood glucose levels, decrease blood pressure, and could possibly interfere with drugs metabolized by cytochrome P450 2C9, cytochrome P450 2C19, and cytochrome P450 3A4. However, these interactions have not been reported in humans.

Vitamins and Minerals

One study examining IM vitamin B_{12} reported no adverse events. High doses of vitamin C (greater than 3000 mg) may increase the half-life of acetaminophen by approximately 50% (from 2.3 to 3.1 hours).[5] Increases in plasma estrogen levels of up to 55% have been reported when vitamin C is taken concurrently with oral contraceptives or hormone replacement therapy. A combination of simvastatin (Zocor) and niacin may raise high density lipoprotein (HDL) cholesterol levels. Antioxidants such as vitamins C and E, beta-carotene, and selenium may blunt this rise in HDL. Vitamin C seems to modestly reduce indinavir (Crixivan) levels, and it is not known whether an interaction could occur with other protease inhibitors, such as amprenavir (Agenerase), nelfinavir (Viracept), ritonavir (Norvir), or saquinavir (Fortovase, Invirase). High doses of vitamin C (up to 16 g) may cause diarrhea and reduce warfarin absorption.[5]

Some data suggest that zinc may stimulate tumor cell production of metallothionein, which inactivates cisplatin.[5] Zinc also forms an insoluble complex with penicillamine, quinolones, tetracyclines, demeclocycline, and minocycline, potentially interfering with their absorption and activity. Theoretically, manganese might reduce the absorption of quinolones. Case reports suggest that chloramphenicol can delay or interrupt the reticulocyte response to supplemental vitamin B_{12} in some patients.[5]

Homeopathic Remedies

Data on adverse events were only available for some of the trials evaluating homeopathy supplements.[14,29] One trial reported that the group who received Spiroflor SRL homeopathic gel had fewer adverse events than the Capsici Compositus FNA group, suggesting that this homeopathic gel is relatively safe.

COSTS

Fees and Third-Party Reimbursement

In the United States, counseling on nutritional supplement use for CLBP that is given by a licensed physician can be delivered in the context of an office or outpatient visit for a new patient using CPT codes 99201 (up to 10 minutes), 99202 (up to 20 minutes), or 99203 (up to 30 minutes). For an established patient, this counseling can likely be provided during an office or outpatient visit using CPT codes 99211 (up to 5 minutes), 99212 (up to 10 minutes), or 99213 (up to 15 minutes). Although time is indicated for the various levels of service and can be a contributing component for selection of the level of office/outpatient visits, the overarching criteria for selection of the level of service should be based on medical necessity and the amount of history, examination, and medical decision making that was required and documented. Counseling provided by other licensed clinicians such as acupuncturists, naturopaths, or chiropractors may be delivered in conjunction with another specific service, such as acupuncture or spinal manipulation therapy, for which a separate fee can be charged.

TABLE 19-5	Medicare Fee Schedule for Related Services	
CPT Code	New York	California
99201	$41	$44
99202	$70	$76
99203	$101	$109
99211	$20	$22
99212	$41	$44
99213	$68	$73

2010 Participating, nonfacility amount.

These procedures are widely covered by other third-party payers such as health insurers and worker's compensation insurance. Although some payers continue to base their reimbursements on usual, customary, and reasonable payment methodology, the majority have developed reimbursement tables based on the Resource Based Relative Value Scale used by Medicare. Reimbursements by other third-party payers are generally higher than Medicare.

The nutritional supplements themselves are rarely reimbursed by third-party payers. The cost of nutritional supplements varies tremendously, from a few pennies per tablet or capsule for common vitamins, minerals, or herbal products, to several dollars per day for rare, proprietary, or mixed products from well-known manufacturers. The costs of nutritional supplements may also vary based on the point of purchase (e.g., from licensed provider, health food store, pharmacy, grocery store, wholesale reseller).

Typical fees reimbursed by Medicare in New York and California for these services are summarized in Table 19-5.

Cost Effectiveness

No cost effectiveness analyses were identified that evaluated the cost effectiveness of nutritional, herbal, or homeopathic supplements as interventions for LBP.

SUMMARY

Description

Nutritional supplements are products used to improve the diet and often contain vitamins, minerals, herbs or amino acids. Nutritional supplements are often associated with CAM, which encompasses a group of diverse medical and health care systems, practices, and products that are not considered part of conventional medicine. The main types of nutritional supplements reviewed here include herbal medicines, vitamins and minerals, and homeopathic remedies. The use of nutritional supplements has gained popularity in recent years among individuals with CLBP and these products are widely available in the United States. Supplements can be purchased from a number of sources, including retail stores such as pharmacies, health food stores, or grocery stores. Nutritional supplements can also be obtained directly from the health care providers who prescribe their use, including some naturopaths, doctors of Chinese medicine, homeopaths, chiropractors, and physicians.

Theory

Herbal medicines are often discovered to contain a variety of active compounds that exhibit different properties, which may explain why some herbs have been used for so many different indications, including CLBP. Various vitamins and minerals have been proposed as beneficial for musculoskeletal conditions such as CLBP. For example, several vitamins and minerals are necessary for the development and repair of connective and muscle tissue, including vitamin C, zinc, manganese, and biotin. The mechanism of action of homeopathy is currently unknown and somewhat controversial. There is little agreement in the scientific community as to how a remedy, when diluted beyond any measurable level, can exert any measurable physiologic effects when taken. Nutritional supplements are indicated for nonspecific mechanical CLBP when other medications are contraindicated or have failed, or based on patient preference. Diagnostic imaging or other forms of advanced testing is generally not required prior to administering nutritional supplements for CLBP.

Efficacy

Three CPGs provide recommendations on nutritional supplements for CLBP. For herbal medicine, one found low-quality evidence supporting the effectiveness of herbals for CLBP, another found that topical capsicum plasters are more effective than placebo, and the third CPG reported small to moderate benefits for capsicum, H. procumbens, and S. alba for acute exacerbations of CLBP. For herbal medicine, an SR conducted by the Cochrane Collaboration concluded that H. procumbens, S. alba, and C. frutescens are treatment options for acute exacerbations of CLBP, while another review concluded that there is moderate evidence that ethanolic willow bark extract is effective for LBP. Three RCTs assessed the efficacy of herbal medicine for CLBP. In one RCT, it was impossible to determine the effects of lavender oil alone because it was combined with other interventions. Two RCTs examined the efficacy of capsicum plaster, both observing a statistically significant improvement in pain versus placebo and one finding a statistically significant improvement in disability versus placebo. No CPGs or SRs were identified for vitamins and minerals, yet one RCT found a statistically significant improvement in disability for IM vitamin B_{12} injections versus placebo. No CPGs, SRs, or RCTs were identified examining homeopathic remedies for CLBP.

Harms

Caution should be exercised when recommending nutritional supplements to patients with CLBP who are concurrently taking over-the-counter or prescription medication, to minimize the risk of harmful interactions. Specific nutritional supplements may also have other contraindications related to renal or hepatic impairment, or other medical conditions that could impact metabolism and excretion. Similarly, each group of supplements has its own set of adverse events. For example, the herb capsicum can cause gastrointestinal discomfort, sweating, headache, and faintness. High doses of vitamin C (up to 16 g) may cause diarrhea and reduce warfarin absorption. Adverse events related to homeopathy are not frequently reported.

Costs

In the United States, costs related to nutritional supplement counseling for CLBP that is given by a licensed physician can range from $20 to $109, depending on the duration of the session. Counseling provided by other licensed clinicians such as acupuncturists, naturopaths, or chiropractors may be delivered in conjunction with other specific services such as acupuncture or spinal manipulation therapy for which a separate fee can be charged. The cost of nutritional supplements varies tremendously, from a few pennies per tablet or capsule for common vitamins, minerals, or herbal products, to several dollars per day for rare, proprietary, or mixed products from well-known manufacturers. The costs of

TABLE 19-6	Summary of Evidence for Nutritional, Herbal, and Homeopathic Supplements for Chronic Low Back Pain
Level of Evidence	**Intervention**
Strong	50 mg harpagoside per dose of an aqueous extract of H. procumbens per day reduces pain more than placebo
Moderate	100 mg harpagoside per dose of an aqueous extract of H. procumbens compared with placebo
	Extract of S. alba yielding 120 mg salicin per day compared with placebo
	240 mg of salicin per day in reducing pain to a greater extent than placebo
	240 mg of salicin per day as equivalent to 120 mg salicin
	60 mg daily harpagoside dose of an aqueous extract of H. procumbens equivalent to 12.5 mg rofecoxib per day
	Spiroflor SRL homeopathic gel (SRL) equivalent to Cremor Capsici Compositus FNA, the capsici oleoresin gel
	Intramuscular B_{12} when compared with placebo
Limited	Topical C. frutescens in the form of Rado-Salil cream or a capsicum plaster for reducing pain more than placebo
	Lavender oil in the treatment of chronic nonspecific LBP homeopathy as equivalent to physiotherapy
None	Any other nutritional supplements, herbal interventions, or homeopathic remedies for NSLBP

nutritional supplements may also vary based on the point of purchase (e.g., from licensed provider, health food store, pharmacy, grocery store, wholesale reseller). In addition, the cost effectiveness of nutritional supplements for CLBP is unknown.

Comments

Evidence from the CPGs, SRs, and RCTs reviewed suggests that some herbal supplements may be effective as interventions for CLBP. However, there was a dearth of evidence examining the efficacy of nutritional and homeopathic supplements for CLBP. As such, health care practitioners giving advice on such products should be qualified, well trained, and have access to the highest quality scientific evidence summarized in Table 19-6.

Although preliminary studies look promising, more data are required to determine whether any nutritional supplements are useful in controlling CLBP. In particular, the data regarding IM vitamin B_{12} should be replicated in future studies. If further research supports these preliminary findings, this could prove to be an inexpensive therapy for CLBP. The relative safety of herbal, nutritional, and homeopathic supplements should be compared with standard medications such as nonsteroidal anti-inflammatory drugs using large observational cohort studies.

CHAPTER REVIEW QUESTIONS

Answers are located on page 451.

1. True or false: Vitamins primarily regulate electrolyte balance in the body.
2. True or false: Minerals are essential for normal cellular function.
3. Which of the following vitamin is not fat soluble?
   a. vitamin A
   b. vitamin C
   c. vitamin D
   d. vitamin K
4. Which of the following is not a method of administering ascorbic acid?
   a. capsule
   b. inhalation
   c. liquid
   d. gel
5. Which of the following may increase the half-life of acetaminophen?
   a. magnesium
   b. vitamin C
   c. devil's claw
   d. *Capsicum frutescens*
   e. niacin
6. Which of the following statement is true with respect to homeopathic potency?
   a. the less a product is diluted, the stronger its potency
   b. the more a product is diluted, the weaker its potency
   c. the more a product is pure, the weaker its potency
   d. the more a product is diluted, the stronger its potency

7. Which of the following herbal supplement was shown to be as effective as a COX-2 inhibitor for LBP?
   a. *Harpagophytum procumbens*
   b. *Thymus officinalis*
   c. *Menthe piperita*
   d. *Arnica montana*

REFERENCES

1. US Food and Drug Administration. Dietary Supplement Health and Education Act of 1994. USFDA 1995 December 1. Available at: http://ods.od.nih.gov/about/dshea_wording.aspx.
2. Her Majesty the Queen in Right of Canada represented by the Minister of Public Works and Government Services. Natural Health Products Regulations. Ottawa, Canada: Gazette Part II; 2007.
3. National Center for Complementary and Alternative Medicine. What is CAM? NCCAM 2007D003. Available at: http://nccam.nih.gov/health/whatiscam/.
4. World Health Organization. General Guidelines for Methodologies on Research and Evaluation of Traditional Medicine. Geneva; 2000, Report No.: WHO/EDM/TRM/2000.1.
5. Natural medicines comprehensive database. Jeff M Jellin, PharmD, Founding Editor, 2007. Available at: www.naturaldatabase.com.
6. Jonas WB, Kaptchuk TJ, Linde K. A critical overview of homeopathy. Ann Intern Med 2003;138:393-399.
7. Tedesco P, Cicchetti J. Like cures like: homeopathy. Am J Nurs 2001;101:43-49.
8. Tyler VE. Herbal medicine: from the past to the future. Public Health Nutr 2000;3:447-452.
9. Muller-Landgraf I. History of vitamins. Ther Umsch 1994; 51:459-461.
10. Groff JL, Gropper SS. Advanced nutrition and human metabolism. 3rd ed. Belmont, CA: Wadsworth Thompson Learning; 2000.
11. Eisenberg DM, Davis RB, Ettner SL, et al. Trends in alternative medicine use in the United States, 1990-1997: results of a follow-up national survey. JAMA 1998;280:1569-1575.
12. Chenot JF, Becker A, Leonhardt C, et al. Use of complementary alternative medicine for low back pain consulting in general practice: a cohort study. BMC Complement Altern Med 2007;7:42.
13. Natural Health Products Directorate. Baseline natural health products survey among consumers. Ottawa: Ipsos Reid; Health Canada; 2005.
14. Millar WJ. Patterns of use—alternative health care practitioners. Health Rep 2001;13:9-21.
15. Vickers A. Recent advances: complementary medicine. BMJ 2000;321:683-686.
16. Mills EJ, Hollyer T, Guyatt G, et al. Teaching evidence-based complementary and alternative medicine: 1. A learning structure for clinical decision changes. J Altern Complement Med 2002;8:207-214.
17. Sierpina VS. Progress notes: a review of educational developments in CAM. Altern Ther Health Med 2002;8:104-106.
18. US Food and Drug Administration. Dietary supplements. FDA 2009 June 18 [cited 2009 Sep 8]. Available at: http://www.fda.gov/Food/DietarySupplements/default.htm.
19. Blumenthal M. The Complete German Commission E Monographs: therapeutic guide to herbal medicines. Austin, TX: American Botanical Council; 1998.

20. Mills S, Bone K. Principles and practice of phytotherapy: modern herbal medicine. Edinburgh: Churchill Livingston; 1999.

21. Al-Zain F, Lemcke J, Killeen T, et al. Minimally invasive spinal surgery using nucleoplasty: a 1-year follow-up study. Acta Neurochir (Wien) 2008;150:1257-1262.

22. Mauro GL, Martorana U, Cataldo P, et al. Vitamin B12 in low back pain: a randomised, double-blind, placebo-controlled study. Eur Rev Med Pharmacol Sci 2000;4:53-58.

23. Nielens H, van Zundert J, Mairiaux P, et al. Chronic low back pain. Good Clinical practice (GCP) Brussels: Belgian Health Care Knowledge Centre (KCE); 2006. KCE reports vol 48C.

24. Airaksinen O, Brox JI, Cedraschi C, et al. European guidelines for the management of chronic nonspecific low back pain. Eur Spine J 2006;15:S192-S300.

25. Chou R, Qaseem A, Snow V, et al. Diagnosis and treatment of low back pain: a joint clinical practice guideline from the American College of Physicians and the American Pain Society. Ann Intern Med 2007;147:478-491.

26. Gagnier JJ, van TM, Berman B, et al. Herbal medicine for low back pain. Cochrane Database Syst Rev 2006;(2):CD004504.

27. Chrubasik S, Zimpfer C, Schutt U, et al. Effectiveness of *Harpagophytum procumbens* in treatment of acute low back pain. Phytomedicine 1996;3:1-10.

28. Chrubasik S, Model A, Black A, et al. A randomized double-blind pilot study comparing Doloteffin and Vioxx in the treatment of low back pain. Rheumatology (Oxford) 2003; 42:141-148.

29. Chrubasik S, Kunzel O, Model A, et al. Treatment of low back pain with a herbal or synthetic anti-rheumatic: a randomized controlled study. Willow bark extract for low back pain. Rheumatology (Oxford) 2001;40:1388-1393.

30. Chrubasik S, Eisenberg E, Balan E, et al. Treatment of low back pain exacerbations with willow bark extract: a randomized double-blind study. Am J Med 2000;109:9-14.

31. Chrubasik S, Junck H, Breitschwerdt H, et al. Effectiveness of *Harpagophytum* extract WS 1531 in the treatment of exacerbation of low back pain: a randomized, placebo-controlled, double-blind study. Eur J Anaesthesiol 1999;16:118-129.

32. Frerick H, Keitel W, Kuhn U, et al. Topical treatment of chronic low back pain with a capsicum plaster. Pain 2003;106:59-64.

33. Keitel W, Frerick H, Kuhn U, et al. Capsicum pain plaster in chronic non-specific low back pain. Arzneimittelforschung 2001;51:896-903.

34. Krivoy N, Pavlotzky E, Chrubasik S, et al. Effect of salicis cortex extract on human platelet aggregation. Planta Med 2001;67:209-212.

35. Vlachojannis JE, Cameron M, Chrubasik S. A systematic review on the effectiveness of willow bark for musculoskeletal pain. Phytother Res 2009;23:897-900.

36. Chrubasik JE, Roufogalis BD, Chrubasik S. Evidence of effectiveness of herbal antiinflammatory drugs in the treatment of painful osteoarthritis and chronic low back pain. Phytother Res 2007;21:675-683.

37. Mason L, Moore RA, Derry S, et al. Systematic review of topical capsaicin for the treatment of chronic pain. BMJ 2004;328:991.

38. Yip YB, Tse SH. The effectiveness of relaxation acupoint stimulation and acupressure with aromatic lavender essential oil for non-specific low back pain in Hong Kong: a randomised controlled trial. Complement Ther Med 2004;12:28-37.

CARLO AMMENDOLIA
ANDREA D. FURLAN
MARTA IMAMURA
EMMA L. IRVIN
MAURITS VAN TULDER

CHAPTER 20

Needle Acupuncture

DESCRIPTION

Terminology and Subtypes

The term *acupuncture* encompasses a variety of different procedures and techniques that involve the stimulation of specific points along the body thought to be related to various bodily functions. Needle acupuncture involves stimulating these points by penetrating the skin with thin, solid, metallic needles that can be further stimulated manually or electrically (Figure 20-1). There are many different types of needle acupuncture used throughout the world, including Japanese Meridian Therapy, French Energetic acupuncture, Korean Constitutional acupuncture, and Lemington Five Elements acupuncture. In recent decades, new forms and styles of needle acupuncture have evolved, including ear (auricular) acupuncture, hand acupuncture, foot acupuncture, and scalp acupuncture.[1] These forms of acupuncture attempt to achieve the same effects as traditional acupuncture by stimulating only points within those targeted areas. Massage acupuncture, also termed *acupressure*, is reviewed in Chapter 16. Acupuncture was traditionally based on the belief that health is maintained in a delicate state of balance by two opposing forces, termed *yin* and *yang*. Yin represents the cold, slow, or passive force, whereas yang represents the hot, excited, or active force. Disease or dysfunction is thought to arise when there is an imbalance of yin and yang, which leads to a blockage in the flow of vital energy (known as *qi*, pronounced chi) along pathways known as *meridians* (Figure 20-2).[2]

History and Frequency of Use

Acupuncture originated in China more than 2000 years ago and is one of the oldest, most commonly used traditional systems of healing in the world. Its popularity in the West has grown rapidly over the past 30 years. Acupuncture gained particular notoriety in 1971 after James Reston, a journalist with *The New York Times*, published an article on his personal experience with the intervention. While traveling in China, he suffered acute appendicitis and required an emergency appendectomy. His postoperative pain was managed with acupuncture by inserting thin needles into his elbows and knees to stimulate and relieve pressure in the intestine and stomach, which were thought to be important in his condition. Having experienced complete relief of symptoms

with acupuncture, Reston is often credited with exposing Americans to this method of healing.[3]

The use of acupuncture appears to be gaining popularity in recent years as increasing numbers of people with chronic low back pain (CLBP) seek complementary and alternative medicine (CAM). A survey of CAM use among the general adult population of the United States conducted in 1991, reported that acupuncture had been used by 0.4% of respondents in the past year, 91% of whom had consulted with a health care provider.[4] When this survey was repeated in 1997, the use of acupuncture in the previous 12 months had grown to 1%.[4] The total number of visits to acupuncture practitioners in 1997 was estimated at five million. A prospective study of CAM use among 1342 patients with low back pain (LBP) who presented to general practitioners (GPs) in Germany reported that 13% received acupuncture in the subsequent 1 year follow-up.[5] The use of acupuncture was statistically significantly higher among those whose GP offered acupuncture, with an odds ratio of 3.0 (95% confidence interval, 2.1 to 4.4). Acupuncture was the third most commonly reported CAM therapy after massage (31%) and spinal manipulation therapy (SMT, 26%).

Practitioner, Setting, and Availability

In North America, acupuncture is widely available and is typically practiced in a private practice setting by a variety of practitioners including acupuncturists and traditional Chinese medicine (TCM) practitioners, as well as some physicians, chiropractors, and physical therapists with additional training. Licensing, credentialing, and regulations to practice acupuncture vary significantly depending on jurisdiction. In 2002, 42 states in the United States had established statutory licensure governing more than 14,000 acupuncture practitioners.[6] In addition, an estimated 3000 physicians had formally studied and incorporated acupuncture into their practices.[6]

Procedure

In order to determine the nature of an illness, an acupuncturist needs to conduct an assessment that may include a brief medical history, history about specific symptoms and bodily functions, traditional physical examination, and examination of the tongue, eyes, peripheral pulses, and odor. The goal of

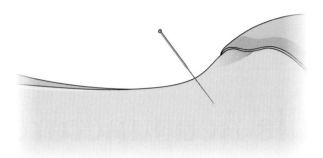

Figure 20-1 Needle acupuncture uses long, thin, metallic needles to penetrate the skin.

the assessment is to help determine which meridians and acupuncture points should be stimulated to address the presenting complaints (see Figure 20-2). Modern acupuncturists typically use a combination of both traditional meridian and extrameridian acupuncture points, which are fixed according to anatomic landmarks and not necessarily associated with meridians (Figures 20-3 and 20-4).

Once appropriate points are selected, the patient usually lies supine or prone on a treatment table while the therapist inserts acupuncture needles. Each needle is typically inserted by holding it over the desired points and gently tapping it into place until it penetrates the skin, after which it is briefly rotated and stimulated; a verbal or physical response may be sought from the patient to help confirm needle placement. A typical session with needle acupuncture may include inserting 20 to 30 needles or more. Needles are generally kept in place for 20 to 30 minutes, during which the therapist may periodically stimulate them manually by rotating the needles (Figure 20-5). Therapists may also use electrical stimulation, in which a transcutaneous electrical nerve stimulation (TENS) device is connected to the acupuncture needles to deliver constant stimulation. Other interventions that may be used in conjunction with needle acupuncture include injection acupuncture (herbal extracts are injected into acupuncture points), heat lamps, or moxibustion (the moxa herb, *Artemisia vulgaris*), which is burned at the end of the needles.[1] The latter interventions are not discussed in this chapter.

Regulatory Status

Not applicable.

THEORY

Mechanism of Action

In traditional needle acupuncture, there are 12 primary meridians, 8 secondary meridians, and more than 2000 associated acupuncture points on the human body; this number varies somewhat, and some texts have described and mapped only the 365 most commonly used points.[7] The goal of traditional acupuncture is to select the appropriate points along different meridians that correspond to a particular illness or bodily

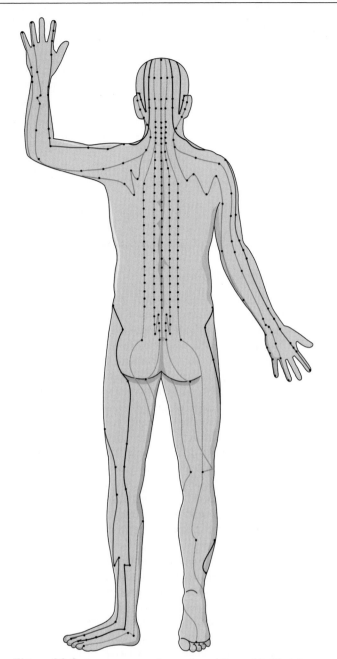

Figure 20-2 Acupuncture points and meridians. (Modified from Anderson SK: The practice of shiatsu. St. Louis, 2008, Mosby.)

dysfunction, and to stimulate those points with needles until balance in the body's energy flow is restored.

In terms of Western scientific principles, it is uncertain how acupuncture functions in general and unclear how it may help CLBP in particular. It is hypothesized that acupuncture produces its effects through the central nervous system (CNS) by stimulating the production of endorphins and neurotransmitters that modulate nociception and other involuntary bodily functions.[8,9] Another theory suggests that acupuncture works through the gate control theory of pain, in which the nociceptive input (e.g., CLBP) is inhibited in the CNS in the presence of another type of input (e.g., acupuncture needle).[10]

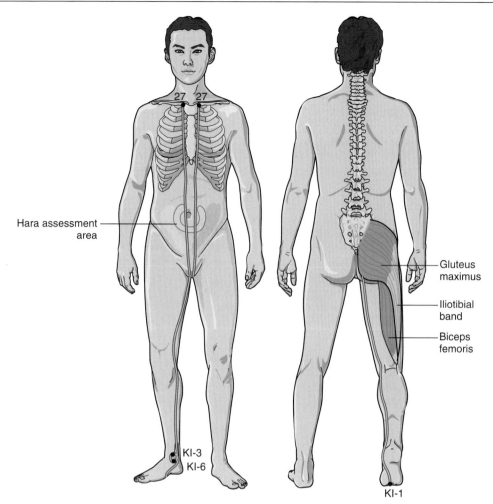

Hara assessment area

Gluteus maximus

Iliotibial band

Biceps femoris

KI-3
KI-6

KI-1

Figure 20-3 Acupuncture points and meridians in the lumbosacral region: anterior and posterior urinary bladder channels. (Modified from Anderson S. The practice of shiatsu. St. Louis, 2008, Mosby.)

It is also postulated that the presence of a foreign substance (e.g., acupuncture needle) within the tissue of the body stimulates vascular and immunomodulatory factors involved as mediators of inflammation.[11] Elevated levels of adrenocorticotropic hormone after acupuncture seem to support this theory.[12] More recently, it was found that active myofascial trigger points at the upper trapezius muscle (corresponding to the GB 21 acupuncture point) had a lower pressure pain threshold (indicating more susceptibility to pain from that region) when compared with controls who had no pain or only latent trigger points.[13] It was also reported that levels of substance P, calcitonin gene–related peptide, bradykinin, tumor necrosis factor-α, interleukin-1β, serotonin, and norepinephrine were elevated in the vicinity of the active myofascial trigger point.[13] It is presumed that stimulating this acupuncture point could impact some of these phenomena, but further research is needed to understand the specific effects of acupuncture on CLBP.

Indication

Acupuncture is typically used for patients with nonspecific mechanical CLBP, with or without radiculopathy.[14] It is uncertain which patient characteristics are associated with improved outcomes when using acupuncture for CLBP. Thomas and colleagues attempted to assess the role of prior expectations in influencing outcomes among patients receiving acupuncture for CLBP. They found that prior expectations of a negative or neutral benefit were associated with better pain outcomes at 24 months among those receiving acupuncture.[15] In contrast, subgroup analysis in another randomized controlled trial (RCT) reported that higher expectations that acupuncture would be beneficial were associated with improved disability scores in CLBP compared with lower expectations.[16] Thomas and colleagues also found that duration of symptoms was negatively associated with better outcomes.[15] However, there is currently insufficient evidence to accurately determine which patient with CLBP would benefit most from needle acupuncture.

Assessment

Before receiving needle acupuncture, patients should first be assessed for LBP using an evidence-based and goal-oriented approach focused on the patient history and neurologic examination, as discussed in Chapter 3. Additional diagnostic imaging or specific diagnostic testing is generally not required before initiating this intervention for CLBP. The

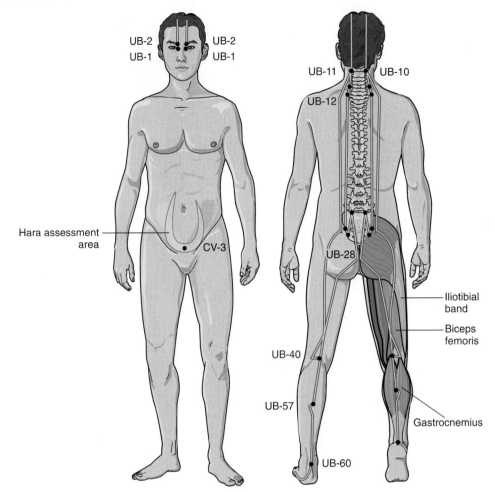

Figure 20-4 Acupuncture points and meridians in the lumbosacral region: anterior and posterior urinary bladder channels. (Modified from Anderson S. The practice of shiatsu. St. Louis, 2008, Mosby.)

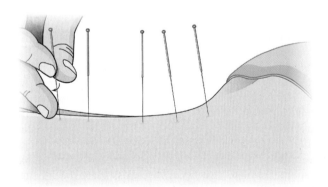

Figure 20-5 Stimulation of acupuncture needle with manual rotation.

clinician should also inquire about general health to identify potential contraindications to this intervention. In order to select the specific acupuncture points to be treated, an additional assessment may be conducted by the clinician. Studies evaluating the consistency of diagnoses and selection of acupuncture points among traditional acupuncturists for CLBP have reported mixed results.[16-18]

EFFICACY

Evidence supporting the efficacy of this intervention for CLBP was summarized from recent clinical practice guidelines (CPGs), systematic reviews (SRs), and RCTs. Observational studies (OBSs) were also summarized where appropriate. Findings are summarized by study design.

Clinical Practice Guidelines

Five of the recent national CPGs on the management of CLBP have assessed and summarized the evidence to make specific recommendations about the efficacy of acupuncture.

The CPG from Belgium in 2006 found conflicting evidence to support the efficacy of acupuncture for CLBP.[19] That CPG found that acupuncture is not more effective than trigger point injections, TENS, or self-care education for CLBP. Acupuncture was less effective than massage or SMT for CLBP, but provided short-term improvements in pain, which might be improved when combined with other interventions.

TABLE 20-1	Clinical Practice Guideline Recommendations on Acupuncture for Chronic Low Back Pain	
Reference	Country	Conclusion
19	Belgium	May provide short-term improvements in pain
20	Europe	Not recommended
21	Italy	Evidence that acupuncture is not effective
22	United Kingdom	Recommended if other options do not obtain adequate pain relief (maximum 10 sessions over 12 weeks)
23	United States	Recommended if self-care alone does not provide pain relief

The CPG from Europe in 2004 found conflicting evidence that acupuncture is more effective than sham acupuncture in the management of CLBP.[20] There was limited evidence that acupuncture combined with other conservative management options, including usual physical therapy (PT), care from a GP, exercise, or back school, is more effective than any of those interventions alone. That CPG also found limited evidence that acupuncture is as effective as brief education or self-care for CLBP. There was moderate evidence that acupuncture is not more effective than trigger point injections or TENS for CLBP, and there was limited evidence that acupuncture is less effective than massage or SMT for CLBP. That CPG did not recommend acupuncture in the management of CLBP.

The CPG from Italy in 2007 found evidence that acupuncture is not effective in the management of CLBP.[21]

The CPG from the United Kingdom in 2009 found evidence to support the efficacy of acupuncture with respect to improvements in pain and function.[22] There was evidence that acupuncture was more effective than usual care for CLBP, and the CPG recommended offering a course of acupuncture when other conservative management options do not obtain adequate pain relief. That CPG recommended a maximum of 10 sessions of acupuncture over a period of up to 12 weeks for CLBP.

The CPG from the United States in 2007 found moderate quality evidence to support the efficacy of acupuncture with respect to improvements in pain.[23] That CPG recommended acupuncture as one management option if patients do not achieve adequate pain relief with self-care alone.

Findings from the CPGs are summarized in Table 20-1.

Systematic Reviews

Cochrane Collaboration

An SR was conducted in 2005 by the Cochrane Collaboration on acupuncture and dry needling for LBP.[14] Of 35 RCTs, 3 examined acute LBP and 32 reported on CLBP.[24-55] For CLBP, two RCTs found a statistically significant difference between acupuncture and no treatment for short-term pain relief and functional improvement.[4,53] One of these RCTs observed significantly decreased pain but not improvement in the intermediate-term for acupuncture versus no treatment.[53] Five RCTs showed that acupuncture was more effective than sham acupuncture for short-term pain relief in CLBP.[44,48-50,52] One small trial failed to reach statistical significance.[30]

For intermediate-term pain relief, three RCTs did not find statistically significant differences between acupuncture and sham acupuncture, and one RCT found this same result for longer-term pain. None of the RCTs found statistically significant differences between acupuncture and sham acupuncture for function in the short- or intermediate-term.[30,49,50] Compared with other interventions, acupuncture was less effective at decreasing pain and improving function than SMT and massage in the long-term and was equally effective as self-education.[40,46] Acupuncture was more effective than TENS at decreasing pain in the short-term, yet another RCT observed no differences.[30,43] Acupuncture and TENS were equally effective at improving function in these two RCTs.[30,43]

Four RCTs assessed the effects of adding acupuncture to other therapies, such as exercise, medication, heat therapy, back education, and behavioral therapy. These trials found that adding acupuncture to these interventions improved pain and function in the short- and intermediate-terms versus the interventions alone. This SR concluded that acupuncture and dry needling improve pain and function in the short-term for CLBP. This review also concluded that acupuncture may not be more effective than other available non-invasive interventions but might be useful to add to other therapies to boost their effectiveness. However, there was insufficient evidence supporting acupuncture and dry needling for acute LBP.[14]

American Pain Society and American College of Physicians

An SR of other published SRs was conducted in 2006 by the American Pain Society and American College of Physicians CPG committee on nonpharmacologic therapies for acute and chronic LBP.[56] That review identified three SRs related to acupuncture for LBP, including the Cochrane Collaboration review mentioned earlier.[14,57,58] Two of these SRs were high quality and concluded that there is insufficient evidence supporting the use of acupuncture for acute LBP but that acupuncture improves pain in the short-term for CLBP.[14,57] These SRs included a total of 51 unique RCTs (references were not provided). Three new trials were also identified (duration of LBP not reported); one did not find any statistically significant differences between acupuncture and sham acupuncture for pain or function, one did not find any clinically meaningful differences between acupuncture and no acupuncture for pain or function, and one found statistically significant differences for pain and medication use for acupuncture versus usual care.[59-61] This SR repeated the results of the Cochrane review mentioned previously and concluded that acupuncture is more effective than sham acupuncture for

CLBP.[14,56] There was insufficient evidence to support acupuncture for acute LBP.

Findings from these SRs are summarized in Table 20-2.

Other

Several other SRs and meta-analyses have been published evaluating the effectiveness of acupuncture for CLBP.[57,58,62-64] Their findings are summarized in Table 20-3. The more recent reviews suggest that acupuncture is equally effective as other active conservative therapies and may be a useful adjunct to some of them.[57] The earlier reviews have similar conclusions to that found in the CPGs on CLBP.[58,62-64]

Randomized Controlled Trials

Nineteen RCTs involving needle acupuncture for CLBP, published in English after 1980 were identified.[30,40,43-55,60,61,65,66] Their methods are summarized in Table 20-4, and their results are briefly described here.

Brinkhaus and colleagues[60] performed an RCT including patients with CLBP. To be included, participants had to experience symptoms lasting longer than 6 months. Participants were randomized to one of three groups: (1) acupuncture, (2) sham acupuncture, or (3) waiting list control. Acupuncture was delivered by an acupuncture physician to both the acupuncture and sham acupuncture groups for

TABLE 20-2	Systematic Review Findings on Acupuncture for Chronic Low Back Pain		
Reference	# RCTs in SR	# RCTs for CLBP	Conclusion
14	36	33	Acupuncture and dry needling improve pain and function in short term for CLBP Acupuncture may not be more useful than other noninvasive therapies but may be a good adjunct to other therapies in the treatment of CLBP
56	3 SRs[14,57,58] with 51 unique RCTs	NR	Acupuncture is more effective than sham acupuncture for CLBP

CLBP, chronic low back pain; NR, not reported; RCT, randomized controlled trial; SR, systematic review.

TABLE 20-3	Other Review Findings on Acupuncture for Chronic Low Back Pain		
Study	Review Features (Search Period)	Total No. RCTs (CLBP RCTs)	Conclusions of Reviewers
57	Meta-analysis (up to August 2004)	33 (22)	Short-term effectiveness on pain: more effective than sham acupuncture, sham TENS, and no additional treatment controls Not more effective than other active treatments Less effective than spinal manipulation therapy Long-term effectiveness on pain: more effective than no additional treatment and sham TENS control Less effective than massage
58	Systematic narrative review (1999-2002)	6	Efficacy remains unclear; recent studies suggest that acupuncture is more effective than no treatment or sham treatment, is as effective as other medical interventions of questionable value, but is less effective than massage
62	Systematic review (1966-1998)	13 (6)	No convincing evidence for the analgesic efficacy of acupuncture for low back pain
63	Best evidence synthesis (1966-1996)	6 (NR)	No evidence that acupuncture is more effective than no treatment Moderate evidence that acupuncture is not more effective than trigger-point injections or transcutaneous electrical nerve stimulation Limited evidence that acupuncture is not more effective than placebo or sham acupuncture
64	Meta-analysis (1969-1996)	12 (8)	Odds ratio of improvement with acupuncture compared with control intervention was 2.30 (95% CI, 1.28 to 4.13) Acupuncture was superior to various control interventions, although there is insufficient evidence to state whether it is superior to placebo

CI, confidence interval; CLBP, chronic low back pain; NR, not reported; RCT, randomized controlled trial; TENS, transcutaneous electrical nerve stimulation.

TABLE 20-4	Randomized Controlled Trials of Acupuncture for Chronic Low Back Pain			
Reference	Indication	Intervention 1	Intervention 2	Intervention 3 or Control
60	CLBP without neurologic involvement, symptoms >6 months	Acupuncture Acupuncture physician 30 min × 12 sessions over 8 weeks Cointervention: analgesic medication n = 120	Sham acupuncture Acupuncture physician 30 min × 12 sessions over 8 weeks Cointervention: analgesic medication n = 58	Waiting list controls Cointervention: analgesic medication n = 64
44	CLBP without neurologic involvement, symptoms >6 months	Manual acupuncture (local and distal points) Clinician 1 session/week × 8 weeks Cointervention: NR n = 18	Manual acupuncture plus electrical stimulation of 4 needles Clinician 1 session/week × 8 weeks Cointervention: NR n = 16	Sham TENS Clinician 1 session/week × 8 weeks Cointervention: NR n = 16
40	CLBP without neurologic involvement, symptoms >6 weeks	TCM acupuncture Licensed acupuncturist 10 sessions over 10 weeks Cointervention: analgesic medication n = 94	Massage Licensed massage therapist 10 sessions over 10 weeks Cointervention: analgesic medication, exercise n = 78	Self-care, education (book, videos), exercise video Cointervention: analgesic medication n = 90
45	CLBP with or without neurologic involvement, symptoms >6 months	Classic Oriental meridian theory (some received electrical acupuncture) Acupuncturists 10 or more sessions over 10 weeks Cointervention: NR n = 25	NA	Waiting list, no treatment 15 weeks Cointervention: NR n = 25
55	CLBP without neurologic involvement, symptoms >13 weeks	Acupuncture (near and far technique, some received electrical acupuncture) Acupuncturist 6 sessions over 3-4 weeks Cointervention: NR n = 46	SMT Chiropractor 6 sessions over 3-4 weeks Cointervention: NR n = 49	Tenoxican (20 mg/day) and ranitidine (50 mg × 2/day) 3-4 weeks Cointervention: NR n = 31
46	CLBP without neurologic involvement, symptoms >6 months	Acupuncture (near and far technique, some received electrical acupuncture) Acupuncturist 2 sessions/week over up to 9 weeks Cointervention: NR n = 36	SMT Chiropractor 2 sessions/week up to 9 weeks Cointervention: NR n = 36	Medication not already tried: Celecoxib (200-400 mg/day), Rofecoxib (12.5 to 25 mg/day), paracetamol (up to 4 g/day) Administrator: NA Cointervention: NR n = 43
47	CLBP, neurologic involvement NR, symptoms >6 months	Manual acupuncture Acupuncturist 2 sessions/week × 4 weeks Cointervention: NR n = 32	TENS at home Administrator: NA 30 minutes/session up to 6 hours/day Cointervention: NR n = 28	NA

Continued

TABLE 20-4	Randomized Controlled Trials of Acupuncture for Chronic Low Back Pain—cont'd			
Reference	Indication	Intervention 1	Intervention 2	Intervention 3 or Control
48	CLBP with or without neurologic involvement, symptoms >6 months	Acupuncture Physical therapist 6 sessions over 6 weeks Cointervention: exercise, education n = 30	NA	Placebo-TENS Investigator 6 sessions over 6 weeks Cointervention: exercise, education n = 30
30	CLBP, neurologic involvement NR, symptoms >3 months	Electroacupuncture with needles Acupuncturist 2 sessions/week × 3 weeks Cointervention: NR n = 18	TENS Physical therapist 15 sessions over 3 weeks Cointervention: NR n = 18	Sham TENS Physical therapist 15 sessions over 3 weeks Cointervention: NR n = 18
49	CLBP without neurologic involvement, symptoms >6 months	Traditional body and ear acupuncture + PT Physician and physical therapist 20 sessions over 12 weeks 26 sessions over 12 weeks PT Cointervention: NR n = 40	PT Physical therapist 26 sessions over 12 weeks Cointervention: NR n = 46	Sham acupuncture + PT Physician and physical therapist 20 sessions over 12 weeks 26 sessions over 12 weeks PT n = 45
50	CLBP, neurologic involvement NR, symptom duration NR	Traditional Chinese acupuncture Surgeon 2 sessions/week × 4 weeks Cointervention: NR n = 36	NA	Sham acupuncture, intradermal injection of 2% lidocaine at nonacupuncture, nontender sites Surgeon 2 sessions/week × 4 weeks Cointervention: NR n = 41
51	CLBP, neurologic involvement NR, symptoms >12 weeks	Acupuncture + standard therapy Anesthesiologist 2 sessions/week × 5 weeks Cointervention: standard therapy (exercise, PT, analgesic medication) n = 28	NA	Standard therapy alone (exercise, PT, analgesic medication) Physician 5 weeks Cointervention: NR n = 23
52	CLBP without neurologic involvement, symptoms >6 weeks	Verum acupuncture + conventional orthopedic therapy Physician 3 sessions/week × 4 weeks Cointervention: orthopedic therapy (daily PT, physical exercises, back school, mud packs, infrared heat therapy, 50 mg diclofenac max 3×/day if demanded) n = 65	Sham acupuncture + conventional orthopedic therapy Physician 3 sessions/week × 4 weeks Cointervention: orthopedic therapy (daily PT, physical exercises, back school, mud packs, infrared heat therapy, 50 mg diclofenac max 3×/day if demanded) n = 61	Conventional orthopedic therapy (daily PT, physical exercises, back school, mud packs, infrared heat therapy, 50 mg diclofenac max 3×/day if demanded) Administrator: NR n = 60

TABLE 20-4	Randomized Controlled Trials of Acupuncture for Chronic Low Back Pain—cont'd			
Reference	Indication	Intervention 1	Intervention 2	Intervention 3 or Control
61	CLBP, neurologic involvement NR, symptoms 4-52 weeks	Acupuncture Acupuncturist 10 sessions over 3 months Cointervention: NR n = 159	NA	Usual care (PT, chiropractic therapy, medication, exercise) Physician Cointervention: NR n = 80
53	CLBP, neurologic involvement NR, symptoms >6 months	Acupuncture (manual, low frequency electrical stimulation, or high frequency electrical stimulation) Physical therapists 10× 30-minute sessions Cointervention: NR n = 10	NA	Waiting list control Administrator: NA Cointervention: NR n = 10
43	CLBP without neurologic involvement, symptoms >2 weeks	Acupuncture (4 points bilaterally, electrical stimulation, press tack needles subsequently left in situ for several days) Acupuncture therapist 2×/week × 2 weeks Cointervention: NR n = 10	TENS Acupuncture therapist 2×/week × 2 weeks Cointervention: poultice containing methyl salicylic acid, menthol, and antihistamine applied at home n = 10	NA
54	CLBP with or without neurologic involvement, symptoms >6 months	Electroacupuncture Physical therapist 3×/week × 4 weeks Cointervention: same exercise program as the control group, analgesic medication n = 25	Standard group exercise program (back strengthening and stretching exercises, education, behavioral modification, ergonomics, home exercise) Physical therapist 1 hour/week × 4 weeks Cointervention: analgesic medication n = 24	NA
65	CLBP with neurologic involvement, symptoms >3 months	Electroacupuncture (6 acupuncture points) Therapist unspecified 2×/week × 4 weeks Cointervention: analgesic medication, same exercise program as control group n = 14	Electroheat acupuncture (6 acupuncture points) Therapist unspecified 2×/week × 4 weeks Cointervention: analgesic medication, same exercise program as control group n = 14	Exercise (6 mobilization plus 1 abdominal stabilization at home) Therapist unspecified 3×/day Cointervention: analgesic medication n = 14
66	CLBP without neurologic involvement, symptoms 6 months	Acupuncture Physician 15 sessions max Cointervention: same routine medical care as the control group n = 1321	NA	Routine medical care Administrator: NA Schedule: NA Cointervention: NR n = 1183

CLBP, chronic low back pain; LBP, low back pain; NA, not applicable; NR, not reported; PT, physical therapy; SMT, spinal manipulation therapy; TCM, traditional Chinese medicine; TENS, transcutaneous electrical nerve stimulation.

twelve 30-minute sessions over 12 weeks. After 8 weeks of follow-up, participants in the acupuncture group experienced a statistically significant improvement in pain compared with those in the sham acupuncture group. However, after 26 and 52 weeks of follow-up, no differences were observed between the acupuncture and sham acupuncture groups.

Carlsson and Sjolund[44] performed an RCT including patients with CLBP. To be included, participants had to experience symptoms lasting longer than 6 months. Participants were randomized to one of three groups: (1) manual acupuncture, (2) manual acupuncture plus electrical stimulation, or (3) sham TENS. A physician delivered acupuncture to all groups once per week over 8 weeks. After 6 months of follow-up, participants in the acupuncture groups experienced a statistically significant improvement in pain compared with baseline. However, those in the sham TENS group did not experience a statistically significant improvement in pain. After 6 months of follow-up, no statistically significant differences were observed between all groups regarding pain in the main analysis. However, when a different analysis was conducted, participants in the acupuncture groups experienced a statistically significant improvement in pain versus the sham TENS group after 6 months.

Cherkin and colleagues[40] performed an RCT including patients with CLBP without neurologic involvement. To be included, participants had to experience symptoms lasting longer than 6 weeks. Participants were randomized to one of three groups: (1) traditional Chinese medical acupuncture, (2) massage, or (3) self-care consisting of education through a book and videos. A licensed acupuncturist delivered acupuncture and a licensed massage therapist administered massage during 10 sessions over 10 weeks. After 1 year of follow-up, participants in the massage group experienced statistically significant improvements in pain and function versus the acupuncture group. However, no statistically significant differences were observed between the massage and self-care groups regarding pain and function after 1 year.

Coan and colleagues[45] performed an RCT including patients with CLBP with or without neurologic involvement. To be included, participants had to experience symptoms lasting longer than 6 months. Participants were randomized to either classical Oriental meridian acupuncture (some received electrical acupuncture) delivered by an acupuncturist during 10 sessions over 10 weeks or to a waiting list control group who received no treatment over 15 weeks. After 40 weeks of follow-up, participants in both groups experienced improvements, with those in the acupuncture group experiencing greater pain reduction, yet no statistically significant differences were reported.

Giles and Müller[55] performed an RCT including patients with CLBP without neurologic involvement. To be included, participants had to experience symptoms lasting longer than 13 weeks. Participants were randomized to one of three groups: (1) acupuncture (using the "near and far" technique), (2) SMT, or (3) medication (tenoxican and ranitidine). Acupuncture was delivered by an acupuncturist and SMT was delivered by a chiropractor during six sessions over 3 to 4 weeks. After a median of 30 days, participants in the SMT group experienced statistically significant improvements in pain and function versus baseline. Comparisons between groups were not reported.

Giles and Müller[46] performed an RCT including patients with CLBP without neurologic involvement. To be included, participants had to experience symptoms lasting longer than 13 weeks. Participants were randomized to one of three groups: (1) acupuncture (using the "near and far" technique), (2) SMT, or (3) medication that had not already been tried (usually celecoxib, rofecoxib, or paracetamol). An acupuncturist delivered acupuncture and SMT was delivered by a chiropractor during two sessions per week delivered over up to 9 weeks. Immediately after the sessions, participants in the SMT group experienced statistically significant improvements in pain and function versus baseline. Comparisons between groups were not reported.

Grant and colleagues[47] performed an RCT including patients with CLBP without neurologic involvement. To be included, participants had to experience symptoms lasting longer than 6 months. Participants were randomized to either manual acupuncture delivered by an acupuncturist over 2 sessions per week up for 4 weeks or to TENS at home for 30 minutes per session up to 6 hours per day. After 3 months of follow-up, participants in the TENS group experienced a statistically significant improvement in pain versus baseline but the acupuncture group experienced a nonsignificant improvement in pain. Comparisons between groups were not reported.

Keir and colleagues[48] performed an RCT including patients with CLBP with or without neurologic involvement. To be included, participants had to experience symptoms lasting longer than 6 months. Participants were randomized to either acupuncture delivered by a physical therapist during six sessions over 6 weeks or to placebo-TENS delivered by the investigator during six sessions over 6 weeks. After 6 months of follow-up, no statistically significant differences between the groups were observed for pain relief.

Lehmann and colleagues[30] performed an RCT including patients with CLBP who experienced symptoms for at least 3 months. Participants were randomized to one of three groups: (1) electroacupuncture, (2) TENS, or (3) sham TENS. An acupuncturist delivered electroacupuncture for 2 sessions per week over 3 weeks, and a physical therapist delivered TENS and sham TENS for 15 sessions over 3 weeks. After 6 months of follow-up, no statistically significant differences between the groups were observed for pain relief.

Leibing and colleagues[49] performed an RCT including patients with CLBP without neurologic involvement, who had experienced symptoms for at least 6 months. Participants were randomized to one of three groups: (1) acupuncture plus PT, (2) PT alone, or (3) sham acupuncture plus PT. A physician delivered acupuncture and sham acupuncture for 20 sessions over 12 weeks, while a physical therapist delivered PT for 26 sessions over 12 weeks. After 9 months of follow-up, participants in the acupuncture group experienced statistically significant improvement in pain versus the PT only group but no differences were observed between the acupuncture group and the sham acupuncture group.

Mendelson and colleagues[50] performed an RCT including patients with CLBP. Participants were randomized to either traditional Chinese acupuncture or sham acupuncture plus an intradermal injection of anesthesia. A surgeon delivered acupuncture and sham acupuncture for two sessions per week over 4 weeks. After 18 weeks of follow-up, no statistically significant differences were observed between the acupuncture group and the sham acupuncture group regarding pain relief.

Meng and colleagues[51] performed an RCT including patients with CLBP. In order to be included, participants had to experience symptoms for at least 12 weeks. Participants were randomized to either acupuncture plus standard therapy or standard therapy alone. An anesthesiologist delivered acupuncture for two sessions per week over 5 weeks, while a physician delivered standard therapy over 5 weeks, which included PT, home exercise, and analgesic medication. After 9 weeks of follow-up, participants in the acupuncture plus standard therapy experienced a statistically significant improvement in pain and disability versus those in the standard therapy only group.

Molsberger and colleagues[52] performed an RCT including patients with CLBP. In order to be included, participants had to experience symptoms for at least 12 weeks. Participants were randomized to one of three groups: (1) verum acupuncture plus conventional orthopedic therapy, (2) sham acupuncture plus conventional orthopedic therapy, or (3) conventional orthopedic therapy. Acupuncture and sham acupuncture were administered by a physician for three sessions per week over 4 weeks, while conventional orthopedic therapy consisted of daily PT, physical exercises, back school, mud packs, infrared heat therapy, as well as diclofenac (50 mg up to three times daily if needed). After 3 months of follow-up, participants in the acupuncture plus orthopedic therapy group experienced a statistically significant improvement in pain versus those in the other two groups.

Thomas and colleagues[61] performed an RCT including patients with LBP lasting 4 to 52 weeks. Participants were randomized to either acupuncture or usual care. An acupuncturist delivered acupuncture for 10 sessions over 3 months, while usual care consisted of PT, chiropractic therapy, medication, and exercise. After 24 months of follow-up, participants in the acupuncture group experienced a statistically significant improvement in pain using the short form 36 (SF-36) bodily pain score, yet no differences were observed for the other outcomes, including function or pain using the Oswestry Disability Index or the McGill Pain Questionnaire.

Thomas and Lundberg[53] performed an RCT including patients with CLBP. In order to be included participants had to experience symptoms for at least 6 months. Participants were randomized to either acupuncture or waiting list control. Physical therapists delivered acupuncture for ten 30-minute sessions. Three different modes of acupuncture were employed: (1) manual acupuncture, (2) low-frequency electrical stimulation, or (3) high-frequency electrical stimulation. After 6 months of follow-up, participants in the acupuncture group who received low-frequency electrical stimulation experienced a statistically significant improvement in pain versus the waiting list control group.

Tsukayama and colleagues[43] performed an RCT including patients with CLBP without neurologic involvement. In order to be included participants had to experience symptoms for at least 2 weeks. Participants were randomized to either acupuncture or TENS. Acupuncture therapists administered acupuncture and TENS twice per week for 2 weeks. Acupuncture consisted of manual acupuncture and electrical stimulation. After 2 weeks of follow-up, no statistically significant differences in pain were observed between the two groups.

Yeung and colleagues[54] performed an RCT including patients with CLBP with or without neurologic involvement. In order to be included, participants had to experience symptoms for at least 6 months. Participants were randomized to either electroacupuncture or a standard exercise program. A physical therapist delivered electroacupuncture three times per week for 4 weeks. Individuals in the electroacupuncture group also received the standard exercise program, consisting of back strengthening and stretching exercises, education, behavioral modification, ergonomics, and home exercise administered by a physical therapist 1 hour per week for 4 weeks. After 3 months of follow-up, participants in the electroacupuncture group experienced statistically significant decreases in pain and disability versus those in the standard exercise program.

Tsui and Cheing[65] performed an RCT including patients with CLBP with neurologic involvement. In order to be included, participants had to experience symptoms for at least 3 months. Participants were randomized to one of three groups: (1) electroacupuncture plus home exercise, (2) electroheat acupuncture plus home exercise, or (3) home exercise only. An unspecified therapist delivered electroacupuncture and electroheat acupuncture twice per week over 4 weeks. The home exercise program consisted of 6 mobilization exercises to be done 20 times and 1 abdominal stabilization exercise to be done 10 times; the exercise program was performed 3 times per day. Immediately after the last session, individuals in every group experienced a statistically significant improvement in pain and disability compared with baseline scores. In addition, the electroacupuncture and electroheat acupuncture groups experienced statistically significant pain relief versus the control group immediately after treatment but no statistically significant differences were observed for disability.

Witt and colleagues[66] performed an RCT including patients with CLBP without neurologic involvement. In order to be included, participants had to experience symptoms for at least 6 months. Participants were randomized to either acupuncture plus routine medical care or routine medical care alone. Physicians delivered acupuncture and participants were allowed to receive a maximum of 15 sessions. After 6 months of follow-up, the acupuncture group experienced a statistically significant improvement in function versus the routine medical care group but no statistically significant differences were observed between groups for pain relief.

SAFETY

Contraindications

Acupuncture for CLBP is contraindicated in those who have hemophilia or other bleeding disorders, septicemia, cellulitis, local skin infections, or regions of hypoesthesia secondary to burns or ulcerations. Those who are afraid of all needles or who are uncooperative because of delusions, hallucinations, or paranoia should also not have needle acupuncture. Electroacupuncture should be avoided over the brain or heart or in an area of an implanted electrical device (e.g., cardiac pacemakers).[67] Extra care should be taken when administering needle acupuncture to individuals who are pregnant, have metal allergies, or are taking anticoagulant drugs.[67]

Adverse Events

CPGs for the management of LBP reported that adverse events associated with acupuncture for CLBP included cardiac trauma, drowsiness, syncope, hepatitis, increased pain, infections, and pneumothorax, although the prevalence of these events is unknown.[20] Twelve trials reported adverse events related to acupuncture for CLBP.[30,40,43,44,48,49,51,52,54,60,61,66] One trial with 10,106 participants reported adverse events in 6%, mostly involving minor local bleeding or hematoma.[66] Among the other 11 trials with 489 participants, 7.8% reported adverse events including increased pain, tiredness, drowsiness, lightheadedness, dizziness, local bleeding, and hematoma.

Similar adverse events have been reported in large studies of needle acupuncture used for other indications.[68,69] The incidence of adverse events among large prospective studies evaluating acupuncture ranged from 0.1% to 23%.[68-73] Serious adverse events were rare and included hepatitis, septicemia, and pneumothorax. In 1996, in an effort to prevent the spread of infectious diseases such as human immunodeficiency virus and hepatitis, the US Food and Drug Administration mandated the use of sterile, disposable needles.[74]

COSTS

Fees and Third-Party Reimbursement

In the United States, treatment with needle acupuncture that is delivered by a licensed health care practitioner such as an acupuncturist, physical therapist, physician, or chiropractor can be delivered using CPT codes 97810 (first 15 minutes), 97811 (each additional 15 minutes), 97813 (with electrical stimulation, first 15 minutes), or 97814 (with electrical stimulation, each additional 15 minutes).

Although relative value units (RVUs) have been established using the Resource Based Relative Value Scale (RBRVS) for these Category 1 CPT codes, there is currently no Medicare reimbursement for those procedures. Medicare has a longstanding national coverage policy that does not consider Medicare reimbursement for acupuncture as reasonable and necessary.[75] However, the RVUs can be used to

TABLE 20-5	Fees for Related Services Based on Medicare RVUs		
CPT	RVU	Value/RVU	Amount
97810	0.98	$36.08	$35
97811	0.75	$36.08	$27
97813	1.05	$36.08	$38
97814	0.85	$36.08	$31

Medicare itself does not cover these services.

assist in establishing a baseline fee schedule, by applying an appropriate conversion factor. In 2010, the Medicare conversion factor was $36.08.

These procedures are often covered by other third-party payers such as health insurers and worker's compensation insurance. Third-party payers will often reimburse a limited number of visits if they are supported by adequate documentation deeming them medically necessary. Prior authorization is recommended. Although acupuncture is not covered by Medicare or Medicaid, an increasing number of commercial health plans and State and Provincial Worker's Compensation Boards now include coverage for acupuncture.[76,77]

Although some payers continue to base their reimbursements on usual, customary, and reasonable payment methodology, the majority have developed reimbursement tables based on the RBRVS used by Medicare. Fees for these services typically range from $50 to $100 per session in the United States.[67]

Fees for related services based on the Medicare RVUs are summarized in Table 20-5.

Cost Effectiveness

Evidence supporting the cost effectiveness of treatment protocols that compared this intervention, often in combination with one or more cointerventions, with control groups who received one or more other interventions, for either acute or chronic LBP, was identified from two SRs on this topic and is summarized here.[78,79] Although many of these study designs are unable to clearly identify the individual contribution of acupuncture, their results provide some insight as to the clinical and economic outcomes associated with this approach.

An RCT in the United States compared two approaches for patients with CLBP.[80] The naturopathic care group included acupuncture, exercise, dietary advice, and relaxation delivered by a naturopath. The control group included brief education from a naturopath given in 30-minute, biweekly sessions over 3 months. Both groups also received an educational booklet, and voluntary crossover was offered to participants after 12 weeks. Clinical outcomes after 6 months favored the naturopathic care group for improvements in utility. Direct medical costs for study interventions over 6 months were $1469 in the naturopathic care group and $337 in the brief education group. Direct medical costs for nonstudy interventions over 6 months, including chiropractic, massage, PT, pain medication, and other interventions, were $1203 lower in the naturopathic care group. Indirect productivity costs associated with lost work days were $1141 lower in the naturopathic care group. Authors concluded that naturopathic care including acupuncture was more cost effective than brief education.

An RCT in the United States compared three approaches for patients with CLBP.[40] The TCM group received needle acupuncture with electrical or manual stimulation of needles, and possibly moxibustion; manual therapy was not permitted. The massage group received a variety of techniques, although acupressure was not permitted. The brief education group received education about LBP from a book and videos. Clinical outcomes after 12 months favored the massage group over the TCM group for improvement in both pain and function; medication use was also lowest in the massage group. Direct medical costs associated with study interventions over 12 months were $352 in the TCM group, $377 in the massage group, and $50 in the brief education group. Direct medical costs associated with nonstudy interventions including provider visits, medication use, and diagnostic imaging over 12 months were $252 in the TCM group, $139 in the massage group, and $200 in the brief education group. Total direct medical costs for both study and nonstudy interventions over 12 months were therefore $604 in the TCM group, $516 in the massage group, and $250 in the brief education group. Indirect productivity costs were not reported. Authors concluded that although cost differences between groups were not significant, massage appeared to be more effective than TCM.

An RCT from Canada compared two approaches for patients who had been injured at work and subsequently suffered from CLBP.[81] The functional restoration group included cognitive behavioral therapy, fear avoidance training, education, biofeedback, group counseling, and strengthening and stretching exercises. The usual care group could receive a variety of interventions, including PT, acupuncture, back school, SMT, medication, or supervised exercise therapy. Clinical outcomes were not reported. Direct medical costs associated with the study intervention were $2507 higher in the functional restoration group. Indirect productivity costs associated with lost work days were $3172 lower in the functional restoration group. Total costs for interventions, lost work days, and disability pensions were $7068 lower in the functional restoration group. These differences were not statistically significant.

An RCT in the United Kingdom compared two approaches for patients with subacute or chronic LBP presenting in general practice.[82] The acupuncture group received treatment according to TCM. The usual care group care consisted of unspecified interventions and was delivered by a GP. Clinical outcomes after 2 years were similar between groups, with the acupuncture group having a slightly greater improvement in utility, though these differences were not significant. Direct medical costs associated with study and nonstudy interventions including provider visits, medication, and other interventions over 2 years were approximately $821 for the acupuncture group and approximately $616 for the usual care group. Indirect productivity costs associated with lost work days were not reported. Because the acupuncture group had marginally better clinical outcomes with greater costs, its

incremental cost effectiveness ratio was estimated at approximately $7591 per quality-adjusted life-year, well within the generally accepted threshold for cost utility analyses.

The CPG from Europe in 2004 found the cost effectiveness of acupuncture for CLBP (>3 months) to be unknown.[20]

Other

An RCT reported no cost savings in back care services after 1 year among groups receiving acupuncture, massage, and self-care.[40] Another RCT concluded that acupuncture when added to usual care was cost effective and only modestly increased the overall treatment costs for LBP.[15] Similar conclusions were made in another RCT.[60]

An observational study reported that acupuncture was found to be cost effective with regard to pain reduction when compared to standard treatment.[83] Nevertheless, the overall costs of acupuncture were higher, despite some savings due to decreased utilization of other care resources.[83]

Findings from these cost-effectiveness analyses are summarized in Table 20-6.

SUMMARY

Description

Needle acupuncture involves stimulating specific points along the body thought to be related to various bodily functions by penetrating the skin with thin, solid, metallic needles. These needles can be further stimulated manually or electrically. There are many different types of needle acupuncture used throughout the world, including Japanese Meridian Therapy and French Energetic acupuncture. Acupuncture originated in China more than 2000 years ago and is one of the oldest, most commonly used systems of traditional healing in the world. Acupuncture is widely available in the United States and is typically practiced in a private practice setting by a variety of practitioners including acupuncturists, TCM practitioners, and some trained physicians, chiropractors, and physical therapists where permitted.

Theory

In traditional needle acupuncture, there are 12 primary meridians, 8 secondary meridians, and more than 2000 associated acupuncture points on the human body. The goal of traditional acupuncture is to select the appropriate points along different meridians that correspond to a particular illness or bodily dysfunction and to stimulate those points with needles until energy balance is restored in the body. There are many Western scientific theories about the mechanism of action for acupuncture. One asserts that acupuncture stimulates the production of endorphins and neurotransmitters that modulate nociception and other involuntary bodily functions. One states that CLBP is inhibited in the system in the presence of another type of input (e.g., acupuncture needle). Yet another asserts that the presence of a foreign substance (e.g., acupuncture needle) within the tissue of the body stimulates an

| TABLE 20-6 | **Cost Effectiveness and Cost Utility Analyses of Acupuncture for Acute or Chronic Low Back Pain** | | | | | |

Reference Country Follow-up	Group	Direct Medical Costs	Indirect Productivity Costs	Total Costs	Conclusion
80 United States 6 months	1. Naturopathic care (including acupuncture) 2. Control	1. $1469 2. $337	1. $1141 lower than group 2	NR	1. More cost effective than 2
40 United States 1 year	1. TCM (including acupuncture) 2. Massage 3. Brief education	1. $604 2. $516 3. $250	NR	NR	No significant difference
81 Canada NR	1. Functional restoration 2. Usual care (inc. acupuncture)	1. $2507 higher than group 2 2. NR	1. $3172 lower than group 2 for lost work days 2. NR	1. $7068 lower than group 2 (lost work days + disability pensions 2. NR	No significant difference
82 United Kingdom 2 years	1. Acupuncture 2. Usual care	1. $821 2. $616	NR	NR	ICER 1 over 2: $7591/QALY

ICER, incremental cost effective ratio; NR, not reported; QALY, quality-adjusted life-years; TCM, traditional Chinese medicine.

inflammatory response. Acupuncture is typically indicated for patients with nonspecific mechanical CLBP with or without neurologic involvement. Diagnostic imaging or other forms of advanced testing is generally not required before administering acupuncture for CLBP.

Efficacy

Five CPGs provided recommendations on acupuncture for CLBP. Two CPGs did not recommend acupuncture for CLBP, one reported conflicting evidence supporting acupuncture, and two others recommended offering a course of acupuncture if other conservative management options did not obtain adequate pain relief. Two high-quality systematic reviews concluded that acupuncture and dry needling improve pain and function in the short-term for CLBP. At least 19 RCTs have assessed the efficacy of acupuncture for CLBP, the majority of which found no significant differences between acupuncture and other comparator groups after the longest period of follow-up available. However, eight RCTs reported some positive results, such as statistically significant improvement in pain or disability versus comparator groups and baseline.

Safety

Acupuncture for CLBP is contraindicated in those who have fear of needles or are uncooperative due to delusions, hallucinations or paranoia, as well as those with hemophilia or other bleeding disorders, septicemia, cellulitis, local skin infections, or regions of hypoesthesia secondary to burns or ulcerations. Electroacupuncture should be avoided over the brain or heart or in an area of an implanted electrical device (e.g., cardiac pacemakers). Precautions are required for those who are pregnant, have metal allergies, or are taking anticoagulant drugs. Adverse events associated with acupuncture for CLBP include drowsiness, lightheadedness, dizziness, local bleeding, hematoma, cardiac trauma, septicemia, syncope, hepatitis, increased pain, infection, and pneumothorax.

Costs

The cost per acupuncture session varies from $50 to $100. At least four studies have assessed the cost associated with acupuncture. One RCT found that acupuncture was cost effective, while another found no differences in cost effectiveness between acupuncture, brief education, and massage. In two other RCTs, the individual contribution of acupuncture to cost effectiveness was unclear because it was combined with other interventions.

Comments

Evidence from the CPGs, SRs, and RCTs reviewed was inconsistent regarding the use of needle acupuncture for CLBP. However, a short course of needle acupuncture may provide short-term pain relief if other conservative management options do not achieve the desired outcomes. The addition of acupuncture to other therapies such as therapeutic exercise may boost the effectiveness of those therapies. These mixed results may be related to an incomplete understanding about the mechanism of action for acupuncture, which makes it difficult to design appropriate clinical studies. Among the eligible studies in this review, many were considered to be of low methodological quality or had fatal flaws in their study design. There is a need for more high-quality studies evaluating the effectiveness of needle acupuncture for CLBP.

More research is also needed to assess the validity of sham acupuncture. It is unknown, for example, whether applying needle acupuncture to nonacupuncture points is associated with a therapeutic benefit beyond that expected with a placebo. There is also a need for better reporting of RCTs for acupuncture. Given the variation in the practice of acupuncture, details regarding specific techniques, use of adjunct treatments, number of needles and/or acupuncture points used, duration of treatment, and experience of the acupuncturists should be reported. Future studies should also report clinically important differences among study groups rather than only statistically significant differences. Inconsistent results were observed for the cost effectiveness of acupuncture. As such, future research evaluating the costs associated with acupuncture in comparison with other interventions is warranted to determine its relative cost effectiveness.

CHAPTER REVIEW QUESTIONS

Answers are located on page 451.

1. In traditional acupuncture, what does *yin* represent?
   a. cold, fast, or passive force
   b. cold, slow, or active force
   c. hot, slow, or passive force
   d. cold, slow, or passive force

2. In traditional acupuncture, what does *yang* represent?
   a. hot, excited, or active force
   b. cold, calm, or active force
   c. hot, calm, or active force
   d. cold, excited, or active force

3. How many main meridians are believed to exist in traditional acupuncture?
   a. 4
   b. 8
   c. 12
   d. 16

4. How many secondary meridians are believed to exist in traditional acupuncture?
   a. 4
   b. 8
   c. 12
   d. 16

5. Which of the following has been proposed as a mechanism of action for acupuncture?
   a. provides an energy release for the muscles
   b. relaxes the muscles by targeting trigger points
   c. stimulates vascular and immunomodulatory factors
   d. stimulates endorphins, which repairs and restores the muscles

6. True or false: Fear of needles may represent a contraindication to needle acupuncture.

7. True or false: CPGs consistently recommend acupuncture for CLBP.

REFERENCES

1. Lao L. Acupuncture techniques and devices. J Altern Complement Med 1996;2:23-25.
2. Kaptchuk TJ. Acupuncture: theory, efficacy, and practice. Ann Intern Med 2002;136:374-383.
3. Reston J. Now, about my operation in Peking. The New York Times 1971 Jul 26.
4. Eisenberg DM, Davis RB, Ettner SL, et al. Trends in alternative medicine use in the United States, 1990-1997: results of a follow-up national survey. JAMA 1998;280:1569-1575.
5. Chenot JF, Becker A, Leonhardt C, et al. Use of complementary alternative medicine for low back pain consulting in general practice: a cohort study. BMC Complement Altern Med 2007;7:42.
6. Eisenberg DM, Cohen MH, Hrbek A, et al. Credentialing complementary and alternative medical providers. Ann Intern Med 2002;137:965-973.
7. National Center for Complementary and Alternative Medicine. Acupuncture. NCCAM 2004. Report No.: D003.
8. Chu LSW, Yeh SDJ, Wood DD. Acupuncture manual: a western approach. New York: Marcel Dekker; 1979.
9. Stux G, Berman B, Pomeranz B. Basics of acupuncture. ed 5. Berlin: Verlag; 2003.
10. Melzack R. Myofascial trigger points: relation to acupuncture and mechanisms of pain. Arch Phys Med Rehabil 1981;62:114-117.
11. Zijlstra FJ, van den Berg-de Lange, Huygen FJ, et al. Anti-inflammatory actions of acupuncture. Mediators Inflamm 2003;12:59-69.
12. Wen HL, Ho WK, Wong HK, et al. Changes in adrenocorticotropic hormone (ACTH) and cortisol levels in drug addicts treated by a new and rapid detoxification procedure using acupuncture and naloxone. Comp Med East West 1979;6:241-245.
13. Shah JP, Phillips TM, Danoff JV, et al. An in vivo microanalytical technique for measuring the local biochemical milieu of human skeletal muscle. J Appl Physiol 2005;99:1977-1984.
14. Furlan AD, van Tulder MW, Cherkin DC, et al. Acupuncture and dry-needling for low back pain. Cochrane Database Syst Rev 2005;(1):CD001351.
15. Thomas KJ, MacPherson H, Ratcliffe J, et al. Longer term clinical and economic benefits of offering acupuncture care to patients with chronic low back pain. Health Technol Assess 2005;9:iii-x
16. Kalauokalani D, Cherkin DC, Sherman KJ, et al. Lessons from a trial of acupuncture and massage for low back pain: patient expectations and treatment effects. Spine 2001;26:1418-1424.
17. MacPherson H, Thorpe L, Thomas K, et al. Acupuncture for low back pain: traditional diagnosis and treatment of 148 patients in a clinical trial. Complement Ther Med 2004;12:38-44.
18. Sherman KJ, Cherkin DC, Hogeboom CJ. The diagnosis and treatment of patients with chronic low-back pain by traditional Chinese medical acupuncturists. J Altern Complem Med 2001;7:641-650.
19. Nielens H, van Zundert J, Mairiaux P, et al. Chronic low back pain. Good Clinical practice (GCP) Brussels: Belgian Health Care Knowledge Centre (KCE); 2006. KCE reports vol 48C.
20. Airaksinen O, Brox JI, Cedraschi C, et al. European guidelines for the management of chronic nonspecific low back pain. Eur Spine J 2006;15:S192-S300.

21. Negrini S, Giovannoni S, Minozzi S, et al. Diagnostic therapeutic flow-charts for low back pain patients: the Italian clinical guidelines. Eura Medicophys 2006;42:151-170.
22. National Institute for Health and Clinical Excellence (NICE). Low back pain: early management of persistent non-specific low back pain. London, 2009, National Institute of Health and Clinical Excellence. Report No.: NICE clinical guideline 88.
23. Chou R, Qaseem A, Snow V, et al. Diagnosis and treatment of low back pain: a joint clinical practice guideline from the American College of Physicians and the American Pain Society. Ann Intern Med 2007;147:478-491.
24. Ceccherelli F, Rigoni MT, Gagliardi G, et al. Comparison of superficial and deep acupuncture in the treatment of lumbar myofascial pain: a double-blind randomized controlled study. Clin J Pain 2002;18:149-153.
25. King YD. Fly-probing-acupoint manipulation as a main treatment for lumbago. Shanghai J Acupuncture Moxibustion 1998;17:25-26.
26. Edelist G, Gross AE, Langer F. Treatment of low back pain with acupuncture. Can Anaesth Soc J 1976;23:303-306.
27. Inoue M, Kitakouji H, Ikeuchi R, et al. Randomized controlled pilot study comparing acupuncture with sham acupuncture for lumbago [Yotsu ni taisuru gishin wo mochiita randamuka hikaku–shiken no kokoromi]. J Jpn Soc Acupuncture Moxibustion 2000;50:356.
28. Inoue M, Kitakouji H, Ikeuchi R, et al. Randomized controlled pilot study comparing manual acupuncture with sham acupuncture for lumbago (2nd report) [Yotsu ni taisuru gishin womochiita randamuka hikaku–shiken no kokoromi]. J Jpn Soc Acupuncture Moxibustion 2001;51:412.
29. Kurosu Y. Comparative experiment of the therapeutic effectiveness of acupuncture and garlic moxibustion. J Jpn Soc Acupuncture Moxibustion 1979;28:31-34.
30. Lehmann TR, Russell DW, Spratt KF, et al. Efficacy of electroacupuncture and TENS in the rehabilitation of chronic low back pain patients. Pain 1986;26:277-290.
31. Li Q, Shang WM. The effect of acupuncture plus cupping on 78 cases with lumbago. Hebei Chinese Traditional Medicine 1997;19:28.
32. Lopacz S, Gralewski Z. Evaluation of the results of treatment of low backache by acupuncture or suggesting (preliminary report). Neurol Neurochir Pol 1979;13:405-409.
33. Macdonald AJ, Macrae KD, Master BR, et al. Superficial acupuncture in the relief of chronic low back pain. Ann R Coll Surg Engl 1983;65:44-46.
34. Sakai T, Tsukayama H, Amagai H, et al. Controlled trial on acupuncture for lumbago. [Yotsu ni taisuru hari no hikaku–taisyo–shiken]. J Jpn Soc Acupuncture Moxibustion 1998;48:110.
35. Sakai T, Tsutani K, Tsukayama H, et al. Multi-center randomized controlled trial of acupuncture with electrical stimulation and acupuncture-like transcutaneous electrical nerve stimulation for lumbago. J Jpn Soc Acupuncture Moxibustion 2001;51:175-184.
36. Tadeda H, Nabeta T. Randomized controlled trial comparing the effect of distal point needling with local point needling for low back pain [RCT ni yoru yotsu–sho ni taisuru enkakubu–sisin to kyokusho–sisin no koka hikaku]. J Jpn Soc Acupuncture Moxibustion 2001;51:411.
37. von Mencke M, Wieden TE, Hoppe M, et al. Akupunktur des Schulter-Arm-Syndroms und der Lumbagie/Ischialgie - zwei prosepktive Doppelblind-Studien (Teil I). Akupunktur 1988;4:204-215.
38. Wang JX. The effect of acupuncture on 492 cases of acute lumbago. Shanghai Acupuncture J 1996;15:28.
39. Wu YC. Acupuncture for 150 cases of acute lumbago. Shanghai J Acupuncture Moxibustion 1991;10:18-19.
40. Cherkin DC, Eisenberg D, Sherman KJ, et al. Randomized trial comparing traditional Chinese medical acupuncture, therapeutic massage, and self-care education for chronic low back pain. Arch Intern Med 2001;161:1081-1088.
41. Garvey TA, Marks MR, Wiesel SW. A prospective, randomized, double-blind evaluation of trigger-point injection therapy for low-back pain. Spine 1989;14:962-964.
42. Gunn CC, Milbrandt WE, Little AS, et al. Dry needling of muscle motor points for chronic low-back pain: a randomized clinical trial with long-term follow-up. Spine 1980;5:279-291.
43. Tsukayama H, Yamashita H, Amagai H, et al. Randomised controlled trial comparing the effectiveness of electroacupuncture and TENS for low back pain: a preliminary study for a pragmatic trial. Acupunct Med 2002;20:175-180.
44. Carlsson CP, Sjolund BH. Acupuncture for chronic low back pain: a randomized placebo-controlled study with long-term follow-up. Clin J Pain 2001;17:296-305.
45. Coan RM, Wong G, Ku SL, et al. The acupuncture treatment of low back pain: a randomized controlled study. Am J Chin Med 1980;8:181-189.
46. Giles LG, Müller R. Chronic spinal pain: a randomized clinical trial comparing medication, acupuncture, and spinal manipulation. Spine 2003;28:1490-1502.
47. Grant DJ, Bishop-Miller J, Winchester DM, et al. A randomized comparative trial of acupuncture versus transcutaneous electrical nerve stimulation for chronic back pain in the elderly. Pain 1999;82:9-13.
48. Kerr DP, Walsh DM, Baxter D. Acupuncture in the management of chronic low back pain: a blinded randomized controlled trial. Clin J Pain 2003;19:364-370.
49. Leibing E, Leonhardt U, Koster G, et al. Acupuncture treatment of chronic low-back pain—a randomized, blinded, placebo-controlled trial with 9-month follow-up. Pain 2002;96:189-196.
50. Mendelson G, Selwood TS, Kranz H, et al. Acupuncture treatment of chronic back pain. A double-blind placebo-controlled trial. Am J Med 1983;74:49-55.
51. Meng CF, Wang D, Ngeow J, et al. Acupuncture for chronic low back pain in older patients: a randomized, controlled trial. Rheumatology (Oxford) 2003;42:1508-1517.
52. Molsberger AF, Mau J, Pawelec DB, et al. Does acupuncture improve the orthopedic management of chronic low back pain—a randomized, blinded, controlled trial with 3 months follow up. Pain 2002;99:579-587.
53. Thomas M, Lundberg T. Importance of modes of acupuncture in the treatment of chronic nociceptive low back pain. Acta Anaesthesiol Scand 1994;38:63-69.
54. Yeung CK, Leung MC, Chow DH. The use of electroacupuncture in conjunction with exercise for the treatment of chronic low-back pain. J Altern Complement Med 2003;9:479-490.
55. Giles LGF, Müller R. Chronic spinal pain syndromes: a clinical pilot trial comparing acupuncture, a nonsteroidal anti-inflammatory drug, and spinal manipulation. J Manipulat Physiol Ther 1999;22:376-381.
56. Chou R, Huffman LH. Nonpharmacologic therapies for acute and chronic low back pain: a review of the evidence for an American Pain Society/American College of Physicians clinical practice guideline. Ann Intern Med 2007;147:492-504.
57. Manheimer E, White A, Berman B, et al. Meta-analysis: acupuncture for low back pain. Ann Intern Med 2005;142:651-663.

58. Cherkin DC, Sherman KJ, Deyo RA, et al. A review of the evidence for the effectiveness, safety, and cost of acupuncture, massage therapy, and spinal manipulation for back pain. Ann Intern Med 2003;138:898-906.

59. Witt CM, Jena S, Selim D, et al. Pragmatic randomized trial evaluating the clinical and economic effectiveness of acupuncture for chronic low back pain. Am J Epidemiol 2006; 164:487-496.

60. Brinkhaus B, Witt CM, Jena S, et al. Acupuncture in patients with chronic low back pain: a randomized controlled trial. Arch Intern Med 2006;166:450-457.

61. Thomas KJ, MacPherson H, Thorpe L, et al. Randomised controlled trial of a short course of traditional acupuncture compared with usual care for persistent non-specific low back pain. BMJ 2006;333:623.

62. Smith LA, Oldman AD, McQuay HJ, et al. Teasing apart quality and validity in systematic reviews: an example from acupuncture trials in chronic neck and back pain. Pain 2000;86(1-2):119-132.

63. van Tulder MW, Cherkin DC, Berman B, et al. Acupuncture for low back pain. Cochrane Database Syst Rev 2000;(2): CD001351.

64. Ernst E, White AR. Acupuncture for back pain: a meta-analysis of randomized controlled trials. Arch Intern Med 1998;158: 2235-2241.

65. Tsui ML, Cheing GL. The effectiveness of electroacupuncture versus electrical heat acupuncture in the management of chronic low-back pain. J Altern Complement Med 2004;10:803-809.

66. Witt CM, Jena S, Selim D, et al. Pragmatic randomized trial evaluating the clinical and economic effectiveness of acupuncture for chronic low back pain. Am J Epidemiol 2006;164: 487-496.

67. Sierpina VS, Frenkel MA. Acupuncture: a clinical review. South Med J 2005;98:330-337.

68. Yamashita H, Tsukayama H, Tanno Y, et al. Adverse events in acupuncture and moxibustion treatment: a six-year survey at a national clinic in Japan. J Altern Complement Med 1999;5: 229-236.

69. MacPherson H, Thomas K, Walters S, et al. The York acupuncture safety study: prospective survey of 34,000 treatments by traditional acupuncturists. BMJ 2001;323:486-487.

70. Melchart D, Weidenhammer W, Streng A, et al. Prospective investigation of adverse effects of acupuncture in 97,733 patients. Arch Intern Med 2004;164:104-105.

71. White A, Hayhoe S, Hart A, et al. Adverse events following acupuncture: prospective survey of 32,000 consultations with doctors and physiotherapists. BMJ 2001;323:485-486.

72. Odsberg A, Schill U, Haker E. Acupuncture treatment: side effects and complications reported by Swedish physiotherapists. Complement Ther Med 2001;9:17-20.

73. Ernst G, Strzyz H, Hagmeister H. Incidence of adverse effects during acupuncture therapy—a multicentre survey. Complement Ther Med 2003;11:93-97.

74. US Food and Drug Administration. FDA Consumer. US Food and Drug Administration, Silver Spring, 1996. Report No.: 5.

75. Centers for Medicare and Medicaid Services. NCD for acupuncture. Centers for Medicare and Medicaid Services, Baltimore, 2009. Report No.: 30.3;4(23).

76. Cleary-Guida MB, Okvat HA, Oz MC, et al. A regional survey of health insurance coverage for complementary and alternative medicine: current status and future ramifications. J Altern Complement Med 2001;7:269-273.

77. Lind BK, Lafferty WE, Tyree PT, et al. The role of alternative medical providers for the outpatient treatment of insured patients with back pain. Spine 2005;30:1454-1459.

78. Dagenais S, Roffey DM, Wai EK, et al. Can cost utility evaluations inform decision making about interventions for low back pain? Spine J 2009;9:944-957.

79. van der Roer N, Goossens MEJB, Evers SMAA, et al. What is the most cost-effective treatment for patients with low back pain? A systematic review. Best Pract Res Clin Rheumatol 2005;19:671-684.

80. Herman PM, Szczurko O, Cooley K, et al. Cost-effectiveness of naturopathic care for chronic low back pain. Alt Ther Health Med 2008;14:32-39.

81. Mitchell RI, Carmen GM. The functional restoration approach to the treatment of chronic pain in patients with soft tissue and back injuries. Spine 1994;19:633-642.

82. Ratcliffe J, Thomas KJ, MacPherson H, et al. A randomised controlled trial of acupuncture care for persistent low back pain: cost effectiveness analysis. BMJ 2006;333:626.

83. Chenot JF, Becker A, Leonhardt C, et al. Determinants for receiving acupuncture for LBP and associated treatments: a prospective cohort study. BMC Health Serv Res 2006; 6:149.

CHAPTER 21

ROBERT J. GATCHEL
KATHRYN H. ROLLINGS

Cognitive Behavioral Therapy

DESCRIPTION

Terminology and Subtypes

Cognitive behavioral therapy (CBT) is a psychosocial intervention approach in which behavioral change is initiated by a therapist helping patients to confront and modify the irrational thoughts and beliefs that are most likely at the root of their maladaptive behaviors. Maladaptive behaviors are those that prevent an individual from adjusting appropriately to normal situations, and which are considered counterproductive or not socially acceptable (Figure 21-1).[1] The primary goal of CBT is to identify these maladaptive behaviors, recognize beliefs associated with those behaviors, correct any inappropriate beliefs, and replace those beliefs with more appropriate ones that will result in greater coping skills and adaptive behaviors (Figure 21-2).

There are several approaches to CBT and various ways of incorporating CBT into the management of chronic low back pain (CLBP). CBT alone does not address all of the contributing factors to CLBP (e.g., anatomic, biologic, physiologic), and it is not intended to replace interventions aimed at correcting those factors when appropriate. The focus of CBT in the context of CLBP is mainly to address psychological comorbidities that may impede recovery. If those factors are solely responsible for CLBP, then CBT may be appropriate as the main intervention. However, patients sometimes find it difficult to perceive the utility of CBT as the sole treatment for CLBP.[2] Use of the term *CBT* varies widely and may be used to denote self-instructions (e.g., distraction, imagery, motivational self-talk), relaxation, biofeedback, development of adaptive coping strategies (e.g., minimizing negative or self-defeating thoughts), changing maladaptive beliefs about pain, and goal setting (Figure 21-3).[3] Patients referred for CBT may be exposed to varying selections of these strategies that are specifically tailored to their needs.

History and Frequency of Use

CBT was pioneered by Aaron Beck and bears some similarities to the rational emotive behavioral therapy developed earlier by Albert Ellis.[4] Beck proposed that people often have two levels of thought that occur simultaneously: (1) automatic thoughts, which are generally evaluative; and (2) maladaptive thoughts, which CBT seeks to challenge and reframe. Many authors trace the origins of CBT farther back in time to Freud's extensive exploration of the unconscious mind, which resembles the CBT concept of "automatic thoughts" and consists of occasional irrational thoughts over which the patient has no control.[5,6]

Regardless of this common genesis, there are important differences between the application of CBT and Freudian psychoanalysis. Whereas Freud focused on the past to discover the root of a patient's psychopathology, CBT focuses on resolving maladaptive behavior in the present without dwelling on its origin.[5] Additionally, whereas Freudian psychoanalysis often requires a lengthy course of treatment during which progressively deeper insight is sought, CBT is widely viewed as a "quick" behavioral therapy intended to achieve long-term results in fewer than 20 sessions.[5]

Others who have contributed to the development of CBT include the American psychologists Albert Bandura and Donald Meichenbaum, who described pain behavior in terms of the learning theories of classic conditioning and operant conditioning.[6,7] For example, classic conditioning may be at play when visiting a doctor's office (e.g., a place where the patient has experienced or focused on their pain in the past) induces tension or fear, thereby increasing the painful experience.[7] Operant conditioning may be occurring when "sick" behavior (e.g., complaining about LBP and decreasing activities) is rewarded by a patient's family (e.g., patient receives care or increased attention), workplace (e.g., patient placed on almost fully paid sick leave or given modified duties), or

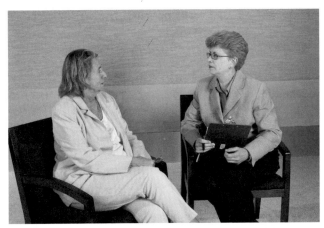

Figure 21-1 Cognitive behavioral therapy first identifies maladaptive behaviors.

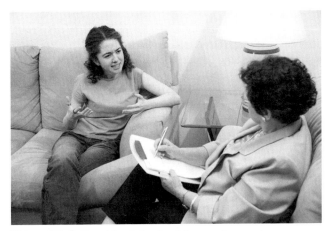

Figure 21-2 Cognitive behavioral therapy then replaces those maladaptive behaviors with appropriate beliefs and coping skills. (© iStockphoto.com / Lisa F. Young.)

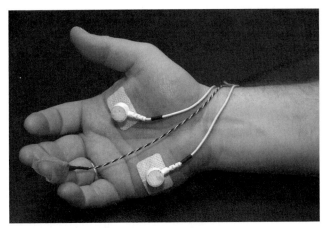

Figure 21-3 Cognitive behavioral therapy may use a variety of instruments to teach mind-body awareness, including biofeedback. (© iStockphoto.com / Francis Twitty.)

physician (e.g., patient receives more attention during a visit if symptoms appear severe). Each of these societal responses to the patient's behaviors may reinforce the patient's perceived worth and prevent them from managing their pain or improving their function.[7]

Practitioner, Setting, and Availability

CBT itself as a sole therapy should only be administered by licensed mental health professionals such as therapists, psychologists, or psychiatrists. However, some of the basic elements of CBT that emphasize the importance of remaining active and participating in self-care may be interspersed throughout the education that should be provided by all clinicians involved in managing CLBP. The CBT intervention itself is usually performed in a private practitioner's office, but it may also take place in a specialized outpatient pain or spine clinic. This intervention is widely available throughout the United States, though the experience of mental health professionals with the management of CLBP varies considerably.

Procedure

Turk and Flor[8] describe CBT as having six distinct phases: (1) assessment, (2) reconceptualization, (3) skills acquisition, (4) skills consolidation and application training, (5) generalization and maintenance, and (6) post-treatment assessment and follow-up. The assessment phase involves a conversation with patients and their families, and a series of self-reported measures that can be used by the practitioner to identify the degree of psychosocial impairment and determine the most appropriate course of action. The reconceptualization phase makes up much of the "cognitive" portion of CBT. A great deal of the psychopathology associated with chronic pain conditions is thought to originate in the automatic thoughts or irrational beliefs that patients with pain may have regarding their pain condition, including thoughts such as "I am never going to get better," "I cannot bear this much pain," "I am a failure in life because I am in pain," and other maladaptive cognitions. The reconceptualization phase of CBT seeks to help patients challenge and question the rationality of such maladaptive thoughts.

In the skills acquisition phase, the therapist teaches patients how to deal with obstacles in their day-to-day lives and how to avoid falling into the pattern of automatic thoughts. In the skills consolidation and application training phase, patients are given homework to reinforce the skills they have acquired during the skills acquisition phase; this is one of the hallmark methods in CBT. In the generalization and maintenance phase, the therapist and patients discuss the future, and how the patients are going to cope once they have left treatment. Finally, patients participate in the post-treatment assessment and follow-up phase, which allows the therapist to monitor and evaluate the patients' application of CBT skills to their lives.

Gatchel and Robinson[9] provided a comprehensive overview of CBT for managing chronic pain, including CLBP, with a session-by-session guide to a typical CBT intervention for a patient with chronic pain. Their approach consists of a short-term, skills-oriented therapy in which new skills are taught at each session to (1) correct negative (distorted) thinking about chronic pain, (2) control emotional reactions to chronic pain, and (3) cope more effectively with chronic pain and other stressors.

Regulatory Status

Not applicable.

THEORY

Mechanism of Action

CBT itself does not attempt to directly address the anatomic or physiologic components of CLBP. Rather, CBT attempts to improve how symptoms of CLBP may be perceived and what impact they may have on a patient's life. By reframing maladaptive thoughts and coping strategies, CBT can decrease distress and promote appropriate self-care, which may in turn reduce the pain experience.[7] CBT interventions must be tailored to each patient because they are intended to address an individual's interpretation, evaluation, and beliefs about his or her health condition and coping repertoire. The exact mechanism of action for CBT may then depend to some degree on the specific behaviors and beliefs it must correct. By improving maladaptive behaviors with respect to CLBP, CBT may affect the degree of emotional and physical disability associated with that condition, if not the underlying symptoms themselves.[10]

The general CBT procedure described earlier by Turk and Flor[8] is used for most psychopathologies encountered, including those that may be active in CLBP. However, there are distinctions in the application of this technique that are specific to the patient's diagnosis. Therefore, when discussing the mechanism of action for CBT, one needs to take into account some of the more prevalent psychosocial diagnoses seen in patients with CLBP. For example, patients with CLBP may experience anxiety associated with activities that may cause pain or increase existing pain. As described in the "medical-symptom stress cycle," such anxiety can lead to behavioral changes that exacerbate the pain.[11] To treat such anxiety, the therapist can use a variety of techniques, including biofeedback and relaxation training. The goal of these techniques is to reduce the anxiety associated with the pain experience and to help ease the patient's tension, thereby decreasing some of the pain symptoms.

In terms of depression, patients with CLBP may have negative cognitions about the present, the future, and the world around them. They may believe that there is nothing that they can do to improve the situation in which they find themselves with regard to pain. The patient may also hold the false cognition that the pain will never go away or will never be palliated. Finally, patients may believe that others do not understand their condition. Therefore when treating depression in CLBP patients, the therapist must actively challenge these negative cognitions and help patients reframe their present and future situations to improve their daily environment.

Indication

Although most patients with CLBP could be diagnosed with a pain disorder, it has also been found that they also have a significantly higher prevalence of psychiatric disorders than the general population.[12] Indeed, spine clinicians must often deal with comorbidities such as the psychiatric sequelae of CLBP. To treat patients with CLBP using CBT, it is often necessary to treat comorbid psychiatric disorders such as anxiety, mood disorders, pain disorders, or depression. However, even though an association between CLBP and certain psychiatric disorders has been noted, this does not indicate a causal relationship. In the absence of a carefully experimentally controlled longitudinal study, no such causal order can be discerned. Clinicians should not assume that comorbid psychiatric disorders were present before developing CLBP.

In fact, development of severe or prolonged CLBP could potentially lead to the development of subsequent psychiatric disorders. For example, persons suffering from a chronic pain disorder may develop alcohol, drug, or medication dependence or addiction in an attempt to obtain some relief.[13] Additionally, withdrawal from regular activities such as work, school, and leisure pursuits due to pain may lead to depression or other affective disorders, and has been shown to be substantially more prevalent in those who suffer from chronic pain.[12,13] Patients suffering from CLBP are also known to suffer from pain-related, rather than generalized, anxiety.[14] The ideal patient with CLBP for CBT is one with average intelligence, who is motivated to learn coping skills to help manage his or her pain, is compliant with the treatment protocol, and is willing to complete "homework" exercises between treatment sessions.

Assessment

Before receiving CBT, patients should first be assessed for CLBP using an evidence-based and goal-oriented approach focused on the patient history and neurologic examination (if necessary), as discussed in Chapter 3. Additional diagnostic imaging or specific diagnostic testing is generally not required before initiating this intervention for CLBP. Certain questionnaires (e.g., Tampa Scale for Kinesiophobia) may be helpful to identify subsets of patients with CLBP who may benefit from specific interventions aimed at addressing those issues (e.g., fear avoidance training, as discussed in Chapter 7).

EFFICACY

Evidence supporting the efficacy of this intervention for CLBP was summarized from recent clinical practice guidelines (CPGs), systematic reviews (SRs), and randomized controlled trials (RCTs). Observational studies (OBSs) were also summarized where appropriate. Findings are summarized by study design.

Clinical Practice Guidelines

Four of the recent national CPGs on the management of CLBP have assessed and summarized the evidence to make specific recommendations about the efficacy of CBT.

The CPG from Belgium in 2006 found high-quality evidence that CBT is more effective than no treatment in patients with CLBP.[15] The same CPG also found moderate evidence to support the efficacy of CBT in the management of CLBP, and no difference in the efficacy of various forms of behavioral interventions for CLBP. That CPG concluded that CBT can be recommended as one management option for CLBP.

The CPG from Europe in 2004 found strong evidence that CBT is more effective than placebo or no treatment with respect to improvements in pain, function, and mental health in patients with CLBP.[16] That CPG also found strong evidence that there is no difference in the efficacy of various forms of behavioral interventions for CLBP. There was limited evidence overall to support the efficacy of CBT in the management of CLBP.

The CPG from the United Kingdom in 2009 found limited evidence to support the efficacy of CBT or other behavioral interventions as sole therapies for the management of CLBP.[17] The same CPG also found no evidence to support the efficacy of longer-term CBT or other behavioral interventions unless they are combined with physical therapy. The CPG recommended CBT or other behavioral interventions as one management option for CLBP, but only when combined with other approaches.

The CPG from the United States in 2007 found moderate-quality evidence to support a moderate benefit for CBT in patients who do not obtain adequate relief with self-care alone.[18]

Findings from these CPGs are summarized in Table 21-1.

Systematic Reviews

Cochrane Collaboration

An SR was conducted in 2003 by the Cochrane Collaboration on CBT for nonspecific CLBP.[19] A total of 21 RCTs were included.[20-40] Two RCTs found that progressive relaxation led to greater improvements in pain, functional, and behavioral

TABLE 21-1	Clinical Practice Guideline Recommendations on Cognitive Behavioral Therapy for Chronic Low Back Pain	
Reference	Country	Conclusion
15	Belgium	Recommended
16	Europe	Evidence of efficacy
17	United Kingdom	Recommended, but only when combined with other approaches
18	United States	Moderate-quality evidence to support moderate benefit

outcomes than in control subjects.[32,33] Seven RCTs examining electromyographic biofeedback found conflicting results and RCTs examining operant therapy versus control found no differences for behavioral or functional outcomes.[23,27,30,32,34,36,40] Combined respondent cognitive therapy showed statistically significant improvement in pain outcomes, however, no differences were found for behavior and functional outcomes.[27,33,34,41] Behavioral therapy was more effective than usual care in one RCT, but was not as effective as exercise in another.[25,40] This review concluded that CBT combined with progressive relaxation is effective in providing short-term relief for CLBP.[19] This SR also concluded that CBT produced the same effects as exercise therapy and that the long-term effects of CBT are unknown.

American Pain Society and American College of Physicians

An SR was conducted in 2006 by the American Pain Society and American College of Physicians CPG committee on non-pharmacologic therapies for acute and chronic LBP.[42] That review identified two SRs related to CBT, including the Cochrane Collaboration review mentioned earlier.[19,43] The other review identified had conclusions consistent with those of the Cochrane review: CBT is effective in the short term for CLBP.[43] These SRs included a total of 35 unique RCTs (references were not provided). No additional trials have been identified. RCTs included in the non-Cochrane review indicated that psychotherapy may not improve outcomes when added to other noninvasive therapies.[43] This SR concluded that psychological therapy is effective for chronic or subacute LBP.[42]

Other

In an earlier review, Gatchel and Bruga concluded that there is now convincing evidence-based data demonstrating the effectiveness and cost effectiveness of multidisciplinary pain management programs for occupational CLBP.[44] Similar findings were reported in the Cochrane Collaboration on multidisciplinary treatment approaches to CLBP, some of which include CBT itself, or at least some of its philosophies.[45]

Multidisciplinary rehabilitation programs are often based on the biopsychosocial approach to chronic pain, which views chronic pain conditions—including CLBP—as complex illnesses requiring consideration of potential complex interactions between biological and psychosocial variables.[46-48] As such, it follows from this perspective that appropriate treatment requires a comprehensive approach designed to address all such factors that cause, mediate, and perpetuate chronic pain and disability.

An influential early review by Morley and colleagues[49] reported the results of their SR and meta-analysis of the existing RCTs of the efficacy of CBT and behavioral therapy for chronic pain in general. Their findings concluded that such treatment is effective for a variety of chronic pain conditions in producing improvement in the following important areas: (1) pain experience; (2) pain behavior and activity level; (3) cognitive coping and appraisal; and (4) social functioning.

TABLE 21-2	Systematic Review Findings on Cognitive Behavioral Therapy for Chronic Low Back Pain or Other Chronic Pain Conditions		
Reference	# RCTs in SR	# RCTs for CLBP	Conclusion
19	21	21	CBT with progressive relaxation is effective in providing short-term relief of CLBP
42	2 SRs, 35 unique RCTs	NR	Psychological therapy in general is effective for CLBP
44	NR	NR	Convincing evidence supporting effectiveness of multidisciplinary/ interdisciplinary pain management programs for occupational CLBP
45	NR	NR	Recommended as a component of multidisciplinary rehabilitation programs
51	NR	NR	Effective for chronic pain conditions
49	NR	NR	CBT is effective for a variety of chronic pain conditions (chronic pain in general)
50	NR	NR	CBT and behavioral treatments for chronic pain reduce patients' pain, distress, pain behavior and improve function (chronic pain in general)

CBT, cognitive behavioral therapy; CLBP, chronic low back pain; NR, not reported; RCT, randomized controlled trial; SR, systematic review.

Subsequently, another review reported numerous controlled clinical trials of CBT and behavioral treatment for chronic pain in general, alone or more commonly in multidisciplinary intervention contexts, that indicated these treatments to be efficacious.[50] Results of many published studies in the scientific literature showed that, overall, CBT and behavioral treatments for chronic pain reduced patients' pain, distress, and pain behavior, and improved daily functioning.

More recently, a review on CBT interventions for chronic pain concluded that "cognitive-behavioral treatment interventions for chronic pain have expanded considerably. It is now well established that these interventions are effective in reducing the enormous suffering that patients with chronic pain have to bear. In addition, these interventions have potential economic benefits in that they appear to be cost effective as well."[51]

Findings from these SRs are summarized in Table 21-2.

Randomized Controlled Trials

Seven RCTs were identified.[38,52-57] Their methods are summarized in Table 21-3 and results are briefly described here.

Mitchell and Carmen[52] conducted an RCT in which patients with soft tissue or back injuries were included if they experienced their symptoms for more than 3 months and exhibited signs of inappropriate illness behavior (e.g., bizarre symptoms, prolonged recovery). Those with serious pathology or those requiring surgery were excluded. Approximately 23% of the included participants had pain originating from structures other than the lower back. Participants were randomized to a functional restoration group or another group who were supervised by their primary care practitioner and received other interventions, such as acupuncture, physical therapy, spinal manipulation, and analgesics. The functional restoration program consisted of up to 8 to 12 weeks of exercise, functional simulation, CBT, biofeedback, relaxation, and group counseling for 7 hours per day, 5 days per week. After 1 year of follow-up, no statistically significant differences were observed between the 2 groups regarding the proportion returning to full-time work. Results for pain or disability were not reported.

Gatchel and colleagues[53] performed an RCT in which patients with acute LBP were categorized into those at high risk or low risk of developing CLBP. Those identified as being at high risk for CLBP were randomized either to a functional restoration program or to a nonintervention group. To be included, participants had to have LBP lasting less than 2 months that did not require surgery. Those with serious pathology or psychiatric conditions were excluded. The functional restoration program was administered by a nurse-physician team and consisted of up to nine 15-minute sessions of individual exercise, nine 30-minute sessions of group exercise, nine sessions of biofeedback or pain management, nine 45-minute sessions of group didactics, CBT, and three clinical team conferences. After 1 year of follow-up, participants in the high risk for CLBP functional restoration group experienced statistically significant improvements in function and pain versus the high risk for CLBP group that did not receive any intervention. Results among the group at low risk for CLPB who did not receive any intervention were similar to those observed among the functional restoration group.

Brox and colleagues[54] performed an RCT in which patients with CLBP due to disc degeneration were included if they were 25 to 60 years old and experienced LBP for at least 1 year. Those with serious pathology or psychiatric conditions were excluded. Participants were randomized to instrumented fusion or an intensive CBT plus therapeutic exercise program. After 1 year of follow-up, no statistically significant differences were observed in pain or disability between the fusion and CBT plus exercise groups.

Fairbank and colleagues[55] performed an RCT in which patients with CLBP due to disc degeneration were included if they were 18 to 55 years old and experienced LBP for at least 1 year. Those with serious pathology, pregnancy, or psychiatric conditions were excluded. Participants were

TABLE 21-3	Randomized Controlled Trials of Cognitive Behavioral Therapy for Chronic Low Back Pain		
Reference	Indication	Intervention 1	Intervention 2/Control
53	Acute LBP, neurologic involvement NR, symptoms <2 months	High risk for CLBP Functional restoration: PT, psychotherapy, occupational therapy, case management Nurse-physician team 3 weeks of up to 9 × 15-minute individual exercise, 9 × 30-minute group exercise, 9 × biofeedback/pain management, 9 × 45-minute group didactic, 3 × team conferences Cointervention: NR n = 22	(1) High risk for CLBP No intervention Cointervention: NR n = 48 (2) Observational group: Low risk for CLBP No treatment Cointervention: NR n = 54
52	Soft tissue or back injury, neurologic involvement NR, symptoms >3 months	Functional restoration: PT, psychotherapy Administrator NR up to 8 to 12 weeks of 7 hours/day × 5 days/week physical exercise, functional simulation, group therapy, CBT, biofeedback, relaxation, group counseling Cointervention: at the discretion of primary care practitioner n = 271	Supervised by primary care practitioner Cointervention: at the discretion of primary care practitioner n = 271
54	CLBP due to disc degeneration, without neurologic involvement, symptoms >1 year	Fusion surgery (with or without instrumentation) Surgeon Cointervention: PT, exercise n = 37	CBT + exercise: education, individual exercise, CBT Administrator NR 1 week supervised, 2 weeks home, 2 weeks supervised × 25 hours/week n = 25
55	CLBP due to disc degeneration, with or without neurologic involvement, symptoms >1 year	Fusion surgery (with or without instrumentation) Surgeon Cointervention: PT, exercise n = 160	Intensive rehabilitation: 60-110 hours of education, exercise, CBT, hydrotherapy Physical therapists, psychologists 5 days/week × 3 weeks n = 159
56	CLBP due to disc degeneration, without neurologic involvement, symptoms >1 year	Fusion surgery (with instrumentation) Surgeon Cointervention: PT, exercise n = 28	CBT + exercise: education, individual exercise, CBT Administrator NR 3 weeks × 25 hours/week n = 27
57	CLBP, neurologic involvement NR, symptoms >8 weeks	Self-care: CBT, education, problem-solving, self-care educational material Psychologists 2 × 2-hour group sessions, 45-minute face-to-face meeting, 3-minute follow-up call Co-intervention: NR n = 113	Usual care Educational book Administrator: NR Cointervention: NR n = 113
38	CLBP, neurologic involvement NR, duration of symptoms NR	Psychoeducational program Psychology graduate 4 × 2-hour therapy: 40-minute video on pain + 7 hours and 20 minutes individual therapy Cointervention: anesthesia, psychiatry, occupational therapy, and PT, plus other consultations as required n = 15	Control Nonspecific program, including a video on balance Research coordinator 8 hours total Cointervention: anesthesia, psychiatry, occupational therapy and PT, plus other consultations as required n = 15

CBT, cognitive behavioral therapy; CLBP, chronic low back pain; LBP, low back pain; NR, not reported; PT, physical therapy.

randomized to fusion or an intensive rehabilitation program including CBT and exercise. After 2 years of follow-up, the fusion group displayed statistically significant improvement in the Oswestry Disability Index (ODI) versus the intensive rehabilitation group, yet no statistically significant differences were observed in pain or any of the other disability outcomes between groups.

Brox and colleagues[56] performed an RCT in which patients with CLBP due to disc degeneration were included if they were 25 to 60 years old and experienced LBP for at least 1 year. Those with serious pathology or psychiatric conditions were excluded. Participants were randomized to fusion with instrumentation or a combined CBT and exercise program. After 1 year of follow-up, both groups experienced statistically significant improvement in the ODI from baseline. However, no differences were observed between groups in the ODI. Participants in the CBT plus exercise group experienced statistically significant improvement in disability after 1 year compared to baseline but this was not observed for pain. Participants in the fusion group experienced statistically significant improvement in pain after 1 year compared to baseline but this was not observed for disability. No differences in pain or disability were observed between groups after 1 year of follow-up.

Moore and colleagues[57] performed an RCT in which patients with CLBP were included if they were 25 to 70 years old and experienced LBP for at least 6 to 8 weeks. Those enrolled in the Group Health plan for less than 1 year were excluded. Participants were randomized to a self-care intervention including CBT and education or to a usual care group including an educational book. After 6 months of follow-up, patients in the self-care intervention experienced statistically significant improvement in pain but no differences were observed in disability. After 1 year of follow-up, no statistically significant differences were observed between groups for pain or disability outcomes.

Strong[38] performed an RCT in patients with CLBP. Participants were randomized to a psychoeducational program including CBT and education or to a control care group who received a nonspecific program, including a video on balance. Both groups also received standard hospital therapy, which included anesthesia, psychiatry, occupational therapy and physical therapy, and other treatment as required. Participants in the psychoeducational group received 7 hours and 20 minutes of psychotherapy from a psychology graduate, while those in the control group received 8 hours of the nonspecific program. After 3 months of follow-up, no statistically significant differences were observed regarding pain relief between the groups.

SAFETY

Contraindications

Contraindications to CBT include CLBP due to potentially serious spinal pathology such as fracture, cancer, infection, or cauda equina syndrome. Because CBT requires cognitive processing skills, it may be contraindicated in patients with major cognitive deficit related to brain trauma or organic pathophysiology, as well as those who refuse to participate.

Adverse Events

CBT is generally considered to be a safe intervention. No adverse events were reported in the studies reviewed. CPGs for the management of CLBP reported that the safety of CBT is currently unknown.[16]

COSTS

Fees and Third-Party Reimbursement

In the United States, CBT for CLBP can initially be delivered by licensed behavioral health professionals using CPT codes for psychiatric diagnostic interview examination, including 90801 or 90802, when the goal is to establish a diagnosis and treatment protocol. Psychotherapy, defined as the treatment for mental illness and behavioral disturbances in which the clinician, through definitive therapeutic communication, attempts to alleviate emotional disturbances, reverse or change maladaptive patterns of behavior, and encourage personality growth and development, can be delivered using CPT codes 90804 (20 to 30 minutes), 90806 (45 to 50 minutes), or 90808 (75 to 80 minutes). If additional evaluation and management services are required, CPT codes 90805 (20 to 30 minutes), 90807 (45 to 50 minutes), or 90809 (75 to 80 minutes) can be used instead. These codes are based on the setting in which the psychotherapy session occurred, the type of psychotherapy provided, and the amount of face-to-face time spent with the patient. The decision regarding the appropriate reporting of individual psychotherapy codes should be based solely on the definition of the codes and the work performed. Alternatively, brief CBT for CLBP may be provided by a clinician in the context of an outpatient visit for a new patient using CPT codes 99201 (up to 10 minutes), 99202 (up to 20 minutes), or 99203 (up to 30 minutes). For an established patient, brief CBT for CLBP may be provided during an outpatient visit using CPT codes 99211 (up to 5 minutes), 99212 (up to 10 minutes), or 99213 (up to 15 minutes).

These procedures are widely covered by other third-party payers such as health insurers and worker's compensation insurance. Although some payers continue to base their reimbursements on usual, customary, and reasonable payment methodology, the majority have developed reimbursement tables based on the Resource Based Relative Value Scale used by Medicare. Reimbursements by other third-party payers are generally higher than Medicare. It should be noted that CPT codes listed in the psychiatry section of the CPT manual (90801-90899) are in fact not limited to psychiatrists or mental health professionals, and may be used to designate the services rendered by any qualified physician or other qualified health care professional. Unfortunately, some third-party payers will not reimburse all providers for these codes.

TABLE 21-4	Medicare Fee Schedule for Related Services	
CPT Code	New York	California
Psychiatric Examination		
90801	$158	$169
90802	$141	$181
Psychotherapy		
90804	$65	$69
90805	$74	$78
90806	$90	$95
90807	$103	$109
90808	$132	$139
90809	$146	$154
Office Visits		
99201	$41	$44
99202	$70	$76
99203	$101	$109
99211	$20	$22
99212	$41	$44
99213	$68	$73

2010 Participating, nonfacility amount.

Typical fees reimbursed by Medicare in New York and California for these services are summarized in Table 21-4.

Cost Effectiveness

Evidence supporting the cost effectiveness of treatment protocols that compared these interventions, often in combination with one or more cointerventions, with control groups who received one or more other interventions, for either acute or chronic LBP, was identified from two SRs on this topic and is summarized here.[58,59] Although many of these study designs are unable to clearly identify the individual contribution of any intervention, their results provide some insight into the clinical and economic outcomes associated with these approaches.

An RCT in Norway compared three approaches for patients with CLBP.[60] Participants received either a light multidisciplinary program consisting of education, fear avoidance training, and advice to remain active given by a physical therapist, nurse, and psychologist, an extensive multidisciplinary program consisting of daily group sessions with CBT, education, fear avoidance training, and strengthening and stabilization exercises for 4 weeks, or usual care by a general practitioner (GP) and possibly a physical therapist or chiropractor. Direct medical costs for the light and extensive multidisciplinary programs were estimated by dividing the total clinic costs for one year by the number of patients treated; direct medical costs were therefore assumed to be equal in both groups, regardless of large differences in time spent by clinic staff with patients in each group. Indirect productivity costs associated with lost work time were evaluated over 24 months. A limited cost benefit analysis for male participants only reported that the light multidisciplinary program would yield average savings of approximately $19,544 per patient

over 2 years, and was therefore cost effective compared to usual care.

An RCT in the United Kingdom compared two approaches for patients with CLBP.[61] The active intervention was delivered by a physical therapist and consisted of back school with education from a book and cassette, group education, advice to remain active, and CBT. Usual care was delivered by a GP and included education from a book and cassette along with other interventions. Clinical outcomes after 15 months were similar between groups, as both improved in pain, function, and utility. Direct medical costs associated with study and nonstudy interventions over 15 months were $47 higher in the active intervention group. Based on nonsignificant differences in utility, the incremental cost effectiveness ratio (ICER) of group training over brief education alone was $8650 per quality-adjusted life-year (QALY), well within the generally accepted threshold for cost utility analyses.

A cluster RCT in The Netherlands compared two approaches for patients with subacute LBP presenting to 60 GPs in 41 offices.[62] The brief education approach was centered on CBT and discussion of psychosocial prognostic factors related to LBP, including fear avoidance beliefs. Usual care included interventions that were not specified. Clinical outcomes after 12 months were largely similar between the two groups. Direct medical costs for study and nonstudy interventions over 12 months were approximately $207 in the brief education group and approximately $202 in the usual care group. Indirect productivity costs associated with absenteeism for both paid and unpaid work over 12 months were approximately $575 in the brief education group and approximately $1059 in the usual care group. Total costs (direct medical and indirect productivity) were therefore approximately $782 in the brief education group and approximately $1261 in the usual care group. The brief education group therefore achieved similar clinical outcomes with lower costs.

An RCT in the United Kingdom compared three approaches for patients with CLBP.[63] The individual physical therapy approach included a maximum of 12 sessions with spinal manipulation therapy (SMT), mobilization, massage, home exercises, and brief education. The spinal stabilization approach included a maximum of eight sessions with abdominal and multifidus exercises. The pain management approach included a maximum of eight sessions with education, exercises, CBT, and fear avoidance training. Clinical outcomes after 18 months were similar for all groups, with improvements noted in pain, function, and utility. Direct medical costs for study and nonstudy interventions paid by the National Health Service over 18 months were approximately $872 for individual physical therapy, approximately $698 for spinal stabilization, and approximately $304 for pain management. Indirect productivity costs were not reported. Over 18 months, the three groups experienced gains in QALY of 0.99, 0.90, and 1.00, respectively. By virtue of having lower direct costs and greater gains in utility, the pain management approach was reported to dominate over both individual physical therapy and spinal stabilization.

An RCT in the United States compared three approaches in patients with acute LBP who had been identified as being at high or low risk for developing chronicity according to a questionnaire.[53] Those at high risk for developing CLBP were randomized to either functional restoration or a nonintervention control; those at low risk for developing CLBP were also monitored in an observational control group. Functional restoration included supervised exercise therapy, CBT, and other interventions as necessary. Clinical outcomes after 1 year reported that the functional restoration group was similar for improvement in pain to the low-risk observational group, and both were superior to the high-risk nonintervention group. Direct medical costs associated with study interventions over 1 year were $3885 for functional restoration and $0 for the nonintervention groups. Direct medical costs associated with nonstudy interventions such as provider visits and medications over 1 year were $1794 for functional restoration and $2892 for the nonintervention group. Indirect productivity costs from lost work days over 1 year were $7072 for functional restoration and $18,951 for the nonintervention group. Total costs (direct medical and indirect productivity) over 1 year were therefore $12,751 in the functional restoration group and $21,843 in the nonintervention group. Authors concluded that functional restoration was cost effective in patients with acute LBP identified as being at high risk of developing CLBP.

An RCT from the Netherlands compared three behavioral approaches in patients with CLBP.[39] The first behavioral intervention included CBT, fear avoidance training, and relaxation. The second behavioral intervention included CBT, fear avoidance training, and group discussion. The third behavioral intervention included fear avoidance training after a 10-week waiting period. Clinical outcomes after 1 year reported no difference in utility scores or global assessment of change between groups. Direct medical costs associated with study interventions after 1 year were $9196 in the relaxation group, $8607 in the group discussion group, and $8795 in the delayed fear avoidance training group. Direct medical costs associated with nonstudy interventions after 1 year were $1088 in the relaxation group, $575 in the group discussion group, and $651 in the delayed fear avoidance training group. Direct medical costs associated with non-healthcare expenditures after 1 year were $2316 in the relaxation group, $1544 in the group discussion group, and $1641 in the delayed fear avoidance training group. Indirect productivity costs associated with lost work days after 1 year were $6522 in the relaxation group, $5938 in the group discussion group, and $8213 in the delayed fear avoidance training group. Total costs (direct medical and indirect productivity) over 1 year were therefore $19,022 in the relaxation group, $16,664 in the group discussion group, and $19,300 in the delayed fear avoidance training group. Authors concluded that neither behavioral intervention was cost effective when compared to fear avoidance training alone.

An RCT from Canada compared two approaches for patients who had been injured at work and subsequently suffered from CLBP.[52] The functional restoration group included CBT, fear avoidance training, education, biofeedback, and group counseling, as well as strengthening and stretching exercises. The usual care group could receive a variety of interventions, including physical therapy, acupuncture, back school, SMT, medication, or supervised exercise therapy. Clinical outcomes were not reported. Direct medical costs associated with the study intervention were $2507 higher in the functional restoration group. Indirect productivity costs associated with lost work days were $3172 lower in the functional restoration group. Total costs for interventions, lost work days, and disability pensions were $7068 lower in the functional restoration group. These differences were not statistically significant.

An RCT in the United Kingdom compared two approaches for patients with acute LBP.[64] The brief pain management group included education, general exercise, and CBT. The physical therapy group included mobilization, SMT, massage, back exercises, and brief education. Clinical outcomes after 1 year were similar between the two groups. Direct medical costs for study and nonstudy interventions over 1 year were approximately $254 in the brief pain management group and approximately $354 in the physical therapy group. Indirect productivity costs were not considered. Because the physical therapy group had marginally better clinical outcomes with higher direct costs, its ICER was estimated at approximately $4710 per QALY, well within the generally accepted threshold for cost utility analyses.

An RCT in Germany compared two approaches for patients with CLBP pain admitted to a three-week inpatient rehabilitation center.[65] The usual care group included group exercise, electrical muscle stimulation, massage, and education. The usual care with CBT group also included both individual and group CBT sessions. Clinical outcomes after 1 year were mostly similar for improvements in pain and function, though greater improvement was noted in utility gains for the usual care with CBT group. Direct medical costs associated with study and nonstudy interventions over 6 months were approximately $2702 in the usual care group and approximately $2809 in the usual care with CBT group. Indirect productivity costs associated with lost work days over 6 months were approximately $6626 in the usual care group and approximately $5061 in the usual care with CBT group. Total costs (direct medical and indirect productivity) over 6 months were therefore approximately $9328 in the usual care group and approximately $7870 in the usual care with CBT group. Since the usual care with CBT group had better clinical outcomes with lower overall costs, authors concluded that it was cost saving and dominated usual care alone.

An RCT in the Netherlands compared two approaches for patients with CLBP.[66] The intensive training group included back school, and both individual and group supervised exercise therapy. The usual physical therapy group included interventions recommended in CPGs, which were not defined. Clinical outcomes after 1 year were similar between groups, which both improved in pain, function, and utility. Direct medical costs associated with study and nonstudy interventions over 1 year were approximately $1468 in the intensive training group and approximately $980 in the usual physical therapy group. Indirect productivity costs associated with lost work days over 1 year were approximately $3797 in the intensive training group and approximately $3969 in the usual physical therapy group. Total costs (direct medical and indirect productivity) over 1 year were therefore approximately $5265 in the intensive training group and approximately $4949 in the usual physical therapy group. Because the intensive training group had marginally better clinical outcomes with higher overall costs, its ICER was estimated at approximately $6957 per QALY, well within the generally accepted threshold for cost utility analyses.

The CPG from Europe in 2004 determined that CBT for CLBP (>3 months) may not be cost effective compared with common individual rehabilitation therapy.[16] That CPG also found from Europe in 2004 found that the same effects could be reached at the same or lower costs with a short and intense standardized group program as with using CBT for CLBP (>3 months).[16]

Findings from cost effectiveness analyses are summarized in Table 21-5.

SUMMARY

Description

CBT is a psychosocial intervention approach in which therapists initiate behavior modifications by helping patients confront and change the irrational thoughts and beliefs that are most likely at the root of maladaptive behaviors (i.e., behaviors that prevent individuals from adjusting appropriately to normal situations). The focus of CBT in the context of CLBP is mainly to address psychological comorbidities that may impede recovery. CBT is widely available throughout the United States and should only be administered by licensed mental health professionals such as therapists, psychologists, or psychiatrists. However, basic elements of CBT emphasizing the importance of remaining active and self-care may be interspersed throughout the education that should be provided by all clinicians involved in managing CLBP. CBT can be performed in a private practitioner's office, specialized outpatient pain clinic, or spine clinic.

Theory

CBT attempts to improve how symptoms of CLBP may be perceived, and what impact they may have on a patient's life. By reframing maladaptive thoughts and using coping strategies, individuals using CBT may experience decreased distress and an increase in appropriate self-care, which may in turn reduce the pain experienced. Evidence suggests that patients with CLBP have a significantly higher prevalence of psychiatric disorders than the general population. The ideal CLBP patient for CBT is one with average intelligence, who is motivated to learn coping skills to help manage his or her pain, is compliant with the treatment protocol, and is willing to complete "homework" exercises between sessions. Diagnostic imaging or other forms of advanced testing is generally not required prior to administering CBT for CLBP.

Efficacy

Four CPGs recommended CBT for CLBP if combined with other therapies. Three SRs concluded that CBT is effective in the short-term for CLBP. At least seven RCTs examined the efficacy of CBT, the majority of which did not find any statistically significant differences in pain or disability versus other comparators after long-term follow-up, though improvements were generally noted over baseline.

Safety

Contraindications to CBT include CLBP due to potentially serious spinal pathology such as fracture, cancer, infection, or cauda equina syndrome. Because CBT requires cognitive processing skills, it may be contraindicated in patients with major cognitive deficit related to brain trauma or organic pathophysiology. CBT is generally considered to be a safe intervention.

Costs

Depending on the setting and duration of the session, the cost of one CBT session can range from $20 to $181. At least ten studies have assessed costs of CBT for CLBP, the majority of which found that multidisciplinary management with a CBT component is within acceptable levels of cost effectiveness. However, one RCT found that a combined approach with CBT was not as cost effective as a fear avoidance program alone.

Comments

Evidence from the CPGs, SRs, and RCTs reviewed suggests that interventions incorporating elements of CBT may be effective for the management of CLBP. As noted earlier, the biopsychosocial approach to chronic pain management has moved away from the outdated view that monotherapy is the best approach to achieve overall therapeutic improvement. Multiple factors—biologic, psychological, and social—must be simultaneously addressed and CBT plays an important role in dealing with the psychosocial component of CLBP. Combining CBT with other therapeutic components, such as therapeutic exercise, may help address other issues, including physical deconditioning.

Currently, there are no studies directly addressing the combination of interventions and subset of patients with CLBP in whom the best therapeutic outcomes will likely be achieved. This is a challenge for future clinical research. For example, a recent study by Molloy and colleagues[67] evaluated whether a combination of CBT and a spinal implantable device was effective in the treatment of a cohort of patients with chronic pain (75% of whom had CLBP). Results demonstrated that this combined approach produced significant improvements in disability, affective distress, self-efficacy, and catastrophizing at long-term follow-up. Previously, this cohort of patients showed a suboptimal response to either of these treatment components when administered alone. This study illustrates the growing perceived need to conduct "component-type" analyses of comprehensive pain management programs to dissect the relative contributions of the various interventions. This will further advance the heuristic value of a biopsychosocial approach to chronic pain management.

TABLE 21-5	Cost Effectiveness and Cost Utility Analyses of Cognitive Behavioral Therapy for Acute or Chronic Low Back Pain				

Ref Country Follow-Up	Group	Direct Medical Costs	Indirect Productivity Costs	Total Costs	Conclusion
60 Norway 2 years	1. Light multidisciplinary program 2. Extensive multidisciplinary program (including CBT) 3. Usual care	NR	NR	NR	Group 1: average savings of $19,544/patient over 2 years
61 United Kingdom 15 months	1. Back school, education, CBT 2. Usual care from GP	1. $47 higher than group 2 2. NR	NR	NR	ICER of 1 over 2: $8650/QALY
62 The Netherlands 1 year	1. Brief education approach (including CBT) 2. Usual care	1. $207 2. $202	1. $575 2. $1059	1. $782 2. $1261	Group 1 achieved similar clinical outcomes with lower costs
63 United Kingdom 18 months	1. Individual PT 2. Spinal stabilization 3. Pain management (including CBT)	1. $872 2. $698 3. $304	NR	NR	Gains in QALY: 1. 0.99 2. 0.90 3. 1.00 Group 3 reported to dominate other interventions
53 United States 1 year	1. Functional restoration (inc. CBT) 2. Nonintervention control 3. Observational control	1. $5679 2. $2892 3. $0	1. $7072 2. $18,951 3. NR	1. $12,751 2. $21,843 3. NR	Group 1 is cost effective
39 The Netherlands 1 year	1. CBT+ fear avoidance training + relaxation 2. CBT + fear avoidance training + group discussion 3. Fear avoidance training after 10 weeks	1. $12,600 2. $10,726 3. $11,087	1. $6522 2. $5938 3. $8213	1. $19,122 2. $16,664 3. $19,300	No significant difference
52 Canada NR	1. Functional restoration (including CBT) 2. Usual care	1. $2507 higher than group 2 2. NR	1. $3172 lower than group 2 for lost work days 2. NR	1. $7068 lower than group 2 (lost work days + disability pensions) 2. NR	No significant difference
64 United Kingdom 1 year	1. Brief pain management (including CBT) 2. PT	1. $254 2. $354	NR	NR	ICER of 1 over 2: $4710/QALY
65 Germany 6 months	1. Usual care 2. Usual care + CBT	1. $2702 2. $2809	1. $6626 2. $5061	1. $9328 2. $7870	Group 2 cost saving and dominated group 1
66 The Netherlands 1 year	1. Intensive training (including behavioral principles) 2. Usual PT	1. $1468 2. $980	1. $3797 2. $3969	1. $5265 2. $4949	ICER of 1 over 2: $6957/QALY

CBT, cognitive behavioral therapy; GP, general practitioner; ICER, incremental cost effectiveness ratio; NR, not report; PT, physical therapy; QALY, quality-adjusted life-year.

CHAPTER REVIEW QUESTIONS

Answers are located on page 451.

1. What is the main goal of cognitive behavioral therapy?
   a. replacing adaptive coping skills with more adaptive ones
   b. replacing maladaptive coping skills with more adaptive ones
   c. increasing maladaptive coping skills with more adaptive ones
   d. decreasing maladaptive coping skills and more adaptive ones

2. Which of the following is not one of the main phases of cognitive behavioral therapy?
   a. reconceptualization
   b. skills consolidation and application training
   c. emotionalization and maintenance
   d. post-treatment assessment follow-up

3. Which of the following is not an example of how a patient's "sick" behavior can be rewarded?
   a. attention from friends
   b. decreased household chores
   c. paid time off
   d. maladaptive coping

4. What is one of the methods a therapist might use to treat pain-related anxiety in patients with CLBP?
   a. acupuncture
   b. biofeedback
   c. TENS
   d. reflexology

5. What type of diagnostic imaging is commonly conducted before CBT?
   a. MRI
   b. CT
   c. discography
   d. none of the above

6. True or false: CBT should be performed as a sole intervention for CLBP.

REFERENCES

1. Feuerstein M, Beattie P. Biobehavioral factors affecting pain and disability in low back pain: mechanisms and assessment. Phys Ther 1995;75:267-280.
2. Jensen IB, Bergstrom G, Ljungquist T, et al. A randomized controlled component analysis of a behavioral medicine rehabilitation program for chronic spinal pain: are the effects dependent on gender? Pain 2001;91:65-78.
3. Gatchel RJ, Okifuji A. Evidence-based scientific data documenting the treatment and cost-effectiveness of comprehensive pain programs for chronic nonmalignant pain. J Pain 2006;7:779-793.
4. Beck JS. In session with Judith S Beck, PhD: cognitive-behavioral therapy. Prim Psychiatry 2006;13:31-34.
5. Javel AF. The Freudian antecedents of cognitive/behavioral therapy. J Psychother Integr 1999;9:397-407.
6. Dowd ET. Cognition and the cognitive revolution in psychotherapy: promises and advances. J Clin Psychol 2004;60:415-428.
7. Turk DC. Cognitive-behavioral approach to the treatment of chronic pain patients. Reg Anesth Pain Med 2003;28:573-579.
8. Turk DC, Flor H. The cognitive-behavioral approach to pain management. In: McMahon SB, Koltzenburg M, editors. Wall and Melzack's textbook of pain. 5th ed. London: Elsevier Churchill Livingstone; 2006.
9. Gatchel R.J, Robinson RC. Pain management. In: O'Donohue W, Fisher JE, Hayes SC, editors. Cognitive behavior therapy: applying empirically supported techniques in your practice. New York: John Wiley & Sons; 2003.
10. Sullivan MJ, Feuerstein M, Gatchel R, et al. Integrating psychosocial and behavioral interventions to achieve optimal rehabilitation outcomes. J Occup Rehabil 2005;15:475-489.
11. Gatchel RJ, Oordt MS. Clinical health psychology and primary care: practical advice and clinical guidance for successful collaboration. Washington, DC: American Psychological Association; 2003.
12. Dersh J, Gatchel RJ, Mayer T, et al. Prevalence of psychiatric disorders in patients with chronic disabling occupational spinal disorders. Spine 2006;31:1156-1162.
13. DSM IV. Diagnostic and statistical manual of mental disorders. Washington, DC: American Psychiatric Association; 1994. p. 527-528.
14. Vowles KE, Zvolensky MJ, Gross RT, et al. Pain-related anxiety in the prediction of chronic low-back pain distress. J Behav Med 2004;27:77-89.
15. Nielens H, van Zundert J, Mairiaux P, et al. Chronic low back pain. Brussels, 2006, Report No.: KCE reports Vol 48C.
16. Airaksinen O, Brox JI, Cedraschi C, et al. European guidelines for the management of chronic nonspecific low back pain. Eur Spine J 2006;15:S192-S300.
17. National Institute for Health and Clinical Excellence (NICE). Low back pain: early management of persistent non-specific low back pain. London: National Institute of Health and Clinical Excellence; 2009. Report No.: NICE clinical guideline 88.
18. Chou R, Qaseem A, Snow V, et al. Diagnosis and treatment of low back pain: a joint clinical practice guideline from the American College of Physicians and the American Pain Society. Ann Intern Med 2007;147:478-491.
19. Ostelo RW, van Tulder MW, Vlaeyen JW, et al. Behavioural treatment for chronic low-back pain. Cochrane Database Syst Rev 2005;(1):CD002014.
20. Vroomen PC, de Krom MC, Slofstra PD, et al. Conservative treatment of sciatica: a systematic review. J Spinal Disord 2000;13:463-469.
21. Basler HD, Jakle C, Kroner-Herwig B. Incorporation of cognitive-behavioral treatment into the medical care of chronic low back patients: a controlled randomized study in German pain treatment centers. Patient Educ Couns 1997;31:113-124.
22. Bru E, Mykletun R, Berge W, et al. Effects of different psychological interventions on neck, shoulder and low back pain in female hospital staff. Psychology Health 1994;9:371-382.
23. Bush C, Ditto B, Feuerstein M. A controlled evaluation of paraspinal EMG biofeedback in the treatment of chronic low back pain. Health Psychol 1985;4:307-321.
24. Donaldson S, Romney D, Donaldson M, et al. Randomized study of the application of single motor unit biofeedback training to chronic low back pain. J Occup Rehabil 1994;4:23-37.
25. Lindstrom I, Ohlund C, Eek C, et al. The effect of graded activity on patients with subacute low back pain: a randomized prospective clinical study with an operant-conditioning behavioral approach. Phys Ther 1992;72:279-290.

26. McCauley JD, Thelen MH, Frank RG, et al. Hypnosis compared to relaxation in the outpatient management of chronic low back pain. Arch Phys Med Rehabil 1983;64:548-552.

27. Newton-John TR, Spence SH, Schotte D. Cognitive-behavioural therapy versus EMG biofeedback in the treatment of chronic low back pain. Behav Res Ther 1995;33:691-697.

28. Nicholas MK, Wilson PH, Goyen J. Operant-behavioural and cognitive-behavioural treatment for chronic low back pain. Behav Res Ther 1991;29:225-238.

29. Nicholas MK, Wilson PH, Goyen J. Comparison of cognitive-behavioral group treatment and an alternative non-psychological treatment for chronic low back pain. Pain 1992;48:339-347.

30. Nouwen A. EMG biofeedback used to reduce standing levels of paraspinal muscle tension in chronic low back pain. Pain 1983;17:353-360.

31. Rose MJ, Reilly JP, Pennie B, et al. Chronic low back pain rehabilitation programs: a study of the optimum duration of treatment and a comparison of group and individual therapy. Spine 1997;22:2246-2251.

32. Stuckey SJ, Jacobs A, Goldfarb J. EMG biofeedback training, relaxation training, and placebo for the relief of chronic back pain. Percept Mot Skills 1986;63:1023-1036.

33. Turner JA. Comparison of group progressive-relaxation training and cognitive-behavioral group therapy for chronic low back pain. J Consult Clin Psychol 1982;50:757-765.

34. Turner JA, Clancy S. Comparison of operant behavioral and cognitive-behavioral group treatment for chronic low back pain. J Consult Clin Psychol 1988;56:261-266.

35. van den Hout JH, Vlaeyen JW, Heuts PH, et al. Secondary prevention of work-related disability in nonspecific low back pain: does problem-solving therapy help? A randomized clinical trial. Clin J Pain 2003;19:87-96.

36. Linton SJ, Bradley LA, Jensen I, et al. The secondary prevention of low back pain: a controlled study with follow-up. Pain 1989;36:197-207.

37. Turner JA, Denny MC. Do antidepressant medications relieve chronic low back pain? J Fam Pract 1993;37:545-553.

38. Strong J. Incorporating cognitive-behavioral therapy with occupational therapy: a comparative study with patients with low back pain. J Occupat Rehab 1998;8:61-71.

39. Goossens ME, Rutten-Van Molken MP, Kole-Snijders AM, et al. Health economic assessment of behavioural rehabilitation in chronic low back pain: a randomised clinical trial. Health Econ 1998;7:39-51.

40. Turner JA, Clancy S, McQuade KJ, et al. Effectiveness of behavioral therapy for chronic low back pain: a component analysis. J Consult Clin Psychol 1990;58:573-579.

41. Watson CP, Evans RJ, Reed K, et al. Amitriptyline versus placebo in postherpetic neuralgia. Neurology 1982;32:671-673.

42. Chou R, Huffman LH. Nonpharmacologic therapies for acute and chronic low back pain: a review of the evidence for an American Pain Society/American College of Physicians clinical practice guideline. Ann Intern Med 2007;147:492-504.

43. Hoffman BM, Papas RK, Chatkoff DK, et al. Meta-analysis of psychological interventions for chronic low back pain. Health Psychol 2007;26:1-9.

44. Gatchel RJ, Bruga D. Multi- and interdisciplinary intervention for injured workers with chronic low back pain. SpineLine 2005;6:8-13.

45. van Tulder M, Koes B, Bombardier C. Low back pain. Best Pract Res Clin Rheumatol 2002;16:761-775.

46. Gatchel RJ. Comorbidity of chronic pain and mental health disorders: the biopsychosocial perspective. Am Psychol 2004;59:795-805.

47. Gatchel RJ. Clinical essentials of pain management. Washington, DC: American Psychological Association; 2005.

48. Turk DC, Monarch ES. Biopsychosocial perspective on chronic pain. In: Turk DC, Gatchel RJ, editors. Psychological approaches to pain management: a practitioner's handbook. 2nd ed. New York: Guilford; 2002.

49. Morley S, Eccleston C, Williams A. Systematic review and meta-analysis of randomized controlled trials of cognitive behaviour therapy and behaviour therapy for chronic pain in adults, excluding headache. Pain 1999;80:1-13.

50. McCracken LM, Turk DC. Behavioral and cognitive-behavioral treatment for chronic pain: outcome, predictors of outcome, and treatment process. Spine 2002;27:2564-2573.

51. Vlaeyen JW, Morley S. Cognitive-behavioral treatments for chronic pain: what works for whom? Clin J Pain 2005;21:1-8.

52. Mitchell RI, Carmen GM. The functional restoration approach to the treatment of chronic pain in patients with soft tissue and back injuries. Spine 1994;19:633-642.

53. Gatchel RJ, Polatin PB, Noe C, et al. Treatment- and cost-effectiveness of early intervention for acute low-back pain patients: a one-year prospective study. J Occup Rehabil 2003;13:1-9.

54. Brox JI, Sorensen R, Friis A, et al. Randomized clinical trial of lumbar instrumented fusion and cognitive intervention and exercises in patients with chronic low back pain and disc degeneration. Spine 2003;28:1913-1921.

55. Fairbank J, Frost H, Wilson-MacDonald J, et al. Randomised controlled trial to compare surgical stabilisation of the lumbar spine with an intensive rehabilitation programme for patients with chronic low back pain: the MRC spine stabilisation trial. BMJ 2005;330:1233.

56. Brox JI, Reikeras O, Nygaard O, et al. Lumbar instrumented fusion compared with cognitive intervention and exercises in patients with chronic back pain after previous surgery for disc herniation: a prospective randomized controlled study. Pain 2006;122:145-155.

57. Moore JE, Von KM, Cherkin D, et al. A randomized trial of a cognitive-behavioral program for enhancing back pain self care in a primary care setting. Pain 2000;88:145-153.

58. Dagenais S, Roffey DM, Wai EK, et al. Can cost utility evaluations inform decision making about interventions for low back pain? Spine J 2009;9:944-957.

59. van der Roer N, Goossens MEJB, Evers SMAA, et al. What is the most cost-effective treatment for patients with low back pain? A systematic review. Best Pract Res Clin Rheumatol 2005;19:671-684.

60. Skouen JS, Grasdal AL, Haldorsen EM, et al. Relative cost-effectiveness of extensive and light multidisciplinary treatment programs versus treatment as usual for patients with chronic low back pain on long-term sick leave: randomized controlled study. Spine (Phila Pa 1976) 2002;27:901-909.

61. Johnson RE, Jones GT, Wiles NJ, et al. Active exercise, education, and cognitive behavioral therapy for persistent disabling low back pain: a randomized controlled trial. Spine 2007;32:1578-1585.

62. Jellema P, van der Roer N, van der Windt DAWM, et al. Low back pain in general practice: cost-effectiveness of a minimal psychosocial intervention versus usual care. Eur Spine J 2007;16:1812-1821.

63. Critchley DJ, Ratcliffe J, Noonan S, et al. Effectiveness and cost-effectiveness of three types of physiotherapy used to reduce chronic low back pain disability: a pragmatic randomized trial with economic evaluation. Spine 2007;32:1474-1481.

64. Whitehurst DGT, Lewis M, Yao GL, et al. A brief pain management program compared with physical therapy for low back pain: results from an economic analysis alongside a randomized clinical trial. Arthrit Rheum 2007;57:466-473.

65. Schweikert B, Jacobi E, Seitz R, et al. Effectiveness and cost-effectiveness of adding a cognitive behavioral treatment to the rehabilitation of chronic low back pain. J Rheumatol 2006;33:2519-2526.

66. van der Roer N, Van Tulder M, van Mechelen W, et al. Economic evaluation of an intensive group training protocol compared with usual care physiotherapy in patients with chronic low back pain. Spine 2008;33:445-451.

67. Molloy AR, Nicholas MK, Asghari A, et al. Does a combination of intensive cognitive-behavioral pain management and a spinal implantable device confer any advantage? A preliminary examination. Pain Pract 2006;6:96-103.

CHAPTER 22

ROBERT J. GATCHEL
TOM G. MAYER

Functional Restoration

| DESCRIPTION

| Terminology and Subtypes

Functional restoration refers not only to a specific intervention for chronic low back pain (CLBP), but also to a wider conceptualization of the challenges facing clinicians and patients dealing with this condition. Functional restoration is based on the biopsychosocial approach to CLBP, which views pain and disability as the result of a complex and dynamic interaction among physiologic, psychological, and socioeconomic factors that can initiate, perpetuate, or exacerbate the clinical presentation.[1,2] Functional restoration is a comprehensive approach that attempts to address these multiple contributing factors by combining interventions aimed at restoring not only physical function, but also behavioral health, and any other occupational or social difficulties that may develop as a result of prolonged disability due to CLBP. Many approaches to functional restoration have been developed by various specialty spine and chronic pain clinics.

The term *multidisciplinary rehabilitation* is often used to designate spine programs in which patients receive concurrent or coordinated care from behavioral, functional, and medical professionals (Figure 22-1). However, that term is not strictly defined. *Multidisciplinary rehabilitation* can also be interpreted narrowly and used to promote spine programs in which patients who fail to obtain adequate relief after physical therapy are then referred to surgery. Similarly, this term can also be used to designate a loose collaboration between surgical and nonsurgical specialists who rely mostly on injections or other invasive approaches aimed at specific anatomic structures. Only multidisciplinary rehabilitation programs using the more comprehensive biopsychosocial approach to CLBP espoused in this chapter can be designated as functional restoration.

| History and Frequency of Use

Functional restoration was developed in the 1980s by the spine surgeon Tom Mayer and psychologist Robert Gatchel through their collaboration in a Dallas clinic that specialized in managing patients with complex, severe, or debilitating CLBP that was not responsive to conventional approaches. This intervention slowly gained popularity in the 1990s as clinicians and third-party payers became increasingly frustrated with the generally poor results observed after patients with CLBP received costly and invasive interventions. The emergence of functional restoration coincided with a wider adoption of the biopsychosocial model of LBP developed by the Scottish surgeon Gordon Waddell, and was well received by those looking for alternative approaches to managing CLBP.[3] Research supporting the principles of functional restoration continues to grow. Researchers recently lauded this approach and indicated that "the concepts underlying functional restoration have been found to be highly relevant to patients with chronic low back pain, medical providers, and disability systems, and continue to gain acceptance and integration into the care of patients throughout the industrialized world."[4]

| Practitioner, Setting, and Availability

Functional restoration requires a multidisciplinary team of clinicians that may include a medical director, pain management specialist, psychologist or psychiatrist, nurse, physical therapist, and occupational therapist, although not all patients with CLBP will require separate interventions from each of those providers when receiving functional restoration (Figure 22-2 and Table 22-1).[3-11] Given the number of health providers involved, effective communication among functional restoration team members is crucial (e.g., a patient's fear of physical activity should be discussed openly to prevent it from interfering with their physical reconditioning program). This intervention is typically offered in specialty spine clinics located in larger cities and is not widely available in the United States.

| Procedure

Functional restoration was developed to overcome the limitations inherent in traditional problem-focused management of CLBP, with medical history taking, evaluation of symptoms and physical function based solely on self-reported pain, and an anatomic diagnosis guided primarily by advanced imaging. To fully understand the nature of CLBP and its complete impact on a patient's life, it was deemed essential to acquire additional (preferably objective) information to arrive at an appropriate diagnosis and make recommendations about multidisciplinary management. This additional information should be collected through structured interviews,

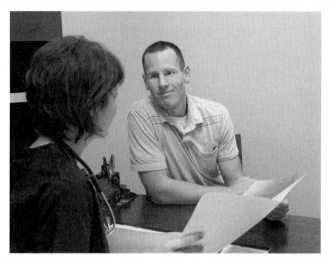

Figure 22-1 Functional restoration requires collaboration and open communication among health care professionals.

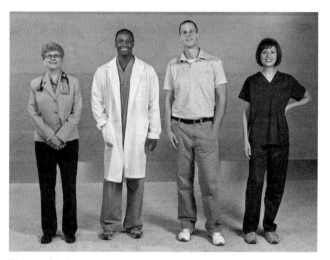

Figure 22-2 Functional restoration requires a multidisciplinary approach and coordination of care.

TABLE 22-1	Health Care Providers Commonly Involved in Functional Restoration for Chronic Low Back Pain
Practitioner	**Role**
Medical director	Most commonly a physician with a complete understanding of the biopsychosocial philosophy of interdisciplinary care and a firm background in providing medical rehabilitation for CLBP
Nurse	Assists the physician, follows up the procedures, and serves as a physician-extender to address patient needs
Occupational therapist	Involved in both the physical and vocational aspects of the patient's rehabilitation because many patients with CLBP will not be working
	Addresses vocational issues such as return to work, work accommodations and training, and may serve as an advocate for the patient with insurers and/or employers
Pain management specialist	Provides anesthesiology services such as injections, nerve blocks, and other medical procedures related to CLBP
Physical therapist	Interacts with the patient on a daily basis to address any issues related to physical deconditioning, educates the patient about the physiologic bases of pain, and teaches methods of reducing the severity of pain through body mechanics and exercise pacing
Psychologist or psychiatrist	Plays the leading role in the day-to-day maintenance of the psychosocial aspects and status of patient care using evaluations to identify potential barriers to recovery and a patient's psychosocial strengths and weaknesses
	A CBT approach can then be used to address important issues such as pain-related depression, anxiety, substance abuse, and other forms of psychopathology that may be encountered in long-standing CLBP
	Such a CBT approach has been found to be the most appropriate and effective modality to use in interdisciplinary programs

CBT, cognitive behavioral therapy; CLBP, chronic low back pain.

quantitative measures, and objective assessment of physical capacity and compared with a normative database. Influenced by a sports medicine approach, this additional information guides the development of treatment programs tailored for each patient and aimed primarily at restoring physical functional capacity and psychosocial performance. The objectives of functional restoration are ambitious and include not only decreasing pain and medication use, but also restoring function in activities of daily living and returning to full employment, with sufficient physical capacity to avoid recurrent injury and limit future health care utilization.

Functional restoration includes the following components: (1) formal, repeated quantification of physical and functional deficits to guide physical therapists in improving "weak-link"

performance of the injured area and guide occupational therapists working to improve activities of daily living; (2) psychosocial and socioeconomic assessment; (3) multimodal disability management; (4) psychopharmacologic interventions; (5) ongoing clinical outcomes assessment; and (6) interdisciplinary, medically directed team approach. The goal of repeated quantification of specific physical deficits (e.g., ability to lift 20 lb to waist level) is to guide and monitor individualized physical training programs designed to correct these deficiencies. A comprehensive psychosocial and socioeconomic assessment is conducted by a behavioral expert to guide and monitor important aspects of recovery, including pain, disability, and mental health. Multidisciplinary disability management programs integrate cognitive behavioral therapy (CBT) approaches into interventions aimed at correcting specific anatomic contributors to CLBP.

The goal of psychopharmacologic interventions is to identify and address addiction or dependence to opioid analgesics or other medications, monitor any required detoxification, and provide psychosocial management to complement pharmaceutical interventions. Medications for symptoms of depression, anxiety, sleep disturbance, or neuropathic pain are routinely provided, at least on a temporary basis, to facilitate rehabilitation and return to work goals. Standardized and validated condition-specific and general health instruments are used to collect objective data about outcomes using questionnaires and structured interviews. The multidisciplinary team critical to functional restoration requires regularly scheduled staff meetings and conferences to discuss the progress of specific patients and suggest any required changes to the current approach.

Regulatory Status

Not applicable.

THEORY

Mechanism of Action

The mechanism of action involved in functional restoration for CLBP is likely complex because it is thought to not only provide the combined beneficial effects of each intervention administered individually, but also derive some synergies from their coordinated and integrated delivery in a multidisciplinary environment. Such synergies are thought to occur as a result of enhanced communication between providers, which may optimize the timing for introducing specific components of the intervention and decrease the likelihood of presenting contradictory information to the patient. This approach also offers practical advantages by combining all providers in one location, thereby facilitating patient access and compliance to what may otherwise be a disparate network of providers. By adopting a comprehensive approach to patient management and simultaneously addressing physical, psychological, and vocational impediments to returning to work, functional restoration may decrease the time necessary to recovery if individual elements were addressed sequentially.

Indication

Functional restoration is an appropriate tertiary care option for those patients with CLBP who have failed to respond to programs such as reactivation and work hardening, have not improved after surgical or other interventional methods, and have no active, objective pathophysiology requiring immediate medical or surgical care. It is well known that significant psychosocial barriers to successful recovery may develop as a patient progresses from acute to chronic pain. Although serious comorbid psychiatric disorders are often a contraindication to many interventions for CLBP, such psychopathology can be effectively managed within the context of a functional restoration program.[12] The ideal CLBP patient for functional restoration is one who is motivated to learn to manage pain more effectively, is compliant with the prescribed rehabilitation regimen, and wishes to return to work and full activities of daily living. Often, there are certain "barriers to recovery," such as secondary gain associated with perceived financial incentives for remaining disabled. However, even these secondary gain issues can be successfully dealt with in a comprehensive functional restoration program.[13]

Assessment

Before receiving functional restoration, patients should first be assessed for LBP using an evidence-based and goal-oriented approach focused on the patient history and neurologic examination, as discussed in Chapter 3. Additional diagnostic imaging or specific diagnostic testing is generally not required before initiating this intervention for CLBP. Certain questionnaires (e.g., Tampa Scale for Kinesiophobia, Fear Avoidance Beliefs Questionnaire) may be helpful to identify subsets of patients with CLBP who may benefit from specific interventions aimed at addressing those issues (e.g., fear avoidance training, as discussed in Chapter 7). Psychological testing is also required for functional restoration to identify coexisting conditions such as depression. An evaluation of medication use and functional capacity may also be indicated to tailor specific recommendations to address any noted deficiencies.

EFFICACY

Evidence supporting the efficacy of this intervention for CLBP was summarized from recent clinical practice guidelines (CPGs), systematic reviews (SRs), and randomized controlled trials (RCTs). Observational studies (OBSs) were also summarized where appropriate. Findings are summarized by study design.

Clinical Practice Guidelines

Six of the recent national CPGs on the management of CLBP have assessed and summarized the evidence to make specific recommendations about the efficacy of functional restoration or other multidisciplinary rehabilitation programs.

The CPG from Belgium in 2006 found high-quality evidence that intensive multidisciplinary rehabilitation programs combining education, exercise, relaxation, behavioral, and other interventions are more effective than conventional interventions alone in patients with CLBP.[14] That CPG also found moderate-quality evidence that intensive multidisciplinary biopsychosocial rehabilitation with a functional restoration approach is more effective than outpatient non-multidisciplinary rehabilitation or usual care with respect to improvements in pain for CLBP. Multidisciplinary rehabilitation programs based on biopsychosocial models for the management of CLBP were recommended.

The CPG from Europe in 2004 found moderate evidence that intensive multidisciplinary biopsychosocial rehabilitation with a functional restoration approach is more effective than outpatient non–multidisciplinary rehabilitation or usual care with respect to improvements in pain for CLBP.[15] That CPG also found strong evidence to support the efficacy of intensive multidisciplinary biopsychosocial rehabilitation with a functional restoration approach with respect to improvements in pain and function for CLBP. There was no evidence comparing the efficacy of multidisciplinary biopsychosocial rehabilitation with a functional restoration approach to sham procedures for CLBP.

The CPG from the United States in 2007 found evidence to support the efficacy of functional restoration with CBT with respect to improvements in work absenteeism.[16]

The CPG from Italy in 2007 recommended that multidisciplinary rehabilitation should include a comprehensive diagnostic assessment and both individual CBT and back exercises when used for the management of CLBP.[17]

The CPG from the United Kingdom in 2009 recommended that multidisciplinary rehabilitation should include CBT, exercise, and some aspect of goal setting or problem solving for CLBP.[18] That CPG also recommended multidisciplinary rehabilitation for patients who continue to have high disability or psychological distress after receiving less intensive interventions, and suggested that the more extensive multidisciplinary rehabilitation approaches were indicated for those with CLBP and a poor prognosis, whereas lower intensity approaches were indicated for those with CLBP and a good prognosis. There was insufficient evidence to determine that any one particular approach to multidisciplinary rehabilitation was superior to others for CLBP.

The CPG from the United States in 2009 found good evidence to support the efficacy of multidisciplinary rehabilitation using a CBT approach in the management of CLBP.[19]

Findings from the above CPGs are summarized in Table 22-2.

Systematic Reviews

Cochrane Collaboration

An SR was conducted in 2003 by the Cochrane Collaboration on functional restoration for acute and chronic LBP and neck pain.[20] A total of 18 RCTs were identified, including 8 that examined the effects of functional restoration with a psychological component for CLBP.[21-28] Three RCTs had no statistically significant differences between exercise combined with psychotherapy and self-exercise or placebo.[22,25,26] In contrast, four RCTs did find that exercise combined with psychotherapy led to statistically significant treatment effects versus physical therapy alone.[23,24,27,28] Results from the final RCT were unclear.[21] This review concluded that functional restoration (i.e., exercise and psychotherapy approaches combined) is effective at reducing time lost from work for CLBP.[20] This SR also concluded that functional restoration is not effective for those with acute LBP.[20]

American Pain Society and American College of Physicians

An SR was conducted in 2006 by the American Pain Society and American College of Physicians CPG committee on nonpharmacologic therapies for acute and chronic LBP.[29] That review identified one SR related to functional restoration, which was the Cochrane Collaboration review mentioned earlier.[20] No additional trials were identified. This SR concluded that functional restoration is effective for chronic or subacute LBP lasting longer than 4 weeks.[29]

Other

A review found strong evidence that intensive interdisciplinary rehabilitation with functional restoration reduces pain and improves function in patients with CLBP significantly more than less intensive programs or usual care.[30]

Similar findings were reported in the Cochrane Collaboration review on multidisciplinary treatment approaches to CLBP, some of which included elements of functional restoration.[31]

Finally, a recent review concluded that a multidisciplinary approach to chronic pain focusing on functional outcomes produced the best outcomes for CLBP.[32]

Findings from the above SRs are summarized in Table 22-3.

Randomized Controlled Trials

Four RCTs were identified.[26,33-35] Their methods are summarized in Table 22-4. Their results are briefly described here.

Gatchel and colleagues[33] performed an RCT in which patients with acute LBP were categorized into those at high risk or low risk of developing CLBP. Patients categorized as being high risk for CLBP were randomized to a functional restoration program or to a non-intervention group. In order to be included, participants had to have LBP lasting less than 2 months and did not require surgery. Those with serious pathology or psychiatric conditions were excluded. The functional restoration program was administered by a nurse-physician team and consisted of up to nine 15-minute sessions of individual exercise, nine 30-minute sessions of group exercise, nine sessions of biofeedback or pain management, nine 45-minute sessions of group didactics, and three team conferences. After 1 year of follow-up, participants in the high risk for CLBP functional restoration group experienced

TABLE 22-2	Clinical Practice Guideline Recommendations on Functional Restoration for Chronic Low Back Pain

Reference	Country	Conclusion
14	Belgium	Recommended
15	Europe	Strong evidence of efficacy
16	United States	Evidence to support efficacy
17	Italy	Recommended for use in conjunction with CBT and back exercises
18	United Kingdom	Recommended
19	United States	Good evidence to support efficacy

CBT, cognitive behavioral therapy.

TABLE 22-3 | **Systematic Review Findings on Functional Restoration for Chronic Low Back Pain**

Reference	# RCTs in SR	# RCTs for CLBP	Conclusion
20	18	8	Functional restoration is effective at reducing time lost from work for CLBP
29	1 SR—Cochrane review above	NR	Functional restoration is effective for CLBP lasting longer than 4 weeks
30	NR	NR	Strong evidence that intensive interdisciplinary rehabilitation with functional restoration reduces pain and improves function in patients with CLBP
31	NR	NR	Recommended as component of multidisciplinary rehabilitation
32	NR	NR	Multidisciplinary approach focusing on functional outcomes had best outcomes

CLBP, chronic low back pain; NR, not reported; RCT, randomized controlled trial; SR, systematic review.

TABLE 22-4 | **Randomized Controlled Trials on Functional Restoration for Chronic Low Back Pain**

Reference	Indication	Intervention 1	Intervention 2	Control
33	Acute LBP, neurologic involvement NR, symptoms <2 months	High risk for CLBP Functional restoration: PT, psychotherapy, occupational therapy, case management Nurse-physician team 3 weeks of up to 9 × 15-minute individual exercise, 9 × 30-minute group exercise, 9 × biofeedback/pain management, 9 × 45-minute group didactic, 3× team conferences Cointervention: NR n = 22	NA	(1) High risk for CLBP No intervention Cointervention: NR n = 48 (2) Observational group: Low risk for CLBP No treatment Cointervention: NR n = 54
26	Soft tissue or back injury, neurologic involvement NR, symptoms >3 months	Functional restoration: PT, psychotherapy Administrator NR Up to 8 to 12 weeks of 7 hours/day × 5 days/week physical exercise, functional simulation, group therapy, cognitive behavioral therapy, biofeedback, relaxation, group counseling Cointervention: at the discretion of primary care practitioner n = 271	NA	Supervised by primary care practitioner Cointervention: at the discretion of primary care practitioner n = 271
34	CLBP with or without neurologic involvement, symptoms >6 months	Functional restoration: behavioral support, exercise, occupational therapy, biofeedback, relaxation Administrator NR 39 hours/week × 3 weeks Cointervention: analgesic medication n = 55	NA	No treatment Cointervention: NR n = 51
35	CLBP, neurologic involvement NR, symptoms >4 months	Functional restoration: behavioral support, PT, balneotherapy, occupational therapy, nutritional advice Physical therapist, physiatrist, psychologist 6 hours/day, 5 days/week for 5 weeks Cointervention: NR n = 43	Active individual therapy: PT, home exercise, Physical therapist 1 hour/day, 3×/week over 5 weeks + 50 minutes/day, 2×/week home exercise Cointervention: NR n = 41	NA

CLBP, chronic low back pain; LBP, low back pain; NA, not applicable; NR, not reported; PT, physical therapy.

statistically significant improvements in function and pain versus the high risk for CLBP group that did not receive any intervention. Results among the low risk for CLBP group who also did not receive any intervention were similar to those observed among the functional restoration group.

Mitchell and Carmen[26] conducted an RCT in which patients with soft tissue or back injuries were included if they experienced their symptoms for more than 3 months and exhibited signs of inappropriate illness behavior (e.g., bizarre symptoms, prolonged recovery). Those with serious pathology or requiring surgery were excluded. Approximately 23% of the included participants had pain originating from structures other than the lower back. Participants were randomized to a functional restoration group or another group who were supervised by their primary care practitioner and received other interventions, such as acupuncture, physical therapy, spinal manipulation, and analgesics. The functional restoration program consisted of up to 8 to 12 weeks of exercise, functional simulation, CBT, biofeedback, relaxation, and group counseling for 7 hours per day, 5 days per week. After 1 year of follow-up, no statistically significant differences were observed between the two groups regarding the proportion returning to full-time work. However, the follow-up rates were not reported in that study. Also, the results for pain or disability were surprisingly not reported. This raises the important question of whether the approach evaluated was clinically appropriate.

Bendix and colleagues[34] performed an RCT including patients with CLBP with or without neurologic involvement. In order to be included, participants had to experience symptoms for more than 6 months. Participants were randomized to either a 3-week intensive functional restoration program including behavioral support or to no treatment. After 4 months of follow-up, individuals who were in the functional restoration group experienced statistically significant functional improvement versus those in the control group. However, no differences between groups were observed for pain relief.

Jousset and colleagues[35] performed an RCT in which patients with CLBP were selected if they failed to improve despite therapy and were aged 18 to 50 years old. Those not willing to participate or those with a psychiatric disorder were excluded. Participants were randomized to either a functional restoration program or an active individual program. The functional restoration program entailed intensive physical therapy, psychiatric support, balneotherapy, occupational therapy, and nutrition advice. The program duration was 6 hours per day, 5 days per week for 5 weeks. The active therapy group received 1 hour of physical therapy per day 3 times per week and were supposed to do 50 minutes of home exercise twice per week for 5 weeks. After 6 months of follow-up, patients in the functional restoration group experienced statistically significant improvement on all measures of disability and pain, while the active individual therapy group experienced statistically significant improvement on some disability measures but not on any pain scales. However, no differences in pain or function were observed between the two groups after 6 months of follow-up.

Observational Studies

The effectiveness of functional restoration programs has been assessed by many observational studies, including Hazard and colleagues[36] and Patrick and colleagues[37] in the United States, Hildebrandt and colleagues[38] in Germany, Corey and colleagues[39] in Canada, Jousset and colleagues[35] in France, and Shirado and colleagues[40] in Japan. Research by Mayer and colleagues demonstrated that functional restoration is associated with substantive improvement in important socioeconomic outcome measures (e.g., return to work and resolution of outstanding legal and medical issues) in chronically disabled patients with spinal disorders after 1 and 2 years of follow-up.[41-43] For example, in the 2-year follow-up study by Mayer and colleagues, 87% of the functional restoration treatment group was actively working compared with only 41% of a nontreatment comparison group which had twice the rate of additional spine surgery and unsettled worker's compensation litigation.[43] The comparison group also had five times more patient visits to health care professionals, and higher rates of recurrence or reinjury. These results were observed in a group consisting primarily of CLBP worker's compensation cases, traditionally the most difficult patients to treat successfully. Many other studies from this group have documented similar high success rates.[12,44-46]

SAFETY

Contraindications

Contraindications to functional restoration include CLBP due to potentially serious spinal pathology such as, cancer, infection, or cauda equina syndrome. Because functional restoration incorporates behavioral therapy that requires cognitive processing skills, it may be contraindicated in patients with major cognitive deficit related to brain trauma or organic disorders. The emphasis on patient education also requires written and oral communication, which may be complicated by language barriers. Many functional restoration programs (e.g., Productive Rehabilitation Institute of Dallas for Ergonomics) have multilingual therapists on staff to overcome this potential contraindication for patients whose primary language is not English.

Adverse Events

Functional restoration is generally considered to be a safe intervention, and involves careful monitoring of symptoms by a multidisciplinary team of health care professionals to avoid severe exacerbation of symptoms or needlessly pursuing interventions that are not effective. One study of functional restoration reported soft tissue injuries and exacerbations of LBP, while another study reported that symptoms were aggravated in 4% of participants.[36,40] However, no serious adverse events have been reported in the studies of functional restoration for CLBP.

COSTS

Fees and Third-Party Reimbursement

Functional restoration involves a collaboration among different types of health providers, including a behavioral therapist, physical therapist, and physician, each of whom can bill separately for their services. Due to the involvement of multiple professionals, the initial cost for functional restoration may be higher than the conventional medical management approach. Therefore, it is recommended that patients contact third-party payers to understand their reimbursement policies. Third-party payers may have nonpayment policies for these programs, based on their cost. Other carriers may have policies which "carve out" reimbursement for specific aspects of the treatment program in an effort to keep costs at a minimum.

The behavioral component of functional restoration can initially be delivered by licensed behavioral health professionals using CPT codes for psychiatric diagnostic interview examination, including 90801 or 90802, when the goal is to establish a diagnosis and treatment protocol. Psychotherapy, defined as the treatment for mental illness and behavioral disturbances in which the clinician, through definitive therapeutic communication, attempts to alleviate emotional disturbances, reverse or change maladaptive patterns of behavior, and encourage personality growth and development, can be delivered using CPT codes 90804 (20 to 30 minutes), 90806 (45 to 50 minutes), or 90808 (75 to 80 minutes). If additional evaluation and management services are required, CPT codes 90805 (20 to 30 minutes), 90807 (45 to 50 minutes), or 90809 (75 to 80 minutes) can be used instead. These codes are based on the setting in which the psychotherapy session occurred, the type of psychotherapy provided and the amount of face-to-face time spent with the patient. The decision regarding the appropriate reporting of individual psychotherapy codes should be based solely on the definition of the codes and the work performed. Alternatively, brief CBT for CLBP may be provided by a clinician in the context of an outpatient visit for a new patient using CPT codes 99201 (up to 10 minutes), 99202 (up to 20 minutes), or 99203 (up to 30 minutes). For an established patient, brief CBT for CLBP may be provided during an outpatient visit using CPT codes 99211 (up to 5 minutes), 99212 (up to 10 minutes), or 99213 (up to 15 minutes).

For the physical therapist, the initial evaluation can be delivered using CPT codes 97001 (physical therapy initial evaluation) or 97750 (physical performance test or measurement, each 15 minutes). Periodic reevaluation can be delivered using CPT codes 97002 (physical therapy reevaluation) or 97750 (physical performance test or measurement, each to 15 minutes). Visits other than evaluations can be delivered using CPT codes 97110 (therapeutic exercises, each 15 minutes) or 97530 (therapeutic activities, each 15 minutes).

For the physician, functional restoration for CLBP may be provided in the context of an office or outpatient visit for a new patient using CPT codes 99201 (up to 10 minutes), 99202 (up to 20 minutes), or 99203 (up to 30 minutes). For an established patient, functional restoration for CLBP may

TABLE 22-5	Medicare Fee Schedule for Related Services	
CPT Code	New York	California
Psychiatric Examination		
90801	$158	$169
90802	$141	$181
Psychotherapy		
90804	$65	$69
90805	$74	$78
90806	$90	$95
90807	$103	$109
90808	$132	$139
90809	$146	$154
Office Visits		
99201	$41	$44
99202	$70	$76
99203	$101	$109
99211	$20	$22
99212	$41	$44
99213	$68	$73
Physical Therapy		
97001	$73	$78
97002	$40	$43
97110	$30	$32
97530	$32	$35
97750	$31	$44

2010 Participating, nonfacility amount.

be provided during an office or outpatient visit using CPT codes 99211 (up to 5 minutes), 99212 (up to 10 minutes), or 99213 (up to 15 minutes).

Although time is indicated for the various levels of service and can be a contributing component for selection of the level of office/outpatient visits, the overarching criteria for selection of the level of service should be based on medical necessity and the amount of history, examination, and medical decision making that was required and documented. These procedures are widely covered by other third-party payers such as health insurers and worker's compensation insurance. Although some payers continue to base their reimbursements on usual, customary, and reasonable payment methodology, the majority have developed reimbursement tables based on the Resource Based Relative Value Scale used by Medicare. Reimbursements by other third-party payers are generally higher than Medicare. It should be noted that CPT codes listed in the psychiatry section of the CPT manual (90801-90899) are in fact not limited to psychiatrists or mental health professionals, and may be used to designate the services rendered by any qualified physician or other qualified health care professional. Unfortunately, some third-party payers will not reimburse all providers for these codes.

Typical fees reimbursed by Medicare in New York and California for these services are summarized in Table 22-5.

Cost Effectiveness

Evidence supporting the cost effectiveness of treatment protocols that compared this intervention, often in combination with one or more cointerventions, with control groups who received one or more other interventions, for either acute or chronic LBP, was identified from two SRs on this topic and is summarized here.[47,48] Although many of these study designs are unable to clearly identify the individual contribution of any intervention, their results provide some insight as to the clinical and economic outcomes associated with this approach.

An RCT in the United States compared three approaches in patients with acute LBP who had been identified as being at high or low risk of developing chronicity according to a questionnaire.[33] Those at high risk of developing CLBP were randomized to either functional restoration or a nonintervention control; those at low risk for developing CLBP were also monitored in an observational control group. Functional restoration included supervised exercise therapy, CBT, and other interventions as necessary. Clinical outcomes after 1 year reported that the functional restoration group was similar for improvement in pain to the low-risk observational group, and both were superior to the high-risk nonintervention group. Direct medical costs associated with study interventions over 1 year were $3885 for functional restoration and $0 for the nonintervention group. Direct medical costs associated with nonstudy interventions such as provider visits and medications over 1 year were $1794 for functional restoration and $2892 for the nonintervention group. Indirect productivity costs from lost work days over 1 year were $7072 for functional restoration and $18,951 for the nonintervention group. Total costs (direct medical and indirect productivity) over 1 year were therefore $12,751 in the functional restoration group and $21,843 in the nonintervention group. Authors concluded that functional restoration was cost effective in patients with acute LBP identified as being at high risk for developing CLBP.

An RCT from Canada compared two approaches for patients who had been injured at work and subsequently suffered from CLBP.[26] The functional restoration group included CBT, fear avoidance training, education, biofeedback, and group counseling, as well as strengthening and stretching exercises. The usual care group could receive a variety of interventions, including physical therapy, acupuncture, back school, spinal manipulation, medication, or supervised exercise therapy. Clinical outcomes were not reported. Direct medical costs associated with the study intervention were $2507 higher in the functional restoration group. Indirect productivity costs associated with lost work days were $3172 lower in the functional restoration group. Total costs for interventions, lost work days, and disability pensions were $7068 lower in the functional restoration group. These differences were not statistically significant.

Other

Because such programs involve the contributions of multiple professionals in a time-intensive manner, the initial cost for such an approach may be higher than that for the conventional medical management approach. Although functional restoration programs have been shown to be both more therapeutic and cost effective than traditional unimodal methods, third-party payers may view them as too costly and resist reimbursement for such programs.[9-11] Despite research suggesting that "carving out" portions of comprehensive, integrated programs (e.g., sending patients to different providers for their various needs outside of the comprehensive pain management programs) may compromise the effectiveness of interdisciplinary pain management programs, some managed care organizations continue to do so in an effort to contain costs.[10,49-52]

In addition, a review of the literature concluded that comprehensive interdisciplinary programs, such as functional restoration, were more therapeutically effective and cost effective than traditional medical treatments for pain conditions such as CLBP.[10] Moreover, in a study analyzing cost utility expressed as quality-adjusted life-years (QALYs), it was found that functional restoration was associated with better QALYs than traditional medical treatments for CLBP, suggesting that such a program was both less costly and more effective than standard care.[53]

Findings from cost effectiveness analyses are summarized in Table 22-6.

TABLE 22-6	Cost Effectiveness and Cost Utility Analyses of Functional Restoration for Chronic Low Back Pain				
Ref Country Follow-Up	Group	Direct Medical Costs	Indirect Productivity Costs	Total Costs	Conclusion
33 United States 1 year	1. Functional restoration 2. Nonintervention control 3. Observational control	1. $5679 2. $2892 3. $0	1. $7072 2. $18,951 3. NR	1. $12,751 2. $21,843 3. NR	Group 1 is cost effective
26 Canada NR	1. Functional restoration 2. Usual care	1. $2507 higher than group 2 2. NR	1. $3172 lower than group 2 for lost work days 2. NR	1. $7068 lower than group 2 (lost work days + disability pensions) 2. NR	No significant difference

NR, not reported.

SUMMARY

Description

Functional restoration is a comprehensive approach that attempts to address physiologic, psychological, and socioeconomic factors that may develop as a result of prolonged CLBP by combining interventions aimed at restoring physical function, behavioral health, and any occupational or social difficulties. Functional restoration requires a multidisciplinary team of clinicians that may include a medical director, pain management specialist, psychologist or psychiatrist, nurse, physical therapist, and occupational therapist, though not all patients with CLBP will require separate interventions from each of those providers. Functional restoration is not widely available in the United States.

Theory

The mechanism of action involved in functional restoration for CLBP is likely complex because it is thought to not only provide the combined beneficial effects of each intervention administered individually, but also derive some synergies from their coordinated and integrated delivery in a multidisciplinary environment. The two major components include a quantitatively-directed exercise progression approach aimed at the injured "weak link" area and subsequently improving activities of daily living relevant to work and recreational demands for that individual, guided by physical and occupational therapists, and a multimodal pain/disability management program providing counseling and education for pain relief, stress control, coping skills, fear avoidance belief training and cognitive behavioral components led by psychologists and other licensed professionals. Outcome-monitoring of subjective change is critical. Functional restoration is indicated as a tertiary care intervention for unspecific CLBP that has not improved with other interventions, such as work hardening, surgery or other interventional methods. Diagnostic imaging or other forms of advanced testing is generally not required before administering this intervention for CLBP.

Efficacy

Six CPGs recommend multidisciplinary rehabilitation with some form of psychotherapy or functional restoration component for CLBP. Furthermore, two recent SRs concluded that functional restoration is effective for CLBP. At least five RCTs assessed the efficacy of functional restoration, two of which found statistically significant improvement in pain or disability versus comparator groups.

Safety

Contraindications to functional restoration include CLBP due to potentially serious spinal pathology such as fracture, cancer, infection, or cauda equina syndrome. Because functional restoration incorporates CBT that requires cognitive processing skills, it may be contraindicated in patients with major cognitive deficit related to brain trauma or organic pathophysiology. Functional restoration is generally considered to be a safe intervention, and involves careful monitoring of symptoms by a multidisciplinary team of health care professionals to avoid severe exacerbation of symptoms or needlessly pursuing interventions that are not effective.

Costs

In the United States, functional restoration involves collaboration among different types of health providers, each of whom bill separately for their services. Because such programs involve the contributions of multiple professionals in a time-intensive manner, the initial cost for such an approach may be higher than that for the conventional medical management approach. At least two studies assessed costs of functional restoration for CLBP, one of which observed that the total costs for interventions, lost workdays, and disability pensions were lower in the functional restoration group, though these differences were not statistically significant.

Comments

Evidence from the CPGs, SRs, and RCTs reviewed suggests that multidisciplinary rehabilitation interventions such as functional restoration that incorporate elements of patient education, behavioral therapy, and exercise therapy may be effective for some patients with CLBP and other comorbidities in whom other therapies have not achieved the desired results. Studies evaluating functional restoration and similar approaches have been conducted among patients with CLBP and known confounders, including worker's compensation and socioeconomic risk factors for chronicity, which speaks highly for the robustness of this approach in patients who may otherwise have a poor prognosis.

An important advantage of functional restoration relative to traditional unimodal medical intervention methods is that it simultaneously addresses multiple outcome measures, including self-reported measures of pain and disability, objective physical functional measures, and socioeconomic outcomes such as return to work. The major deterrent to the wider use of this approach is the reluctance of third-party payers to authorize its use because of its perceived high initial costs. However, such perceptions may be misguided if this approach is able to yield the potential long-term cost savings through decreased health utilization and reduced work absence.

CHAPTER REVIEW QUESTIONS

Answers are located on page 451.
1. On what approach is functional restoration based?
   a. biogenetic approach, which views pain and disability as a complex and dynamic interaction among genetic and physiological factors that perpetuate or worsen the clinical presentation

b. biopsychosocial approach, which views pain and disability as a complex and dynamic interaction among physiological, psychological, and social factors that perpetuate or worsen the clinical presentation

c. biopharmaceutical approach, which views pain and disability as a complex and dynamic interaction among pharmaceuticals and chemical mediators that perpetuate or worsen the clinical presentation

d. biosurgical approach, which views pain and disability as a complex and dynamic interaction among anatomical structures and osseous pathologies that perpetuate or worsen the clinical presentation

2. Which of the following is not an important component of functional restoration?
   a. formal quantification of physical deficits
   b. psychosocial and socioeconomic assessment
   c. incorporating yoga and pilates into daily work routine
   d. psychopharmacological interventions for required detoxification and psychosocial management
   e. ongoing outcome assessment
   f. interdisciplinary medically directed team approach

3. True or false? It has previously been reported that functional restoration is cost effective.

4. What type of diagnostic imaging is commonly conducted prior to functional restoration?
   a. x-rays
   b. MRI
   c. CT
   d. discography
   e. none of the above

5. Which of the following components are usually addressed in a functional restoration program?
   a. physiologic
   b. psychological
   c. social
   d. economic
   e. all of the above

6. True or false: All comprehensive functional restoration programs should require involvement of the following individuals: medical director, pain management specialist, psychologist or psychiatrist, nurse, physical therapist, and occupational therapist.

7. What is the opposite approach to functional restoration?
   a. holistic
   b. uniform
   c. atomistic
   d. singular
   e. none of the above

REFERENCES

1. Gatchel RJ. Comorbidity of chronic pain and mental health disorders: the biopsychosocial perspective. Am Psychol 2004;59:795-805.

2. Turk DC, Monarch ES. Biopsychosocial perspective on chronic pain. In: Turk DC, Gatchel RJ, editors. Psychological approaches to pain management: a practitioner's handbook. 2nd ed. New York: Guilford; 2002.

3. Mayer TG, Gatchel RJ. Functional restoration for spinal disorders: the sports medicine approach. Philadelphia: Lea & Febiger; 1988.

4. Rainville J, Kim RS, Katz JN. A review of 1985 Volvo Award winner in clinical science: objective assessment of spine function following industrial injury: a prospective study with comparison group and 1-year follow-up. Spine 2007;32: 2031-2034.

5. Deschner M, Polatin PB. Interdisciplinary programs: chronic pain management. Occupational musculoskeletal disorders: function, outcomes and evidence. Philadelphia: Lippincott Williams & Wilkins; 2000. p. 629-637.

6. Mayer TG, Polatin PB. Tertiary nonoperative interdisciplinary programs: the functional restoration variant of the outpatient chronic pain management program. Occupational musculoskeletal disorders function, outcomes, and evidence. Philadelphia: Lippincott Williams & Wilkins; 2000. p. 639-650.

7. Turk DC, Gatchel RJ. Psychosocial factors and pain: revolution and evolution. In: Gatchel RJ, Turk DC, editors. Psychosocial factors in pain: critical perspectives. New York: Guilford; 1999. p. 481-494.

8. Wright AR, Gatchel RJ. Occupational musculoskeletal pain and disability. In: Turk DC, Gatchel RJ, editors. Psychological approaches to pain management: a practitioner's handbook. 2nd ed. New York: Guilford; 2002. p. 349-364.

9. Gatchel RJ, Kishino N, Noe C. "Carving-out" services from multidisciplinary chronic pain management programs: negative impact on therapeutic efficacy. In: Schatman ME, Campbell A, editors. Chronic pain management: guidelines for multidisciplinary program development. New York: Informa Health Care; 2007.

10. Gatchel RJ, Okifuji A. Evidence-based scientific data documenting the treatment and cost-effectiveness of comprehensive pain programs for chronic nonmalignant pain. J Pain 2006;7:779-793.

11. Gatchel RJ, Rollings KH. Evidence-informed management of chronic low back pain with cognitive behavioral therapy. Spine J 2008;8:40-44.

12. Gatchel RJ, Polatin PB, Mayer TG, et al. Psychopathology and the rehabilitation of patients with chronic low back pain disability. Arch Phys Med Rehabil 1994;75:666-670.

13. Leeman G, Polatin PB, Gatchel RJ, et al. Managing secondary gain in patients with pain-associated disability: a clinical perspective. J Workers Compens 2000;9:25-43.

14. Nielens H, van Zundert J, Mairiaux P, et al. Chronic low back pain. Brussels, 2006, Report No.: KCE reports Vol 48C.

15. Airaksinen O, Brox JI, Cedraschi C, et al. European guidelines for the management of chronic nonspecific low back pain. Eur Spine J 2006;15:S192-S300.

16. Chou R, Qaseem A, Snow V, et al. Diagnosis and treatment of low back pain: a joint clinical practice guideline from the American College of Physicians and the American Pain Society. Ann Intern Med 2007;147:478-491.

17. Negrini S, Giovannoni S, Minozzi S, et al. Diagnostic therapeutic flow-charts for low back pain patients: the Italian clinical guidelines. Eura Medicophys 2006;42:151-170.

18. National Institute for Health and Clinical Excellence (NICE). Low back pain: early management of persistent non-specific low back pain. London: National Institute of Health and Clinical Excellence; 2009. Report No.: NICE clinical guideline 88.

19. Chou R, Loeser JD, Owens DK, et al. Interventional therapies, surgery, and interdisciplinary rehabilitation for low back pain: an evidence-based clinical practice guideline from the American Pain Society. Spine 2009;34:1066-1077.

20. Schonstein E, Kenny DT, Keating J, et al. Work conditioning, work hardening and functional restoration for workers with back and neck pain. Cochrane Database Syst Rev 2003; (1):CD001822.

21. Alaranta H, Rytokoski U, Rissanen A, et al. Intensive physical and psychosocial training program for patients with chronic low back pain. A controlled clinical trial. Spine 1994;19: 1339-1349.

22. Altmaier EM, Lehmann TR, Russell DW, et al. The effectiveness of psychological interventions for the rehabilitation of low back pain: a randomized controlled trial evaluation. Pain 1992;49:329-335.

23. Bendix AF, Bendix T, Lund C, et al. Comparison of three intensive programs for chronic low back pain patients: a prospective, randomized, observer-blinded study with one-year follow-up. Scand J Rehabil Med 1997;29:81-89.

24. Bendix A, Bendix T, Vaegter K, et al. Intensive work rehabilitation [Intensiv tvaerfaglig rygbehandling]. Videnskab og praksis 1994;156:2388-2395.

25. Friedrich M, Gittler G, Halberstadt Y, et al. Combined exercise and motivation program: effect on the compliance and level of disability of patients with chronic low back pain: a randomized controlled trial. Arch Phys Med Rehabil 1998;79:475-487.

26. Mitchell RI, Carmen GM. The functional restoration approach to the treatment of chronic pain in patients with soft tissue and back injuries. Spine 1994;19:633-642.

27. Lindstrom I, Ohlund C, Eek C, et al. The effect of graded activity on patients with subacute low back pain: a randomized prospective clinical study with an operant-conditioning behavioral approach. Phys Ther 1992;72:279-290.

28. Loisel P, Abenhaim L, Durand P, et al. A population-based, randomized clinical trial on back pain management. Spine 1997;22:2911-2918.

29. Chou R, Huffman LH. Nonpharmacologic therapies for acute and chronic low back pain: a review of the evidence for an American Pain Society/American College of Physicians clinical practice guideline. Ann Intern Med 2007;147:492-504.

30. Guzman J, Esmail R, Karjalainen K, et al. Multidisciplinary rehabilitation for chronic low back pain: systematic review. BMJ 2001;322:1511-1516.

31. van Tulder M, Koes B, Bombardier C. Low back pain. Best Pract Res Clin Rheumatol 2002;16:761-775.

32. Carragee EJ. Clinical practice. Persistent low back pain. N Engl J Med 2005;352:1891-1898.

33. Gatchel RJ, Polatin PB, Noe C, et al. Treatment- and cost-effectiveness of early intervention for acute low-back pain patients: a one-year prospective study. J Occup Rehabil 2003; 13:1-9.

34. Bendix AF, Bendix T, Vaegter K, et al. Multidisciplinary intensive treatment for chronic low back pain: a randomized, prospective study. Cleve Clin J Med 1996;63:62-69.

35. Jousset N, Fanello S, Bontoux L, et al. Effects of functional restoration versus 3 hours per week physical therapy: a randomized controlled study. Spine 2004;29:487-493.

36. Hazard RG, Fenwick JW, Kalisch SM, et al. Functional restoration with behavioral support. A one-year prospective study of patients with chronic low-back pain. Spine 1989;14: 157-161.

37. Patrick LE, Altmaier EM, Found EM. Long-term outcomes in multidisciplinary treatment of chronic low back pain: results of a 13-year follow-up. Spine 2004;29:850-855.

38. Hildebrandt J, Pfingsten M, Saur P, et al. Prediction of success from a multidisciplinary treatment program for chronic low back pain. Spine 1997;22:990-1001.

39. Corey DT, Koepfler LE, Etlin D, et al. A limited functional restoration program for injured workers: a randomized trial. J Occupat Rehabil 1996;6:239-249.

40. Shirado O, Ito T, Kikumoto T, et al. A novel back school using a multidisciplinary team approach featuring quantitative functional evaluation and therapeutic exercises for patients with chronic low back pain: the Japanese experience in the general setting. Spine 2005;30:1219-1225.

41. Mayer TG, Gatchel RJ, Kishino N, et al. Objective assessment of spine function following industrial injury. A prospective study with comparison group and one-year follow-up. Spine 1985;10:482-493.

42. Mayer TG, Gatchel RJ, Kishino N, et al. A prospective short-term study of chronic low back pain patients utilizing novel objective functional measurement. Pain 1986;25:53-68.

43. Mayer TG, Gatchel RJ, Mayer H, et al. A prospective two-year study of functional restoration in industrial low back injury. An objective assessment procedure. JAMA 1987;258:1763-1767.

44. Garcy P, Mayer T, Gatchel RJ. Recurrent or new injury outcomes after return to work in chronic disabling spinal disorders. Tertiary prevention efficacy of functional restoration treatment. Spine 1996;21:952-959.

45. Jordan KD, Mayer TG, Gatchel RJ. Should extended disability be an exclusion criterion for tertiary rehabilitation? Socioeconomic outcomes of early versus late functional restoration in compensation spinal disorders. Spine 1998;23:2110-2116.

46. Mayer T, McMahon MJ, Gatchel RJ, et al. Socioeconomic outcomes of combined spine surgery and functional restoration in workers' compensation spinal disorders with matched controls. Spine 1998;23:598-605.

47. Dagenais S, Roffey DM, Wai EK, et al. Can cost utility evaluations inform decision making about interventions for low back pain? Spine J 2009;9:944-957.

48. van der Roer N, Goossens MEJB, Evers SMAA, et al. What is the most cost-effective treatment for patients with low back pain? A systematic review. Best Pract Res Clin Rheumatol 2005;19:671-684.

49. Gatchel RJ, Noe C, Gajraj N, et al. The negative impact on an interdisciplinary pain management program of insurance "treatment carve out" practices. J Workers Compensation 2001;10:50-63.

50. Keel PJ, Wittig R, Deutschmann R, et al. Effectiveness of in-patient rehabilitation for sub-chronic and chronic low back pain by an integrative group treatment program (Swiss Multicentre Study). Scand J Rehabil Med 1998;30:211-219.

51. Robbins H, Gatchel RJ, Noe C, et al. A prospective one-year outcome study of interdisciplinary chronic pain management: compromising its efficacy by managed care policies. Anesth Analg 2003;97:156-162.

52. U.S. Department of Health and Human Services. 1997 National hospital discharge survey. Washington, DC: National Center for Health Statistics; 1997.

53. Hatten AL, Gatchel RJ, Polatin PB, et al. A cost-utility analysis of chronic spinal pain treatment outcomes: converting SF-36 data into quality-adjusted life years. Clin J Pain 2006;22: 700-711.

MICHAEL J. DEPALMA
CURTIS W. SLIPMAN

CHAPTER 23

Epidural Steroid Injections

DESCRIPTION

Terminology and Subtypes

Epidural steroid injection (ESI) is a generic term used to indicate various types of injections that attempt to introduce one or more medications into the epidural space; not all ESIs involve corticosteroids. There are three main subtypes of ESIs that are named according to the method used to introduce therapeutic agents into the epidural space: (1) caudal ESI (CESI), (2) interlaminar ESI (ILESI), and (3) transforaminal ESI (TFESI) (Figure 23-1).[1,2] ILESI is also termed *translaminar ESI*. TFESI is also termed *selective nerve root injection* or *selective nerve root block*. However, because the latter targets the spinal nerve root rather than the intervertebral disc, selective nerve root injections are typically performed to treat specific radicular symptoms rather than axial CLBP.

The term *ESI* is generic and can also apply to injections administered to the cervical spine. ESIs for chronic low back pain (CLBP) are referred to as lumbar or lumbosacral ESIs. The CESI and ILESI approaches are the most commonly used as they can generally be performed without fluoroscopy (also called image guided); there is a substantial likelihood of needle misplacement when administering CESI or ILESI without fluoroscopy (also called a blind approach).[3,4] Whereas TFESIs often place medication around the posterolateral perimeter of the affected spinal level, CESIs and ILESIs are often unable to do so with accuracy. CESI and ILESI are consequently termed *nonspecific ESI*, whereas TFESI may be termed *specific ESI*.

History and Frequency of Use

Conventional medicine has commonly upheld the notion that 80% to 90% of low back pain (LBP) does not have any identifiable etiology and is thus termed *nonspecific LBP*. This belief has been predicated on the early work of Dillane and colleagues who could not detect an identifiable cause of LBP in 79% of males and 89% of females in a general clinical practice.[5,6] Similar findings were presented by Nachemson, who could not identify a demonstrable pathoanatomic explanation for 85% of those with LBP.[7] Valkenburg and Haanen reported finding objective evidence of disc prolapse in only 2% of patients with LBP, whereas 6% had objective findings of lumbago.[8] Additional research conducted in the general asymptomatic adult population reported that lumbosacral spine abnormalities were routinely discovered by myelography, computed tomography (CT), and magnetic resonance imaging (MRI).[9-11] The prevalence of lumbar degenerative findings generally increases with age.

It should be noted that Dillane and colleagues conducted their research before the advent of advanced diagnostic modalities. Studies using fluoroscopically guided, diagnostic spinal procedures have reported being able to differentiate the various sources of LBP. It has been reported that 30% to 50% of LBP is due to internal disc disruption syndrome, 13% to 19% can be attributed to sacroiliac (SI) joint dysfunction, and 15% to 17% is related to painful zygapophysial joints.[12-15] If these findings are mutually exclusive, these results might suggest that 58% to 86% of LBP cases could potentially be attributed to specific diagnoses involving discs, SI joints, or facets. These findings also suggest that local injections of anesthetic, analgesic, or anti-inflammatory medication targeted at lumbosacral anatomic structures involved in the genesis of LBP may provide at least temporary symptomatic relief if successful.

The CESI approach was first described in 1901 by a French radiologist who injected diluted solutions of cocaine (commonly used as an anesthetic at the time) through the sacral hiatus to treat intractable LBP or sciatica.[16] Half a century later, in 1957, Cappio investigated the therapeutic benefit of injecting corticosteroid into the epidural space using a caudal approach.[17] The ILESI technique was first described by Pages in Spain in 1921, and the therapeutic benefits of this approach for LBP were investigated 40 years later.[18-20] The first report of a lumbosacral TFESI appeared in the Italian literature when Robechhi and Capra reported using this approach to successfully treat lumbar and sciatic pain.[21]

ESIs are commonly used to manage CLBP in the United States.[22] In fact, it has been reported that they are the single most commonly used injection procedure for CLBP by interventional pain specialists.[23] TFESIs are widely used to

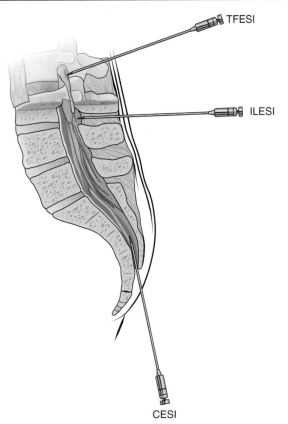

Figure 23-1 Three main methods of epidural steroid injection (ESI): (1) caudal ESI (CESI), (2) interlaminar ESI (ILESI), and (3) transforaminal ESI (TFESI). (Modified from Kirkaldy-Willis WH, Bernard TH. Managing low back pain, ed 4, Philadelphia, 1999, Churchill Livingstone.)

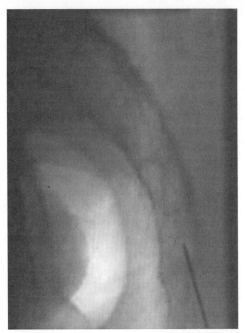

Figure 23-2 Caudal epidural steroid injection. Lateral view of the sacrum demonstrates the needle tip at the opening of the sacral hiatus. (Modified from Pope T et al. Imaging of the musculoskeletal system, 2-volume set: expert radiology series. Philadelphia, 2008, Saunders.)

manage symptoms of radiculopathy related to LBP.[24] A study examining the prevalence of ESIs in Medicare patients reported an increase of 271% between 1994 and 2001, from 0.6% of the population to 2.1%.[25] A related study reported substantial variations in the use of ESIs across various states, varying from 0.5% of Medicare enrollees in Hawaii to 4.0% in Alabama.[26] Larger variations were noted between cities, ranging from 0.6% in Honolulu to 10.4% in Palm Springs.

Practitioner, Setting, and Availability

ESIs should only be performed by a physician trained in the safe and competent administration of these procedures, with advanced training in life support to address potential complications that could result from such injections. Weekend cadaver workshops may also be useful during medical residency before deciding to pursue additional fellowship training. CESI and ILESI have traditionally been taught with hands-on workshops. TFESIs are best learned during a rigorous, comprehensive 1-year interventional pain or spine fellowship. All ESIs should be performed in a setting with ready access to intravenous fluids, cardiac and pulse oximetry monitoring, and code carts, such as a private practice, ambulatory surgery center, or hospital-based surgery center. ILESIs and CESIs can be performed without fluoroscopic guidance and require fewer staff and support personnel. However, TFESIs require specialized equipment typically available only in specialized surgical centers or hospitals. Although ultrasonography has been used

to guide injections in preclinical trials, further investigation is required to examine ultrasonography's capacity to detect intravascular uptake of the injectate.[27,28]

Procedure

Most lumbosacral ESIs are conducted with the patient lying prone on a treatment table, sometimes dressed in a medical gown. The skin in the area surrounding the injection site is first cleaned with sequential alcohol or iodine wipes. CESIs and ILESIs may be conducted without imaging guidance and require the physician to estimate needle placement using available anatomic landmarks and tactile feedback. The addition of fluoroscopy using standalone contrast agents or mixed into the injected medication has allowed visualization of targeted structures and monitoring of whether the medication reaches the potential pain generator, maximizing the chance of therapeutic benefit.

CESI is performed by placing a spinal needle through the skin and subcutaneous tissue, oriented almost vertically into the sacral hiatus (Figure 23-2). This technique can be performed with relative ease, by an experienced clinician, in relatively thin individuals. Because the sacral epidural space must be filled completely before the injected medication is distributed cephalad to eventually reach the lumbar epidural space, a relatively large volume of medication must be injected. Even when using a large volume, medication injected with CESIs rarely reaches the ventral epidural space or progresses cephalad beyond the L5-S1 segmental level.[29]

ILESI is performed by placing a spinal needle through the skin, subcutaneous tissue, and muscle, oriented inferior to superior and between adjacent spinous processes in order to reach the epidural space (Figure 23-3). This approach offers

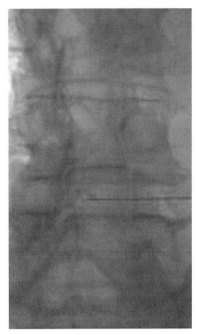

Figure 23-3 Interlaminar epidural steroid injection. Posteroanterior oblique view reveals the tip of the spinal needle marking the dome-shaped space beneath the junction of the spinous process and lamina. This region is used to gain access into the epidural space. (From Pope T et al. Imaging of the musculoskeletal system, 2-volume set: expert radiology series. Philadelphia, 2008, Saunders.)

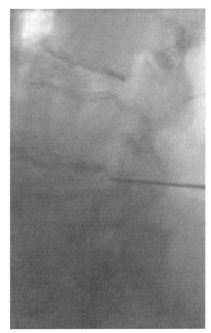

Figure 23-4 Transforaminal epidural steroid injection. After injection of the medications the contrast agent has been diluted, tracking along the nerve root sheath and spreading both proximally and distally within the epidural space. (Modified from Pope T et al. Imaging of the musculoskeletal system, 2-volume set: expert radiology series. Philadelphia, 2008, Saunders.)

the potential advantage of delivering medication directly into the lumbar region rather than introducing it in the sacral region and hoping it will reach intended target cephalad. However, the ILESI approach is technically more demanding than the CESI. The medication is injected into the posterior epidural space without any assurances it will flow anteriorly to the ventral epidural space.[30]

TFESI is typically performed under fluoroscopy by placing a spinal needle through the skin, subcutaneous tissue, and muscle, oriented from lateral to medial, in order to reach the lateral foramen of the targeted spinal nerve root (Figure 23-4). In contrast to CESI and ILESI, the medication injected with TFESI will reach the ventral epidural space in virtually every case.[31] The instillation of therapeutic doses of corticosteroid into the anterior epidural space to maximally reach the targeted intervertebral disc is best accomplished by TFESIs rather than with ILESIs or CESIs.

Regulatory Status

The medications commonly injected during ESIs are regulated by the US Food and Drug Administration and approved for these indications.

THEORY

Mechanism of Action

Evidence suggests that there is an increased production of proinflammatory mediators and cytokines because of disc herniation and higher levels of interleukin (IL)-6, IL-8, and prostaglandin E_2 (PGE_2) in degenerative, nonherniated painful discs.[32-39] Cyclical mechanical loading of the disc coupled with inflammatory stimuli have increased PGE_2 production by nuclear and annular disc cells in vitro, with a stronger reactivity in the latter models.[40] Painful degenerative lumbar intervertebral discs have higher concentrations of sensory fibers—located in the end plate and nucleus—than nonpainful discs, and both IL-8 and PGE_2 induce hyperalgesia.[41-43]

The combination of the abundant innervation of the disc and increased production of proinflammatory mediators suggests that discogenic pain may involve hyperalgesia.[38] Injection of corticosteroids into the anterior epidural space has long been used to bathe the posterolateral periphery of the annulus to help curtail the biochemical stimulation of the intervertebral disc. The main goals of this approach are to improve pain and function and allow the patient to participate in a comprehensive physical therapy program addressing biomechanical deficiencies after this reduction of hyperalgesia is achieved. Before using ESIs, the target disc may be confirmed as the source of pain. To ensure the success of this approach, the appropriate therapeutic medication deposited into the anterior epidural space must also gain access to sensitized nerve endings.

The instillation of corticosteroid and anesthetic into the anterior epidural space introduces therapeutic agents with potent anti-inflammatory properties adjacent to suspected painful intervertebral discs. Local anesthetics help curtail inflammation by inhibiting phagocytosis, decreasing phagocytic oxygen consumption, reducing polymorphonuclear leukocyte lysosomal enzyme release, and diminishing super-oxide anion production.[44-48] Additionally, local anesthetics improve neural blood flow and function.[49,50] Corticosteroids are well known for their anti-inflammatory properties, and also stabilize neural membranes, suppress ectopic neural discharges, and may have direct anesthetic effect on small unmyelinated nociceptive C-fibers.[51-54] Painful lumbar intervertebral discs are innervated by substance-P containing nerve fibers, unmyelinated C-fibers, and thinly myelinated A delta fibers that provide a substrate on which corticosteroids and local anesthetics exert therapeutic benefit.[41,42,55] The nucleus pulposus of the lumbar intervertebral disc is biologically active, responds to proinflammatory cytokines most sensitively after degeneration, and, once painful, produces further proinflammatory mediators.[38,56] Hence, corticosteroids and local anesthetics may exert a therapeutic benefit by bathing the posterolateral annular fibers, which are most prone to injury, in solutions with anti-inflammatory and neural stabilizing effects.[57-59]

Indication

The primary indication for ESIs is CLBP with radicular pain. Despite minimal work having been completed investigating the efficacy of these interventions solely for axial lumbar spine pain, ESIs are routinely offered to patients presenting with axial CLBP presumed to be discogenic in origin based on a comprehensive evaluation of the patient.[60] However, the role of ESIs to treat axial CLBP has not been well defined and is currently supported largely by conjecture and expert opinion. Deciding which level to inject is influenced by imaging findings and pain referral zones, but is more commonly determined by initially targeting the levels most likely to be responsible for discogenic CLBP (L4-5 and L5-S1).[12,61] If the patient experiences only short-term or no improvement with S1 TFESIs adequately targeting the L4-5 and L5-S1 discs, lumbar discography would be warranted to determine whether one or both of the lowest two discs, or perhaps an upper level disc, is painful.

The ideal patient for ESIs would have CLBP with discogenic pain, provocative discography to demonstrate outer annular disruption causing the patient's usual symptoms, and internally sound, nonpainful adjacent discs serving as internal controls. A reasonable algorithmic approach to a patient presenting with CLBP most consistent with a discogenic etiology is to perform TFESIs to empirically target the L4-5 and L5-S1 discs and monitor outcomes.[61,62]

Assessment

Before receiving ESIs, patients should first be assessed for LBP using an evidence-based and goal-oriented approach focused on the patient history and neurologic examination, as discussed in Chapter 3. Clinicians should also inquire about medication history to note prior hypersensitivity/allergy or adverse events (AEs) with drugs similar to those being considered, and evaluate contraindications for these types of drugs. Diagnostic imaging is often required before administering ESIs for CLBP. At minimum, plain film radiography of the lumbar spine is required to identify anatomic variations that may impact needle placement, as well as a general assessment of alignment, disc height, and stability.

In addition, advanced imaging such as MRI or CT can be used to help guide the spine specialist to target the appropriate spinal levels involved in a patient's CLBP. Findings on advanced imaging that may influence the clinician's recommendation of ESIs include degenerative endplate changes and high-intensity zone lesions, which may help to differentiate painful from nonpainful segments.[63-65]

Interventional diagnostic testing is also used occasionally before recommending or performing TFESIs, especially in cases of symptoms that persist for more than 6 months and prove recalcitrant to exhaustive conservative treatment measures. The use of provocative discography for CLBP remains controversial, but is used by some clinicians to identify painful annular fissures that may subsequently be targeted with other interventions such as ESIs. When interpreting provocative discography, extension of isotopic dye into or beyond the outer annulus has been shown to be the strongest predictor of concordant pain.[61] Findings of concordantly painful outer annular disruption on discography would indicate to the clinician which discs may be targeted with TFESIs to achieve maximum impact. However, such a strategy has not been critically evaluated and further study is required.

EFFICACY

Evidence supporting the efficacy of these interventions for CLBP was summarized from recent clinical practice guidelines (CPGs), systematic reviews (SRs), and randomized controlled trials (RCTs). Observational studies (OBSs) were also summarized where appropriate. Findings are summarized by study design for each injection approach.

It should be noted that CPGs and SRs often lack the critical evaluation of the clinical methodology of the ESIs employed in the underlying RCTs on which their recommendations are based. These RCTs have often evaluated mixed cohorts of patients with CLBP with or without radicular pain for whom clinicians may not have had a definitive diagnosis, did not use a clinically appropriate ESI technique, used non-radiographically guided injections or techniques without contrast confirmation of needle placement. Additional comments on these RCTs are provided below.

Clinical Practice Guidelines

Six of the recent national CPGs on the management of CLBP have assessed and summarized the evidence to make specific recommendations about the efficacy of ESIs.

The CPG from Belgium in 2006 found low-quality and conflicting evidence to support the efficacy of ESIs for the management of CLBP with radicular pain.[66] That CPG also found no evidence to support the efficacy of ESIs for the management of CLBP without radicular pain. There was low-quality evidence to support the efficacy of TFESIs for the management of CLBP with radicular pain.

TABLE 23-1	Clinical Practice Guideline Recommendations on Epidural Steroid Injections for Chronic Low Back Pain	
Reference	**Country**	**Conclusion**
66	Belgium	Low-quality and conflicting evidence of efficacy of ESIs and no evidence of efficacy of ESIs in CLBP without radicular pain
		Low-quality evidence to support efficacy of TFESIs in CLBP with radicular pain
67	Europe	Not recommended
68	Italy	Consider if adequate relief not obtained with medication
69	United States	Consider if adequate relief not obtained with other conservative interventions
70	United States	Poor evidence to support efficacy
71	United Kingdom	Not recommended

CLBP, chronic low back pain; ESI, epidural steroid injection; TFESI, transforaminal epidural steroid injection.

The CPG from Europe in 2004 found conflicting evidence to support the efficacy of ESIs when compared with sham or other procedures for the management of CLBP with radicular pain.[67] That CPG also found no evidence to support the efficacy of ESIs for the management of CLBP without radicular pain. ESIs for CLBP were not recommended.

The CPG from Italy in 2007 reported that ESIs could be considered as one management option for CLBP with radicular pain when adequate relief is not obtained with medication alone.[68]

The CPG from the United States in 2007 reported that ESIs could be considered as one management option for CLBP with radicular pain associated with a prolapsed disc when adequate relief is not obtained with other conservative interventions.[69]

The CPG from the United States in 2009 found poor evidence to support the efficacy of ESIs in the management of CLBP.[70]

The CPG from the United Kingdom in 2009 did not recommend ESIs for the management of CLBP.[71]

Findings from the above CPGs are summarized in Table 23-1.

Systematic Reviews

Cochrane Collaboration

The Cochrane Collaboration conducted an SR in 2007 on injection therapy for subacute and chronic LBP without neurologic involvement.[72] A total of 18 RCTs were identified, including RCTs related to ESIs for patients with LBP and neurologic involvement, LBP without neurologic involvement, failed back surgery syndrome, CLBP, and degenerative spinal disease.[73-79] Two RCTs did not find any statistically significant differences between ESIs and placebo for pain, disability, and general improvement.[73,74] In two RCTs of failed back surgery syndrome, no statistically significant differences were observed between ESIs and nonsteroidal anti-inflammatory drugs or morphine.[76,77] In one RCT including LBP without neurologic involvement, no statistically significant differences were observed for ESIs versus intrathecal benzodiazepine for pain relief or general improvement.[75] Two RCTs did not find any statistically significant differences between ESIs combined with ropivacaine versus ESIs combined with bupivacaine for CLBP or degenerative spinal disease.[78,79] This review concluded that there is insufficient evidence supporting the use of ESIs for subacute and chronic LBP without neurologic involvement.[72] This SR also recommended that future RCTs be conducted to determine patient subgroups who are most likely to benefit from ESIs.

American Pain Society and American College of Physicians

The American Pain Society (APS) and American College of Physicians (ACP) CPG committee conducted an SR in 2008 on nonsurgical therapies for acute and chronic LBP.[80] That review identified seven SRs related to ESIs, one of which was the Cochrane Collaboration review mentioned earlier.[72,81-86] Two high-quality SRs concluded that ESIs were not significantly different than placebo, yet another higher-quality SR concluded that ESIs were more effective at improving symptoms than placebo for LBP with neurologic involvement.[72,82,86] In addition, two lower-quality SRs concluded that there was short-term pain relief from ESIs for LBP with neurologic involvement.[81,85] The conclusions of two of the SRs were not reported.[83,84] These SRs included 19 RCTs examining LBP with neurologic involvement of acute and subacute duration, mixed subacute and chronic, chronic, mixed duration LBP, and unknown duration.[73,74,87-103] The rest of the RCTs examined LBP without neurologic involvement of unknown duration, including seven additional RCTs identified by the APS and ACP.[1,24,75-77,104-122]

RCTs comparing ESIs with nonepidural placebo injections for LBP with neurologic involvement generally found short-term benefits in pain and function (n = 5/6 RCTs). However, RCTs that compared ESIs with epidural placebo injections generally did not find any statistically significant improvement for LBP with neurologic involvement (n = 9/11). Three RCTs had unclear results for LBP with neurologic involvement. Long-term benefits for ESIs were not commonly observed among the RCTs (n = 4/18). ESIs were not consistently associated with lower rates of surgery versus placebo injections (n = 2/7). RCTs examining LBP without neurologic involvement, spinal stenosis, and failed back surgery did not find consistent benefits with ESIs. This SR concluded that ESIs are moderately beneficial in the short-term for LBP with neurologic involvement.[80] It also concluded that there is insufficient evidence for ESIs among those with spinal stenosis or LBP without radiculopathy. The SR recommended that future RCTs should examine the long-term benefits of ESIs as well as compare ESIs with saline or local anesthetic versus a nonepidural placebo injections to determine the utility of ESIs.

Other

In 1994, a review was published by the Australian Working Party of the National Health and Medical Research Council summarizing recommendations for ESIs in the management of LBP.[60] This review referenced a body of evidence endorsing ILESIs and CESIs as viable treatment options for LBP with radicular pain but cited a minimal body of literature evaluating the use of ESIs for nonradicular LBP.

Another review conducted a meta-analysis of RCTs which reported that both CESIs and ILESIs were effective for radicular, but not axial, LBP.[123]

A review identified 15 RCTs evaluating CESIs and ILESIs for LBP with or without sciatica.[124] Although studies generally supported the use of ESIs in LBP with sciatica, there was no clear evidence supporting their use for CLBP without radicular pain. Review authors did not evaluate the clinical utility of the ESI techniques used by each study and were thus unable to comment on the possible effects of RCTs without fluoroscopic guidance and contrast confirmation of accurate needle placement.

A more recent review assessed the efficacy and safety of TFESIs and selective nerve root blocks for LBP with radiculopathy.[125] That review was based on six clinical trials, including five RCTs and one OBS. It concluded that there was moderate evidence to support the use of TFESIs for LBP with radicular pain.

Findings from these SRs are summarized in Table 23-2.

Randomized Controlled Trials

Caudal Epidural Steroid Injections

Two RCTs were identified.[74,126] Their methods are summarized in Table 23-3. Their results are briefly described here.

The critical features of each study that must be assessed are the route of injection (fluoroscopic control), number of injections, clinical presentation (axial LBP vs. radicular pain), diagnostic evaluation (provocative discography), length of follow-up, and outcome measures.

Breivik and colleagues[74] in a prospective, double-blind, crossover study, assessed improvement in CLBP and sciatic pain in 35 patients treated with up to 3 blind, CESIs of either bupivicaine and methylprednisolone or bupivicaine and normal saline. The study followed a parallel, cohort design allowing patients not benefiting from their randomized treatment to then undergo treatment in the reciprocal arm. Initially, 56% of patients receiving methylprednisolone experienced significant relief compared with 26% treated with bupivicaine and saline. In the crossover, 14% of the methylprednisolone group obtained relief from subsequent bupivicaine and saline injections, whereas 73% of the bupivicaine and saline group reported satisfactory relief after the methylprednisolone injection. Fifty percent of the steroid group and 20% of the bupivicaine group returned to work at a range of 3 to 17 months after treatment. Up to three injections were performed in each arm. Thirty-two patients had undergone radiculography demonstrating disc prolapse, arachnoiditis, or inconclusive findings. However, the CESIs were performed without fluoroscopic guidance, and no further diagnostic testing had been conducted.

In a subsequent study, Yates performed caudal injections of saline, lidocaine, saline and triamcinolone, and lidocaine and triamcinolone in random order in 20 consecutive patients with LBP.[126] Each patient was assessed at 30 minutes and again 1 week after each injection. Outcome measures were improvement in straight leg raising and lumbar range of motion, which both improved more so after the injections of steroid. Patients reporting more than 50% improvement demonstrated significant improvement in lumbar range of motion and straight leg raising. Yet, no specific diagnostic criteria were used in selecting patients for the trial, the follow-up interval was short, and limited injections were completed.

Only one study has prospectively evaluated the efficacy of CESIs in patients diagnosed with discogenic LBP by

TABLE 23-2	Systematic Review Findings on Epidural Steroid Injections for Chronic Low Back Pain		
Reference	# RCTs in SR	# RCTs for CLBP	Conclusion
72	18	NR	Insufficient evidence supporting the use of ESIs for CLBP without neurologic involvement
80	7 SRs, 19 RCTs	NR	Moderately beneficial in the short term for LBP with neurologic involvement Insufficient evidence for spinal stenosis or LBP without radiculopathy
60	NR	NR	Viable treatment option for radicular pain Insufficient evidence for nonradicular LBP
123	NR	NR	CESIs and ILESIs effective for radicular LBP only
124	NR	NR	CESIs and ILESIs effective for radicular LBP only
125	5	NR	Moderate evidence supporting TFESIs for LBP with radicular pain

CESI, caudal epidural steroid injection; CLBP, chronic low back pain; ESI, epidural steroid injection; ILESI, interlaminar epidural steroid injection; LBP, low back pain; NR, not reported; RCT, randomized controlled trial; SR, systematic review.

TABLE 23-3	Randomized Controlled Trials of Caudal Epidural Steroid Injections for Chronic Low Back Pain				
Reference	Indication	Intervention 1	Intervention 2	Intervention 3	Control
74	CLBP with neurologic involvement	CESI: 20 mL bupivacaine 0.25% with 80 mg depo-methylprednisolone Clinician 3 injections (1 week apart) then cross over to the other intervention Cointervention: NR n = 16	CESI: 20 mL bupivacaine 0.25% + 100 mL saline Clinician 3 injections (1 week apart) then cross over to the other intervention Cointervention: NR n = 19	NA	
126	LBP with neurologic involvement, mixed duration LBP	CESI: 47 mL 0.5% lignocaine + 3 mL triamcinolone hexacetonide Clinician 1 (1 week apart) then cross over to the other interventions Cointervention: NR n = 20 total	Anesthetic injection: 47 mL saline + 3 mL triamcinolone hexacetonide Clinician 1 (1 week apart) then cross over to the other interventions Cointervention: NR n = 20 total	CESI: 50 mL 0.5 % lignocaine Clinician 1 (1 week apart) then cross over to the other interventions Cointervention: NR n = 20 total	Placebo injection: 50 mL saline Clinician 1 (1 week apart) then cross over to the other interventions Cointervention: NR n = 20 total

CLBP, chronic low back pain; CESI, caudal epidural steroid injection; LBP, low back pain; NA, not applicable; NR, not reported.

provocative discography.[23] Greater than 50% reduction in pain was achieved at 6 months after completing one to three CESIs in 60% of patients with negative discogram results and in 64% of patients with positive discogram results. Although each patient had undergone negative diagnostic facet joint and SI joint blocks with local comparative anesthetic, the investigators did not assess for concordantly painful outer annular disruption. A small number of patients comprised the discogram-positive group. Neither the positive discogram levels nor the immediate postinjection improvement in LBP were reported. Reporting whether or not patients experienced immediate improvement might help confirm whether the CESI adequately reached the putatively painful disc. The results of this study, despite its use of discography, do not confirm that CESIs are effective for discogenic LBP.

Interlaminar Epidural Steroid Injections
Nine RCTs were identified, including two that investigated ILESIs for CLBP with primarily radicular pain and seven that investigated their use for axial CLBP.[75,77,90-96,100-102] Their methods are summarized in Table 23-4. The results are briefly described here.

Radicular CLBP. In a prospective, double-blind, randomized fashion, Serrao and colleagues[75]studied the therapeutic effects of single injections of methylprednisolone (80 mg) administered epidurally compared with intrathecal midazolam (2 mg) in 28 patients with CLBP. No statistically significant difference in pain or analgesic use was observed between the two groups at 2 months. The authors did not

report their diagnostic evaluation of these patients or the segmental level at which each injection was performed, and fluoroscopic guidance was not used.

Years previously, Helliwel and colleagues[96] studied 39 patients with LBP and radicular leg pain in a single-blind investigation. Twenty subjects underwent a single extradural injection of methylprednisolone (80 mg) in 10-mL normal saline. These patients reported statistically significant reduction in pain levels at 1 and 3 months compared with 19 control patients who underwent an interspinous injection of 5 mL normal saline. However, the authors did not report at what level each injection was performed and did not clarify whether the pain scores were recorded for lumbar pain or radicular pain primarily.

The results of these RCTs can only weakly clarify the efficacy of lumbar ILESIs for axial LBP and suggest that these injections may afford a patient some short-term improvement in lumbar pain. However, ILESIs are not target-specific, especially in the absence of fluoroscopy, and definitive diagnostic measures were not taken in these studies.

Axial CLBP. Cuckler and colleagues[95] performed an RCT in which patients with LBP with neurologic involvement due to herniated disc or spinal stenosis were selected when they failed to improve despite therapy and their symptoms were confirmed by diagnostic tests. Those with serious pathology or pain 6 months after a previous back surgery were excluded. Participants were randomized to either ILESIs with methylprednisolone plus procaine or saline plus procaine injections. One to 2 injections were administered by a clinician to each group 24 hours apart. After an average of 20 months,

TABLE 23-4	Randomized Controlled Trials of Interlaminar Epidural Steroid Injections for Chronic Low Back Pain				
Reference	Indication	Intervention 1	Intervention 2	Intervention 3	Control
75	Mechanical LBP, neurologic involvement NR, symptoms >1 year	ILESI: 3 mL (5%) dextrose solution prednisolone (80 mg) in 10 mL saline Clinician 1 injection Cointervention: analgesic medication n = 28 total	ILESI: 10 mL normal saline (epidural) and 2 mg midazolam in 3 mL (5%) dextrose Clinician 1 injection Cointervention: analgesic medication n = 28 total	NA	NA
96	CLBP with neurologic involvement	ILESI: methylprednisolone (80 mg) in 10 mL normal saline n = 20	NA	NA	Placebo injection: saline n = 19
90	LBP with neurologic involvement due to herniated disc, symptoms >4 months but <1 year	ILESI: methylprednisolone (80 mg) Clinician 1-3 injections (3 weeks apart) Cointervention: acetaminophen n = 78	NA	NA	Placebo injection: 1 mL isotonic saline Clinician 1-3 injections (3 weeks apart) Cointervention: acetaminophen n = 80
95	CLBP with neurologic involvement due to herniated disc or spinal stenosis	ILESI: 2 mL sterile water with methylprednisolone (80 mg) plus 5 mL 5% procaine Clinician 1-2 injections (24 hours apart) Cointervention: NR n = 42	NA	NA	Placebo injection: 2 mL saline plus 5 mL 1% procaine Clinician 1-2 injections (24 hours apart) Cointervention: NR n = 31
91	LBP with neurologic involvement due to lumbar disc disease, mixed subacute LBP and CLBP	ILESI: methylprednisolone (80 mg) in 10 mL saline Clinician 1-2 injections (7 days apart) Cointervention: bed rest, exercise, hydrotherapy, analgesics n = 42	NA	NA	Placebo injection: 1 mL saline Clinician 1-2 injections (7 days apart) Cointervention: bed rest, exercise, hydrotherapy, analgesics n = 38
102	LBP with neurologic involvement, symptoms <6 months	IL ESI: Depomedrone (80 mg) in 20 mL saline Anesthesiologist 1 injection Cointervention: NR n = 19	20 mL 0.25% bupivacaine solution in normal saline Anesthesiologist 1 injection Cointervention: NR n = 16	Needling with a standard Touhy needle (no injection) Anesthesiologist 1 session Cointervention: NR n = 12	Placebo injection: 20 mL saline Administrator: Anesthesiologist 1 injection Cointervention: NR n = 16

TABLE 23-4 | **Randomized Controlled Trials of Interlaminar Epidural Steroid Injections for Chronic Low Back Pain—cont'd**

Reference	Indication	Intervention 1	Intervention 2	Intervention 3	Control
100	LBP with neurologic involvement, mixed duration LBP	ILESI: methylprednisolone (80 mg) in 10 mL saline Clinician 2 injections max, 1 week apart Cointervention: rest n = 19	NA	NA	Placebo injection: 2 mL saline Clinician 2 injections max, 1 week apart; if no improvement then cross over to receive active treatment Cointervention: rest n = 16
77	Failed back surgery, without neurologic involvement, duration LBP NR	ILESI: triamcinolone diacetate (75 mg) plus lidocaine (50 mg) Administrator: NR 3 (1 month apart) Cointervention: NR n = 8	ILESI: morphine (8 mg) plus lidocaine (50 mg) Administrator: NR 3 (1 month apart) Cointervention: NR n = 7	ILESI: triamcinolone diacetate (75 mg) plus lidocaine (50 mg) plus morphine (8 mg) Administrator: NR 3 (1 month apart) Cointervention: NR n = 7	NA
101	LBP with neurologic involvement, mixed duration LBP	ILESI: methylprednisolone acetate (80 mg) Clinician 1 injection Cointervention: bed rest, PT, analgesics n = 27	NA	NA	Placebo injection: 2 mL saline Clinician 1 injection Cointervention: bed rest, PT, analgesics n = 24

CLBP, chronic low back pain; LBP, low back pain; ILESI, interlaminar epidural steroid injection; NA, not applicable; NR, not reported; PT, physical therapy.

there were no statistically significant differences between the groups in symptom improvement.

Dilke and colleagues[91] performed an RCT in which patients with LBP and neurologic involvement due to lumbar disc disease were selected if they had limitation of sciatic or femoral nerve stretch or sciatic scoliosis or appropriate neurologic deficit. Those with previous back surgery or diagnostic uncertainty were excluded. Participants were randomized to either ILESIs with methylprednisolone plus saline or saline injections. One to two injections were administered by a clinician to each group 7 days apart. Immediately after the injections, participants in the treatment group experienced statistically significant pain improvement versus the control group. However, no differences between groups were observed after 3 months of follow-up. Those in the treatment group were significantly more likely to be back at work than those in the control group after 3 months of follow-up.

Klenerman and colleagues[102] performed an RCT in which patients with LBP and neurologic involvement were selected when their unilateral sciatica and symptoms lasted less than 6 months. Those with previous in-patient LBP treatment were

excluded. Participants were randomized to one of four groups: (1) ILESI depomedrone plus saline, (2) bupivacaine solution, (3) saline solution, or (4) dry needling. The injections were administered by an anesthesiologist to all groups. After 2 months of follow-up, participants in all groups improved, yet no statistically significant differences in pain relief between groups were observed.

Ridley and colleagues[100] performed an RCT including patients with LBP and neurologic involvement. Participants were randomized to either ILESIs with methylprednisolone or placebo saline injections. A clinician administered a maximum of two injections to each group 7 days apart. After two injections the placebo group had the opportunity to receive the active injection, 1 week after the second injection. After 24 weeks of follow-up, no differences in pain were observed between groups.

Rocco and colleagues[77] performed an RCT including patients with LBP after undergoing laminectomy (i.e., failed back surgery). Participants were randomized to one of three groups: (1) ILESI with triamcinolone diacetate plus lidocaine, (2) morphine plus lidocaine, and (3) ILESI with triamcinolone diacetate plus lidocaine plus morphine. Each participant received one injection per month for 3 months. One to 30 days after treatment, no differences in pain were observed between the groups. This lack of a statistically significant finding between groups was also observed beyond the 1 month of follow-up.

Snoek and colleagues[101] performed an RCT in which patients with LBP and neurologic involvement were included if their symptoms were confirmed with myelography. Those who had previous back surgery and an uncertain diagnosis were excluded. Participants were randomized to methylprednisolone acetate or a placebo injection with saline solution. One injection was administered to both groups by a clinician. One to 2 days after injection, each group improved but there was a lack of statistical significance in pain relief between the two groups.

Buttermann[118] performed an RCT in which patients with LPB due to degenerative disc disease were included if their symptoms were confirmed with MRI and they failed to improve despite conservative therapy. Those who were pregnant or who had comorbidities were excluded. Participants were randomized to fluoroscopically guided ILESI or intradiscal steroid injection. One to three injections were administered to the ILESI group by a clinician and the injection schedule was unclear for the intradiscal steroid injection group. Both groups experienced statistically significant pain relief after one year of follow-up, yet no differences were observed between the two groups.

Transforaminal Epidural Steroid Injections

Two RCTs were identified that evaluated the efficacy of TFESIs primarily for radicular LBP, although data pertaining to axial CLBP were also provided.[92,97] Their methods are summarized in Table 23-5. Their results are briefly described here.

Karppinen and colleagues[92] completed a double-blind RCT of patients with lumbar radiculopathy due to a corroborative disc herniation who underwent a single TFESI at the indicated level. Although the study was designed to assess the efficacy of a TFESI for nerve root pain, the authors did evaluate lumbar pain. Each injection was performed under fluoroscopy using 2 to 3 mL of injectate at the level of clinical involvement. Only one injection was performed in each patient, with the treatment arm undergoing injection of 1 mL of 40 mg/mL methylprednisolone and 1 mL of 5 mg/mL bupivicaine, and the control group underwent injection of 2 mL of isotonic saline. Eighty patients were enrolled into each group after a power analysis revealed a need for 68 patients in each study arm. No difference in immediate improvement in lumbar pain occurred between the groups. At the 2-week, 4-week, and 12-month follow-up, lumbar pain intensity was subtly less in the steroid group, and did not reach statistical significance. In contrast, at 3 and 6 months, statistically greater improvement in lumbar pain occurred in the saline group.

Although the Karppinen study used an appropriate number of subjects, the investigation did not ideally address the question of whether or not TFESIs are effective for discogenic LBP. Each patient's LBP was presumably due to the disc herniation, whose posterolateral annular fibers were reached by the injectate affecting the treated nerve root.[30] However, further diagnostic interventions such as provocative discography were not performed; the side of the annular disruption may not have corresponded to the side of symptom manifestation and the axial pain symptoms may have actually represented proximal nerve root pain.[127] Only one injection was completed in each patient. Frequently more than one injection may be necessary to adequately treat radicular pain, but evidence suggesting how many injections may be necessary to adequately treat discogenic lumbar pain is lacking.[106,128] Epidural saline may have a greater therapeutic benefit than placebo, thus underestimating a treatment effect in Karppinen's study.[129-131] Long-term benefit may not have

TABLE 23-5	Randomized Controlled Trials of Transforaminal Epidural Steroid Injections for Chronic Low Back Pain		
Reference	Indication	Intervention 1	Control
92	LBP with neurologic involvement due to disc herniation, symptoms 1-6 months	TFESI: 1 mL of 40 mg/mL methylprednisolone plus 1 mL of 5 mg/mL bupivicaine Clinician 1 injection Cointervention: NR n = 80	Placebo injection: 2 mL isotonic saline Clinician 1 injection Cointervention: NR n = 80
97	CLBP with neurologic involvement due to disc herniation and peripheral foraminal stenosis	TFESI: 2 mL 0.25% bupivacaine and methylprednisolone (40 mg) Surgeon 1 injection Cointervention: not allowed to change current oral analgesic medication during study n = 80	Anesthetic injection: 2 mL 0.25% bupivacaine Surgeon 1 injection Cointervention: not allowed to change current oral analgesic medication during study n = 80

CLBP, chronic low back pain; LBP, low back pain; TFESI, transforaminal epidural steroid injection; NR, not reported.

been achieved due to a subtherapeutic number of TFESIs performed in the treatment arm, lack of true placebo control (sham injection), and improperly targeting the correct level of axial pain generation.

Ng and colleagues[97] randomized 86 lumbar radicular pain patients in a double-blind manner to either periradicular infiltration of 2 mL of 0.25% bupivicaine or 2 mL of bupivicaine and methylprednisolone (40 mg). To be included, patients had to have lower limb pain equal to or greater than back pain and MRI evidence of a corroborative disc herniation or foraminal stenosis. Each patient underwent only one injection, and visual analog scale rating and Oswestry Disability Index were measured at weekly intervals up to 12 weeks with 100% follow-up rate. No difference was observed for lumbar pain or disability at 12 weeks after one injection. It is difficult to derive conclusions from this study regarding the efficacy of one TFESI to treat axial lumbar pain. Corroborative diagnostic evaluation such as discography was not performed. Patients with foraminal stenosis were included. These two factors may have diminished the likelihood of discogenic lumbar pain in a portion of enrolled patients. Patients requiring repeat injections were deemed treatment failures and removed from study follow-up. Therefore, a subtherapeutic number of TFESIs may have been undertaken.

Observational Studies

In an OBS with 292 participants, Buttermann observed significant improvement in pain and function in 25% to 35% of patients with CLBP (>1-year duration) after performing one fluoroscopically guided epidural steroid injection (either ILESI or TFESI).[118] Follow-up was carried out to 1 to 2 years. There was no indication regarding at which level each injection was performed. In addition to the absence of a control group, a high number of dropouts occurred as patients went on to other treatment interventions, including discography with corticosteroids and fusion surgery. Hence, the treatment effect reported may have been overestimated.

SAFETY

Contraindications

Absolute contraindications to ESIs include bleeding diathesis and lack of coagulation because of the risk of epidural hematoma. Generally, patients taking anticoagulants must stop their medication until their coagulation profile is normalized before undergoing any injection, if it is deemed medically prudent to do so. Patients taking warfarin should not take this medication for 3-5 days and undergo laboratory analysis of their clotting factors immediately before any scheduled injection procedure.[132] If the risks associated with a thromboembolic event are too great, low-dose heparin or low-molecular-weight heparin may be substituted while stopping the warfarin for 5 to 7 days before the injection, resuming warfarin within 6 to 12 hours after the injection.[132] Other medications that may inhibit clot formation, including nonsteroidal anti-inflammatory agents and aspirin, generally do not pose a contraindication to an injection procedure.[133] The safety of ticlopidine (Ticlid) and clopidogrel (Plavix) has not been established for this indication, and these medications should be withheld for 5 to 7 days and 7 to 14 days, respectively, before an injection.[132]

Additional contraindications to ESIs include local infection at the injection site, sepsis, hypovolemia, pregnancy, uncontrolled diabetes, uncontrolled glaucoma, and high concentrations of local anesthetics in patients with multiple sclerosis.[132] Corticosteroid use during ESIs is contraindicated for patients with spinal infection, malignancy, or acute or non-healed fracture. Healed spinal fractures may not represent a contraindication to ESI.

Predictors of negative outcomes after ILESIs have been studied when treating lumbar radicular pain.[134,135] In an OBS with 209 participants who received two to three ILESIs with methylprednisolone (120 mg), poor outcomes after 2 weeks were associated with the following variables: (1) lower levels of education, (2) smoking, (3) unemployment, (4) constant pain, (5) chronic pain, (6) psychological disturbances, and (7) nonradicular diagnoses. Upon further analysis, only prolonged duration of pain, nonradicular diagnosis, unemployment, and smoking were independently associated with poor outcomes.[134] However, only 6% of the participants presented with primarily nonradicular pain. In a study of 249 participants with CLBP, the following factors were associated with a poor outcome at 2 weeks after one ILESI with triamcinolone (50 mg): (1) increased number of previous treatments for pain, (2) more medication taken, (3) pain not increased by activities, and (4) pain increased by coughing.[135] As participants with psychiatric disorders were excluded, these could not be evaluated as prognostic indicators. Poor outcomes after one year were associated with pain not interfering with activities, unemployment because of pain, normal straight leg raise test before treatment, and pain not decreased by medication. However, only 53% of participants were followed for one year.

Adverse Events

AEs associated with ESIs have been well studied and tend to be relatively minor and transient.[136-138] They may arise as a consequence of incorrect needle placement, the type of medication injected, and use of x-ray guidance or fluoroscopy for TFESIs. The overall prevalence of AEs associated with ESIs ranges from 5.5% to 9.6% with TFESIs to 15.6% with CESIs.[137,139] The most commonly reported AEs include increased pain at the injection site (17.1%), increased radicular pain (0.6% to 8.8%), increased spinal pain (2.4% to 5.1%), light-headedness (6.5%), nausea (3.7%), nonpositional headache (1.4% to 3.1%), vomiting (0.5%), facial flushing (1.2%), vasovagal reaction (0.3%), increased blood glucose (0.3%), and intraoperative hypertension (0.3%).[136,138,139] In addition, anecdotal evidence indicates that CESIs result in considerably more discomfort than ILESIs and TFESIs.

If the needle is misplaced, the therapeutic agent will likely not reach the anterior epidural space, regardless of the operator's clinical experience.[140] It has been estimated that ILESIs achieve ventral epidural contrast spread in only 36% of attempts.[30] Furthermore, vascular evacuation of the therapeutic medication occurs in 11% of CESIs and TFESIs, and in 2% of ILESIs, thus preventing the therapeutic agent from reaching its target.[141,142]

Serious AEs associated with ESIs are rare. Although any percutaneous procedure involving a needle carries the risk of infection, large case series have not reported such complications with ESIs.[93,136,137] Spinal injections carry the additional risk of inadvertent dural puncture, neural trauma, vascular injury, or central nervous system injury. Dural puncture occurs in 5% of ILESIs, 0% to 0.6% of CESIs, and 0% to 0.1% of TFESIs, and may result in positional headache related to leakage of cerebrospinal fluid.[60,136-138] More persistent or severe dural puncture headaches can be managed with bed rest while the puncture wound heals, increased fluid intake, or an autologous blood injection into the epidural space to stop the leak with a blood patch.

Injection of corticosteroids and anesthetics into the subarachnoid space can also cause spinal anesthesia or arachnoiditis. Intravascular injection has been demonstrated to occur in 6.4% to 10.9% of CESIs, 1.9% of ILESIs, and 10.8% to 11.2% of TFESIs; the prevalence is generally increased when injections occur at the S1 level.[140-143] A positive blood aspirate during TFESIs is 97.9% specific but only 44.7% sensitive for predicting intravascular injection.[142] Intravascular injection can potentially result in serious AEs, including spinal cord injury because of injection into the artery of Adamkiewicz and subsequent arteriole vasospasm or embolization of corticosteroid particulate–induced ischemic injury.[144] Therefore, fluoroscopic control using contrast confirmation of needle placement is mandatory to ensure safe and effective needle placement as evidenced by safe performance of large numbers of TFESIs.[136-138]

CPGs for the management of LBP have reported that minor AEs associated with ESIs are relatively frequent but transient, while serious AEs are very uncommon.[66] Minor AEs include suppression of adrenocorticotropic hormone and symptoms of Cushing's disease, while more serious AEs include accidental dural puncture, epidural hematoma, epidural abscess, chemical meningitis, and arachnoiditis.[66]

Some AEs associated with ESIs are summarized in Table 23-6.

COSTS

Fees and Third-Party Reimbursement

In the United States, ESIs for CLBP can be delivered by physicians using CPT codes 62311 (injection, single; epidural or subarachnoid, lumbar spine), 64483 (injection, anesthetic and/or steroid agent, transforaminal [single level]), or 64484 (injection, anesthetic and/or steroid agent, transforaminal [each additional level]). If radiologic guidance is used, CPT code 77003 (fluoroscopic guidance) or 77012 (CT guidance) may also be appropriate. Disposable medical equipment, needles and syringes, used in conjunction with ESI are included in the practice expense for these procedures.

TABLE 23-6	Adverse Events Associated with Epidural Steroid Injections for Low Back Pain		
Reference	Intervention	Event	% of Study Population Affected
136, 137	CESI	Dural puncture	0%-0.1%
140, 141, 143	CESI	Intravascular injection	6.4%-10.9%
60, 138	ILESI	Dural puncture	5%
141, 142	ILESI	Intravascular injection	1.9%
141, 142	TFESI	Intravascular injection	10.8%-11.2%

CESI, caudal epidural steroid injection; ILESI, interlaminar epidural steroid injection; TFESI, transforaminal epidural steroid injection.

Additional fees will apply for the medications injected and should be reported using the appropriate Healthcare Common Procedure Coding System drug code to be submitted on the same claim. The outpatient surgical center in which the procedure takes place will also charge facility fees for use of its operating room, recovery room, other disposable medical equipment, nurses, radiology, and other services. Because of these ancillary fees, the total cost of an ESI can reach $3000 or more, although there is wide variation in fees.

These procedures are widely covered by other third-party payers such as health insurers and worker's compensation insurance. Medicare has coverage guidelines that are supported by Local Coverage Determination (LCD) policies implemented by the Medicare Administrative Contractors in each locality. It is recommended that these policies be referenced for the most current information. The most current LCD referenced (effective 1/1/2010) provides a list of approximately 50 ICD-9 codes that support medical necessity for ESIs. The patient's medical record must contain documentation that fully supports the medical necessity of these services. Although some payers continue to base their reimbursements on usual, customary, and reasonable payment methodology, the majority have developed reimbursement tables based on the Resource Based Relative Value Scale used by Medicare. Reimbursements by other third-party payers are generally higher than Medicare. Reimbursement of multiple ESIs may require documented improvement with the previous injections.

Typical fees reimbursed by Medicare in New York and California for these services are summarized in Table 23-7.

Cost Effectiveness

No cost effective analyses or cost utility analyses were identified which evaluated the cost effectiveness of ESIs as an intervention for LBP.

Other

The CPG from Europe in 2004 found that ESIs might be cost effective for patients with unilateral sciatica.[67]

TABLE 23-7	Medicare Fee Schedule for Related Services	
CPT Code	New York	California
62311	$191	$210
64483	$266	$294
64484	$135	$147
77003	$61	$66
77012	$180	$200

2010 Participating, nonfacility amount.

SUMMARY

Description

ESI is a generic term used to indicate various types of injections that attempt to introduce one or more medications into the epidural space; not all ESIs involve corticosteroids. There are three main subtypes of ESIs that are named according to the method used to introduce therapeutic agents into the epidural space: (1) CESI; (2) ILESI, also called *translaminar ESI*; and (3) TFESI, also called *selective nerve root injection* or *selective nerve root block*. ESIs are commonly used to manage CLBP in the United States and should only be performed by a physician trained in the safe and competent administration of these procedures, with adequate life support training to address potential complications that could result from ESIs can be performed in private practices, ambulatory surgery centers, or hospital-based surgery centers depending on the equipment required.

Theory

Disc herniation can lead to increased production of proinflammatory mediators and cytokines, as well as higher levels of IL-6, IL-8, and prostaglandin E_2 (PGE_2), which can induce hyperalgesia. Injection of corticosteroids into the anterior epidural space has long been used to bathe the posterolateral periphery of the annulus to help curtail the biochemical stimulation of the intervertebral disc. As such, ESIs can improve pain and function and allow the patient to participate in a comprehensive physical therapy program addressing biomechanical deficiencies after this reduction of hyperalgesia. The primary indication for ESIs is radicular CLBP. Prior to ESI, plain film radiography of the lumbar spine is required to identify anatomic variations that may impact needle placement, as well as a general assessment of alignment, disc height, and stability. In addition, advanced imaging such as MRI or CT can be used to help guide the spine specialist to target the appropriate spinal levels involved in a patient's CLBP. Finally, some clinicians use provocative discography to identify painful annular defects that may subsequently be targeted with other interventions, although this procedure is controversial for CLBP.

Efficacy

Six CPGs provide recommendations for ESIs. For LBP with neurologic involvement, one CPG found conflicting evidence of efficacy, two did not recommend ESIs for CLBP, one reported poor evidence supporting efficacy, and two recommend ESIs if adequate relief was not obtained with other conservative interventions. None of the CPGs recommended ESIs for LBP without neurologic involvement. Two high-quality SRs concluded that ESIs were not significantly different than placebo, yet another higher-quality SR concluded that ESIs were more effective at improving symptoms than placebo for LBP with neurologic involvement. In addition, two lower-quality SRs concluded that there was short-term pain relief from ESIs for LBP with neurologic involvement. At least eleven RCTs have been conducted, and most did not report statistically significant differences between the ESI group and comparators regarding pain relief or disability improvement.

Safety

Contraindications to ESIs include concurrent use of anticoagulants, blood thinners (e.g., warfarin), local infection at the injection site, sepsis, hypovolemia, pregnancy, uncontrolled diabetes, uncontrolled glaucoma, high concentrations of local anesthetics in patients with multiple sclerosis, spinal infection, malignancy, and fracture. Minor AEs associated with ESIs include headache (sometimes associated with dural puncture), dizziness, transient local pain, tingling and numbness, nausea, increased radicular, spine, or leg pain, vomiting, facial flushing, fever, vasovagal reaction, increased blood glucose, increased pain, insomnia, voiding difficulty, and intraoperative hypertension. Rare but potentially serious AEs associated with ESIs include infection, cauda equina syndrome, dural puncture, arachnoiditis, conus medullaris, epidural abscess, bleeding, paraplegia, emergence of new neurologic symptoms, respiratory depression, spinal cord trauma, hematoma formation, intracranial air injection, epidural lipomatosis, pneumothorax, death, brain damage, vascular injury, cerebral vascular or pulmonary embolus, ophthalmologic changes (e.g., transient blindness, retinal hemorrhage), persistent recurrent intractable hiccups, chemical meningitis, nerve damage, and discitis. AEs related to steroid administration include pituitary-adrenal axis suppression, hypercorticism, Cushing's disease, osteoporosis, avascular necrosis of bone, steroid myopathy, epidural lipomatosis, weight gain, fluid retention, and hyperglycemia.

Costs

The cost per ESI varies according to the type of procedure and clinical setting, but can be as high as $3000 with facility fees. The cost effectiveness for ESIs is unknown.

Comments

Evidence from the CPGs, SRs, and RCTs reviewed was mixed regarding the use of ESIs for CLBP. However, this intervention may be beneficial to offer short-term relief for a subgroup of patients with CLBP and radicular symptoms who fail to improve after conservative therapy. If patients are interested in trying ESIs, they should be advised about the potential AEs associated with this intervention. The judicious use of fluoroscopically guided, contrast-enhanced, controlled diagnostic spinal procedures provides better direction for the use of target-specific therapeutic interventions such as TFESIs.

Injury of an anterior column component such as the intervertebral disc would suggest that instillation of a therapeutic agent into the anterior epidural space would maximize therapeutic benefit if such benefit is feasible. The most direct means by which to achieve anterior epidural spread is via a transforaminal approach. Hence, TFESIs are most appropriate in targeting discogenic pain after confirmation that the source of CLBP is an intervertebral disc. TFESIs may also be useful in instilling corticosteroid into the anterior epidural space to treat painful lumbosacral intervertebral discs.

Performing one to three injections would be clinically reasonable before deeming the treatment a failure, though evidence to support this is mostly anecdotal in nature and requires additional investigation. The timing of ESIs may have a bearing on successful outcomes and should be independently evaluated. Outcome measures should include measurement of pain, disability, analgesic intake, return to previous level of function or work, and avoidance of more aggressive treatment options such as surgery. Only a stringent protocol controlling for concurrent structural abnormalities (spondylolisthesis) while assuring proper identification of the discogenic source of pain will allow proper and accurate evaluation of the efficacy of ESIs in treating axial lumbar pain. Reporting whether or not patients experienced immediate improvements might help confirm if the ESIs adequately reached the putatively painful disc in future studies.

Few well-designed studies have been constructed to thoroughly assess the efficacy of TFESIs in treating discogenic CLBP. This is an area where future research is warranted. Furthermore, a definitive study protocol aimed at assessing the utility of ESIs for axial LBP has not been engineered. Such a protocol must use target-specific injections to adequately reach the diagnostically proven intervertebral discs responsible for clinical symptoms. Patients could be enrolled who have CLBP that is recalcitrant to physical therapy, nonsteroidal anti-inflammatory medications, and adjunctive analgesics.

CHAPTER REVIEW QUESTIONS

Answers are located on pages 451–452.

1. Which of the following is not a type of ESI?
   a. caudal
   b. interlaminar
   c. intradiscal
   d. transforaminal

2. Which of the following is a possible disadvantage to CESI?
   a. may cause considerably more discomfort to patient
   b. technically more demanding
   c. must be performed under fluoroscopy
   d. requires advanced equipment

3. Which of the following is not a proposed mechanism of action for local anesthetics used with ESIs to ease inflammation?
   a. inhibiting phagocytosis
   b. decreasing phagocytic oxygen consumption
   c. increasing polymorphonuclear leukocyte lysosomal enzyme release
   d. diminishing superoxide anion production

4. True or false: MRI or CT must be performed before ESIs.

5. Which of the following was a key milestone in the history of ESIs?
   a. discovery that cocaine could be injected as an anesthetic
   b. development of proper needle care by Cappio
   c. Robechhi and Capra's method of injecting into the caudal space
   d. advent of fluoroscopy

6. Which of the following is currently the most promising indication for ESIs?
   a. spinal stenosis
   b. degenerative disc disorder
   c. spinal fracture
   d. LBP with neurologic involvement

7. Which of the following ingredients is not commonly used for ESIs?
   a. lidocaine
   b. cocaine
   c. bupivacaine
   d. methylprednisolone

8. Which type of ESI is generally thought to be safer?
   a. caudal
   b. interlaminar
   c. intradiscal
   d. transforminal

REFERENCES

1. Ackerman WE III, Ahmad M. The efficacy of lumbar epidural steroid injections in patients with lumbar disc herniations. Anesth Analg 2007;104:1217-1222.
2. Weinstein SM, Herring SA, Derby R. Contemporary concepts in spine care. Epidural steroid injections. Spine (Phila Pa 1976) 1995;20:1842-1846.
3. Furman MB, Giovanniello MT, O'Brien EM. Incidence of intravascular penetration in transforaminal cervical epidural steroid injections. Spine 2003;28:21-25.
4. Renfrew DL, Moore TE, Kathol MH, et al. Correct placement of epidural steroid injections: fluoroscopic guidance and contrast administration. AJNR Am J Neuroradiol 1991;12:1003-1007.
5. Dillane JB, Fry J, Kalton G. Acute back syndrome: a study from general practice. BMJ 1966;2:82-84.

6. Spratt KF, Lehmann TR, Weinstein JN, et al. A new approach to the low-back physical examination. Behavioral assessment of mechanical signs. Spine 1990;15:96-102.

7. Nachemson AL. The natural course of low back pain. Symposium on idiopathic low back pain. St Louis, MO: Mosby; 1982. p. 46-51.

8. Valkenburg HA, Haanen HCM. The epidemiology of low back pain. Symposium on Idiopathic Low Back Pain. St Louis, MO: Mosby; 1982. p. 9-22.

9. Hitselberger WE, Witten RM. Abnormal myelograms in asymptomatic patients. J Neurosurg 1968;28:204-206.

10. Boden SD, Davis DO, Dina TS, et al. Abnormal magnetic-resonance scans of the lumbar spine in asymptomatic subjects. A prospective investigation. J Bone Joint Surg Am 1990; 72:403-408.

11. Wiesel SW, Tsourmas N, Feffer HL, et al. A study of computer-assisted tomography. I. The incidence of positive CAT scans in an asymptomatic group of patients. Spine 1984;9: 549-551.

12. Schwarzer AC, Aprill CN, Derby R, et al. The prevalence and clinical features of internal disc disruption in patients with chronic low back pain. Spine 1995;20:1878-1883.

13. Maigne JY, Aivaliklis A, Pfefer F. Results of sacroiliac joint double block and value of sacroiliac pain provocation tests in 54 patients with low back pain. Spine 1996;21: 1889-1892.

14. Schwarzer AC, Aprill CN, Bogduk N. The sacroiliac joint in chronic low back pain. Spine 1995;20:31-37.

15. Schwarzer AC, Aprill CN, Derby R, et al. The false-positive rate of uncontrolled diagnostic blocks of the lumbar zyg-apophysial joints. Pain 1994;58:195-200.

16. Sicard MA. Les injections medicamenteuse extraduraqles per voie saracoccygiene. Comptes Renues des Senances de la Societe de Biolgie et de ses Filliales 1901;53:396.

17. Cappio M. [Sacral epidural administration of hydrocortisone in therapy of lumbar sciatica; study of 80 cases.]. Reumatismo 1957;9:60-70.

18. Pages E. Anesthesia metamerica. Rev Sanid Mil Madr 1921;11:351-385.

19. Goebert Jr HW, Jallo SJ, Gardner WJ, et al. Painful radiculopathy treated with epidural injections of procaine and hydrocortisone acetate: results in 113 patients. Anesth Analg 1961;40:130-134.

20. Brown J. Pressure caudal anesthesia and back manipulation. Conservative method for treatment of sciatica. Northwest Med 1960;59:905-909.

21. Robechhi A, Capra R. Prime esperienze cliniche in campo reumatologico. Minerva Med 1952;98:1259-1263.

22. Conn A, Buenaventura RM, Datta S, et al. Systematic review of caudal epidural injections in the management of chronic low back pain. Pain Physician 2009;12:109-135.

23. Manchikanti L, Singh V, Rivera JJ, et al. Effectiveness of caudal epidural injections in discogram positive and negative chronic low back pain. Pain Physician 2002;5:18-29.

24. Jeong HS, Lee JW, Kim SH, et al. Effectiveness of transforaminal epidural steroid injection by using a preganglionic approach: a prospective randomized controlled study. Radiology 2007;245:584-590.

25. Friedly J, Chan L, Deyo R. Increases in lumbosacral injections in the Medicare population: 1994 to 2001. Spine 2007;32: 1754-1760.

26. Friedly J, Chan L, Deyo R. Geographic variation in epidural steroid injection use in Medicare patients. J Bone Joint Surg Am 2008;90:1730-1737.

27. Chen CP, Tang SF, Hsu TC, et al. Ultrasound guidance in caudal epidural needle placement. Anesthesiology 2004; 101:181-184.

28. Galiano K, Obwegeser AA, Bodner G, et al. Real-time sonographic imaging for periradicular injections in the lumbar spine: a sonographic anatomic study of a new technique. J Ultrasound Med 2005;24:33-38.

29. Bryan BM, Lutz C, Lutz GE. Fluoroscopic assessment of epidural contrast spread after caudal injection. ISIS, 7th annual scientific meeting, Las Vegas, Nevada, August 1999.

30. Botwin KP, Natalicchio J, Hanna A. Fluoroscopic guided lumbar interlaminar epidural injections: a prospective evaluation of epidurography contrast patterns and anatomical review of the epidural space. Pain Physician 2004;7:77-80.

31. Botwin K, Natalicchio J, Brown LA. Epidurography contrast patterns with fluoroscopic guided lumbar transforaminal epidural injections: a prospective evaluation. Pain Physician 2004;7:211-215.

32. Saal JS, Franson RC, Dobrow R, et al. High levels of inflammatory phospholipase A2 activity in lumbar disc herniations. Spine 1990;15:674-678.

33. Kang JD, Georgescu HI, Intyre-Larkin L, et al. Herniated lumbar intervertebral discs spontaneously produce matrix metalloproteinases, nitric oxide, interleukin-6, and prostaglandin E2. Spine 1996;21:271-277.

34. Kang JD, Stefanovic-Racic M, McIntyre LA, et al. Toward a biochemical understanding of human intervertebral disc degeneration and herniation. Contributions of nitric oxide, interleukins, prostaglandin E2, and matrix metalloproteinases. Spine 1997;22:1065-1073.

35. O'Donnell JL, O'Donnell AL. Prostaglandin E2 content in herniated lumbar disc disease. Spine 1996;21:1653-1655.

36. Takahashi H, Suguro T, Okazima Y, et al. Inflammatory cytokines in the herniated disc of the lumbar spine. Spine 1996;21:218-224.

37. Nygaard OP, Mellgren SI, Osterud B. The inflammatory properties of contained and noncontained lumbar disc herniation. Spine 1997;22:2484-2488.

38. Burke JG, Watson RW, McCormack D, et al. Intervertebral discs which cause low back pain secrete high levels of proinflammatory mediators. J Bone Joint Surg Br 2002;84: 196-201.

39. Weiler C, Nerlich AG, Bachmeier BE, et al. Expression and distribution of tumor necrosis factor alpha in human lumbar intervertebral discs: a study in surgical specimen and autopsy controls. Spine 2005;30:44-53.

40. Miyamoto H, Doita M, Nishida K, et al Effects of cyclic mechanical stress on the production of inflammatory agents by nucleus pulposus and anulus fibrosus derived cells in vitro. Spine 2006;31:4-9.

41. Coppes MH, Marani E, Thomeer RT, et al. Innervation of "painful" lumbar discs. Spine 1997;22:2342-2349.

42. Brown MF, Hukkanen MV, McCarthy ID, et al. Sensory and sympathetic innervation of the vertebral endplate in patients with degenerative disc disease. J Bone Joint Surg Br 1997; 79:147-153.

43. Cunha JM, Cunha FQ, Poole S, et al. Cytokine-mediated inflammatory hyperalgesia limited by interleukin-1 receptor antagonist. Br J Pharmacol 2000;130:1418-1424.

44. Hasue M. Pain and the nerve root. An interdisciplinary approach. Spine 1993;18:2053-2058.

45. MacGregor RR, Thorner RE, Wright DM. Lidocaine inhibits granulocyte adherence and prevents granulocyte delivery to inflammatory sites. Blood 1980;56:203-209.

46. Cullen BF, Haschke RH. Local anesthetic inhibition of phago-cytosis and metabolism of human leukocytes. Anesthesiology 1974;40:142-146.

47. Hoidal JR, White JG, Repine JE. Influence of cationic local anesthetics on the metabolism and ultrastructure of human alveolar macrophages. J Lab Clin Med 1979;93:857-866.

48. Goldstein IM, Lind S, Hoffstein S, et al. Influence of local anesthetics upon human polymorphonuclear leukocyte function in vitro. Reduction of lysosomal enzyme release and superoxide anion production. J Exp Med 1977;146:483-494.

49. Yabuki S, Kikuchi S. Nerve root infiltration and sympathetic block. An experimental study of intraradicular blood flow. Spine 1995;20:901-906.

50. Yabuki S, Kawaguchi Y, Nordborg C, et al. Effects of lidocaine on nucleus pulposus-induced nerve root injury. A neurophysiologic and histologic study of the pig cauda equina. Spine 1998;23:2383-2389.

51. Flower RJ, Blackwell GJ. Anti-inflammatory steroids induce biosynthesis of a phospholipase A2 inhibitor which prevents prostaglandin generation. Nature 1979;278:456-459.

52. Devor M, Govrin-Lippmann R, Raber P. Corticosteroids suppress ectopic neural discharge originating in experimental neuromas. Pain 1985;22:127-137.

53. Johansson A, Hao J, Sjolund B. Local corticosteroid application blocks transmission in normal nociceptive C-fibres. Acta Anaesthesiol Scand 1990;34:335-338.

54. Woodward JL, Weinstein SM. Epidural injections for the diagnosis and management of axial and radicular pain syndromes. In: Physical Medicine and Rehabilitation Clinics of North America. Philadelphia: Saunders; 1995. p. 691-714.

55. Freemont AJ, Peacock TE, Goupille P, et al. Nerve ingrowth into diseased intervertebral disc in chronic back pain. Lancet 1997;350:178-181.

56. Burke JG, Watson RW, Conhyea D, et al. Human nucleus pulposus can respond to a pro-inflammatory stimulus. Spine 2003;28:2685-2693.

57. Shirazi-Adl A. Strain in fibers of a lumbar disc. Analysis of the role of lifting in producing disc prolapse. Spine 1989;14:96-103.

58. Tsantrizos A, Ito K, Aebi M, et al. Internal strains in healthy and degenerated lumbar intervertebral discs. Spine 2005;30:2129-2137.

59. Marchand F, Ahmed AM. Investigation of the laminate structure of lumbar disc anulus fibrosus. Spine 1990;15:402-410.

60. Bogduk N. Epidural steroids for low back pain and sciatica. Pain Digest 1999;9:226-227.

61. Moneta GB, Videman T, Kaivanto K, et al. Reported pain during lumbar discography as a function of anular ruptures and disc degeneration. A re-analysis of 833 discograms. Spine 1994;19:1968-1974.

62. Schwarzer AC, Wang SC, O'Driscoll D, et al. The ability of computed tomography to identify a painful zygapophysial joint in patients with chronic low back pain. Spine 1995;20:907-912.

63. Milette PC, Fontaine S, Lepanto L, et al. Differentiating lumbar disc protrusions, disc bulges, and discs with normal contour but abnormal signal intensity. Magnetic resonance imaging with discographic correlations. Spine 1999;24:44-53.

64. Aprill C, Bogduk N. High-intensity zone: a diagnostic sign of painful lumbar disc on magnetic resonance imaging. Br J Radiol 1992;65:361-369.

65. Schellhas KP, Pollei SR, Gundry CR, et al. Lumbar disc high-intensity zone. Correlation of magnetic resonance imaging and discography. Spine 1996;21:79-86.

66. Nielens H, van Zundert J, Mairiaux P, et al. Chronic low back pain. Brussels, 2006, Report No.: KCE reports Vol 48C.

67. Airaksinen O, Brox JI, Cedraschi C, et al. European guidelines for the management of chronic nonspecific low back pain. Eur Spine J 2006;15:S192-S300.

68. Negrini S, Giovannoni S, Minozzi S, et al. Diagnostic therapeutic flow-charts for low back pain patients: the Italian clinical guidelines. Eura Medicophys 2006;42:151-170.

69. Chou R, Qaseem A, Snow V, et al. Diagnosis and treatment of low back pain: a joint clinical practice guideline from the American College of Physicians and the American Pain Society. Ann Intern Med 2007;147:478-491.

70. Chou R, Loeser JD, Owens DK, et al. Interventional therapies, surgery, and interdisciplinary rehabilitation for low back pain: an evidence-based clinical practice guideline from the American Pain Society. Spine 2009;34:1066-1077.

71. National Institute for Health and Clinical Excellence (NICE). Low back pain: early management of persistent non-specific low back pain. London: National Institute of Health and Clinical Excellence; 2009. Report No.: NICE clinical guideline 88.

72. Staal JB, de BR, de Vet HC, et al. Injection therapy for subacute and chronic low-back pain. Cochrane Database Syst Rev 2008;(3):CD001824.

73. Beliveau P. A comparison between epidural anaesthesia with and without corticosteroid in the treatment of sciatica. Rheumatol Phys Med 1971;11:40-43.

74. Breivik H, Hesla PE, Molnar I, et al. Treatment of chronic low back pain and sciatica. Comparison of caudal epidural injections of bupivacaine and methylprednisolone with bupivacaine followed by saline. Adv Pain Res Ther 1976;1:927-932.

75. Serrao JM, Marks RL, Morley SJ, et al. Intrathecal midazolam for the treatment of chronic mechanical low back pain: a controlled comparison with epidural steroid in a pilot study. Pain 1992;48:5-12.

76. Aldrete JA. Epidural injections of indomethacin for postlaminectomy syndrome: a preliminary report. Anesth Analg 2003;96:463-468.

77. Rocco AG, Frank E, Kaul AF, et al. Epidural steroids, epidural morphine and epidural steroids combined with morphine in the treatment of post-laminectomy syndrome. Pain 1989;36:297-303.

78. Lierz P, Gustorff B, Markow G, et al. Comparison between bupivacaine 0.125% and ropivacaine 0.2% for epidural administration to outpatients with chronic low back pain. Eur J Anaesthesiol 2004;21:32-37.

79. Takada M, Fukusaki M, Terao Y, et al. Comparative efficacy of ropivaciane and bupivacaine for epidural block in outpatients with degenerative spinal disease and low back pain. Pain Clin 2005;17:275-281.

80. Chou R, Atlas SJ, Stanos SP, et al. Nonsurgical interventional therapies for low back pain: a review of the evidence for an American Pain Society clinical practice guideline. Spine 2009;34:1078-1093.

81. Abdi S, Datta S, Trescot AM, et al. Epidural steroids in the management of chronic spinal pain: a systematic review. Pain Physician 2007;10:185-212.

82. Luijsterburg PA, Verhagen AP, Ostelo RW, et al. Effectiveness of conservative treatments for the lumbosacral radicular syndrome: a systematic review. Eur Spine J 2007;16:881-899.

83. Slipman CW, Bhat AL, Gilchrist RV, et al. A critical review of the evidence for the use of zygapophysial injections and radiofrequency denervation in the treatment of low back pain. Spine J 2003;3:310-316.

84. DePalma MJ, Slipman CW. Evidence-informed management of chronic low back pain with epidural steroid injections. Spine J 2008;8:45-55.

85. Tonkovich-Quaranta LA, Winkler SR. Use of epidural corticosteroids in low back pain. Ann Pharmacother 2000;34:1165-1172.

86. Vroomen PC, de Krom MC, Slofstra PD, et al. Conservative treatment of sciatica: a systematic review. J Spin Disord 2000;13:463-469.

87. Mathews JA, Mills SB, Jenkins VM, et al. Back pain and sciatica: controlled trials of manipulation, traction, sclerosant and epidural injections. Br J Rheumatol 1987;26:416-423.

88. Arden NK, Price C, Reading I, et al. A multicentre randomized controlled trial of epidural corticosteroid injections for sciatica: the WEST study. Rheumatology (Oxford) 2005;44:1399-1406.

89. Bush K, Hillier S. A controlled study of caudal epidural injections of triamcinolone plus procaine for the management of intractable sciatica. Spine 1991;16:572-575.

90. Carette S, Leclaire R, Marcoux S, et al. Epidural corticosteroid injections for sciatica due to herniated nucleus pulposus. N Engl J Med 1997;336:1634-1640.

91. Dilke TF, Burry HC, Grahame R. Extradural corticosteroid injection in management of lumbar nerve root compression. Br Med J 1973;2:635-637.

92. Karppinen J, Malmivaara A, Kurunlahti M, et al. Periradicular infiltration for sciatica: a randomized controlled trial. Spine 2001;26:1059-1067.

93. Riew KD, Yin Y, Gilula L, et al. The effect of nerve-root injections on the need for operative treatment of lumbar radicular pain. A prospective, randomized, controlled, double-blind study. J Bone Joint Surg Am 2000;82:1589-1593.

94. Wilson-MacDonald J, Burt G, Griffin D, et al. Epidural steroid injection for nerve root compression. A randomised, controlled trial. J Bone Joint Surg Br 2005;87:352-355.

95. Cuckler JM, Bernini PA, Wiesel SW, et al. The use of epidural steroids in the treatment of lumbar radicular pain. A prospective, randomized, double-blind study. J Bone Joint Surg Am 1985;67:63-66.

96. Helliwell M, Robertson JC, Ellia RM. Outpatient treatment of low back pain and sciatica by a single extradural corticosteroid injection. Br J Clin Pract 1985;39:228-231.

97. Ng L, Chaudhary N, Sell P. The efficacy of corticosteroids in periradicular infiltration for chronic radicular pain: a randomized, double-blind, controlled trial. Spine 2005;30:857-862.

98. Rogers P, Nash T, Schiller D, et al. Epidural steroids for sciatica. Pain Clinic 1992;5:67-72.

99. Zahaar M. The value of caudal epidural steroids in the treatment of lumbar neural compression syndromes. J Neurol Orthop Med Surg 1991;12:181-184.

100. Ridley MG, Kingsley GH, Gibson T, et al. Outpatient lumbar epidural corticosteroid injection in the management of sciatica. Br J Rheumatol 1988;27:295-299.

101. Snoek W, Weber H, Jorgensen B. Double blind evaluation of extradural methyl prednisolone for herniated lumbar discs. Acta Orthop Scand 1977;48:635-641.

102. Klenerman L, Greenwood R, Davenport HT, et al. Lumbar epidural injections in the treatment of sciatica. Br J Rheumatol 1984;23:35-38.

103. Kraemer J, Ludwig J, Bickert U, et al. Lumbar epidural perineural injection: a new technique. Eur Spine J 1997;6:357-361.

104. Klenerman L, Greenwood R, Davenport HT, et al. Lumbar epidural injections in the treatment of sciatica. Br J Rheumatol 1984;23:35-38.

105. Kraemer J, Ludwig J, Bickert U, et al. Lumbar epidural perineural injection: a new technique. Eur Spine J 1997;6:357-361.

106. Riew KD, Yin Y, Gilula L, et al. The effect of nerve-root injections on the need for operative treatment of lumbar radicular pain. A prospective, randomized, controlled, double-blind study. J Bone Joint Surg Am 2000;82:1589-1593.

107. Buchner M, Zeifang F, Brocai DR, et al. Epidural corticosteroid injection in the conservative management of sciatica. Clin Orthop Relat Res 2000;(375):149-156.

108. Dashfield AK, Taylor MB, Cleaver JS, et al. Comparison of caudal steroid epidural with targeted steroid placement during spinal endoscopy for chronic sciatica: a prospective, randomized, double-blind trial. Br J Anaesth 2005;94:514-519.

109. Devulder J, Deene P, De Laat M, et al. Nerve root sleeve injections in patients with failed back surgery syndrome: a comparison of three solutions. Clin J Pain 1999;15:132-135.

110. Hesla E, Breivik H. [Epidural analgesia and epidural steroid injection for treatment of chronic low back pain and sciatica.] Tidsskr Nor Laegeforen 1979;99:936-939.

111. Kolsi I, Delecrin J, Berthelot JM, et al. Efficacy of nerve root versus interspinous injections of glucocorticoids in the treatment of disk-related sciatica. A pilot, prospective, randomized, double-blind study. Joint Bone Spine 2000;67:113-118.

112. McGregor AH, Anjarwalla NK, Stambach T. Does the method of injection alter the outcome of epidural injections? J Spinal Disord 2001;14:507-510.

113. Meadeb J, Rozenberg S, Duquesnoy B, et al. Forceful sacrococcygeal injections in the treatment of postdiscectomy sciatica. A controlled study versus glucocorticoid injections. Joint Bone Spine 2001;68:43-49.

114. Pirbudak L, Karakurum G, Onder U. Epidural corticosteroid injection and amitriptyline for the treatment of chronic low back pain associated with radiculopathy. Pain Clin 2003;15:247-253.

115. Pirbudak L, Karakurum G, Satana T. Epidural steroid injection and amitriptyline in the management of acute low back pain originating from lumbar disc herniation. Artroplasti Artroskopik Cerrahi 2003;14:89-93.

116. Revel M, Auleley GR, Alaoui S, et al. Forceful epidural injections for the treatment of lumbosciatic pain with postoperative lumbar spinal fibrosis. Rev Rhum Engl Ed 1996;63:270-277.

117. Thomas E, Cyteval C, Abiad L, et al. Efficacy of transforaminal versus interspinous corticosteroid injection in discal radiculalgia—a prospective, randomised, double-blind study. Clin Rheumatol 2003;22:299-304.

118. Buttermann GR. The effect of spinal steroid injections for degenerative disc disease. Spine J 2004;4:495-505.

119. Bonetti M, Fontana A, Cotticelli B, et al. Intraforaminal O(2)-O(3) versus periradicular steroidal infiltrations in lower back pain: randomized controlled study. AJNR Am J Neuroradiol 2005;26:996-1000.

120. Fukusaki M, Miyako M, Miyoshi H, et al. Prostaglandin E1 but not corticosteroid increases nerve root blood flow velocity after lumbar diskectomy in surgical patients. J Neurosurg Anesthesiol 2003;15:76-81.

121. Gallucci M, Limbucci N, Zugaro L, et al. Sciatica: treatment with intradiscal and intraforaminal injections of steroid and oxygen-ozone versus steroid only. Radiology 2007;242:907-913.

122. Manchikanti L, Rivera JJ, Pampati V, et al. One day lumbar epidural adhesiolysis and hypertonic saline neurolysis in treatment of chronic low back pain: a randomized, double-blind trial. Pain Physician 2004;7:177-186.

123. Watts RW, Silagy CA. A meta-analysis on the efficacy of epidural corticosteroids in the treatment of sciatica. Anaesth Intensive Care 1995;23:564-569.

124. Koes BW, Scholten R, Mens JMA, et al. Epidural steroid injections for low back pain and sciatica: an updated systemtic review of randomized clinical trials. Pain Digest 1999;9: 241-247.

125. DePalma MJ, Bhargava A, Slipman CW. A critical appraisal of the evidence for selective nerve root injection in the treatment of lumbosacral radiculopathy. Arch Phys Med Rehabil 2005;86:1477-1483.

126. Yates DW. A comparison of the types of epidural injection commonly used in the treatment of low back pain and sciatica. Rheumatol Rehabil 1978;17:181-186.

127. Slipman CW, Patel RK, Zhang L, et al. Side of symptomatic annular tear and site of low back pain: is there a correlation? Spine 2001;26:E165-E169.

128. Lutz GE, Vad VB, Wisneski RJ. Fluoroscopic transforaminal lumbar epidural steroids: an outcome study. Arch Phys Med Rehabil 1998;79:1362-1366.

129. Bhatia MT, Parikh CJ. Epidural-saline therapy in lumbosciatic syndrome. J Indian Med Assoc 1966;47:537-542.

130. Gupta AK, Mital VK, Azmi RU. Observations on the management of lumbosciatic syndrome (sciatica) by epidural saline injection. J Indian Med Assoc 1970;54:194-196.

131. Wittenberg RH, Greskotter KR, Steffen R, et al. [Is epidural injection treatment with hypertonic saline solution in intervertebral disk displacement useful? (The effect of NaCl solution on intervertebral disk tissue).] Z Orthop Ihre Grenzgeb 1990;128:223-226.

132. Atluri SL. Interlaminar epidural use of steroids. In: Manchikanti L, Slipman B, Fellows C, editors. Low back pain: diagnosis and treatment. Paduka, KY: ASIPP Publishing; 2002. p. 314-326.

133. Horlocker TT, Wedel DJ, Offord KP. Does preoperative antiplatelet therapy increase the risk of hemorrhagic complications associated with regional anesthesia? Anesth Analg 1990;70:631-634.

134. Hopwood MB, Abram SE. Factors associated with failure of lumbar epidural steroids. Reg Anesth 1993;18:238-243.

135. Jamison RN, VadeBoncouer T, Ferrante FM. Low back pain patients unresponsive to an epidural steroid injection: identifying predictive factors. Clin J Pain 1991;7: 311-317.

136. Huston CW, Slipman CW, Garvin C. Complications and side effects of cervical and lumbosacral selective nerve root injections. Arch Phys Med Rehabil 2005;86:277-283.

137. Stalcup ST, Crall TS, Gilula L, et al. Influence of needle-tip position on the incidence of immediate complications in 2,217 selective lumbar nerve root blocks. Spine J 2006;6: 170-176.

138. Botwin KP, Gruber RD, Bouchlas CG, et al. Complications of fluoroscopically guided caudal epidural injections. Am J Phys Med Rehabil 2001;80:416-424.

139. Botwin KP, Gruber RD, Bouchlas CG, et al. Complications of fluoroscopically guided transforaminal lumbar epidural injections. Arch Phys Med Rehabil 2000;81:1045-1050.

140. Renfrew DL, Moore TE, Kathol MH, et al. Correct placement of epidural steroid injections: fluoroscopic guidance and contrast administration. AJNR Am J Neuroradiol 1991;12: 1003-1007.

141. Sullivan WJ, Willick SE, Chira-Adisai W, et al. Incidence of intravascular uptake in lumbar spinal injection procedures. Spine 2000;25:481-486.

142. Furman MB, O'Brien EM, Zgleszewski TM. Incidence of intravascular penetration in transforaminal lumbosacral epidural steroid injections. Spine 2000;25:2628-2632.

143. White AH, Derby R, Wynne G. Epidural injections for the diagnosis and treatment of low-back pain. Spine 1980;5: 78-86.

144. Houten JK, Errico TJ. Paraplegia after lumbosacral nerve root block: report of three cases. Spine J 2002;2:70-75.

CHAPTER 24

Trigger Point Injections

DESCRIPTION

Terminology and Subtypes

Trigger point injections (TPIs) refer to the injection of medication directly into trigger points. Trigger points are defined as firm, hyperirritable loci of muscle tissue located within a "taut band" in which external pressure can cause an involuntary local twitch response termed a "jump sign", which in turn provokes referred pain to distant structures.[1] Establishing a diagnosis of trigger points often includes a history of regional pain, with muscular overload from sustained contraction in one position or repetitive activity, presence of a taut band with exquisite spot tenderness, reproduction of the patient's pain complaint, and a painful limit to muscle stretch.[2-4] Despite being an integral component to the definition of trigger points, it has been reported that the twitch response cannot reliably be established.[5]

The two main types of trigger points are active and latent. Active trigger points can cause spontaneous pain or pain with movement, whereas latent trigger points cause pain only in response to direct compression.[6] A pressure threshold meter, also termed an *algometer* or *dolorimeter,* is often used in clinical research to measure the amount of compression required to elicit a painful response in trigger points.[7] Trigger points can be classified as *central* if they occur within a taut band, or *attachment* if they occur at a musculotendinous junction (Figure 24-1). When accompanied by other symptoms, trigger points may also constitute myofascial pain syndrome, one of the most frequent causes of musculoskeletal pain (Figure 24-2).[8] Many often inaccurate terms have been used to denote trigger points, including Travell points, myofascial pain syndrome, myofascitis, fibrositis, myofibrositis, myalgia, muscular rheumatism, idiopathic myalgia, regional fibromyalgia, nonarthritic rheumatism, tendinomyopathy nonarticular rheumatism, local fibromyalgia, and regional soft-tissue pain.[1,9]

TPIs may be classified according to the substances injected, which may include local anesthetic, saline, sterile water, steroids, nonsteroidal anti-inflammatory drugs, botulinum toxin, 5-HT3 receptor antagonists, or even dry needling.[10-38] Although this chapter focuses on TPIs for chronic low back pain (CLBP), trigger points may occur elsewhere in the body.

History and Frequency of Use

The German anatomist Froriep referred to tender spots occurring in muscles as muscle calluses in 1843; these points were called "myalgic spots" by Gutstein in 1938.[39] Many other eponyms have been used to describe the same phenomenon. Studies have reported that 14.4% of the population of the United States has experienced myofascial pain, and suggested that 21% to 93% of all pain complaints were myofascial in origin.[40,41] Although long thought to be separate entities, there was no clear delineation between myofascial pain syndrome and fibromyalgia until the American College of Rheumatology published diagnostic criteria for fibromyalgia in 1990.[42] This milestone was not universally celebrated within the medical profession, and some have contended that both myofascial pain syndrome and fibromyalgia were the products of "junk medicine," supported by poorly designed trials and unfounded theories, with the aim of legitimizing somewhat vague psychosomatic illnesses.[39] Trigger points may also be present in fibromyalgia, osteoarthritis, rheumatoid arthritis, or connective tissue disorders.[43]

The term *myofascial trigger point* was coined and popularized by Janet Travell, who was the personal physician to President John F. Kennedy. Her contribution to medical pain management was primarily the study and description of myofascial pain with the publication, along with coauthor and physician David Simons, of the text *Myofascial Pain and Dysfunction: The Trigger Point Manual* in 1983.[44] Travell and Simons continued to advance their proposed understanding of myofascial pain treatment and published a second edition of their manual in 1992.[2] Although the method proposed by Travell and Simons for identifying and injecting trigger points became prominent, it was based largely on anecdotal observations and their personal clinical experience.[39,45] The use of injection therapy for trigger points had previously been reported almost four decades earlier in 1955 by Sola and Kuitert, who noted that "Procaine and pontocaine have been most commonly used but Martin has reported success with injections of benzyl salicylate, camphor, and arachis oil."[46]

Practitioner, Setting, and Availability

Any physician familiar with the localization of trigger points and the use of therapeutic musculoskeletal injections may perform TPIs. However, these injections are probably best

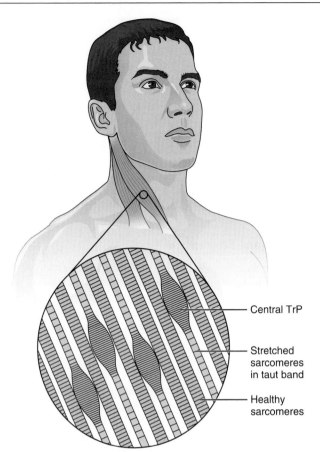

Figure 24-1 A central trigger point (TrP) located within a taut band of muscle. (Modified from Muscolino JE: The muscle and bone palpation manual with trigger points, referral patterns, and stretching. St. Louis, Mosby, 2009.)

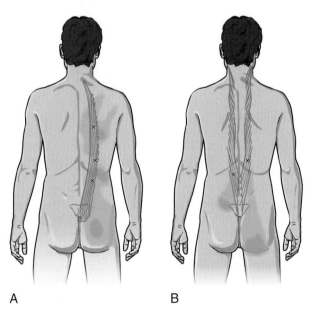

A   B

Figure 24-2 Locations of trigger points in the iliocostalis (**A**) and longissimus (**B**) muscles and their common referral zones. (Modified from Muscolino JE: The muscle and bone palpation manual with trigger points, referral patterns, and stretching. St. Louis, Mosby, 2009.)

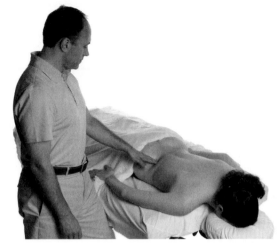

Figure 24-3 Palpation of trigger points prior to injections. (From Muscolino JE: The muscle and bone palpation manual with trigger points, referral patterns, and stretching. St. Louis, Mosby, 2009.)

performed by physicians with postgraduate education in musculoskeletal anatomy, and a greater understanding of orthopedic and neurologic disorders. Although a few states currently allow physical therapists or naturopaths to perform dry needling, most states do not permit such injections by nonphysicians.[47] This intervention is typically performed in private outpatient clinics, but can also be offered in specialty pain management or spine clinics. TPIs are widely available throughout the United States.

Procedure

TPIs usually require that the patient wear a medical gown and lie prone on a treatment table. Patient positioning should be comfortable to minimize involuntary muscle contractions and facilitate access to the painful areas. Trigger points are first located by manual palpation with a variety of techniques (Figure 24-3). The highest inter- and intra-examiner reliability for locating trigger points was achieved with pressure threshold algometry.[48,49] Once trigger points are located and marked with a skin pen, the skin is generally prepared with a standard antibacterial agent such as isopropyl alcohol or betadine solution. The needle size used for TPIs is typically quite small, frequently 25 or 27 gauge (G), but needles as large as 21G have been reported.[10-12,14,18-20,24,26,32,50] The length of needle used is dependent on the depth of the trigger point through subcutaneous tissue, but is commonly from 0.75 inches to 2.5 inches.[10,12,14,18,20,46,50-52] Acupuncture needles may be used for dry needling of trigger points, using 0.16 × 13 mm for facial muscles to 0.30 × 75 mm for larger or deeper muscles.

The number of trigger points injected at each session varies, as does the volume of solution injected at each trigger point and in total. A common practice is to use 0.5 to 2 mL per trigger point, which may depend on the pharmacologic dosing limits of the injected mixture.[11,12,14,15,19-21,26,32,33,50] For example, the total dose of Botox A administered during TPIs ranged from 5 to 100 units/site, for 10-20 sites, up to a total

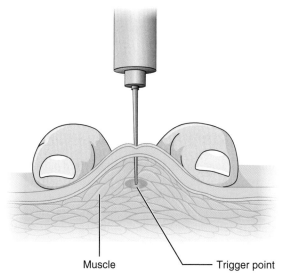

Figure 24-4 Trigger point injection technique. (Courtesy of Kopecky Campbell Associates as found on http://www.kcadocs.com/trigger_point.html)

of 250 units.[18,22,24,25] Lidocaine is a frequently used local anesthetic for TPIs; a dilution to 0.2% to 0.25% with sterile water has been suggested as the least painful on injection.[11,13-15,18,26] Other studies have used ropivacaine or bupivacaine 0.5% with or without dexamethasone.[12]

The injection technique recommended by Hong and Hsueh for trigger points was modified from that proposed by Travell and Simons.[13,50] It described holding the syringe in the dominant hand while palpating the trigger point with the thumb or index finger of the opposite hand (Figure 24-4). Needle insertion was into the subcutaneous tissue adjacent to the trigger point at an angle of 50 to 70 degrees to the skin, aiming at the taut band. Multiple insertions in different directions from the subcutaneous layer were "fast in" and "fast out" to probe for latent trigger points. Each thrust coincided with the injection of 0.02 to 0.05 mL of injectate, up to a total of 0.5 to 1 mL in each trigger point. Compression of the point for 2 minutes allowed hemostasis, which was followed by stretching of the muscle. They noted that the best responses to injection were found when the "local twitch response" was provoked by impaling the active point.[13]

Regulatory Status

The US Food and Drug Administration regulates the medications commonly administered during TPIs and most are approved for these indications. Specific medications such as Botox are only approved for other indications and are thus used off-label for TPIs with CLBP.

THEORY

Mechanism of Action

The physiology of trigger points themselves is controversial, and therefore the mechanism of action through which injections aimed at trigger points may relieve pain is unknown.[39] In 1979, a theory of "diffuse noxious inhibitory control" was suggested where noxious input from nociceptive afferent fibers inhibited dorsal horn efferents as a "counter irritant" from a distant location.[53] Some support was given to this theory when subcutaneous sterile water improved myofascial pain scores after a brief period of severe burning pain at that site.[54] Spontaneous electrical activity was found more frequently in rabbit and human trigger points.[9,55] Simons[56] theorized that the spontaneous electrical activity found in active trigger point loci was abnormal end-plate potentials from excessive acetylcholine leakage. This acetylcholine was thought to depolarize the postjunctional membrane, resulting in prolonged Ca^{++} release, continuous muscle fiber shortening, and increased metabolism.

Additionally, local circulation was thought to be compromised, thus reducing available oxygen and nutrient supply to the affected area, impairing the healing process. A muscle fiber "energy crisis" was hypothesized to produce taut bands. The concept of abnormal end-plate potentials was used to justify injection of botulinum toxin to block acetylcholine release in trigger points.[57] McPartland has expanded on the idea of excessive acetylcholine by suggesting that congenital or acquired genetic defects in presynaptic, synaptic, or postsynaptic structures may contribute to an individual's susceptibility to myofascial pain.[45]

Animal and human models suggest that the local twitch responses and referred pain associated with trigger points are related to spinal cord reflexes.[34] Simons and Hong suggested that there are multiple trigger point loci in a region that consist of sensory (nociceptors) and motor (abnormal end-plates) components.[63] By modifying the peripheral nociceptive response (desensitization), the nociceptive input to higher neurologic centers of pain and resulting increased muscle fiber contraction are blocked. The desensitization or antinociceptive effects by pressure, cold, heat, electricity, acupuncture, or chemical irritation relies on "gate-control theory" from Melzack.[58,59] Local anesthetic also blocks nociceptors by reversible action on sodium channels.

Endogenous opioid release may play a role in TPIs. Fine and colleagues reported that the analgesic effects of TPIs could be reversed with intravenous naloxone.[60] Mechanical disruption may play some role in breaking up trigger points.[38,61] Spontaneous electrical activity, as originally observed, was later confirmed to be end-plate potentials.[62] This finding was used to show that many traditional "ah-shi" acupuncture points corresponded to trigger points.[63] Animal models also suggest the role of the autonomic nervous system related to phentolamine, an alpha-adrenergic agonist that inhibits sympathetic activation and decreases spontaneous electrical activity in rabbit myofascial trigger spots.[64]

Thermographic imaging evaluation has previously demonstrated elevated temperatures in the referral pain pattern of trigger points, suggesting increased local heat production from increased metabolism or neural activity.[65] Gerwin and colleagues recently expanded on Simons' integrated hypothesis for trigger point formation and proposed a complex molecular pathway whereby unconditioned muscle undergoes eccentric exercise or trauma, which results in muscle fiber injury and hypoperfusion from capillary constriction.[66] Sympathetic nervous system activation further enhances this constriction and creates a hypoxic and acidic environment, facilitating the release of calcitonin gene-related peptide and acetylcholine. Additional proinflammatory mediators (e.g., adenosine triphosphate, serotonin, tumor necrosis factor-1a, interleukin 1, substance P, and Hþ ions) are then released from damaged muscle fibers, leading to activation of nociceptors and end-plate activity. Acetylcholine receptors are then up-regulated, resulting in more efficient binding, and producing taut bands. Neuroplastic changes in the dorsal horn may also activate neighboring neurons at lower thresholds, resulting in allodynia, hypersensitivity, and referred pain. The calcitonin gene-related peptide may be associated with this condition becoming chronic, as is hypothesized to occur in some patients with CLBP.

Indication

The indication for TPIs is CLBP with active trigger points in patients who also have myofascial pain syndrome that has failed to respond to analgesics and therapeutic exercise, or when a joint is deemed to be mechanically blocked due to trigger points and is unresponsive to other interventions.[67] The best outcomes with TPIs are thought to occur in CLBP patients who demonstrate the local twitch response on palpation or dry needling.[13,68] Patients with CLBP who also had fibromyalgia reported greater post-injection soreness and a slower response time than those with myofascial pain syndrome, but had similar clinical outcomes.[50,69,70]

Assessment

Before receiving TPIs, patients should first be assessed for LBP using an evidence-based and goal-oriented approach focused on the patient history and neurologic examination, as discussed in Chapter 3. Clinicians should also inquire about medication history to note prior hypersensitivity/ allergy or adverse events (AEs) with drugs similar to those being considered, and evaluate contraindications for these types of drugs. Diagnostic imaging or other forms of advanced testing is generally not required before administering this intervention for CLBP.

Identification of trigger points is required before performing these injections and is generally performed with a thorough manual and orthopedic examination. However, insufficient training in trigger point examination likely impedes recognition of myofascial pain, and palpation generally has poor interrater reliability.[2,44,71] Hsieh and colleagues reported difficulties when attempting to reproduce findings of taut bands and local twitch responses, both characteristics of trigger points, in the lower back.[72] In a study of intra-rater reliability, local twitch response and referred pain varied from one session to the next while taut bands, tender points, and "jump sign" remained consistent.[73] Likewise, Njoo and van der Does found that "jump sign" and "reproduction of pain" were much more reliable than "referred pain" in identifying myofascial pain.[74] It is interesting to note that when Hong and colleagues compared referred pain response from needling and palpation, they found that only 53.9% of their patients had referred pain from palpation, compared with 87.6% when needling.[35]

Differentiating between the trigger points of myofascial pain syndrome and the tender points of fibromyalgia syndrome has also proven problematic. When clinicians were asked to examine patients with either myofascial pain, fibromyalgia, or healthy controls, the number of tender points identified was generally consistent.[43] Even among experts in myofascial pain and fibromyalgia there was inconsistency in the number of taut bands, presence of referred pain, and local twitch responses reported. Asymptomatic subjects were reported to have as many latent trigger points as those with myofascial pain or fibromyalgia. This study prompted some clinicians to abandon the local twitch response to more reliably quantify tenderness with pressure thresholds, as reflected in the most current diagnostic criteria for trigger points.[2-4]

Pressure threshold is the minimum pressure that reproduces pain (or tenderness) in a suspected trigger point, and has been claimed to be an objective, reproducible, and reliable method for their detection.[48,50,75-77] Fischer attempted to establish standard, normal pressure thresholds, which were found to be different for each gender and each muscle.[76] A follow-up study declared that observing a 2-kg difference between the left and right sides in the same patient was more reliable than relying on published normative values.[77] Anecdotal evidence was offered to support this conclusion, but no account was taken of the nonnociceptive components to pain threshold. Pressure threshold also cannot differentiate between trigger points and tender points, for which a patient history and referred pain are necessary. Electromyography localization of trigger points has also been proposed, but evidence to suggest more reliability or efficacy than the previously described methods is currently lacking.[23,78]

EFFICACY

Evidence supporting the efficacy of this intervention for CLBP was summarized from recent clinical practice guidelines (CPGs), systematic reviews (SRs), and randomized controlled trials (RCTs). Observational studies (OBSs) were also summarized where appropriate. Findings are summarized by study design.

Clinical Practice Guidelines

Three of the recent national CPGs on the management of CLBP have assessed and summarized the evidence to make specific recommendations about the efficacy of TPIs.

The CPG from Belgium in 2006 found insufficient evidence to make a recommendation about the efficacy of TPIs in the management of CLBP.[79] That CPG also found insufficient evidence to support the efficacy of intramuscular botulinum toxin injections in the management of CLBP.

The CPG from Europe in 2004 found no evidence to support the efficacy of intramuscular injections, including TPIs, for the management of CLBP.[80] That CPG did not recommend TPIs for CLBP.

The CPG from the United States in 2009 found poor evidence to support the efficacy of local injections, including TPIs, in the management of CLBP.[81]

Findings from the above CPGs are summarized in Table 24-1.

Systematic Reviews

Cochrane Collaboration

An SR was conducted in 2007 by the Cochrane Collaboration on injection therapy for subacute and chronic LBP without neurologic involvement.[82] A total of 18 RCTs were identified, including 3 RCTs related to TPIs for patients with persistent LBP without neurologic involvement, iliac crest pain, and nonspecific LBP.[14,83,84] One RCT found no statistically significant differences between TPIs and active control for self-reported outcomes.[14] However, the second RCT did find statistically significant decreased pain among those receiving TPIs into the iliac crest versus placebo after 2 weeks of follow-up.[83] The third RCT did not find statistically significant decreased pain among those receiving TPIs into the iliolumbar ligament versus placebo but did find that self-reported pain was statistically significantly improved after 2 weeks of follow-up for those receiving the TPIs.[84] This review concluded that there is insufficient evidence supporting the use of TPIs for subacute and chronic LBP without neurologic involvement.[82] This SR review also recommended that future RCTs be conducted to determine patient subgroups who are most likely to benefit from TPIs.

American Pain Society and American College of Physicians

An SR was conducted in 2008 by the American Pain Society and American College of Physicians CPG committee on nonsurgical therapies for acute and chronic LBP.[85] That review identified one SR related to TPIs, which was the Cochrane Collaboration review mentioned earlier.[82] This SR also identified one additional RCT excluded from the Cochrane review and which examined both cervical and lower back TPIs for myofascial pain syndrome.[20] This RCT found that TPIs were superior to placebo after 2 weeks of follow-up.[20] This SR was unable to make any definitive conclusions about the effectiveness of TPIs because of the methodologic shortcomings and clinical heterogeneity of the included RCTs.[85] The SR recommended that higher quality RCTs be conducted in the future to assess the effects of TPIs for LBP.

Other

Nelemans and colleagues[86] conducted a review of all injection therapies for CLBP. The review combined all studies of local injections, whether they were directed at ligaments or muscles. This review concluded that there was insufficient evidence to make any recommendations about local injections for CLBP. Four of the five studies involving local injections in that review reported results that were superior to placebo, whereas one study showed no difference. Myofascial pain was not always a requirement for study participants.

Findings from the above SRs are summarized in Table 24-2.

Randomized Controlled Trials

Four RCTs were identified.[10,14,20,87] Their methods are summarized in Table 24-3. Their results are briefly described here.

Hameroff and colleagues[20] performed an RCT in which patients with chronic pain conditions were selected if they had an initial favorable response to a TPI. Those participants were then randomized to (1) TPIs with bupivacaine, (2) TPIs with etidacaine, or (3) saline injections. Each group received three injections administered by a clinician 1 to 3 weeks apart. After 1 week, both TPI groups experienced statistically significant improvements in average pain but there was no difference in outcomes between these two TPI groups.

Garvey and colleagues[14] performed an RCT in which patients with low back strain were selected if they had more than 4 weeks of LBP and failed to improve despite conservative treatment. LBP with neurologic involvement or signs of tension was excluded. Participants were randomized to (1) TPIs with lidocaine, (2) TPIs with lidocaine plus steroid, (3) dry needling, or (4) acupressure plus one sham

TABLE 24-1	Clinical Practice Guideline Recommendations on Trigger Point Injections for Chronic Low Back Pain	
Reference	Country	Conclusion
79	Belgium	Insufficient evidence to make a recommendation
80	Europe	Not recommended
81	United States	Poor evidence to support efficacy

TABLE 24-2	Systematic Review Findings on Trigger Point Injections For Chronic Low Back Pain		
Reference	# RCTs in SR	# RCTs for CLBP	Conclusion
82	18	NR	Insufficient evidence for CLBP without neurologic involvement
85	1 SR	NR	Unable to make definitive conclusions because of the methodological shortcomings and clinical heterogeneity of the included RCTs
86	NR	NR	Insufficient evidence to make any recommendations about local injections into muscles or ligaments for CLBP

CLBP, chronic low back pain; NR, not reported; RCT, randomized controlled trial; SR, systematic review.

TABLE 24-3	Randomized Controlled Trials of Trigger Point Injections for Chronic Low Back Pain				
Reference	Indication	Intervention 1	Intervention 2	Intervention 3	Control
20	Chronic pain conditions, neurologic involvement NR, duration LBP NR	TPI: bupivacaine 0.5% Clinician 3 injections (1-3 weeks apart) Cointervention: patient's regular medication and therapy n = 13	TPI: etidacaine 1% Clinician 3 injections (1-3 weeks apart) Cointervention: patient's regular medication and therapy n = 14	NA	Saline injection Clinician 1 injection Cointervention: patient's regular medication and therapy n = 20
14	Low back strain, LBP without neurologic involvement, symptoms >4 weeks	TPI: lidocaine 1% Clinicians 1 injection Cointervention: hot shower 2×/day, restricted physical activity, told not to begin a new exercise program n = 13	TPI: lidocaine + steroid Clinicians 1 injection Cointervention: hot shower 2×/day, restricted physical activity, told not to begin a new exercise program n = 14	Dry needling Clinicians 1 injection Cointervention: hot shower 2×/day, restricted physical activity, told not to begin a new exercise program n = 20	Acupressure + 1 sham injection Clinicians 1 injection Cointervention: hot shower 2×/day, restricted physical activity, told not to begin a new exercise program n = 16
10	Pain in neck, shoulder, hip, neurologic involvement NR, duration LBP NR	TPI: Botox A Physiatrist Max 8×/subject Cointervention: allowed to continue taking pain medication, education on self-heat therapy and ergonomics, home exercise n = 9	TPI: bupivacaine 0.5% Physiatrist Max 8×/subject Cointervention: exercise program, allowed to continue taking pain medication, education on self-heat therapy and ergonomics, home exercise n = 8	NA	NA
87	CLBP with or without neurologic involvement, symptoms >12 weeks	TPI: NR Clinician 1-2×/week (max 15 injections) Cointervention: continued with usual clinical regimen n = 29	NA	NA	No treatment Cointervention: continued with usual clinical regimen n = 27

CLBP, chronic low back pain; LBP, low back pain; NA, not applicable; NR, not reported; TPI, trigger point injection.

injection. One injection (or dry needling session) was administered by a clinician to each group. After 1 month, all groups improved when compared to baseline, yet no statistically significant differences were observed between the groups for pain improvement.

Gunn and colleagues[87] performed an RCT in which patients with CLBP were selected if they had more than 12 weeks of LBP and failed to improve despite conservative treatment. Those with psychiatric conditions were excluded. Participants were randomized to TPIs or to a control group, which did not receive any intervention. Both groups continued with the study clinic's usual regime, which included

workplace modifications and physical therapy. For the TPI group, up to 15 injections were administered by a clinician. After an average of 27.3 weeks, the TPI group experienced statistically significant improvements in pain and function versus the control group.

Graboski and colleagues[10] performed an RCT in which adults with pain in their neck, shoulder, hip, or lower back were selected if they had an initial favorable response to TPIs. Those who were pregnant or had comorbidities were excluded. The duration of pain was not reported and the results were not categorized by type of pain. Participants were randomized to TPIs with botulinum toxin or bupivacaine and up to eight injections were administered by a physiatrist. After 10 weeks, both groups experienced statistically significant improvements in pain, yet there were no statistically significant differences between TPI groups.

SAFETY

Contraindications

Contraindications to TPIs are commonly thought to be the same as any other injection procedure, and include spinal infection, malignancy, and fracture, as well as anticoagulation therapy or bleeding diathesis. There is limited evidence to suggest that concurrent aspirin or nonsteroidal anti-inflammatory drug use may also represent relative contraindications to TPIs.[88]

An observational study analyzed 31 baseline factors in 193 participants who underwent TPIs.[89] Factors associated with poor outcomes included unemployment due to pain, no relief from analgesic medications, constant pain, prolonged pain duration, high levels of pain at its worst and pain at its least, change in social activity, and poor coping ability. Upon further analysis using logistic regression, only unemployment, change in social activity, and prolonged pain duration were independently associated with poor outcomes. Factors that were not associated with poor outcomes included the number and types of previous interventions, age, sex, ethnicity, marital status, compensation, and smoking.

Adverse Events

AEs associated with TPIs include local post-injection soreness, vasovagal depression, negative reaction to the medication injected, hematoma formation, or development of an abscess. If corticosteroids are injected, AEs may also include local muscle necrosis. Observational studies of TPIs using botulinum toxin have reported soreness, excessive weakness, flu-like symptoms, transient numbness or heaviness of the ipsilateral limb, as well as a shift in pain patterns.[25,31] There have also been case reports of serious AEs such as pneumothorax, cervical epidural abscess, and intrathecal injection following TPIs.[90,91]

The CPG from Europe in 2004 found that intramuscular injections to treat CLBP (>3 months) can weaken the muscles if repeated injections are given over a long period of time.[80]

COSTS

Fees and Third-Party Reimbursement

In the United States, TPIs for CLBP can be delivered by physicians using CPT codes 20552 (injection, one to two muscles) or 20553 (injection, three or more muscles); only one code should be reported on any particular day, no matter how many sites or regions are injected. Disposable medical equipment, needles and syringes, used in conjunction with

TABLE 24-4	Medicare Fee Schedule for Related Services	
CPT Code	New York	California
20552	$56	$55
20553	$58	$63

2010 Participating, nonfacility amount.

TPIs are included in the practice expense for these procedures. Additional fees will apply for the medications injected and should be reported using the appropriate Health Care Common Procedure Coding drug code to be submitted on the same claim. Local anesthetics are considered inclusive of the procedure.

Third-party payer coverage is widespread but variable. Medicare has coverage guidelines that are supported by Local Coverage Determination (LCD) policies implemented by the Medicare Administrative Contractors for each locality; these policies should be referenced for the most current information. The most current LCD referenced (effective 1/1/2010) indicates that the only ICD-9 code which supports medical necessity for TPIs is 729.1 (myalgia and myositis, unspecified). The patient's medical record must contain documentation that fully supports the medical necessity for services. Proper documentation is required of the evaluation, muscles selected, reasoning for treatment strategy (initial vs. subsequent therapy), and proper diagnosis determination. Oxford Medicare suggests up to 3 injection sessions in 12 months, but no closer than 7 days apart, whereas Empire Medicare allows up to 12 injection sessions in a year.[67,92] Individual insurance carriers should be consulted for coverage of neurotoxic agents that may be used for TPIs (e.g., botulinum toxin). Although some payers continue to base their reimbursements on usual, customary, and reasonable payment methodology, the majority have developed reimbursement tables based on the Resource Based Relative Value Scale used by Medicare. Reimbursements by other third-party payers are generally higher than Medicare.

Typical fees reimbursed by Medicare in New York and California for these services are summarized in Table 24-4.

Cost Effectiveness

No cost effectiveness analyses or cost utility analyses were identified that evaluated the cost effectiveness of TPIs as an intervention for LBP.

The CPG from Europe in 2004 indicates that the cost effectiveness of intramuscular injections to treat CLBP (>3 months) is unknown.[80]

Other

A study by Graboski and colleagues[10] in 2005 showed that the overall cost of care did not differ significantly between injections of 0.5% bupivacaine and Botox A, except for the extreme difference in the cost of the medication injected.

SUMMARY

Description

TPIs refer to the injection of medication directly into trigger points. Trigger points are firm, hyperirritable loci of muscle tissue located within a "taut band" in which external pressure can cause an involuntary local twitch response termed a "jump sign," which in turn provokes referred pain to distant structures. TPIs may be classified according to the substances injected, which include local anesthetic, saline, sterile water, steroids, nonsteroidal anti-inflammatory drugs, botulinum toxin, 5-HT3 receptor antagonists, or dry needling. Any physician familiar with the localization of trigger points and the use of therapeutic musculoskeletal injections may perform TPIs. They are widely available throughout the United States and are usually performed in private outpatient clinics, specialty pain management or spine clinics.

Theory

The physiology of trigger points themselves is controversial, and therefore the mechanism of action through which injections aimed at trigger points may relieve pain is unknown. The indication for TPIs is CLBP with active trigger points in patients who also have myofascial pain syndrome that has failed to respond to medications and exercise, or when a joint is deemed to be mechanically blocked due to trigger points and is unresponsive to other interventions. Diagnostic imaging or other forms of advanced testing is generally not required before administering this intervention for CLBP.

Efficacy

Three CPGs and two SRs found insufficient evidence supporting TPIs. At least four RCTs have assessed TPIs, three of which found no statistically significant improvements versus other groups and another which found statistically significant improvement in pain and function versus a non-treatment control group.

Harms

Contraindications to TPIs include spinal infection, malignancy, fracture, anticoagulation therapy, and bleeding diathesis. There is limited evidence suggesting that concurrent aspirin or nonsteroidal anti-inflammatory drug use may also be contraindications to TPIs. AEs associated with TPIs may include local post-injection soreness, vasovagal depression, negative reaction to the medication injected, hematoma formation, and development of an abscess. If corticosteroids are injected, AEs may also include local muscle necrosis.

Costs

The cost per TPI for one to two muscles is approximately $56 and it increases to approximately $63 for three or more muscles. One study reported that the overall cost of care did not differ significantly between injections of 0.5% bupivacaine and Botox A, except for the extreme difference in the cost of the medication. However, the cost effectiveness for TPIs for CLBP is unknown.

Comments

Evidence from the CPGs, SRs, and RCTs reviewed to support the use of TPIs for CLBP is conflicting. However, this intervention may be beneficial for a small subgroup of patients with CLBP and myofascial pain who fail to improve after more conservative therapy. If patients are interested in trying TPIs, they should be advised about the potential AEs associated with this intervention.

The conflicting results observed across the included RCTs may be due to methodologic differences. For example, previous injection trials using saline injection controls may have inadvertently administered TPIs to study participants, thereby confounding results. The first step in administering appropriate treatment is careful and accurate diagnosis. From there, treatment should be based on safety (first do no harm), as well as scientific evidence supporting the efficacy of this treatment to both control pain and improve function. Furthermore, the saline often used as a control in RCTs may contain (unless preservative-free) 0.9% benzyl alcohol, which, in addition to being bacteriostatic, has some local anesthetic properties that could confound study outcomes.[93] Specifying the use of preservative-free saline may reduce this potential confounding factor in future studies.

Because it appears that most patients improve regardless of the type of needling procedure, it would be interesting to determine if there is an optimal volume of injectate, frequency of injection, injection depth, and number of muscles injected with TPIs. Perhaps those who fail to improve in one injectate may respond more favorably with another substance. An investigation into the long-term pain and functional outcomes of myofascial pain in CLBP is also needed. In addition, continued study of the pathophysiology of myofascial pain in general will lead to novel approaches for better and longer-acting treatments as our understanding advances. A look into the psychological contributions proposed by Bohr may also lead to better approaches to myofascial pain in CLBP.[39]

CHAPTER REVIEW QUESTIONS

Answers are located on page 452.

1. What was the initial term used by Gutstein in 1938 to denote "trigger points"?
   a. myalgic spots
   b. Travell points
   c. myalgia
   d. regional soft tissue pain
2. What type of advanced diagnostic imaging is required prior to TPIs?
   a. MRI
   b. CT
   c. discography
   d. none of the above

3. Which of the following has been suggested as the least painful concentration for lidocaine injections?
 a. 0.4% to 0.5%
 b. 0.05% to 0.15%
 c. 0.2% to 0.25%
 d. 0.5% to 0.75%

4. Who coined the term *myofascial trigger point?*
 a. John F. Kennedy
 b. David Simons
 c. Janet Travell
 d. Robert Gutstein

5. Which of the following is not a characteristic of trigger points?
 a. firm, hyperirritable loci of muscle tissue
 b. located within a taut band
 c. external pressure causes a local twitch response and jump sign
 d. provokes radicular pain to distant structures

6. What is the indication for TPIs?
 a. spondylolisthesis
 b. spinal stenosis
 c. unresolved CLBP
 d. myofascial pain

7. What types of ingredients are frequently used for TPIs?
 a. local anesthetic
 b. sterile saline
 c. paracetamol
 d. opioids

8. What was a key milestone in the development of TPIs?
 a. discovery that saline solution could be injected
 b. creation of diagnostic criteria for fibromyalgia
 c. coining of the term myofascial trigger point
 d. invention of the discograph

REFERENCES

1. Bronfort G, Nilsson N, Haas M, et al. Non-invasive physical treatments for chronic/recurrent headache. Cochrane Database Syst Rev 2004;(3):CD001878.
2. David G. Travell & Simons' myofascial pain and dysfunction: the trigger point manual. Philadelphia: Williams & Wilkins; 1999.
3. Simons DG. Review of enigmatic MTrPs as a common cause of enigmatic musculoskeletal pain and dysfunction. J Electromyogr Kinesiol 2004;14:95-107.
4. Kilkenny MB, Deane K, Smith KA, et al. Non-invasive physical treatments of myofascial pain. Cochrane Database of Systematic Reviews 2006;(3).
5. Gerwin RD, Shannon S, Hong CZ, et al. Interrater reliability in myofascial trigger point examination. Pain 1997;69:65-73.
6. Alvarez DJ, Rockwell PG. Trigger points: diagnosis and management. Am Fam Physician 2002;65:653-660.
7. Reeves JL, Jaeger B, Graff-Radford SB. Reliability of the pressure algometer as a measure of myofascial trigger point sensitivity. Pain 1986;24:313-321.
8. Lavelle ED, Lavelle W, Smith HS. Myofascial trigger points. Med Clin North Am 2007;91:229-239.
9. Fricton JR, Auvinen MD, Dykstra D, et al. Myofascial pain syndrome: electromyographic changes associated with local twitch response. Arch Phys Med Rehabil 1985;66:314-317.
10. Graboski CL, Gray DS, Burnham RS. Botulinum toxin A versus bupivacaine trigger point injections for the treatment of myofascial pain syndrome: a randomised double blind crossover study. Pain 2005;118:170-175.
11. Iwama H, Ohmori S, Kaneko T, et al. Water-diluted local anesthetic for trigger-point injection in chronic myofascial pain syndrome: evaluation of types of local anesthetic and concentrations in water. Reg Anesth Pain Med 2001;26:333-336.
12. Krishnan SK, Benzon HT, Siddiqui T, et al. Pain on intramuscular injection of bupivacaine, ropivacaine, with and without dexamethasone. Reg Anesth Pain Med 2000;25:615-619.
13. Hong CZ. Lidocaine injection versus dry needling to myofascial trigger point. The importance of the local twitch response. Am J Phys Med Rehabil 1994;73:256-263.
14. Garvey TA, Marks MR, Wiesel SW. A prospective, randomized, double-blind evaluation of trigger-point injection therapy for low-back pain. Spine 1989;14:962-964.
15. Frost A. Diclofenac versus lidocaine as injection therapy in myofascial pain. Scand J Rheumatol 1986;15:153-156.
16. Frost FA, Jessen B, Siggaard-Andersen J. A control, double-blind comparison of mepivacaine injection versus saline injection for myofascial pain. Lancet 1980;315:499-500.
17. Esenyel M, Caglar N, Aldemir T. Treatment of myofascial pain. Am J Phys Med Rehabil 2000;79:48-52.
18. Kamanli A, Kaya A, Ardicoglu O, et al. Comparison of lidocaine injection, botulinum toxin injection, and dry needling to trigger points in myofascial pain syndrome. Rheumatol Int 2005;25:604-611.
19. McMillan AS, Nolan A, Kelly PJ. The efficacy of dry needling and procaine in the treatment of myofascial pain in the jaw muscles. J Orofac Pain 1997;11:307-314.
20. Hameroff SR, Crago BR, Blitt CD, et al. Comparison of bupivacaine, etidocaine, and saline for trigger-point therapy. Anesth Analg 1981;60:752-755.
21. Tschopp KP, Gysin C. Local injection therapy in 107 patients with myofascial pain syndrome of the head and neck. ORL J Otorhinolaryngol Relat Spec 1996;58:306-310.
22. Ferrante FM, Bearn L, Rothrock R, et al. Evidence against trigger point injection technique for the treatment of cervicothoracic myofascial pain with botulinum toxin type A. Anesthesiology 2005;103:377-383.
23. Qerama E, Fuglsang-Frederiksen A, Kasch H, et al. A double-blind, controlled study of botulinum toxin A in chronic myofascial pain. Neurology 2006;67:241-245.
24. Ojala T, Arokoski JP, Partanen J. The effect of small doses of botulinum toxin a on neck-shoulder myofascial pain syndrome: a double-blind, randomized, and controlled crossover trial. Clin J Pain 2006;22:90-96.
25. Wheeler AH, Goolkasian P, Gretz SS. A randomized, double-blind, prospective pilot study of botulinum toxin injection for refractory, unilateral, cervicothoracic, paraspinal, myofascial pain syndrome. Spine 1998;23:1662-1666.
26. Iwama H, Akama Y. The superiority of water-diluted 0.25% to neat 1% lidocaine for trigger-point injections in myofascial pain syndrome: a prospective, randomized, double-blinded trial. Anesth Analg 2000;91:408-409.
27. Cheshire WP, Abashian SW, Mann JD. Botulinum toxin in the treatment of myofascial pain syndrome. Pain 1994;59:65-69.
28. Guttu RL, Page DG, Laskin DM. Delayed healing of muscle after injection of bupivicaine and steroid. Ann Dent 1990;49:5-8.
29. Freund BJ, Schwartz M. Treatment of whiplash associated neck pain [corrected] with botulinum toxin-A: a pilot study. J Rheumatol 2000;27:481-484.

30. Schnider P, Moraru E, Vigl M, et al. Physical therapy and adjunctive botulinum toxin type A in the treatment of cervical headache: a double-blind, randomised, placebo-controlled study. J Headache Pain 2002;3:93-99.

31. Wheeler AH, Goolkasian P, Gretz SS. Botulinum toxin A for the treatment of chronic neck pain. Pain 2001;94:255-260.

32. Ettlin T. Trigger point injection treatment with the 5-HT3 receptor antagonist tropisetron in patients with late whiplash-associated disorder. First results of a multiple case study. Scand J Rheumatol Suppl 2004;(119):49-50.

33. Muller W, Stratz T. Local treatment of tendinopathies and myofascial pain syndromes with the 5-HT3 receptor antagonist tropisetron. Scand J Rheumatol Suppl 2004;(119):44-48.

34. Hesse J, Mogelvang B, Simonsen H. Acupuncture versus metoprolol in migraine prophylaxis: a randomized trial of trigger point inactivation. J Intern Med 1994;235:451-456.

35. Hong CZ, Kuan TS, Chen JT, et al. Referred pain elicited by palpation and by needling of myofascial trigger points: a comparison. Arch Phys Med Rehabil 1997;78:957-960.

36. Itoh K, Katsumi Y, Kitakoji H. Trigger point acupuncture treatment of chronic low back pain in elderly patients—a blinded RCT. Acupunct Med 2004;22:170-177.

37. Irnich D, Behrens N, Gleditsch JM, et al. Immediate effects of dry needling and acupuncture at distant points in chronic neck pain: results of a randomized, double-blind, sham-controlled crossover trial. Pain 2002;99:83-89.

38. Chen JT, Chung KC, Hou CR, et al. Inhibitory effect of dry needling on the spontaneous electrical activity recorded from myofascial trigger spots of rabbit skeletal muscle. Am J Phys Med Rehabil 2001;80:729-735.

39. Bohr TW. Fibromyalgia syndrome and myofascial pain syndrome. Do they exist? Neurol Clin 1995;13:365-384.

40. Magni G, Caldieron C, Rigatti-Luchini S, et al. Chronic musculoskeletal pain and depressive symptoms in the general population. An analysis of the 1st National Health and Nutrition Examination Survey data. Pain 1990;43:299-307.

41. Finley JE. Myofascial pain. Available at: http://emedicine.medscape.com/article/313007-overview.

42. Wolfe F, Smythe HA, Yunus MB, et al. The American College of Rheumatology 1990 Criteria for the Classification of Fibromyalgia. Report of the Multicenter Criteria Committee. Arthritis Rheum 1990;33:160-172.

43. Wolfe F, Simons DG, Fricton J, et al. The fibromyalgia and myofascial pain syndromes: a preliminary study of tender points and trigger points in persons with fibromyalgia, myofascial pain syndrome and no disease. J Rheumatol 1992;19:944-951.

44. Travell JG, Simons DG. Myofascial pain and dysfunction: the trigger point manual. Baltimore: Williams & Wilkins. 1983. p. 276-277.

45. McPartland JM. Travell trigger points–molecular and osteopathic perspectives. J Am Osteopath Assoc 2004;104:244-249.

46. Sola AE, Kuitert JH. Myofascial trigger point pain in the neck and shoulder girdle; report of 100 cases treated by injection of normal saline. Northwest Med 1955;54:980-984.

47. Simons DG, Dommerholt J. Myofascial pain syndromes—trigger points (literature reviews). J Musculoskel Pain 2005;13:53-64.

48. Delaney GA, McKee AC. Inter- and intra-rater reliability of the pressure threshold meter in measurement of myofascial trigger point sensitivity. Am J Phys Med Rehabil 1993;72:136-139.

49. Sciotti VM, Mittak VL, DiMarco L, et al. Clinical precision of myofascial trigger point location in the trapezius muscle. Pain 2001;93:259-266.

50. Hong CZ, Hsueh TC. Difference in pain relief after trigger point injections in myofascial pain patients with and without fibromyalgia. Arch Phys Med Rehabil 1996;77:1161-1166.

51. Cooper AL. Trigger-point injection: its place in physical medicine. Arch Phys Med Rehabil 1961;42:704-709.

52. Simons DG, Dommerholt J. Myofascial pain syndromes—trigger points. J Musculoskel Pain 2005;13:51-62.

53. Le Bars D., Dickenson AH, Besson JM. Diffuse noxious inhibitory controls (DNIC). I. Effects on dorsal horn convergent neurones in the rat. Pain 1979;6:283-304.

54. Byrn C, Olsson I, Falkheden L, et al. Subcutaneous sterile water injections for chronic neck and shoulder pain following whiplash injuries. Lancet 1993;341:449-452.

55. Simons DG, Hong CZ, Simons LS. Spontaneous electrical activity of trigger points. J Musculoskel Pain 1995;3:124.

56. Simons DG. Clinical and etiological update of myofascial pain from trigger points. J Musculoskel Pain 1996;4:93-121.

57. Kuan TS, Chen JT, Chen SM, et al. Effect of botulinum toxin on endplate noise in myofascial trigger spots of rabbit skeletal muscle. Am J Phys Med Rehabil 2002;81:512-520.

58. Melzack R. Myofascial trigger points: relation to acupuncture and mechanisms of pain. Arch Phys Med Rehabil 1981;62:114-117.

59. Melzack R, Wall PD. Pain mechanisms: a new theory. Science 1965;150:971-979.

60. Fine PG, Milano R, Hare BD. The effects of myofascial trigger point injections are naloxone reversible. Pain 1988;32:15-20.

61. Jaeger B, Skootsky SA. Double blind, controlled study of different myofascial trigger point injection techniques. Pain 1987;4:S292.

62. Simons DG, Hong CZ, Simons LS. Endplate potentials are common to midfiber myofacial trigger points. Am J Phys Med Rehabil 2002;81:212-222.

63. Kao MJ, Hsieh YL, Kuo FJ, et al. Electrophysiological assessment of acupuncture points. Am J Phys Med Rehabil 2006;85:443-448.

64. Chen JT, Chen SM, Kuan TS, et al. Phentolamine effect on the spontaneous electrical activity of active loci in a myofascial trigger spot of rabbit skeletal muscle. Arch Phys Med Rehabil 1998;79:790-794.

65. Kruse RA Jr, Christiansen JA. Thermographic imaging of myofascial trigger points: a follow-up study. Arch Phys Med Rehabil 1992;73:819-823.

66. Gerwin RD, Dommerholt J, Shah JP. An expansion of Simons' integrated hypothesis of trigger point formation. Curr Pain Headache Rep 2004;8:468-475.

67. American Medical Association. Article for trigger point injections—coding guidelines for LCD L19485. Centers for Medicare and Medicaid Services 2007. Available at: http://www.empiremedicare.com/newjpolicy/policy/l19485_final.htm.

68. Chu J, Schwartz I. The muscle twitch in myofascial pain relief: effects of acupuncture and other needling methods. Electromyogr Clin Neurophysiol 2002;42:307-311.

69. Staud R. Are tender point injections beneficial: the role of tonic nociception in fibromyalgia. Curr Pharm Des 2006;12:23-27.

70. Reddy SS, Yunus MB, Inanici F, et al. Tender point injections are beneficial in fibromyalgia syndrome: a descriptive, open study. J Musculoskeletal Pain 2000;8:7-18.

71. Nice DA, Riddle DL, Lamb RL, Mayhew TP, et al. Intertester reliability of judgments of the presence of trigger points in patients with low back pain. Arch Phys Med Rehabil 1992;73:893-898.

72. Hsieh CY, Hong CZ, Adams AH, et al. Interexaminer reliability of the palpation of trigger points in the trunk and lower limb muscles. Arch Phys Med Rehabil 2000;81:258-264.

73. Al-Shenqiti AM, Oldham JA. Test-retest reliability of myofascial trigger point detection in patients with rotator cuff tendonitis. Clin Rehabil 2005;19:482-487.

74. Njoo KH, van der Dose E. The occurrence and inter-rater reliability of myofascial trigger points in the quadratus lumborum and gluteus medius: a prospective study in non-specific low back pain patients and controls in general practice. Pain 1994; 58:317-323.

75. Jaeger B, Reeves JL. Quantification of changes in myofascial trigger point sensitivity with the pressure algometer following passive stretch. Pain 1986;27:203-210.

76. Fischer AA. Pressure algometry over normal muscles. Standard values, validity and reproducibility of pressure threshold. Pain 1987;30:115-126.

77. Fischer AA. Documentation of myofascial trigger points. Arch Phys Med Rehabil 1988;69:286-291.

78. Porta M, Maggioni G. Botulinum toxin (BoNT) and back pain. J Neurol 2004;251:I15-I18.

79. Nielens H, van Zundert J, Mairiaux P, et al. Chronic low back pain. Brussels, 2006, Report No.: KCE reports Vol 48C.

80. Airaksinen O, Brox JI, Cedraschi C, et al. European guidelines for the management of chronic nonspecific low back pain. Eur Spine J 2006;(Suppl 2):192-300.

81. Chou R, Loeser JD, Owens DK, et al. Interventional therapies, surgery, and interdisciplinary rehabilitation for low back pain: an evidence-based clinical practice guideline from the American Pain Society. Spine 2009;34:1066-1077.

82. Staal JB, de Bie RA, de Vet HC, et al. Injection therapy for subacute and chronic low-back pain. Cochrane Database Syst Rev 2008;(3):CD001824.

83. Collee G, Dijkmans BA, Vandenbroucke JP, et al. Iliac crest pain syndrome in low back pain. A double blind, randomized study of local injection therapy. J Rheumatol 1991;18: 1060-1063.

84. Sonne M, Christensen K, Hansen SE, et al. Injection of steroids and local anaesthetics as therapy for low-back pain. Scand J Rheumatol 1985;14:343-345.

85. Chou R, Atlas SJ, Stanos SP, et al. Nonsurgical interventional therapies for low back pain: a review of the evidence for an American Pain Society clinical practice guideline. Spine 2009;34:1078-1093.

86. Nelemans PJ, de Bie R, de Vet HC, et al. Injection therapy for subacute and chronic benign low-back pain. Cochrane Database of Systematic Reviews 2006;(2).

87. Gunn CC, Milbrandt WE, Little AS, et al. Dry needling of muscle motor points for chronic low-back pain: a randomized clinical trial with long-term follow-up. Spine 1980;5: 279-291.

88. Weiss BD. Why is aspirin a contraindication for trigger-point injections? Am Fam Physician 2003;67:32.

89. Hopwood MB, Abram SE. Factors associated with failure of trigger point injections. Clin J Pain 1994;10:227-234.

90. Shafer N. Pneumothorax following "trigger point" injection. JAMA 1970;213:1193.

91. Elias M. Cervical epidural abscess following trigger point injection. J Pain Symptom Manage 1994;9:71-72.

92. American Medical Association. Healthcare Common Procedure Coding System. American Medical Association Healthcare Common Procedure Coding System Medicare's National Level II Codes HCPCS 2006. Available at: https://www.oxhp.com/secure/policy/trigger_point_injections_709.html.

93. Cummings TM, White AR. Needling therapies in the management of myofascial trigger point pain: a systematic review. Arch Phys Med Rehabil 2001;82:986-992.

CHAPTER 25

SIMON DAGENAIS
JOHN MAYER
SCOTT HALDEMAN
JOANNE BORG-STEIN

Prolotherapy

DESCRIPTION

Terminology and Subtypes

Intraligamentous injection of solutions aimed at promoting connective tissue repair is commonly known as prolotherapy, which has been defined as "the rehabilitation of an incompetent structure (such as a ligament or tendon) by the induced proliferation of new cells."[1] Common synonyms for this intervention include regenerative injection therapy, growth factor stimulation injection, nonsurgical tendon, ligament and joint reconstruction, proliferant injection, prolo, and joint sclerotherapy.[2] Proponents of this intervention generally dislike the term sclerotherapy, which is associated with the formation of unorganized scar tissue rather than the organized connective tissue that prolotherapy is intended to generate.[3,4]

Although there are no formal subtypes of prolotherapy, there is substantial heterogeneity in the treatment protocols used by different practitioners. The approaches to prolotherapy generally differ according to the type of solution injected, the volume and frequency of injections, and use of cointerventions. The method used in studies by Ongley and colleagues typically involves six weekly injections of 20 to 30 mL of a solution containing dextrose 12.5%, glycerin 12.5%, phenol 1%, and lidocaine 0.25% into multiple preselected lumbosacral ligaments.[5,6] Injections are usually accompanied by spinal manipulation therapy (SMT) and instructions for the patient to perform repeated standing lumbar flexion-extension exercises for several weeks. This approach may also use corticosteroid injections into tender lumbosacral areas before the first session of prolotherapy. This approach has occasionally been termed the Ongley approach or West Coast approach.

Prolotherapy methods used in other studies involved a greater number of injections at longer intervals (biweekly to monthly) with a smaller gauge needle, a lower injected volume (10 to 20 mL), and a solution containing only dextrose 10% to 20% and lidocaine 0.2% to 0.5%.[5-10] The rationale provided by proponents of this latter method is that it minimizes the inflammatory reaction and is therefore more easily tolerated by patients with severe pain. It should be noted that all methods of prolotherapy were developed clinically based largely on anecdotal evidence. Practitioners often further modify these interventions and cointerventions according to perceived patient needs.

History and Frequency of Use

Prolotherapy has been used to treat chronic low back pain (CLBP) for more than 60 years and was originally adapted from sclerotherapy, which involves injection of irritant solutions to induce acute inflammation, stimulate connective tissue growth, and promote formation of collagen tissue.[7,11] Sclerotherapy was commonly used to close the lumen in varicose veins, and in nonsurgical abdominal hernia repair.[8] Based on the hypothesis that joint hypermobility could be attributed to incomplete connective tissue repair after an injury (similar to hernias), this treatment approach was later applied to chronic musculoskeletal conditions suspected of being related to ligament or connective tissue laxity. The use of prolotherapy for CLBP was promoted in the 1950s by a surgeon named George S. Hackett, who published large case series claiming very high rates of success for a condition that had few effective surgical options at that time. A survey of 908 primary care patients receiving opioids for chronic pain, most commonly CLBP (38.4%), reported that 8.3% had used prolotherapy in their lifetime and that 5.9% had used it in the past year.[9] Those who reported using prolotherapy had an average of 3.5 injections in the past year, which corresponds with some of the commonly used protocols recommending injections every few months to achieve maximum benefits.

Practitioner, Setting, and Availability

Prolotherapy is mainly administered by medical or osteopathic physicians, although in rare instances a physician's assistant, nurse practitioner, or naturopath can administer injections where state licensure permits.[12] Practitioners who perform this treatment are expected to have advanced knowledge of spinal anatomy, including the attachment points for all connective tissue structures that may be injected, and the locations of any surrounding blood vessels or nerves that may be inadvertently injected. Extensive experience with spinal injections is usually recommended before learning prolotherapy and many clinicians who perform these treatments also have specialized training in anesthesiology, pain management, or physical medicine and rehabilitation.[12]

Additional postgraduate training specifically in prolotherapy is typically offered through continuing medical education courses sponsored by related organizations and medical schools, including the University of Wisconsin. Organizations involved in prolotherapy training include the American

Association of Orthopaedic Medicine (AAOM), American College of Osteopathic Sclerotherapeutic Pain Management (ACOSPM), Hackett Hemwall Foundation, and American Institute of Prolotherapy.[13-16]

In general, this treatment is performed in private clinics. It may occasionally be performed in an outpatient facility if radiologic guidance is required. Some practitioners prefer to administer oral or intravenous (IV) sedation before treatment to calm the patients and facilitate an otherwise uncomfortable procedure, which requires an ambulatory surgical center. Prophylactic oral analgesics may also be administered before the treatment instead of, or in addition to, sedation. This procedure is rarely performed in hospitals. Based on membership in related associations, it is estimated that there are approximately 500 to 1000 practitioners offering this treatment in private practices in various cities throughout the United States. Groups such as the AAOM and ACOSPM maintain on-line membership directories with contact information of practitioners who offer this treatment.

Procedure

The treatment procedure for prolotherapy varies a great deal among practitioners. The treatment typically begins with a thoroughly focused musculoskeletal history and physical, neurologic, and provocative manual examination of the area of complaint and surrounding joints and muscles. Once the assessment is completed and target structures are identified as amenable to prolotherapy injections, treatment may begin. For CLBP, treatment is usually conducted while the patient wears a medical gown and lies prone on a treatment table. Through manual palpation, the physician first identifies—and possibly indicates with a skin marker—anatomic landmarks in the lumbosacral spine area such as the iliac crest, sacroiliac (SI) joints, and intervertebral spaces to use as reference points for the injections. The skin is then cleaned with alcohol and betadine to minimize the risk of infection. Some practitioners first inject subcutaneous wheals of local anesthetic into the targeted areas to minimize patient discomfort.[6]

Prolotherapy injections are often administered with a fairly large 2.5- to 3-inch, 20 gauge spinal needle. This size of needle is preferred in order to deliver a bolus of somewhat viscous solution into targeted deep anatomic structures. The following areas are commonly injected for CLBP: posterior SI ligaments, iliolumbar ligaments, interspinous ligaments, supraspinous ligaments, and posterior intervertebral facet capsules (Figures 25-1 through 25-3). Some practitioners target ligaments that are tender to manual palpation or otherwise suspected of causing pain, whereas others prefer to inject all of the larger posterior ligaments that are easily accessible by injection and potentially associated with CLBP.[5,10]

To access these ligaments, the needle is typically inserted in the midline directly above an intervertebral space and oriented laterally to avoid accidentally injecting into the spinal canal (Figure 25-4). The needle is then inserted until the tip contacts bone and the plunger is partially withdrawn to confirm the absence of blood in the aspirate that would indicate possible blood vessel puncture. The desired bolus of solution, typically 0.5 to 2.0 mL, is then injected at each site.[6]

Practitioners often target several ligaments from a single needle insertion point by reorienting the needle in situ. The total amount of solution injected during one session of prolotherapy depends on the number of structures that are targeted and the bolus delivered to each structure; 10 to 30 mL is common. Radiologic guidance (e.g., fluoroscopy) is seldom used in prolotherapy.

After the injection procedure, the patient is briefly observed and then sent home with instructions to perform repetitive spinal range of motion (ROM) exercises, such as standing lumbar flexion and extension to maintain flexibility if the acute inflammation produced by the injections results in lumbosacral stiffness and soreness over the next few days. Patients are also advised to use over-the-counter (e.g., acetaminophen) or prescription (e.g., hydrocodone) analgesics as needed to control pain in the few days after the injections. Instructions are also instructed to avoid anti-inflammatory medication, because the acute inflammatory reaction provoked by this treatment is considered beneficial.[10]

This injection procedure is typically repeated weekly, biweekly, or monthly until six to eight treatments have been administered. Treatment intervals are dictated partially by patient response to treatment, partially by the recovery time required for any resulting acute inflammation to diminish before the next injection, and partially by practitioner preference. Patients may also require periodic injections beyond the initial course of six to eight treatments if their symptoms relapse or a reinjury occurs.

Regulatory Status

Drug solutions injected during prolotherapy are typically prepared by compound pharmacies or individual practitioners for specific patients; since they are not intended for resale or sold across state lines, they are generally not subject to close regulatory scrutiny by the US Food and Drug Administration (FDA). Although individual drug ingredients such as dextrose or lidocaine are approved for injection by the FDA, they are not approved specifically for this indication.

THEORY

Mechanism of Action

As with many other treatments available for CLBP, the mechanism of action for prolotherapy is not well understood. This treatment was derived from sclerotherapy for varicose veins, where injected irritants provoke a localized acute inflammatory reaction, connective tissue proliferation, and lumen closure. In prolotherapy, four types of solutions have been identified according to their suspected mechanism of action: (1) osmotic (e.g., hypertonic dextrose); (2) irritant/hapten (e.g., phenol); (3) particulate (e.g., pumice flour); and (4) chemotactic (e.g., sodium morrhuate).[17] Osmotics are thought to dehydrate cells, leading to cell lysis and release of cellular fragments, which attracts granulocytes and macrophages; dextrose may also cause direct glycosylation of cellular proteins.[17] Irritants possess phenolic hydroxyl groups that are

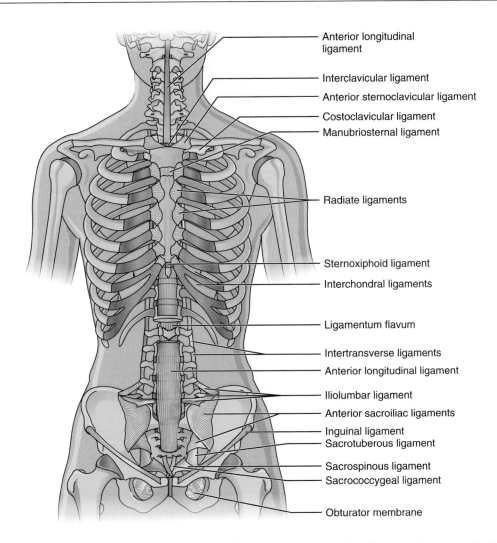

Figure 25-1 Lumbosacral ligaments targeted with prolotherapy injections: anterior view. (Modified from Muscolino JE. The muscle and bone palpation manual with trigger points, referral patterns, and stretching. St. Louis, 2009, Mosby.)

believed to alkylate surface proteins, which renders them antigenic or damages them directly, attracting granulocytes and macrophages.[17] Particulates are also believed to attract macrophages, leading to phagocytosis.[17] Chemotactics are structurally related to inflammatory mediators such as prostaglandins, leukotrienes, and thromboxanes, and are believed to undergo conversion to these compounds.[17]

Other mechanisms of action for prolotherapy that do not involve localized acute inflammation have also been proposed. For instance, macrophages that respond to particulates are believed to secrete polypeptide growth factor, leading to fibroplasia.[17] Other hypotheses include neurolysis of nociceptive fibers (denervation) associated with phenol, lysis of connective tissue adhesions because of the large volume of solution injected, and neovasculogenesis or neoneurogenesis during the inflammatory cascade.[18] A number of studies have been conducted in animals to elucidate the mechanism of action for solutions used in prolotherapy, including rat, guinea pig, and rabbit models.[2] In general, these studies involved ligament or tendon injections and histological or biomechanical examination of connective tissue.

For example, rabbit medial collateral ligament mass, thickness, and weight-to-length ratio increased significantly 7 weeks after 5% sodium morrhuate injections.[19] However, there were no differences in traumatized rat Achilles tendon tensile strength 7 weeks after injection of various solutions used in prolotherapy (e.g., dextrose, sodium morrhuate).[20] Other studies reported changes consistent with local acute inflammation.[2] In three patients with CLBP of suspected ligamentous origin, biopsies of posterior SI ligaments were taken 3 months after six weekly injections with dextrose 12.5%, glycerin 12.5%, phenol 1.25%, lidocaine 0.25%, SMT, and repeated trunk flexion exercises.[21] Electron microscopy revealed a significant increase in cellularity and active fibroblasts, with a 60% increase in average fiber diameter.[21]

Indication

This treatment is generally used for nonspecific mechanical CLBP resulting from suspected ligament or tendon injury due to trauma, repetitive sprain injury, or collagen deficiency.[21] It is challenging to identify this subgroup of CLBP patients, as

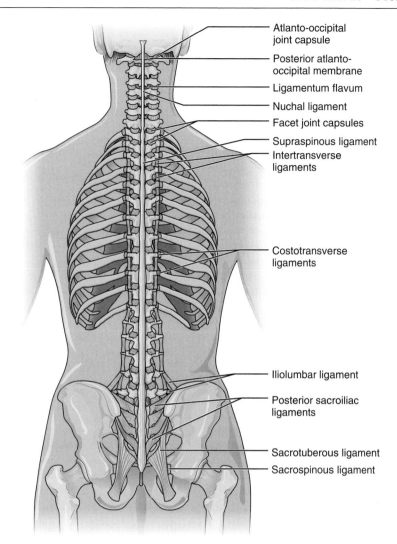

Atlanto-occipital
joint capsule

Posterior atlanto-
occipital membrane

Ligamentum flavum

Nuchal ligament

Facet joint capsules

Supraspinous ligament

Intertransverse
ligaments

Costotransverse
ligaments

Iliolumbar ligament

Posterior sacroiliac
ligaments

Sacrotuberous ligament

Sacrospinous ligament

Figure 25-2 Lumbosacral ligaments targeted with prolotherapy injections: posterior view. (Modified from Muscolino JE. The muscle and bone palpation manual with trigger points, referral patterns, and stretching. St. Louis, 2009, Mosby.)

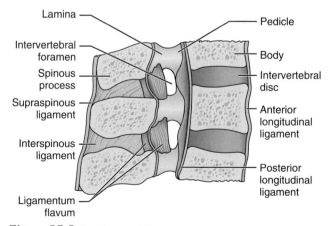

Lamina

Pedicle

Intervertebral
foramen

Body

Spinous
process

Intervertebral
disc

Supraspinous
ligament

Anterior
longitudinal
ligament

Interspinous
ligament

Posterior
longitudinal
ligament

Ligamentum
flavum

Figure 25-3 Lumbosacral ligament targeted with prolotherapy injections: lateral view. (Modified from Muscolino JE. Kinesiology: the skeletal system and muscle function, ed. 2. St. Louis, 2011, Mosby.)

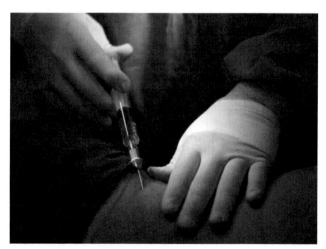

Figure 25-4 Prolotherapy injection technique requires careful needle placement. (© iStockphoto.com / Juanmonino.)

there are no direct, noninvasive methods of assessing lumbosacral ligament health. Diagnosis is therefore made on a clinical basis according to pain referral patterns, superficial ligament palpation, joint palpation, or history (e.g., pain aggravated by maintaining a position for extended periods). The identity of anatomic structures responsible for nociception may be confirmed by observing temporary pain relief after local anesthetic injections, although the presumption that these findings can be used to identify structures to be injected with prolotherapy has yet to be validated. As is often the case with other interventions, the indication for prolotherapy may be CLBP that has failed to respond to other, more conservative treatments. The ideal patient for this treatment, purely on the basis of anecdotal evidence, is an otherwise healthy adult aged 30 to 50 years with mechanical CLBP, no serious comorbidities, no psychopathology, signs and symptoms of lumbosacral ligament or tendon involvement, confirmation of pain structures by local anesthetic, and a positive but temporary response to manual therapy.

Assessment

Before receiving prolotherapy, patients should first be assessed for LBP using an evidence-based and goal-oriented approach focused on the patient history and neurologic examination, as discussed in Chapter 3. Clinicians should also inquire about medication history to note prior hypersensitivity/allergy or adverse events (AEs) with drugs similar to those being considered, and evaluate contraindications for these types of drugs. Diagnostic imaging or other forms of advanced testing is generally not required before administering prolotherapy for CLBP, although plain film radiography is often used to evaluate spinal anatomy and pathology before these injections.

EFFICACY

Evidence supporting the efficacy of this intervention for CLBP was summarized from recent clinical practice guidelines (CPGs), systematic reviews (SRs), and randomized controlled trials (RCTs). Observational studies (OBSs) were also summarized where appropriate. Findings are summarized by study design.

Clinical Practice Guidelines

Five of the recent national CPGs on the management of CLBP have assessed and summarized the evidence to make specific recommendations about the efficacy of prolotherapy injections.

The CPG from Belgium in 2006 did not recommend prolotherapy injections for the management of CLBP because the evidence of effectiveness is conflicting.[22]

The CPG from Europe in 2004 found strong evidence that prolotherapy injections into the ligaments of the lower back are not effective for managing CLBP.[23]

The CPG from Italy in 2007 did not recommend prolotherapy for CLBP, due to evidence of nonefficacy.[24]

TABLE 25-1	Clinical Practice Guideline Recommendations on Prolotherapy for Chronic Low Back Pain	
Reference	Country	Conclusion
22	Belgium	Conflicting evidence of benefit
23	Europe	Strong evidence that it is not effective
24	Italy	Not recommended
32	United Kingdom	Not recommended
25	United States	Strong evidence of no benefit

The CPG from the United Kingdom in 2009 did not recommend any injections for the management of CLBP, including prolotherapy injections.[32]

The CPG from the United States in 2009 found good evidence that prolotherapy injections are not effective for the management of CLBP.[25]

Findings from the above CPGs are summarized in Table 25-1.

Systematic Reviews

Cochrane Collaboration

Two reviews on prolotherapy injections for CLBP have been published by the Cochrane Collaboration, one by Yelland and colleagues[10] in 2004 and an update by Dagenais and colleagues[26] in 2007. Study eligibility for both reviews included RCTs and quasi-RCTs on prolotherapy for CLBP, and both reviews assessed study quality using Cochrane Back Review Group criteria. The efficacy results of prolotherapy for CLBP reported in the updated review were as follows: study protocols vary a great deal and results cannot easily be combined; there is a possible dose-response relationship with prolotherapy, because negative results were noted in two RCTs with lower doses of the administered drug (e.g., 3×10 mL) compared with three studies with higher doses (e.g., 6×20 to 30 mL); two RCTs with prolotherapy administered with cointerventions had positive results, whereas three RCTs with prolotherapy administered alone had negative results. Thus the authors concluded that there is no evidence of efficacy for prolotherapy alone, whereas there is some evidence of prolonged partial pain relief for prolotherapy combined with exercise, SMT, and other interventions.[26]

American Pain Society and American College of Physicians

An SR was conducted in 2008 by the American Pain Society and American College of Physicians CPG committee on nonsurgical therapies for acute and chronic LBP.[27] That review identified one SR related to prolotherapy, which was the Cochrane Collaboration review mentioned earlier.[26] No additional RCTs were identified. This SR concluded that there is good evidence that prolotherapy injections are not effective in managing CLBP.[27]

Other Reviews

A review was published in *The Spine Journal* by our group in 2005 and identified the same five RCTs that were uncovered in the updated review by the Cochrane Collaboration described earlier.[2] Two of those RCTs had positive results and noted improvements in pain or disability with 6 weekly sessions injecting 20 to 30 mL of solutions containing dextrose/glycerin/phenol/lidocaine, SMT, exercise, and other cointerventions.[5,6] Three RCTs had negative results and reported improvements but no differences between the prolotherapy and control groups: one study used only dextrose/lidocaine, one used only three sessions of dextrose/glycerin/phenol/lidocaine, and one study with a small sample size used dextrose/glycerin/phenol/procaine without SMT.[10] The review concluded that there was no evidence to support prolotherapy with dextrose alone. Furthermore, a dose-response relationship was postulated for solutions containing dextrose/glycerin/phenol/lidocaine, in which the lower doses (e.g., 3×10 mL) appeared to be less effective than the larger doses (e.g., 6×20 mL).

Findings from the above SRs are summarized in Table 25-2.

Randomized Controlled Trials

Five RCTs were identified.[5,6,10,28,29] Their methods are summarized in Table 25-3. Their results are briefly described here.

TABLE 25-2	Systematic Review Findings on Prolotherapy for Chronic Low Back Pain		
Reference	# RCTs in SR	# RCTs for CLBP	Conclusion
26	5	5	No evidence of efficacy for prolotherapy alone Evidence of partial pain relief when prolotherapy is combined with exercise, spinal manipulation therapy, and other interventions
27	1 SR, 5 RCTs	NR	Good evidence that prolotherapy is not effective in managing CLBP
2	5	5	No evidence to support prolotherapy with dextrose alone

CLBP, chronic low back pain; NR, not reported; RCT, randomized controlled trial; SR, systematic review.

In an RCT by Mathews and colleagues,[28] 22 individuals with CLBP were randomly assigned to receive prolotherapy (n = 16) or control (n = 6) injections. Prolotherapy injections consisted of a solution containing dextrose 10%, glycerin 10%, phenol 1%, and procaine 0.3%. There were 3 sessions injecting 10 mL every 2 weeks into lumbosacral ligaments. Control injections consisted of a solution containing 0.05% procaine, also with 3 sessions injecting 10 mL every 2 weeks into tender spots. Outcomes were assessed at 2 weeks and 1, 3, 6, and 12 months and included a 6-point numerical rating scale (1 to 4 designated as "not recovered" and 5 to 6 designated as "recovered"), pain intensity (visual analog scale [VAS]), and medication use. At 3 months, 10 out of 16 patients in the experimental group (63%) were recovered, compared with 2 out of 6 (33%) in the control group. There were no significant differences between the groups at the other follow-up points.

In an RCT by Ongley and colleagues,[5] 82 individuals with CLBP were randomly assigned to receive prolotherapy (n = 40) or control (n = 42) injections, along with various cointerventions. Prolotherapy injections for the experimental group consisted of a solution containing dextrose 12.5%, glycerin 12.5%, phenol 1.25%, and lidocaine 0.25%. There were 6 sessions injecting 20 mL every week into lumbosacral ligaments with IV sedation. Cointerventions included triamcinolone (50 mg) injection into the gluteus medius and SMT for the experimental group, lidocaine 0.5% injection and sham SMT for the control group, and standing lumbar flexion-extension stretching exercises for both groups. At 6 months, there were statistically significant differences ($P < .05$) for all outcomes in favor of the experimental group. Additionally, 35 of 40 (88%) patients in the experimental group had greater than 50% improvement in disability score at 6 months, compared with 16 of 41 (39%) patients in the control group ($P < .05$). Fifteen of 40 (38%) patients in the experimental group versus 4 of 41 (10%) patients in the control group had a disability score of 0 at 6 months ($P < .05$). Radiating leg pain present at baseline was resolved in 10 of 12 (83%) patients in the experimental group versus 2 of 12 (17%) patients in the control group ($P < .05$) at 6 months. Given the various cointerventions, however, it is difficult to attribute the positive outcomes of the experimental group to the prolotherapy injections rather than any other cointervention.

In an RCT by Klein and colleagues,[6] 79 individuals with CLBP were randomly assigned to receive prolotherapy (n = 39) or control (n = 40) injections. Prolotherapy injections for the experimental group consisted of a solution containing dextrose 12.5%, glycerin 12.5%, phenol 1.2%, and lidocaine 0.5%. There were 6 weekly sessions injecting 30 mL into lumbosacral ligaments, facet joints and SI joints, along with IV sedation and lidocaine wheals. Control injections consisted of a solution containing saline 0.45% and lidocaine 0.25%, along with IV sedation. Outcomes were assessed at 6 months and included the Roland Morris Disability Questionnaire, pain intensity (VAS), pain grid, lumbar ROM, lumbar isometric strength, and the proportion of subjects with greater than 50% improvement in disability and pain intensity. Both groups had significant improvement ($P < .05$) in pain intensity, pain grid scores, and disability at 6 months.

TABLE 25-3	Randomized Controlled Trials on Prolotherapy for Chronic Low Back Pain		
Reference	Indication	Intervention 1	Control
28	Local backache and local tenderness, LBP with neurologic involvement, symptoms >3 months	Injection prolotherapy: Dextrose 10% Glycerin 10% Phenol 1% Procaine 0.3% Administrator: NR 3 × 10 mL every 2 weeks into lumbosacral ligaments Cointervention: paracetamol 500 mg, spinal corset, posture/back care education n = 16	Injection trigger point: Procaine 0.5% Administrator: NR 3 × 10 mL every 2 weeks into tender spot Cointervention: paracetamol 500 mg, spinal corset, posture/back care education n = 6
5	CLBP, neurologic involvement NR, symptoms >1 year	Injection prolotherapy: Dextrose 12.5% Glycerin 12.5% Phenol 1.25% Lidocaine 0.25% Administrator: NR 6 × 20 mL weekly into lumbosacral ligaments IV sedation Cointervention: max 60 mL lidocaine into lumbosacral ligaments 50 mg triamcinolone in gluteus medius, SMT, standing lumbar flexion/extension 150×/day, return to full ADL, standing lumbar flexion/extension 4×/day, walking 1 mile 5×/week n = 40	Placebo injection: Saline 0.9% Administrator: NR 6 × 20 mL weekly into lumbosacral ligaments Cointervention: 10 mL lidocaine into lumbosacral ligaments, sham SMT, standing lumbar flexion/extension 150×/day, return to full ADL, standing lumbar flexion/extension 4×/day, walking 1 mile 5×/week n = 42
6	CLBP, neurologic involvement NR, symptoms >6 months	Injection prolotherapy: Dextrose 12.5% Glycerin 12.5% Phenol 1.2% Lidocaine 0.5% Administrator: NR 6 × 30 mL (max) weekly into lumbosacral ligaments, facets, sacroiliac joints, IV sedation Lidocaine wheals Cointervention: first intervention was triamcinolone injections into irritable foci if needed, NSAIDs/analgesics, acetaminophen/ice as needed n = 39	Placebo injection: Saline 0.45% Lidocaine 0.25% IV sedation Administrator: NR 6 × 30 mL (max) Cointervention: first intervention was triamcinolone injections into irritable foci if needed, NSAIDs/analgesics, acetaminophen/ice as needed n = 40
29	CLBP without neurologic involvement, symptoms >6 months	Injection prolotherapy: Dextrose 12.5% Glycerin 12.5% Phenol 1.2% Lidocaine 0.5% Administrator: NR 3 ×10 mL weekly into L4-L5 ligaments with single needle insertion point IV sedation Cointervention: NR n = 36	Placebo injection: Saline 0.45% Lidocaine 0.5% 3× weekly Administrator: NR Cointervention: NR n = 38
10	CLBP without neurologic involvement, symptoms >50% days past 6 months	Injection prolotherapy: Dextrose 20% Lidocaine 0.2% Administrator: NR 6 × 30 mL every 2 weeks into lumbosacral ligaments Cointervention: analgesics, heat, general activity, daily zinc, manganese, beta carotene, pyridoxine, vitamin C, no NSAIDs Exercise subgroup: standing lumbar flexion/extension 4×/day n = 54	Placebo injection: Saline 0.9% Administrator: NR 6 × 30 mL (max) every 2 weeks into lumbosacral ligaments Cointervention: analgesics, heat, general activity, daily zinc, manganese, beta carotene, pyridoxine, vitamin C, no NSAIDs Exercise subgroup: standing lumbar flexion/extension 4×/day n = 56

ADL, activities of daily living; CLBP, chronic low back pain; IV, intravenous; LBP, low back pain; NA, not applicable; NR, not reported; NSAIDs, nonsteroidal anti-inflammatory drugs; SMT, spinal manipulation therapy

When defining success with treatment as a 50% improvement in pain intensity or disability, 30 of 39 (77%) patients in the experimental group versus 21 of 40 (53%) patients in the control group were successful ($P < .05$).

In an RCT by Dechow and colleagues,[29] 74 individuals with CLBP who were referred by a general practitioner were randomly assigned to receive prolotherapy (n = 36) or control (n = 38) injections. Prolotherapy injections for the experimental group consisted of a solution containing dextrose 12.5%, glycerin 12.5%, phenol 1.2%, and lidocaine 0.5%. There were 3 sessions injecting 10 mL every week into L4-L5 ligaments with single needle insertion point, along with IV sedation. Control injections consisted of a solution containing saline 0.45% and lidocaine 0.5%. Outcomes were assessed at 1, 3, and 6 months and included the McGill Pain Questionnaire, ROM (modified Schober test), modified somatic perception questionnaire, modified Zung questionnaire, Oswestry Disability Index, pain grid, and pain intensity (VAS). At each follow-up time point, there were no significant differences between the treatment and control groups in any of the outcomes.

An RCT by Yelland and colleagues[10] was designed to concurrently assess the efficacy of prolotherapy and exercise. In this study, 110 individuals with CLBP were randomly assigned to one of four groups: prolotherapy injections with exercise (n = 28) or without exercise (n = 26), or control injection with exercise (n = 27) or without exercise (n = 29). Prolotherapy injections consisted of a solution containing dextrose 20% and lidocaine 0.2%. There were 6 sessions injecting a maximum of 30 mL every 2 weeks into lumbosacral ligaments. Control injections consisted of a solution containing saline 0.9%. Exercise consisted of standing lumbar flexion/extension stretches four times daily, whereas the nonexercise groups continued normal activity. Outcomes were assessed at 2.5, 4, 6, 12, and 24 months. At each follow-up time point, there were no significant differences in any of the outcomes between the study groups. In their analysis, the authors disregarded subgroup assignment to exercise or normal activity and compared groups who received prolotherapy with those who received saline injections.

SAFETY

Contraindications

Contraindications to prolotherapy include patients with nonmusculoskeletal CLBP (e.g., referred visceral pain), metastatic cancer, systemic inflammation, spinal anatomic defects that preclude deep injections (e.g., spina bifida), morbid obesity, inability to perform post-treatment ROM exercises, bleeding disorders, low pain threshold, chemical dependency, or whole body pain.[2] In addition, there is some indication from preclinical studies that very high doses of a prolotherapy solution containing dextrose 12.5%, glycerin 12.5%, phenol 1.0%, and lidocaine 0.25% may produce a temporary increase in hepatic enzymes such as alanine transaminase and aspartate aminotransferase.[30] Although these findings are preliminary, it may be prudent to not administer high doses of these solutions to patients with preexisting hepatic impairment. Practitioners often report that the predictors of negative outcomes with prolotherapy are similar to other treatments for CLBP, including tobacco use, obesity, unwillingness to perform back exercises, serious comorbidities, psychopathology, and an incorrect diagnosis.

Adverse Events

The most common AE related to prolotherapy is a temporary (12 to 96 hours postinjection) increase in pain and/or stiffness, which is consistent with the drug's purported mechanism of action involving acute inflammation.[12] In a recent survey of practitioners who performed prolotherapy (n = 171), AEs with the highest median estimated prevalence were pain (70%), stiffness (25%), and bruising (5%). Other AEs reported in the literature include transient leg pain, headache, nausea, diarrhea, minor allergic reactions, and other transient symptoms.[12]

Needlestick injuries associated with prolotherapy are similar to those reported with other spinal injection procedures.[12] There are previous reports of severe headache indicative of lumbar puncture, leg pain with neurologic features, disturbed sleep because of psychological trauma from injections, and severe cough.[12] A survey of practitioners who had each provided a median of 2000 prolotherapy treatments for spinal pain uncovered 470 AEs.[12] Of these, 70 were considered severe, including 65 that required hospitalization and 5 that resulted in permanent injury. The vast majority (80%) of AEs were related to needle injuries rather than drug toxicity. They included spinal headache (n = 164), pneumothorax (n = 123), nerve damage (n = 54), hemorrhage (n = 27), spinal cord insult (n = 7), and disc injury (n = 2). No fatalities related to this treatment have been reported in the literature since previous cases almost 50 years ago in which unspecified substances were inadvertently injected intrathecally.[2]

COSTS

Fees and Third-Party Reimbursement

In the United States, there is no CPT code designated specifically for prolotherapy. The Healthcare Common Procedure Coding System (HCPCS) code M0076 is available for reporting prolotherapy, defined as injection of sclerosing solutions into the joints, muscles, or ligaments in an attempt to increase joint stability. However, Medicare does not cover the service and states that the medical effectiveness of the therapy has not been verified by scientifically controlled studies; services are therefore denied on the grounds that they are not reasonable and necessary treatment.[31] An Advance Beneficiary Notice must be executed for a Medicare patient to pay for the service out of pocket. Other third-party payers may also consider prolotherapy to be investigational and should be contacted before billing to determine their policy for this service. The unlisted procedure CPT code 20999 with a description of the procedure clearly indicated on the claim may also be used for billing purposes.

Physicians who offer prolotherapy may choose not to bill third-party payers and simply charge a fee that must be paid out-of-pocket by the patient. A single treatment session typically costs $250 to $500. Other physicians who offer prolotherapy may choose to deliver it using related injection codes that describe various aspects of this procedure, including CPT code 20550 (injection, single tendon sheath or ligament), 20551 (injection, single tendon origin/insertion), 20552 (injection, trigger points in one to two muscles), or 27096 (injection, sacroiliac joint, unilateral). Anecdotally, the validity of this billing method has been questioned by some third-party payers as an attempt to circumvent noncoverage policies for HCPCS code M0076.

In some cases, prolotherapy may be covered by automobile insurance medical payment riders. A survey of patients with chronic pain (including CLBP) who had used prolotherapy reported that insurance coverage paid part of the cost in 88% of cases; the billing methods used by physicians for those patients were not reported.[9] Patients had paid some cost out-of-pocket in 19% of cases; mean out-of-pocket costs in the past year for prolotherapy were $365.[9]

Cost Effectiveness

No cost effectiveness analyses or cost utility analyses were identified which evaluated the cost effectiveness of prolotherapy as an intervention for LBP.

SUMMARY

Description

Prolotherapy is a procedure in which connective tissue repair is induced by injecting solutions into the ligaments, proliferating the growth of new cells. The treatment protocol used for prolotherapy is heterogeneous but one method commonly used in studies involves 6 weekly injections of 20 to 30 mL of a solution containing dextrose 12.5%, glycerin 12.5%, phenol 1%, and lidocaine 0.25% into multiple preselected lumbosacral ligaments. Prolotherapy has been used to treat CLBP for more than 60 years and is usually administered by medical or osteopathic physicians in private clinics. Physician assistants, nurse practitioners, or naturopaths may rarely perform prolotherapy where permitted, and these injections are typically performed in private practices.

Theory

As with many other treatments available for CLBP, the mechanism of action for prolotherapy is not well understood. This treatment was derived from sclerotherapy for varicose veins, where injected irritants provoke a localized acute inflammatory reaction, connective tissue proliferation, and lumen closure. In prolotherapy, four types of solutions have been identified according to their suspected mechanism of action: (1) osmotic (dehydrates cells), (2) irritant (alkylates surface proteins), (3) particulate (attracts macrophages), and (4) chemotactic (undergoes conversion to inflammatory mediators

such as prostaglandins, leukotrienes, and thromboxanes). Indications for prolotherapy include nonspecific mechanical CLBP resulting from ligament or tendon injury from trauma, repetitive sprain injury, or collagen deficiency. Diagnostic imaging or other forms of advanced testing is generally not required before administering prolotherapy for CLBP, although plain film radiography is often used to evaluate spinal anatomy and pathology before the injections.

Efficacy

Five CPGs assessed prolotherapy. One found conflicting evidence, one did not recommend any form of injection therapy, and three reported evidence of non-efficacy for CLBP. A Cochrane review concluded that the there is no evidence of efficacy for prolotherapy alone, whereas there is evidence of partial prolonged pain relief for prolotherapy combined with exercise, SMT, and other interventions. Another review concluded that there is good evidence that prolotherapy injections are not effective in managing CLBP. A third review concluded that there was no evidence to support prolotherapy with dextrose alone and that higher doses of prolotherapy solutions containing dextrose, glycerin, phenol, and lidocaine might be more effective than lower doses. At least five RCTs examined the efficacy of prolotherapy. Three of these observed no statistically significant differences between prolotherapy and comparator groups. However, one found a statistically significant improvement in pain versus comparator groups and another observed a statistically significant improvement in pain and function versus comparator groups.

Safety

Contraindications to prolotherapy include patients with nonmusculoskeletal CLBP (e.g., referred visceral pain), metastatic cancer, systemic inflammation, spinal anatomic defects that preclude deep injections (e.g., spina bifida), morbid obesity, inability to perform posttreatment ROM exercises, bleeding disorders, low pain threshold, chemical dependency, or whole body pain. In addition, there is some indication from preclinical studies that very high doses of a prolotherapy solution may produce a temporary increase in hepatic enzymes. AEs include increase in pain and/or stiffness, bruising, transient leg pain, headache, nausea, diarrhea, minor allergic reactions, and needlestick injuries (e.g., spinal headache, pneumothorax, nerve damage, hemorrhage, spinal cord insult, disc injury).

Costs

The cost per prolotherapy session ranges from $250 to $500. The cost effectiveness of prolotherapy is unknown.

Comments

Evidence from the CPGs, SRs, and RCTs reviewed is conflicting regarding the use of prolotherapy for CLBP. However, this intervention has a prolonged history of use, a reasonable but not proven theoretical basis, and generally favorable results in several OBSs. Prolotherapy may be beneficial for a small subgroup of patients with CLBP who fail to improve after conservative therapy, although this group remains difficult to define. If patients with CLBP are interested in trying prolotherapy, they should be advised about the potential AEs associated with this intervention.

A possible dose-response effect or the combination with other interventions such as SMT may explain the conflicting results of RCTs. Two of the RCTs in which prolotherapy was administered using 6 weekly injections of 20 to 30 mL dextrose/glycerin/phenol/lidocaine with SMT and exercise had positive results, suggesting that this particular intervention protocol is worth considering for patients with CLBP who are refractory to other approaches. Future studies are needed to support or refute the positive results obtained in some of the prior RCTs while addressing some of the methodologic weaknesses by minimizing differences between the intervention and control groups. Other studies are needed to establish the safety of common prolotherapy solutions and to determine the optimal dose and number of injection sessions required.

CHAPTER REVIEW QUESTIONS

Answers are located on page 452.

1. Which of the following ingredients is not generally used for prolotherapy?
   a. methylprednisone
   b. phenol
   c. dextrose
   d. glycerin
2. Which of the following is not a type of ingredient used in prolotherapy?
   a. osmotic
   b. particulate
   c. chemotactic
   d. analgesic
3. Which of the following is not a proposed mechanism of action for a prolotherapy ingredient?
   a. dehydrates cells
   b. attracts macrophages
   c. methylates surface proteins
   d. undergoes conversion to inflammatory mediators
4. True or false? Patients who wish to undergo prolotherapy treatments must first be tested for allergies to the injection ingredients.
5. Which of the following is generally not a contraindication to prolotherapy?
   a. chronic pain
   b. bleeding disorder
   c. morbid obesity
   d. spinal cord injury
6. For how many years has prolotherapy been used to treat CLBP?
   a. 10 years
   b. 25 years
   c. 50 years
   d. 60 years
7. True or false: Fluoroscopy is commonly used in prolotherapy.

REFERENCES

1. Gove P. Webster's Third new international dictionary, unabridged. Springfield, MA: Merriam-Webster; 2002.
2. Dagenais S, Haldeman S, Wooley JR. Intraligamentous injection of sclerosing solutions (prolotherapy) for spinal pain: a critical review of the literature. Spine J 2005;5:310-328.
3. Munavalli GS, Weiss RA. Complications of sclerotherapy. Semin Cutan Med Surg 2007;26:22-28.
4. Kim SR, Stitik TP, Foye PM, et al. Critical review of prolotherapy for osteoarthritis, low back pain, and other musculoskeletal conditions: a physiatric perspective. Am J Phys Med Rehabil 2004;83:379-389.
5. Ongley MJ, Klein RG, Dorman TA, et al. A new approach to the treatment of chronic low back pain. Lancet 1987;2:143-146.
6. Klein RG, Eek BC, DeLong WB, et al. A randomized double-blind trial of dextrose-glycerine-phenol injections for chronic, low back pain. J Spinal Disord 1993;6:23-33.
7. Hackett GS. Prolotherapy in whiplash and low back pain. Postgrad Med 1960;27:214-219.
8. Tisi PV, Beverley C, Rees A. Injection sclerotherapy for varicose veins. Cochrane Database Syst Rev 2006;(4):CD001732.
9. Fleming S, Rabago DP, Mundt MP, et al. CAM therapies among primary care patients using opioid therapy for chronic pain. BMC Complement Altern Med 2007;7:15.
10. Yelland MJ, Glasziou PP, Bogduk N, et al. Prolotherapy injections, saline injections, and exercises for chronic low-back pain: a randomized trial. Spine 2004;29:9-16.
11. Gedney EH. Hypermobile joint. Osteopathic Profession 1937;4.
12. Dagenais S, Ogunseitan O, Haldeman S, et al. Side effects and adverse events related to intraligamentous injection of sclerosing solutions (prolotherapy) for back and neck pain: a survey of practitioners. Arch Phys Med Rehabil 2006;87:909-913.
13. American Association of Orthopaedic Medicine. AAOM Organizational Statement. AAOM 2007. Available at: http://www.aaomed.org/Mission-Vision.php.
14. American College of Osteopathic Sclerotherapeutic Pain Management. What is sclerotherapy? ACOSPM 2007. Available at: http://www.acopms.com/.
15. The Hackett Hemwall Foundation. Welcome to the Hackett Hemwall Foundation. The Hackett Hemwall Foundation 2005. Available at: www.prolotherapy-hhf.org.
16. The American Institute of Prolotherapy. The American Institute of Prolotherapy 2007. Available at: www.prolotherapy-training.com.
17. Banks AR. A rationale for prolotherapy. J Orthop Med 1991;13:54-59.
18. Linetsky FS, Miguel R, Torres F. Treatment of cervicothoracic pain and cervicogenic headaches with regenerative injection therapy. Curr Pain Headache Rep 2004;8:41-48.
19. Liu YK, Tipton CM, Matthes RD, et al. An in situ study of the influence of a sclerosing solution in rabbit medial collateral ligaments and its junction strength. Connect Tissue Res 1983;11:95-102.
20. Harrison ME. The biomechanical effects of prolotherapy on traumatized Achilles tendons of male rats. Provo, UT: Brigham Young University; 1995.

21. Klein RG, Dorman TA, Johnson CE. Proliferant injections for low back pain: histologic changes of injected ligaments and objective measurements of lumbar spinal mobility before and after treatment. J Neurol Orthop Med Surg 1989;10: 123-126.

22. Nielens H, van Zundert J, Mairiaux P, et al. Chronic low back pain. Brussels, 2006, Report No.: KCE reports Vol 48C.

23. Airaksinen O, Brox JI, Cedraschi C, et al. European guidelines for the management of chronic nonspecific low back pain. Eur Spine J 2006;15:S192-S300.

24. Negrini S, Giovannoni S, Minozzi S, et al. Diagnostic therapeutic flow-charts for low back pain patients: the Italian clinical guidelines. Eura Medicophys 2006;42:151-170.

25. Chou R, Loeser JD, Owens DK, et al. Interventional therapies, surgery, and interdisciplinary rehabilitation for low back pain: an evidence-based clinical practice guideline from the American Pain Society. Spine 2009;34:1066-1077.

26. Dagenais S, Yelland MJ, Del MC, et al. Prolotherapy injections for chronic low-back pain. Cochrane Database Syst Rev 2007;(2):CD004059.

27. Chou R, Atlas SJ, Stanos SP, et al. Nonsurgical interventional therapies for low back pain: a review of the evidence for an American Pain Society clinical practice guideline. Spine 2009;34:1078-1093.

28. Mathews JA, Mills SB, Jenkins VM, et al. Back pain and sciatica: controlled trials of manipulation, traction, sclerosant and epidural injections. Br J Rheumatol 1987;26:416-423.

29. Dechow E, Davies RK, Carr AJ, et al. A randomized, double-blind, placebo-controlled trial of sclerosing injections in patients with chronic low back pain. Rheumatology (Oxford) 1999;38:1255-1259.

30. Dagenais S, Ogunseitan O, Haldeman S, et al. Acute toxicity pilot evaluation of proliferol in rats and swine. Int J Toxicol 2006;25:171-181.

31. Centers for Medicare and Medicaid Services. Decision memo for prolotherapy for chronic low back pain. 2010. Report No.: CAG-00045N, 2(4).

32. National Institute for Health and Clinical Excellence (NICE). Low back pain: early management of persistent non-specific low back pain. London: National Institute of Health and Clinical Excellence; 2009. Report No.: NICE clinical guideline 88.

NIKOLAI BOGDUK

CHAPTER 26

Lumbar Medial Branch Neurotomy

DESCRIPTION

Terminology and Subtypes

Lumbar medial branch neurotomy (LMBN) involves inserting a radiofrequency electrode onto particular lumbar medial branches to deliver an electric current that will coagulate sensory nerves, stop their conduction of nociceptive impulses, and thereby relieve pain thought to originate from the zygapophysial joints. Other terms have been used to describe LMBN, including *facet radiofrequency neurotomy, facet rhizotomy,* and *facet denervation;* these terms are incorrect because they refer to a different procedure with a discredited anatomic basis.[1,2] The two main types of LMBN are the Dutch technique and the Interventional Spine Intervention Society (ISIS) technique; each is briefly described below.

Lumbar medial branch blocks (LMBBs) are a diagnostic procedure used to identify candidates who may benefit from LMBN. Various terms are used to denote LMBBs, including *facet joint injections*, *facet intra-articular injections*, *facet intra-articular blocks*, *zygapophysial blocks*, and *zygapophysial injections.*

The term *facet joint* is an American neologism, coined in the 1970s when surgeons became interested in the small joints of the lumbar spine as a potential source of low back pain (LBP). However, these joints had already been given a formal name which had been in use for centuries and was endorsed by the International Anatomical Nomenclature Committee: *zygapophysial joints.*[3] That term was derived from the Greek words *zygos* (meaning yoke, connection, or bridge) and *physis* (meaning growth) because these joints are formed by the small growths that bridge consecutive vertebrae posteriorly.[4] A contraction for "zygapophysial joint" that has gained some popularity is "Z-joint." Although sometimes spelled "zygapophyseal," the correct spelling is "zygapophysial."[4]

History and Frequency of Use

Goldthwaite is sometimes credited for initiating interest in the lumbar Z-joints as a source of pain, but his study actually focused on their role in protecting the L5 vertebra from spondylolisthesis.[5] Other physicians and researchers early in the 20th century alluded to these joints indirectly when they attributed LBP to arthritis of the spine.[6,7] It was Ghormley who, in 1933, raised the clinical profile of the lumbar Z-joints by introducing oblique view x-rays of the lumbar spine to visualize these structures and observe degenerative changes that may occur as a result of osteoarthritis.[8] Interest in the Z-joints faded shortly thereafter when Mixter and Barr proposed that lumbar disc herniations were likely the cause of LBP.[9] Others tried to resurrect interest in the lumbar Z-joints during the 1940s, but the concept lay mostly dormant for another 30 years.[10]

Hirsch and colleagues then reported experiments in which noxious stimulation applied to the lumbar Z-joints produced pain in volunteers, but that work attracted little clinical interest.[11] More attention was paid in 1971 when Rees reported a success rate of 99.9% in treating LBP using an operation in which the nerves from the lumbar Z-joints could be transected percutaneously with a special scalpel blade.[12,13] Other surgeons attempted to reproduce these results but were unable to do so.[14-17] Anatomic studies eventually proved that the Rees procedure could not possibly denervate the Z-joints because their nerves were not located where the scalpel had been inserted.[18,19]

Nevertheless, Shealy became intrigued by the proposition that LBP arising from the Z-joints could be treated by denervating them, and developed a procedure by which the nerves from these joints could be coagulated percutaneously using a radiofrequency electrode similar to that used to treat trigeminal neuralgia. This procedure was called facet denervation, and several descriptive studies were published and reported generally successful results.[20-23] Others successfully adopted the Shealy procedure with equally positive outcomes.[24-40] However, subsequent anatomic studies reported that the anatomic basis of this procedure was flawed as there were no sensory nerves where the electrode was placed; this raised serious questions about the validity of the procedure.[1,2] These reports did not deter clinicians interested in using this procedure, and reports of its efficacy have continued to emerge even as recently as 1997.[41] Even a controlled trial purportedly showed positive results for a procedure with no anatomic basis.[42]

Notwithstanding the uncertainties about how to treat LBP associated with lumbar Z-joints, Mooney and Robertson demonstrated that these joints could be a source of LBP in normal volunteers and that certain patients could be relieved of their pain by anesthetizing these joints.[43] Other important findings in the history of this procedure were that pain from the Z-joints could be referred distally into the lower extremity and accompanied by hamstring tightness that limited straight-leg-raising, mimicking some of the features of sciatica. Findings of LBP being induced by Z-joint stimulation in normal volunteers were reproduced, with subsequent pain relief achieved by anesthetizing the joints.[44,45] These studies formed the basis for the concept of "facet syndrome" in LBP, which should more properly be referred to as "zygapophysial joint pain" or "Z-joint pain."

These developments prompted interest in the clinical diagnosis of lumbar Z-joint pain, the use of injection techniques for its diagnosis, and appropriate means of treatment in selected patients. Some investigators claimed that certain clinical features were indicative of lumbar Z-joint pain while others disagreed, but these studies used only single diagnostic blocks that did not control for false-positive responses.[46,47] Other studies using controlled diagnostic blocks reported that no clinical features were pathognomonic for the diagnosis of lumbar Z-joint pain, and that computed tomography (CT) was not able to make this diagnosis.[48-50] More recently, a set of decision rules was designed to diagnose lumbar Z-joint pain, but the positive predictive value of the rules was weak and achieved only weak diagnostic confidence.[51-53] Subsequent studies refuted these rules, which were also based on single diagnostic blocks.[54,55]

The failure of multiple studies to identify any clinical features that are indicative of lumbar Z-joint pain leaves LMBBs as the only reliable and valid method of identifying this entity in those with LBP. Although some physicians, particularly interventional radiologists, have advocated that Z-joint intra-articular injections could serve both diagnostic and therapeutic purposes, this procedure has never been tested for its validity as a diagnostic test.[56-70] In contrast, controlled diagnostic LMBBs have been validated and now constitute the best available method to identify lumbar Z-joint pain.

Practitioner, Setting, and Availability

LMBBs should only be performed by a trained physician able to interpret the patient's response in the context of the presenting complaint, history, and current psychosocial circumstances to determine if the patient is an appropriate candidate for LMBN. Physicians performing both LMBBs and LMBN should also be trained to recognize and deal with possible complications promptly. This training requires extensive knowledge of spinal anatomy to correctly guide and interpret the various radiographic views before and during the placement of the needle or electrode, and knowledge of how to adapt to local variations in anatomy to recognize procedural errors before incurring complications. ISIS has prescribed guidelines for how LMBBs and LMBN should be performed and regularly conducts postgraduate courses based on these guidelines.[71,72] These procedures can be performed in any facility that has a fluoroscopy suite, which is mandatory for the procedures to be accurate and valid. This limits the availability of LMBN to specialty spine clinics, pain management clinics, or hospitals.

Procedure

LMBN first requires that diagnostic LMBBs be conducted in order to identify patients with LBP who may benefit from this procedure; blocks are described below. LMBN requires placing a radiofrequency electrode parallel to the target nerve. This involves inserting the electrode from below, so that it crosses the neck of the superior articular process at the target level (Figure 26-1). A thermal lesion is generated by maintaining a temperature of 80° C to 85° C at tip of the electrode for 90 seconds. Depending on the gauge of the electrode used, and the length of its active tip, two or more lesions may need to be placed in various locations to accommodate possible variations in the exact location of the nerve. Details concerning how to place the electrode and perform

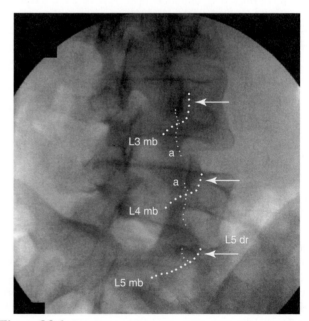

Figure 26-1 An oblique fluoroscopy view of the lower lumbar spine, on which have been depicted the courses of the L5 dorsal ramus (dr), the medial branches (mb) of L3, L4, and L5, and their articular branches (a). *Arrows* indicate the target points for medial branch blocks.

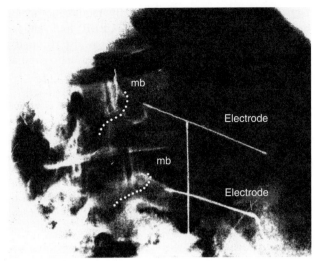

Figure 26-2 A reproduction of an illustration of electrodes in position for lumbar radiofrequency denervation, as depicted by Sluijter and Mehta.[73] The electrode position is as depicted in the original. Added are the courses of the medial branches (mb) at the levels targeted.

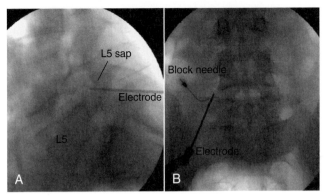

Figure 26-4 Radiographs of an electrode accurately placed on the L4 medial branch. The electrode crosses the neck of the superior articular process of L5.

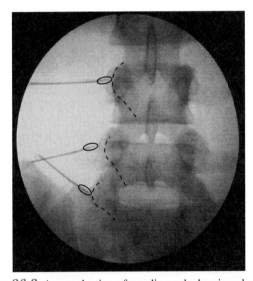

Figure 26-3 A reproduction of a radiograph showing electrodes in position for lumbar radiofrequency denervation, as depicted by van Wijk, et al.[74] Added to the illustration are the courses of the lumbar medial branches at the target levels and ellipses that estimate the size and location of the lesions made by the electrodes.

the procedure accurately and safely are described later in this chapter.[71]

Dutch Technique

Although the Dutch technique is widely practiced, materials to describe the procedure are unclear. For example, one illustration depicts electrodes placed on the tips of the transverse processes, nowhere near the target nerve (Figure 26-2). Another shows electrodes in positions where lesions would likely fail to incorporate the target nerve fully (Figure 26-3).

One version of the Dutch technique that appears anatomically accurate is that of van Kleef and colleagues,[75] but in this technique, the electrodes are placed perpendicular to the lumbar medial branches, which lessens the effectiveness of the procedure.

ISIS Technique

The technique promoted by the ISIS evolved from "facet denervation" through two modifications: (1) the electrodes are placed accurately on the target nerves; and (2) the electrodes are placed parallel to those nerves, rather than perpendicular (Figure 26-4).[71] Radiographic anatomy studies have shown that when placed in this manner the electrodes coagulate a substantial length of the target nerves, which correlates with the duration of relief obtained.[76]

Regulatory Status

The local anesthetics injected during LMBBs are regulated by the US Food and Drug Administration (FDA) and approved for related indications. The electrodes used during LMBN are generally regulated by the FDA as class II medical devices. Obtaining this approval mainly requires that the manufacturer submits evidence that the new device is substantially equivalent to a currently approved similar device.

THEORY

Mechanism of Action

LMBBs relieve pain through the action of local anesthetic on the sodium channels of the target nerve. The effect is temporary, and relates to the duration of action of the agent used. LMBN exerts a far more lasting effect because the nerve is physically altered. Histologically and physiologically, thermal coagulation at temperatures greater than 80° C affects motor fibers and sensory fibers of all calibers in a nonselective manner.[77,78] Coagulation denatures the nerve, and stops conduction of nociceptive traffic, thereby relieving pain. Although the nerve eventually regenerates, the rate of regeneration is slower following LMBN than after traumatic nerve injuries.

When nerves are transected, axon tubules regenerate within hours of the injury, cross the gap, and grow into the distal segment at a rate of 1 mm per day. In contrast, radiofrequency thermal coagulation (as performed in LMBN) seals the nerve in situ, providing no gap across which the nerve can regenerate. Before regeneration can occur into the distal segment, the coagulated segment must be repaired by endocellular processes, which may take several months. Because the time for repair is proportional to the length of segment coagulated, the duration of relief from pain is much longer if a longer length of nerve is coagulated. Because radiofrequency electrodes make small lesions beyond their tip but long lesions along their tip, longer pain relief occurs if electrodes are placed parallel to the nerve than if they are placed perpendicular to the nerve.[79]

Indication

The clinical indication for LMBBs is unresolved CLBP requiring further investigation, as determined by the physician, patient, and third-party payers (if any). This indication is tempered by the variable prevalence of Z-joint pain. Among injured workers with LBP, its prevalence was 15%, but other studies place the figure at less than 5%.[47,48,54,55,80] In older patients without a history of injury, the prevalence is higher, with approximately 30% of patients with LBP reporting at least 90% relief after placebo-controlled LMBBs.[81]

ISIS guidelines recommend that younger patients are far less likely to respond to LMBBs than older patients, and that physicians first consider discogenic pain or sacroiliac joint pain as an etiology for CLBP.[82] Furthermore, the protocol recommends that once LMBBs are initiated, a screening block of all levels liable to be symptomatic first be performed. This is intended promote efficiency and cost effectiveness. The pretest probability is that blocks at all levels will be negative. A single screening block will identify negative patients in one step, and obviates performing repeated blocks at multiple levels only to discover that all are negative. If a screening block is positive, repeat blocks at individual levels can be justified to establish one or more symptomatic joints. For LMBN, the singular indication is complete relief of pain after controlled, diagnostic LMBBs. The ideal patient for LMBBs is one with CLBP worthy of investigation, who has no other sources of pain, is older, and does not have any psychosocial comorbidity. The ideal patient for LMBN is one who tests positive to LMBBs.

Assessment

Before receiving LMBN, patients should first be assessed for LBP using an evidence-based and goal-oriented approach focused on the patient history and neurologic examination, as discussed in Chapter 3. Clinicians should also inquire about medication history to note prior hypersensitivity/allergy or adverse events (AEs) with drugs similar to those being considered, and evaluate contraindications for these types of drugs. Advanced diagnostic imaging such as CT or magnetic resonance imaging is typically required to rule out other potential anatomic causes of CLBP. Interventional diagnostic testing in the form of LMBBs is also required to identify appropriate candidates for this intervention and are described below.

Lumbar Medial Branch Blocks

LMBBs require depositing a small volume of local anesthetic accurately and safely onto each of the two nerves that innervate the target joint. A volume of 0.3 mL is sufficient and larger volumes do not improve the accuracy of the block; excess injectate leaves the vicinity of the target nerve. At typical lumbar levels, the target point lies on the neck of the superior articular process, which the medial branch crosses (see Figure 26-4B). At the L5 level, it is the L5 dorsal ramus, rather than the medial branch, that crosses the neck of the superior articular process of S1; and the dorsal ramus is the target nerve, not its medial branch. Two medial branches innervate each Z-joint but the segmental nomenclature is post-fixed.[83,84] For example, the L4-5 Z-joint is innervated by the L3 and L4 medial branches, and the L5-S1 joint by the L4,5 nerves. To avoid confusion in communications and records, ISIS recommends that hyphens between numbers (e.g., L2-3) be used to refer to joints, whereas commas (e.g., L2,3) refer to nerves.[85]

The technique for LMBBs has been described in detail elsewhere.[71] Essentially, under fluoroscopic guidance, a needle is introduced directly onto the target point for the nerve (Figure 26-5). Once the needle has been correctly placed, a test dose of contrast medium is injected to test for venous uptake. In the absence of venous uptake, 0.3 mL of local anesthetic agent is injected. The procedure is repeated for each of the nerves that need to be blocked. For blocks to be valid, they must be performed under controlled conditions in each and every patient. Single diagnostic blocks are not

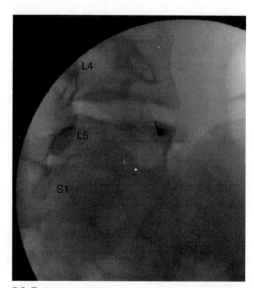

Figure 26-5 Oblique fluoroscopy view showing a needle in position to block the L4 medial branch where it crosses the L5 transverse process. The white dot marks the target point for an L5 dorsal ramus block.

valid and carry a false-positive rate of between 25% and 41%.[86-89]

In the past, comparative local anesthetic blocks have been used to serve as controlled blocks; this involves performing the same block on two separate occasions but using a different local anesthetic agent on each occasion. A positive response is defined as complete relief of pain after each block for the duration of action of the agent used.[72,86,87] A recent analysis, however, has shown that comparative local anesthetic blocks are not valid for the diagnosis of lumbar Z-joint pain.[90] Comparative blocks have a sensitivity of 100% but a specificity of only 65%.[86,90] When the prevalence of lumbar Z-joint pain is low, a specificity of 65% results in a prohibitively high incidence of false-positive responses, far in excess of the prevalence of the condition. Depending on the exact prevalence, for every true-positive response there will be two, three, or more false-positive responses, and the operator cannot tell which is which.[90] In effect, operators who rely on comparative blocks will be wrong in their diagnosis far more often than they will be correct.

Placebo-controlled LMBBs are the only means by which to secure confidence in a diagnosis of lumbar Z-joint pain.[90] These require blocks on each of three occasions. On the first occasion, a local anesthetic agent is used, in order to establish, prima facie, that the target joint is symptomatic. The second block should use either a local anesthetic agent or a placebo, randomly assigned on a double-blind basis. The third block uses the agent not used for the second block. A positive response is complete relief whenever a local anesthetic is used, and no relief when placebo is used.

ISIS guidelines require that patients be evaluated for a minimum of 2 hours after the block, or until pain relief ceases, whichever occurs first.[72] Relief of pain must be recorded in terms of a visual analog scale (VAS) or numerical pain rating scale. Moreover, the relief should be corroborated by the restoration of activities that previously were precluded or limited by pain. Optimally, the physical response should be accompanied by a narrative record of how the patient described and valued the relief.

The optimal criterion for a positive response is complete relief of pain, though anecdotal experience suggests this rarely happens in practice in patients with CLBP in the United States. As an alternative, 80% pain relief is generally accepted, provided that it is corroborated by restoration of activities, and the patient is spontaneously complimentary about the relief that they obtain. Although some clinicians accept only 50% pain relief as a positive response, this is not recommended and may falsely identify candidates for LMBN when the patient's pain in fact arises from other sources.

It has never been shown that patients commonly have multiple sources of pain, and that a 50% relief after LMBB can be a valid sign of lumbar Z-joint pain. Studies have indicated that in patients with CLBP, the prevalence of combined discogenic and Z-joint pain, or sacroiliac joint and Z-joint pain, is less than 5%.[91,92] When a pain source can be detected, it is typically one or the other of these structures. Under those conditions, 50% relief of pain is at best a spurious response, and cannot be held as a positive response. The notion of multiple, simultaneous sources of pain can be

TABLE 26-1	Clinical Practice Guideline Recommendations on Lumbar Medial Branch Neurotomy for Chronic Low Back Pain	
Reference	Country	Conclusion
93	Belgium	Low-quality and conflicting evidence to support efficacy
94	Europe	Not recommended
95	United Kingdom	Not recommended
96	United States	Insufficient evidence to make a recommendation

sustained only if simultaneous anesthetization of the Z-joints and the other source of pain completely relieves the patient's pain.

EFFICACY

Evidence supporting the efficacy of this intervention for CLBP was summarized from recent clinical practice guidelines (CPGs), systematic reviews (SRs), and randomized controlled trials (RCTs). Observational studies (OBSs) were also summarized where appropriate. Findings are summarized by study design.

Clinical Practice Guidelines

Four of the recent national CPGs on the management of CLBP have assessed and summarized the evidence to make specific recommendations about the efficacy of facet rhizotomy.

The CPG from Belgium in 2006 found low-quality and conflicting evidence to support the efficacy of facet rhizotomy for the management of CLBP.[93]

The CPG from Europe in 2004 found conflicting evidence that facet rhizotomy is more effective than placebo for the management of CLBP.[94] That CPG also found limited evidence that intra-articular facet rhizotomy is more effective than extra-articular facet rhizotomy. That CPG did not recommend facet rhizotomy in the management of CLBP.

The CPG from the UK in 2009 found limited and conflicting evidence to support the efficacy of facet rhizotomy in the management of CLBP.[95] That CPG did not recommend facet rhizotomy for CLBP.

The CPG from the US in 2009 found insufficient evidence to make a recommendation about the use of facet rhizotomy in the management of CLBP.[96]

Findings from these CPGs are summarized in Table 26-1.

Systematic Reviews

Cochrane Collaboration

In 2002, the Cochrane Collaboration conducted an SR on radiofrequency denervation for neck pain and LBP.[97] It identified three RCTs related to lumbar medial branch radiofrequency denervation for patients with CLBP.[42,75,98] This Cochrane review concluded that there is conflicting evidence for short-term pain relief and improvement in disability for radiofrequency denervation in CLBP presumed to originate from the facet joints.[97] The review recommended that more RCTs be conducted in the future with larger samples to examine the long-term effectiveness of radiofrequency denervation for CLBP.

American Pain Society and American College of Physicians

In 2008, the American Pain Society and the American College of Physicians committee on nonsurgical therapies conducted a SR for acute and chronic LBP.[99] That review identified six SRs related to radiofrequency denervation, including the Cochrane Collaboration review mentioned earlier.[94,100-104] Four of the SRs concluded that there was inconsistent evidence supporting facet neurotomy, whereas one SR concluded that moderate evidence supports facet neurotomy.[100-104] These SRs included the three RCTs identified in the Cochrane review described earlier and two additional RCTs that pertained to LMBN.[42,75,98,105,106] Owing to conflicting results, this SR was unable to make definitive conclusions about radiofrequency denervation for patients with CLBP.

Other

Two other reviews have also been conducted on this topic.[100,101] These reviews were based on three randomized controlled studies.[42,75,98] Both reviews concluded that there was insufficient evidence to make any recommendations about the efficacy of LMBN.

A narrative review had previously pointed out that previous reviews did not take into account patient selection and accuracy of surgical technique when evaluating evidence from RCTs, a view also articulated by others.[107-110] Reviews based on the negative results of studies that used inadequate, erroneous, or discredited surgical techniques can lead to conflicting or inconclusive findings. A different evaluation arises if only those RCTs where appropriately selected patients who responded to LMBBs, and subsequently used correct surgical techniques to perform LMBN. Under those conditions, the eligible RCTs generally corroborate the favorable outcomes reported by eligible OBSs.[73,105,106,111-113]

Findings from the above SRs are summarized in Table 26-2.

Randomized Controlled Trials

Five RCTs were identified.[42,75,98,105,106] The methods of these RCTs are summarized in Table 26-3 and their results are briefly described here. However, two of these RCTs are not valid tests of LMBN as mentioned above.[42,98]

Using Incorrect Technique

Leclaire and colleagues conducted an RCT of radiofrequency joint denervation for CLBP.[98] In order to be included, participants had to have LBP for more than 3 months, and a good response to LMBB, defined as significant relief of LBP for at least 24 hours the week after their diagnostic block. Percutaneous radiofrequency neurotomy was compared to a

TABLE 26-2	Systematic Review Findings on Lumbar Medial Branch Neurotomy for Chronic Low Back Pain		
Reference	# RCTs in SR	# RCTs for CLBP	Conclusion
97	9	NR	Conflicting evidence for short-term pain relief and improvement in disability for radiofrequency denervation in CLBP
99	6 SRs	NR	Due to conflicting results, this SR was unable to make definitive conclusions about radiofrequency denervation for patients with CLBP

CLBP, chronic low back pain; NR, not reported; RCT, randomized controlled trial; SR, systematic review.

sham procedure in which the electrode was placed at the desired location but its temperature was not elevated. After 12 weeks, there were no differences between the two groups in pain (VAS) or physical function (Roland Morris Disability Questionnaire, Oswestry Disability Index). However, participants in this study were not selected on the basis of appropriate diagnostic LMBB as described above, and the intervention used an anatomically inaccurate surgical technique.[107]

Gallagher and colleagues[42] conducted an RCT of radiofrequency joint denervation for individuals with lumbar Z-joint pain. To be included, participants were required to experience LBP, with or without neurologic involvement, for more than 3 months. Patients in the intervention group included those experiencing a good or equivocal response to a diagnostic block who were then treated with radiofrequency joint denervation. The control group received sham radiofrequency denervation. After 6 months of follow-up, no statistically significant improvement in pain relief was observed between the intervention and control groups. However, the intervention in this study used the discredited facet denervation technique of Shealy described above.[107]

Using Correct Technique

The study of van Kleef and colleagues used a suboptimal surgical technique that was not inaccurate but which would limit the duration of effect because the electrode was placed perpendicular rather than parallel to the targeted nerve.[75,107] Nevertheless, it did show that at 8 weeks, active LMBN reduced pain, improved disability, and reduced use of analgesics significantly more than sham LMBN. More convincingly, survival analysis showed that a significantly greater proportion of patients had prolonged relief of pain beyond 8 weeks after active LMBN than the sham approach.

Using a meticulous surgical technique, the study of Nath and colleagues[105] addressed the treatment of LBP in

TABLE 26-3	Randomized Controlled Trials of Lumbar Medial Branch Neurotomy for Chronic Low Back Pain		
Reference	Indication	Intervention	Control
Using Incorrect Technique			
98	CLBP with positive lumbar medial branch block, with or without neurologic involvement, symptoms >3 months	Radiofrequency denervation Physiatrist 1 session Cointervention: medication, physical or manual therapy n = 36	Sham denervation Physiatrist 1 session Cointervention: medication, physical or manual therapy n = 34
42	Lumbar zygapophysial joint pain, with or without neurologic involvement, symptoms >3 months	Radiofrequency denervation Administrator: NR 1 session Cointervention: NR n = 24	Sham radiofrequency denervation Administrator: NR 1 session Cointervention: NR n = 17
Using Correct Technique			
75	CLBP without neurologic involvement, symptoms >1 year; relief from a single medial branch block	Radiofrequency neurotomy Specialist pain Anesthesiologist 1 session Cointervention: NR n = 15	Sham denervation Specialist pain Anesthesiologist 1 session Cointervention: NR n = 16
105	CLBP with or without neurologic involvement, symptoms >2 years; relief from controlled medial branch blocks	Radiofrequency denervation Specialist pain Anesthesiologist 1 session Cointervention: medication n = 20	Sham denervation Specialist pain Anesthesiologist 1 session Cointervention: medication n = 20
106	CLBP without neurologic involvement, symptoms >6 months; relief from single medial branch block	Thermal medial branch neurotomy Anesthesiologist 1 session Cointervention: NSAIDs n = 20	Pulsed radiofrequency Anesthesiologist 1 session Cointervention: NSAIDs n = 20

CLBP, chronic low back pain; NR, not reported; NSAIDs, nonsteroidal anti-inflammatory drugs.

patients who had other, concurrent pain problems. These comorbitities likely interfered with reported improvements in disability and other outcomes. Nevertheless, active LMBN achieved significantly greater improvements in LBP, and greater reductions in use of analgesics than sham LMBN.

Tekin and colleagues[106] compared the outcomes of thermal radiofrequency LMBN with those of pulsed radiofrequency LMBN, for which there is no evidence of efficacy and which constitutes a suitable sham treatment. Thermal radiofrequency LMBN achieved significantly greater improvements in pain, disability, and reduced use of analgesics than the sham approach.

Among the three studies described above,[75,105-107] there is no inconsistency in their results. To various degrees, all reported that active LMBN was superior to sham treatment. No other study using correct LMBN technique can refute these consistent results.

Observational Studies

Medial Branch Blocks
LMBBs are the single most validated diagnostic test in interventional pain medicine. It has been shown that the injectate does not spread to other adjacent structures, provided that correct techniques are used.[114] LMBBs protect normal volunteers from experimentally induced lumbar Z-joint pain.[111] Controlled blocks can be used to minimize the possibility of false-positive responses.[87]

Medial Branch Neurotomy
One study in which anatomically accurate technique was used showed that 80% of patients obtained at least 60% relief of their pain, and 60% of patients obtained at least 80% relief, lasting at least 12 months after treatment.[115] These data in isolation do not establish that LMBN is effective, but they do indicate what the outcomes can be when patients are correctly selected using controlled LMBBs, and when anatomically accurate technique is used. Relief after LMBN typically lasts between 6 and 12 months.[116] Pain recurs when the nerves regenerate, but relief can be reinstated by repeat LMBN.[116] Successful treatment repeated two and three times has been reported, and no limit has yet been established as to the number of times that the procedure can be successfully repeated to maintain relief of pain.[116]

Other OBSs attest to long-term success rates of about 50%.[112,113] Relief of pain is accompanied by reduced disability and reduced use of analgesics.

SAFETY

Contraindications

Contraindications to LMBBs and LMBN include allergy to the local anesthetic, any anatomic abnormality that precludes safe administration of the needle or electrode, pregnancy, and concurrent illness that renders the procedure unsafe.

Poor outcomes for LMBN can likely be anticipated in patients who do not achieve complete or substantial pain relief following properly conducted LMBBs.

Adverse Events

If correctly performed by highly skilled and experienced practitioners in well selected patients, LMBBs should not result in any AEs.[117] Potential AEs that could occur as a result of incorrect needle placement during LMBBs may lead to the types of injuries commonly reported with other injection procedures performed in the lumbar spine, such as dural puncture, spinal cord injury, infection, intravascular injection, spinal anesthesia, chemical meningitis, nerve injury, facet capsule rupture, hematoma formation, and facet joint septic arthritis. However, it should be stated that such serious AEs have previously been misattributed to LMBBs when they were in fact related to other procedures, such as intra-articular Z-joint injections.[94,118] Although guided LMBBs involve ionizing radiation, the amount of radiation exposure is quite small.

For LMBN, minor and major AEs may occur. Even when electrodes are correctly placed, some patients may experience temporarily increased postoperative pain. Variously this has been attributed to neuritis or inflammation around the site of the lesion. Its actual basis has never been established. Major AEs can rarely arise if electrodes are not correctly placed. Such AEs have occurred when the procedure was performed under general anesthesia, under which conditions the patient cannot warn of impending misadventure, when the electrodes were placed in grossly erroneous positions, such as onto a dorsal root ganglion, and when the electrode position was not monitored during coagulation and allowed to slip over the transverse process where it contacted a ventral ramus, resulting in weakness and numbness in the lower limb.[117]

COSTS

Fees and Third-Party Reimbursement

In the United States, LMBBs may be delivered by physicians using CPT codes 64493 (injections, paravertebral facet joint with image guidance; single level), 64494 (injections, paravertebral facet joint with image guidance; second level, to be listed in addition to 64493 code for primary procedure), or 64495 (injections, paravertebral facet joint with image guidance; third level, to be listed in addition to 64493 and 64494 codes). CPT guidelines were modified in 2010 and now state that image guidance (fluoroscopy or CT) and any injection of contrast are inclusive components of 64493-64495. If ultrasound guidance is used, the CPT code 64999 may be used. LMBN may be delivered by physicians using CPT codes 64622 (destruction by neurolytic agent, paravertebral facet joint, single level), or 64623 (destruction by neurolytic agent, paravertebral facet joint nerve; additional level, to be listed in addition to 64622 code for primary procedure); CPT code 77003 (fluoroscopic guidance) may also be used.

Disposable medical equipment, needles and syringes, used in conjunction with these procedures are included in the practice expense for these procedures. Additional fees will apply for the medications injected and should be reported using the appropriate Healthcare Common Procedure Coding System drug code to be submitted on the same claim.[119] The outpatient surgical center in which the procedure takes place will also charge facility fees for use of their operating room, recovery room, other disposable medical equipment, nurses, radiology, and other services. Because of these ancillary fees, the total cost of LMBN can reach $3000 or more, although there is wide variation in fees.

These procedures may be covered by other third-party payers such as health insurers and worker's compensation insurance. Medicare has coverage guidelines which are supported by Local Coverage Determination (LCD) policies implemented by Medicare Administrative Contractors. It is recommended that these policies be referenced for the most current information. The most current LCD referenced (effective 1/1/2010) provides a list of ICD-9 codes that support medical necessity of these procedures.[120] The patient's medical record must contain documentation that fully supports the medical necessity of these services.

Although some payers continue to base their reimbursements on usual, customary, and reasonable payment methodology, the majority have developed reimbursement tables based on the Resource Based Relative Value Scale used by Medicare. Reimbursement by other third-party payers is generally higher than Medicare. Pre-authorization may be required to obtain reimbursement from third-party payers, which generally indicates that patients and physicians must adhere to specific criteria in order to deem the procedure medically necessary.

By way of comparison, the fee for LMBB in Australia is $94.50 under its Medicare program and $225 under the Australian Medical Association fee schedule. The fee in Australia for LMBN is $258 under its Medicare program and $655 under the Australian Medical Association fee schedule. In both cases, additional fees apply for fluoroscopy.

Typical fees reimbursed by Medicare in New York and California for these services are summarized in Table 26-4.

Cost Effectiveness

No cost effectiveness analyses or cost utility analyses were identified which evaluated the cost effectiveness of LMBN as an intervention for LBP.

TABLE 26-4	Medicare Fee Schedule for Related Services	
CPT Code	New York	California
Lumbar Medial Branch Blocks		
64493	$171	$188
64494	$87	$94
64495	$88	$96
Lumbar Medial Branch Neurotomy		
64622	$323	$354
64623	$120	$132
77003	$61	$66

2010 Participating, nonfacility amount.

The CPG from Europe in 2004 indicates that the cost effectiveness of facet joint injections for CLBP (>3 months) is unknown.[94]

Other

Some practitioners, and many insurers, argue that multiple controlled blocks are not cost effective and refuse reimbursement. However, a modeling study has shown that controlled LMBBs are indeed cost effective by helping to avoid the short term and long term direct and indirect costs of a false-positive diagnosis and subsequent LMBN.[121]

SUMMARY

Description

LMBN involves inserting a radiofrequency electrode onto particular lumbar medial branches to deliver an electric current that will coagulate sensory nerves, stop the conduction of nociceptive impulses, and thereby relieve pain thought to originate from the Z-joints. This procedure should only be performed by a trained physician in a facility that has a fluoroscopy suite, such as specialty spine clinics, pain management clinics, or hospitals.

Theory

The clinical indication for LMBB is unresolved CLBP requiring further investigation, as determined by the physician, patient, and third-party payers. The indication for LMBN is patients whose pain has been relieved by controlled, diagnostic LMBBs. Concerns have been raised about the validity of single and comparative LMBBs. Placebo-controlled LMBBs are the optimal means of securing a firm diagnosis of lumbar Z-joint pain.

Efficacy

Four CPGs found conflicting, limited, or insufficient evidence supporting the use of LMBN. A Cochrane review and three other SRs reached the same conclusion. Only one SR concluded that there is moderate evidence supporting LMBN. However, these CPGs and SRs included studies that used inappropriately selected patients or incorrect surgical techniques for LMBN and consequently reported negative results. When considering only those studies that used adequately selected participants and correct LMBN techniques, results have shown that LMBN achieves statistically greater improvements in pain, disability, and use of analgesics than sham treatment both in the short-term and for up to 1 year after treatment.

Safety

Contraindications to LMBBs and LMBN include pregnancy, allergy to local anesthetic, any anatomic abnormality that precludes safe placement of a needle or electrode, or concurrent illness that renders the procedure unsafe. Potential AEs may occur during LMBBs or LMBN if the needle or electrodes are misplaced, which could result in injury to a spinal nerve root or ventral ramus.

Costs

The costs of LMBBs and LMBN vary, but can be as high as $3000 per procedure owing to facility fees. The cost effectiveness of LMBN is unknown.

Comments

LMBN is the only intervention that has been tested for pain shown to originate from the lumbar Z-joints through controlled diagnostic LMBBs, and is the only treatment shown to be able to eliminate or substantially reduce this pain, improve disability, and reduce the use of analgesics. No other intervention has been shown to achieve similar outcomes for that small subgroup of patients with CLBP shown to arise from the Z-joints. Not all practitioners use LMBBs correctly, and not all use the correct surgical techniques that have been validated in the literature for LMBN. Patients interested in trying LMBN should be advised as to whether the procedure will be performed in accordance with the best available published evidence.

CHAPTER REVIEW QUESTIONS

Answers are located on page 452.
1. Which of the following is generally required before performing LMBN?
   a. epidural steroid injection
   b. opioid analgesics
   c. lumbar medial branch block
   d. radicular pain
2. What is the estimated rate of false-positive results with single medial branch blocks?
   a. 10% to 15%
   b. 15% to 26%
   c. 25% to 41%
   d. 44% to 56%

3. Which of the following outcome measures is often used after a medial branch block?
   a. brief pain inventory
   b. VAS
   c. McGill pain questionnaire
   d. pain diagram

4. Historically, which event was critical to raising the concept that the zygapophysial joints might be a source of LBP?
   a. Mixter and Barr's introduction of disc herniation as a cause of LBP
   b. Ghormley's introduction of the oblique view of the lumbar spine
   c. Shealy's invention of radiofrequency neurotomy
   d. the perfection of the Dutch technique

5. Which of the following is critical in order for diagnostic blocks to be considered valid?
   a. they must be cost effective
   b. they must be delivered at L4 and L5
   c. they must be administered according to the protocols outlined in the Dutch technique
   d. they must be very specific and controlled

6. What diagnostic test is generally ordered before lumbar medial branch neurotomy?
   a. MRI or CT
   b. discography
   c. EMG or NCV
   d. x-rays

7. True or false: Fluoroscopy should be used to guide the diagnostic medial branch blocks?

8. True or false: CPGs consistently recommend LMBN.

REFERENCES

1. Bogduk N, Long DM. The anatomy of the so-called "articular nerves" and their relationship to facet denervation in the treatment of low-back pain. J Neurosurg 1979;51: 172-177.
2. Bogduk N, Long DM. Percutaneous lumbar medial branch neurotomy: a modification of facet denervation. Spine 1980;5:193-200.
3. Warwick R. Nomina anatomica. Edinburgh: Churchill Livingstone; 1989.
4. Bogduk N. On the spelling of zygapophysial and of anulus. Spine 1994;19:1771.
5. Goldthwait JE. The lumbosacral articulation: an explanation of many cases of lumbago, sciatica, and paraplegia. Boston Med Surg J 1911;164:365-372.
6. Key JA. Low back pain as seen in an orthopedic clinic. Am J Med Sci 1924;169:526.
7. Ayers CE. Lumbo-sacral backache. N Engl J Med 1929;200: 592-608.
8. Ghormley RK. Low back pain with special reference to the articular facets with presentation of an operative procedure. JAMA 1933;101:1773-1777.
9. Mixter WJ, Barr JS. Rupture of the intervertebral disc with involvement of the spinal canal. N Engl J Med 1934;211: 210-215.
10. Badgley CE. The articular facets in relation to low-back pain and sciatic radiation. J Bone Joint Surg 1941;23:481.
11. Hirsch C, Ingelmark BE, Miller M. The anatomical basis for low back pain. Studies on the presence of sensory nerve endings in ligamentous, capsular and intervertebral disc structures in the human lumbar spine. Acta Orthop Scand 1963;33:1-17.
12. Rees WES. Multiple bilateral subcutaneous rhizolysis of segmental nerves in the treatment of the intervertebral disc syndrome. Ann Gen Pract 1971;16:126.
13. Rees WS. Multiple bilateral percutaneous rhizolysis. Med J Aust 1975;1:536-537.
14. Brenner L. Report on a pilot study of percutaneous rhizolysis. Bulletin of the Postgraduate Committee in Medicine 1973;29:203-206.
15. Toakley JG. Subcutaneous lumbar "rhizolysis"—an assessment of 200 cases. Med J Aust 1973;2:490-492.
16. Houston JR. A study of subcutaneous rhizolysis in the treatment of chronic backache. J R Coll Gen Pract 1975;25: 692-697.
17. Collier BB. Treatment for lumbar sciatic pain in posterior articular lumbar joint syndrome. Anaesthesia 1979;34: 202-209.
18. Bogduk N, Colman RR, Winer CE. An anatomical assessment of the "percutaneous rhizolysis" procedure. Med J Aust 1977;1397-1399.
19. Bogduk N. "Rhizolysis" and low back pain. Med J Aust 1977;1:504.
20. Shealy CN. Facets in back and sciatic pain. A new approach to a major pain syndrome. Minn Med 1974;57:199-203.
21. Shealy CN. The role of the spinal facets in back and sciatic pain. Headache 1974;14:101-104.
22. Shealy CN. Percutaneous radiofrequency denervation of spinal facets. Treatment for chronic back pain and sciatica. J Neurosurg 1975;43:448-451.
23. Shealy CN. Facet denervation in the management of back and sciatic pain. Clin Orthop Relat Res 1976;(115):157-164.
24. Pawl RP. Results in the treatment of low back syndrome from sensory neurolysis of the lumbar facets (facet rhizotomy) by thermal coagulation. Proc Inst Med Chic 1974;30:151-152.
25. Oudenhoven RC. Articular rhizotomy. Surg Neurol 1974; 2:275-278.
26. Banerjee T, Pittman HH. Facet rhizotomy. Another armamentarium for treatment of low backache. N C Med J 1976; 37:354-360.
27. Lora J, Long D. So-called facet denervation in the management of intractable back pain. Spine 1976;1:121-126.
28. Burton CV. Percutaneous radiofrequency facet denervation. Appl Neurophysiol 1976;39:80-86.
29. McCulloch JA. Percutaneous radiofrequency lumbar rhizolysis (rhizotomy). Appl Neurophysiol 1976;39:87-96.
30. McCulloch JA, Organ LW. Percutaneous radiofrequency lumbar rhizolysis (rhizotomy). Can Med Assoc J 1977; 116:28-30.
31. Ogsbury JS III, Simon RH, Lehman RA. Facet "denervation" in the treatment of low back syndrome. Pain 1977;3: 257-263.
32. Florez G, Eiras J, Ucar S. Percutaneous rhizotomy of the articular nerve of Luschka for low back and sciatic pain. Acta Neurochir (Wien) 1977;(Suppl 24):67-71.
33. Oudenhoven RC. Paraspinal electromyography following facet rhizotomy. Spine 1977;2:299-304.
34. Fuentes E. La neurotomia apofisaria transcutanea en el tratamento de la lumbalgia cronica. Rev Med Chile 1978;106:440.

35. Schaerer JP. Radiofrequency facet rhizotomy in the treatment of chronic neck and low back pain. Int Surg 1978;63: 53-59.

36. Oudenhoven RC. The role of laminectomy, facet rhizotomy, and epidural steroids. Spine 1979;4:145-147.

37. Fassio B, Bouvier JP, Ginestie JF. Denervation articulaire posterieure percutanqe et chirurgicale: Sa place dans le traitement des lombalgies. Rev Chir Orthop 1980;67:131.

38. Drevet JG, Chirossel JP, Phelip X. Lombalgies-lomboradiculalgies et articulations vertebrales posterieures. Lyon Med 1981;245:781.

39. Uyttendaele D, Verhamme J, Vercauteren M, et al. Local block of lumbar facet joints and percutaneous radiofrequency denervation. Preliminary results. Acta Orthop Belg 1981;47: 135-139.

40. Andersen KH, Mosdal C, Vaernet K. Percutaneous radiofrequency facet denervation in low-back and extremity pain. Acta Neurochir (Wien) 1987;87:48-51.

41. Cho J, Park YG, Chung SS. Percutaneous radiofrequency lumbar facet rhizotomy in mechanical low back pain syndrome. Stereotact Funct Neurosurg 1997;68:212-217.

42. Gallagher J, Vadi PLP, Wesley JR. Radiofrequency facet joint denervation in the treatment of low back pain: a prospective controlled double-blind study to assess its efficacy. Pain Clinic 1994;7:193-198.

43. Mooney V, Robertson J. The facet syndrome. Clin Orthop Relat Res 1976;115:149-156.

44. McCall IW, Park WM, O'Brien JP. Induced pain referral from posterior lumbar elements in normal subjects. Spine 1979;4:441-446.

45. Fairbank JC, Park WM, McCall IW, et al. Apophyseal injection of local anesthetic as a diagnostic aid in primary low-back pain syndromes. Spine 1981;6:598-605.

46. Helbig T, Lee CK. The lumbar facet syndrome. Spine 1988;13:61-64.

47. Jackson RP, Jacobs RR, Montesano PX. 1988 Volvo award in clinical sciences. Facet joint injection in low-back pain. A prospective statistical study. Spine 1988;13:966-971.

48. Schwarzer AC, Aprill CN, Derby R, et al. Clinical features of patients with pain stemming from the lumbar zygapophysial joints. Is the lumbar facet syndrome a clinical entity? Spine 1994;19:1132-1137.

49. Schwarzer AC, Derby R, Aprill CN, et al. Pain from the lumbar zygapophysial joints: a test of two models. J Spinal Disord 1994;7:331-336.

50. Schwarzer AC, Wang SC, O'Driscoll D, et al. The ability of computed tomography to identify a painful zygapophysial joint in patients with chronic low back pain. Spine 1995;20: 907-912.

51. Revel M, Poiraudeau S, Auleley GR, et al. Capacity of the clinical picture to characterize low back pain relieved by facet joint anesthesia. Proposed criteria to identify patients with painful facet joints. Spine 1998;23:1972-1976.

52. de Sèze MP, Poiraudeau S, de Sèze M, et al. [Interest of the criteria of Cochin to select patients with significant relief of low back pain after corticosteroid facet joint injections: a prospective study.] Ann Readapt Med Phys 2004; 47:1-6.

53. Bogduk N. Commentary on the capacity of the clinical picture to characterize low back pain relieved by facet joint anesthesia. Pain Medicine J Club J 1998;4:221-222.

54. Laslett M, Oberg B, Aprill CN, et al. Zygapophysial joint blocks in chronic low back pain: a test of Revel's model as a screening test. BMC Musculoskelet Disord 2004;5:43.

55. Laslett M, McDonald B, Aprill CN, et al. Clinical predictors of screening lumbar zygapophyseal joint blocks: development of clinical prediction rules. Spine J 2006;6:370-379.

56. Glover JR. Arthrography of the joints of the lumbar vertebral arches. Orthop Clin North Am 1977;8:37-42.

57. Carrera GF. Lumbar facet arthrography and injection in low back pain. Wisc Med J 1979;78:35-37.

58. Carrera GF. Lumbar facet joint injection in low back pain and sciatica: preliminary results. Radiology 1980;137: 665-667.

59. Carrera GF. Lumbar facet joint injection in low back pain and sciatica: description of technique. Radiology 1980;137: 661-664.

60. Carrera GF, Williams AL. Current concepts in evaluation of the lumbar facet joints. Crit Rev Diagn Imaging 1984; 21:85-104.

61. Destouet JM, Gilula LA, Murphy WA, et al. Lumbar facet joint injection: indication, technique, clinical correlation, and preliminary results. Radiology 1982;145:321-325.

62. Dory MA. Arthrography of the lumbar facet joints. Radiology 1981;140:23-27.

63. Eisenstein SM, Parry CR. The lumbar facet arthrosis syndrome. Clinical presentation and articular surface changes. J Bone Joint Surg Br 1987;69:3-7.

64. Bough B, Thakore J, Davies M, et al. Degeneration of the lumbar facet joints. Arthrography and pathology. J Bone Joint Surg Br 1990;72:275-276.

65. Lau LS, Littlejohn GO, Miller MH. Clinical evaluation of intra-articular injections for lumbar facet joint pain. Med J Aust 1985;143:563-565.

66. Lewinnek GE, Warfield CA. Facet joint degeneration as a cause of low back pain. Clin Orthop Relat Res 1986;213:216-222.

67. Lippitt AB. The facet joint and its role in spine pain. Management with facet joint injections. Spine 1984;9:746-750.

68. Lynch M, Taylor J. Facet joint injection for low back pain. A clinical study. J Bone Joint Surg Br 1986;68:138-141.

69. Moran R, O'Connell D, Walsh MG. The diagnostic value of facet joint injections. Spine 1988;13:1407-1410.

70. Murtagh FR. Computed tomography and fluoroscopy guided anesthesia and steroid injection in facet syndrome. Spine 1988;13:686-689.

71. International Spine Intervention Society. Lumbar medial neurotomy. In: Bogduk N, editor. Practice guidelines for spinal diagnostic and treatment procedures. San Francisco: International Spinal Intervention Society; 2004. p. 188-218.

72 International Spine Intervention Society. Lumbar medial neurotomy. In: Bogduk N, editor. Practice guidelines for spinal diagnostic and treatment procedures. San Francisco: International Spinal Intervention Society; 2004. p. 47-65.

73. Sluijter ME, Mehta M. Treatment of chronic back and neck pain by percutaneous thermal lesions. In: Lipton S, Miles J, editors, Persistent pain. Modern methods of treatment, Vol. 3. London: Academic Press; 1981. p. 141-179.

74. van Wijk RMA, Geurts JWM, Wynne HJ, et al. Radiofrequency denervation of lumbar facet joints in the treatment of chronic low back pain. A randomized, double-blind sham lesion-controlled trial. Clin J Pain 2004;21:335-344.

75. van Kleef M., Barendse GA, Kessels A, et al. Randomized trial of radiofrequency lumbar facet denervation for chronic low back pain. Spine 1999;24:1937-1942.

76. Lau P, Mercer S, Govind J, et al. The surgical anatomy of lumbar medial branch neurotomy (facet denervation). Pain Med 2004;5:289-298.

77. Letcher FS, Goldring S. The effect of radiofrequency current and heat on peripheral nerve action potential in the cat. J Neurosurg 1968;29:42-47.

78. Frohling MA, Schlote W, Wolburg-Buchholz K. Nonselective nerve fibre damage in peripheral nerves after experimental thermocoagulation. Acta Neurochir (Wien) 1998;140:1297-1302.

79. Bogduk N, Macintosh J, Marsland A. Technical limitations to the efficacy of radiofrequency neurotomy for spinal pain. Neurosurgery 1987;20:529-535.

80. Carette S, Marcoux S, Truchon R, et al. A controlled trial of corticosteroid injections into facet joints for chronic low back pain. N Engl J Med 1991;325:1002-1007.

81. Schwarzer AC, Wang SC, Bogduk N, et al. Prevalence and clinical features of lumbar zygapophysial joint pain: a study in an Australian population with chronic low back pain. Ann Rheum Dis 1995;54:100-106.

82. International Spine Intervention Society. Lumbar medial neurotomy. In: Bogduk N, editor. Practice guidelines for spinal diagnostic and treatment procedures. San Francisco: International Spinal Intervention Society; 2004.

83. Bogduk N, Wilson AS, Tynan W. The human lumbar dorsal rami. J Anat 1982;134:383-397.

84. Bogduk N. The innervation of the lumbar spine. Spine 1983;8:286-293.

85. Cooper AL. Trigger-point injection: its place in physical medicine. Arch Phys Med Rehabil 1961;42:704-709.

86. Bogduk N. Diagnostic nerve blocks in chronic pain. Best Pract Res Clin Anaesthesiol 2002;16:565-578.

87. Schwarzer AC, Aprill CN, Derby R, et al. The false-positive rate of uncontrolled diagnostic blocks of the lumbar zygapophysial joints. Pain 1994;58:195-200.

88. Manchikanti L, Pampati V, Fellows B, et al. Prevalence of lumbar facet joint pain in chronic low back pain. Pain Physician 1999;2:59-64.

89. Manchikanti L, Pampati V, Fellows B, et al. The diagnostic validity and therapeutic value of lumbar facet joint nerve blocks with or without adjuvant agents. Curr Rev Pain 2000;4:337-344.

90. Bogduk N. On the rational use of diagnostic blocks for spinal pain. Neurosurg Q 2009;19:88-100.

91. Schwarzer AC, Aprill CN, Derby R, et al. The relative contributions of the disc and zygapophyseal joint in chronic low back pain. Spine 1994;19:801-806.

92. Schwarzer AC, Aprill CN, Bogduk N. The sacroiliac joint in chronic low back pain. Spine 1995;20:31-37.

93. Nielens H, van Zundert J, Mairiaux P, et al. Chronic low back pain. Brussels, 2006, Report No.: KCE reports Vol 48C.

94. Airaksinen O, Brox JI, Cedraschi C, et al. European guidelines for the management of chronic nonspecific low back pain. Eur Spine J 2006;15:192-300.

95. National Institute for Health and Clinical Excellence (NICE). Low back pain: early management of persistent nonspecific low back pain. London, 2009, National Institute of Health and Clinical Excellence. Report No.: NICE clinical guideline 88.

96. Chou R, Loeser JD, Owens DK, et al. Interventional therapies, surgery, and interdisciplinary rehabilitation for low back pain: an evidence-based clinical practice guideline from the American Pain Society. Spine 2009;34:1066-1077.

97. Niemisto L, Kalso E, Malmivaara A, et al. Radiofrequency denervation for neck and back pain. A systematic review of randomized controlled trials. Cochrane Database Syst Rev 2003;(1):CD004058.

98. Leclaire R, Fortin L, Lambert R, et al. Radiofrequency facet joint denervation in the treatment of low back pain: a placebo-controlled clinical trial to assess efficacy. Spine 2001;26:1411-1416.

99. Chou R, Atlas SJ, Stanos SP, et al. Nonsurgical interventional therapies for low back pain: a review of the evidence for an American Pain Society clinical practice guideline. Spine 2009;34:1078-1093.

100. Geurts JW, van Wijk RM, Stolker RJ, et al. Efficacy of radiofrequency procedures for the treatment of spinal pain: a systematic review of randomized clinical trials. Reg Anesth Pain Med 2001;26:394-400.

101. Niemisto L, Kalso E, Malmivaara A, et al. Radiofrequency denervation for neck and back pain: a systematic review within the framework of the Cochrane collaboration back review group. Spine 2003;28:1877-1888.

102. Boswell MV, Colson JD, Sehgal N, et al. A systematic review of therapeutic facet joint interventions in chronic spinal pain. Pain Physician 2007;10:229-253.

103. Slipman CW, Bhat AL, Gilchrist RV, et al. A critical review of the evidence for the use of zygapophysial injections and radiofrequency denervation in the treatment of low back pain. Spine J 2003;3:310-316.

104. Resnick DK, Choudhri TF, Dailey AT, et al. Guidelines for the performance of fusion procedures for degenerative disease of the lumbar spine. Part 13: injection therapies, low-back pain, and lumbar fusion. J Neurosurg Spine 2005;2:707-715.

105. Nath S, Nath CA, Pettersson K. Percutaneous lumbar zygapophysial (facet) joint neurotomy using radiofrequency current, in the management of chronic low back pain: a randomized double-blind trial. Spine 2008;33:1291-1297.

106. Tekin I, Mirzai H, Ok G, et al. A comparison of conventional and pulsed radiofrequency denervation in the treatment of chronic facet joint pain. Clin J Pain 2007;23:524-529.

107. Bogduk N, Dreyfuss P, Govind J. A narrative review of lumbar medial branch neurotomy for the treatment of back pain. Pain Med 2009;10:1035-1045.

108. Hooten WM, Martin DP, Huntoon MA. Radiofrequency neurotomy for low back pain: evidence-based procedural guidelines. Pain Med 2005;6:129-138.

109. Bogduk N. In defense of radiofrequency neurotomy. Reg Anesth Pain Med 2002;27:439-441.

110. Bogduk N. Lumbar radiofrequency neurotomy. Clin J Pain 2006;22:409.

111. Dreyfuss P, Halbrook B, Pauza K, et al. Efficacy and validity of radiofrequency neurotomy for chronic lumbar zygapophysial joint pain. Spine 2000;25:1270-1277.

112. Gofeld M, Jitendra J, Faclier G. Radiofrequency denervation of the lumbar zygapophysial joints: 10-year prospective clinical audit. Pain Physician 2007;10:291-300.

113. Burnham RS, Holitski S, Dinu I. A prospective outcome study on the effects of facet joint radiofrequency denervation on pain, analgesic intake, disability, satisfaction, cost, and employment. Arch Phys Med Rehabil 2009;90:201-205.

114. Dreyfuss P, Schwarzer AC, Lau P, et al. Specificity of lumbar medial branch and L5 dorsal ramus blocks. A computed tomography study. Spine 1997;22:895-902.

115. Kaplan M, Dreyfuss P, Halbrook B, et al. The ability of lumbar medial branch blocks to anesthetize the zygapophysial joint. A physiologic challenge. Spine 1998;23:1847-1852.

116. Schofferman J, Kine G. Effectiveness of repeated radiofrequency neurotomy for lumbar facet pain. Spine 2004;29:2471-2473.

117. Bogduk N, Dreyfuss P, Baker R, et al. Complications of spinal diagnostic and treatment procedures. Pain Med 2008;6: 11-34.

118. Datta S, Lee M, Falco FJ, et al. Systematic assessment of diagnostic accuracy and therapeutic utility of lumbar facet joint interventions. Pain Physician 2009;12:437-460.

119. Centers for Medicare and Medicaid Services. Article for pain management: Supplemental instructions article. Baltimore, 2009. Report No.: A48042.

120. Centers for Medicare and Medicaid Services. LCD for pain management. Baltimore, 2009. Report No.: L28529.

121. Bogduk N, Holmes S. Controlled zygapophysial joint blocks: the travesty of cost-effectiveness. Pain Med 2000;1:24-34.

RICHARD DERBY
RAY M. BAKER
IRINA L. MELNIK
JEONG-EUN LEE
CHANG-HYUNG LEE
PAUL A. ANDERSON

CHAPTER 27

Intradiscal Thermal Therapies

DESCRIPTION

Terminology and Subtypes

Intradiscal thermal therapies encompass a group of interventions that deliver heat energy to the intervertebral disc (IVD) with the goal of reducing discogenic pain by a variety of proposed mechanisms, including shrinking subannular disc protrusions, destroying nociceptors, sealing annular tears by collagen modification, and stimulating a healing response.[1,2] The original intradiscal thermal therapies delivered heat to the nucleus using the same radiofrequency device used in lumbar medial branch neurotomy (LMBN), discussed in Chapter 26. Subsequently, the more widely used intradiscal electrothermal therapy (IDET) procedure used a catheter inserted into the nucleus and advanced circumferentially to the outer annulus. A later modification of the device used the same technique but a shorter active heating length using radiofrequency rather than electrothermal energy to heat the adjacent annulus. This procedure is also termed *intradiscal electrothermal annuloplasty* (IDEA) or *intradiscal thermal annuloplasty* (IDTA).

The heat delivered with IDET can be generated through a variety of means, including electrocautery, thermal cautery, laser, and radiofrequency energy (RFE). IDET using RFE may also be termed *intradiscal radiofrequency treatment* or *intradiscal radiofrequency thermocoagulation* (IRFT). That procedure is also termed *percutaneous intradiscal radiofrequency thermocoagulation* (PIRFT). Another device also using radiofrequency and termed *intradiscal radiofrequency treatment* (IDRT) targets the outer annulus using an electrode passed through an introducer needle inserted into the outer posterior lateral annulus and passed across the posterior annulus.

The most recent advance is termed *cooled bipolar RFE* or *intradiscal biacuplasty* (IDB), and actively cools a radiofrequency probe using circulating water pumped through a cannula. IDB uses a bipolar system that includes two cooled RFE electrodes placed on the posterolateral sides of the annulus fibrosus portion of the IVD. Cooled RFE electrodes are thought to increase the lesion size and facilitate ablation when compared with standard RFE electrodes, whereas linear placement of the two electrodes makes the procedure less complicated. This cooling is thought to create a more uniform heating profile across the disc annulus between two bilateral introducer needles placed into the outer annulus.

Most intradiscal thermal treatments are performed using RFE, which may be applied with unipolar or bipolar probes. Unipolar RFE is similar to electrocautery and involves an electric current that passes through the probe to the IVD, and then to a grounding pad. Bipolar RFE allows an electric current to pass from the positive pole directly to the negative pole, theoretically decreasing collateral damage that may be incurred as the energy travels through the body to the grounding pad. Bipolar probes are thought to allow for greater control and focus of the RFE. A modification of the bipolar probe has been termed "coblation," which involves creating plasma of high-energy ionized particles in the tissues surrounding the probe rather than a traditional heat lesion. This plasma is thought to disrupt organic bonds, thus allowing debridement and effective treatment of soft tissues.

An overview of the various methods of intradiscal thermal therapies is presented in Table 27-1 and illustrated in Figures 27-1 through 27-5.

History and Frequency of Use

The rationale for heating IVDs was strongly influenced by preclinical and clinical studies investigating the application of heat to stabilize joints by modifying collagen. The intervention thermal capsulorrhaphy, which involves using laser or radiofrequency heating devices to denature the collagen of the shoulder capsule to cause shrinkage, has been used to treat shoulder instability since 1994.[3] Type I collagen in the shoulder capsule has a triple-helical configuration that is responsible for the molecule's ability to resist tensile forces, and is similar to the collagen found in the outer annulus of the IVD.

The biologic effects of laser thermal modification were investigated by Hayashi and colleagues, who used a YAG laser to deliver 250 J to the glenohumeral and patellofemoral joint capsules.[4,5] Joint capsule thickness immediately increased but normalized after 60 days, while stiffness and strength initially decreased but normalized after 30 days. Histologically, collagen hyalinization and cell death was noted at the application site, but the surrounding tissues were normal. Healing was thought to be the result of an active reparative process initiated by acute inflammation resulting in fibroblast proliferation and migration, neovascularization, and eventual collagen repair. Biochemical analysis revealed that the laser treatment had denatured collagen by disrupting

TABLE 27-1	Categories and Subcategories of Intradiscal Thermal Therapies for Chronic Low Back Pain			
Category/Subcategory	Equipment	Description		Figure
Intranuclear				
	Radionics RF Disc Catheter System	The radiofrequency probe is placed into the center of the disc rather than around the annulus. The device is activated for only 90 seconds at a temperature of 70° C with direct application of RFE with no coagulation or burning of tissue.		27-1A, B
Intra-Annular				
IDET IDTA IDEA	IDET catheter, (Smith & Nephew)	Following posterolateral puncture of the annulus, the introducer needle is positioned in the nucleus. A temperature-controlled thermal resistive coil is navigated circumferentially so that the 5 cm active heating element is positioned within the posterior annulus. The electrothermal coagulation starts at 65° C to final 80° C to 90° C, maintained for 4 to 5 minutes for total of 15 minutes of treatment time.		27-2A, B
	Decompression Catheter (Smith & Nephew)	Similar technique performed with a short 1.5-cm active tip using Decompression Catheter wherein the most active heating occurs within 2 mm of the outer annulus on the opposite side of the disc.		27-3A, B
IDRT PIRFT RFA	DiscTRODE RF Catheter (Radionics)	The introducer needle is directed into the outer posterior lateral annulus, rather than nucleus, and the active electrode is advanced across the posterior annulus. Using RFE, the temperature is incrementally elevated beginning at 65° C, and is maintained for 4 minutes. The final temperature is determined by measuring contralateral outer annulus using a temperature monitoring needle that can be placed into the outer posterior annulus.		27-4A, B
Biacuplasty Cooled bipolar RFE IDB	RF electrodes (Baylis Medical)	Two water-cooled straight radiofrequency electrodes with a 6-mm active tip placed on the posterolateral sides of the intervertebral annulus fibrosus. Bipolar heating with tissue ablation occurs using RFE, up to 55° C maintained for 4 minutes. Total 15 minutes of treatment time.		27-5A, B

IDB, intradiscal biacuplasty; IDEA, intradiscal electrothermal annuloplasty; IDET, intradiscal electrothermal therapy; IDRT, intradiscal radiofrequency treatment; IDTA, intradiscal thermal annuloplasty; PIRFT, percutaneous intradiscal radiofrequency thermocoagulation; RFA, radiofrequency annuloplasty; RFE, radiofrequency energy.

alpha bands, resulting in unwinding of the triple helix. Because the initial effects of laser energy were deleterious, recovery was dependent on a subsequent healing response. It should be noted that although cartilaginous tissue regained most of its preinjury strength, long-term weakness remained during creep strain.

The US Food and Drug Administration (FDA) gave clearance to the medical device used during IDET—the Spine-CATH intradiscal catheter—in March 1998. It has been estimated that more than 40,000 procedures were performed in the first 5 years after IDET was approved for marketing.[6] The manufacturer of the IDET device, Smith & Nephew (Memphis, Tennessee) has estimated that 60,000 procedures have been performed worldwide as of June 2005.[6]

Practitioner, Setting, and Availability

IDET is typically performed in secondary care settings by nonsurgical or surgical spine specialists, including physiatrists, anesthesiologists, orthopedic surgeons, or interventional pain management specialists. Because this intervention must be conducted under fluoroscopy, it is typically limited to specialty spine or pain management clinics in outpatient centers or hospitals. IDET is available throughout the United States, but mostly in larger cities.

Procedure

The IDET procedure begins with the patient wearing a medical gown and lying prone on a treatment table. The area to be treated is typically cleaned with sequential alcohol or betadine wipes. The procedure can be performed under conscious sedation to minimize patient discomfort or anxiety. IDET is performed under image guidance using fluoroscopy. The IDET procedure usually consists of the following stages: (1) catheter placement, (2) heating protocol, and (3) postprocedure care. Each stage is briefly described here, as is a variant of IDET using a different instrument.

Catheter Placement

The IDET procedure uses a navigable intradiscal catheter with a thermal-resistive coil, the SpineCATH intradiscal catheter or decompression catheter. A 17-gauge introducer needle is first inserted through the skin, subcutaneous tissue, and muscle, and advanced circuitously to the posterior annulus; catheter position is critical to IDET.[7,8] Using a standard posterolateral

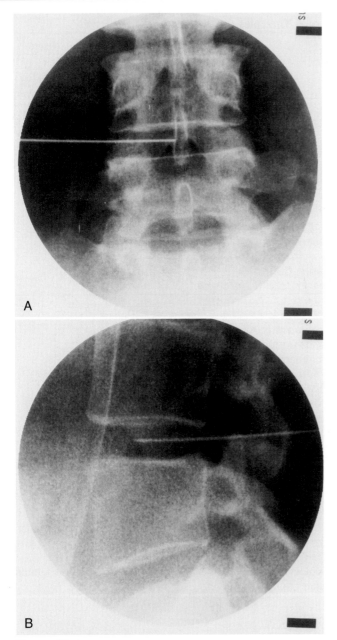

Figure 27-1 The radiofrequency probe (Radionics RF Disc Catheter System) is placed into the center of the disc rather that around the annulus (**A** anterior view, **B** lateral view). The device is activated for only 90 seconds at a temperature of 70° C with direct application of radiofrequency energy with no coagulation or burning of tissue. (From Barendse GAM, van den Berg SGM, Kessels AHF, Weber WEJ, van Kleef M. Randomized controlled trial of percutaneous intradiscal radiofrequency thermocoagulation for chronic discogenic back pain. SPINE, Volume 26, Number 3, pp 287-292, 2001.)

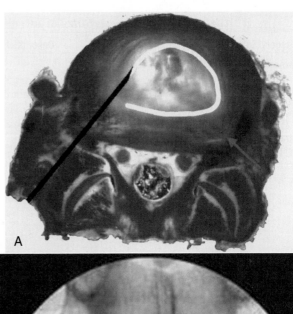

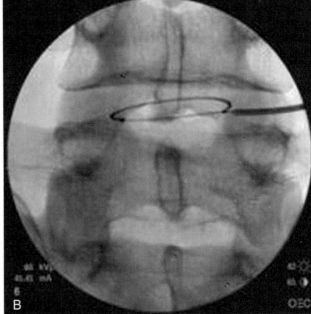

Figure 27-2 Following posterolateral puncture of the annulus, the introducer needle is positioned in the nucleus (**A** axial view, **B** anterior view). A temperature-controlled thermal resistive coil (IDET catheter, Smith & Nephew, London, UK) is navigated circumferentially so that the 5 cm active heating element is positioned within the posterior annulus. The electrothermal coagulation starts at 65° C to final 80° C to 90° C, maintained for 4 to 5 minutes for total of 15 minutes of treatment time. (**A** from: Finch PM, Price LM, Drummond PD. Radiofrequency heating of painful annular disruptions: one-year outcomes. J Spinal Disord Tech, Volume 18, Number 1, February 2005, pp 6-13. Courtesy Professor JA Taylor. **B** Courtesy of Baylis Medical Company, Inc. Images found at www.baylismedical.com/images/PDF%20pain/PM1007_TD.pdf.)

discogram technique, a 30-cm catheter with a 5- or 1.5-cm active electrothermal tip is then inserted through the introducer needle (Figure 27-6). One catheter is usually enough, but in some cases two catheters may be used in a bilateral deployment to treat the entire posterior annular wall.[7] Ideally, the active length of the catheter should cross the "symptomatic" annular fissure and lie close enough (approximately 5 mm) to

the outer annulus to allow sufficient heat to spread to both the outer and inner annulus (Figure 27-7).[9]

Interestingly, the original brochure for the IDET procedure published by the Oratec company showed the catheter lying incorrectly within the nuclear-annular junction. Many of the original clinical studies investigating the efficacy of IDET reproduced this catheter position, thereby preventing adequate spread of heat to the outer annular fibers. This problem is rarely noted in clinical practice, where the tip of

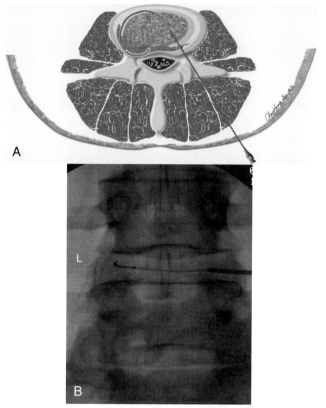

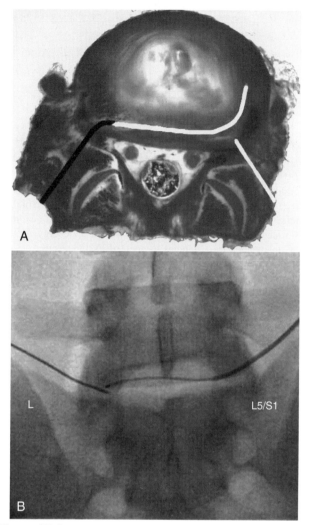

Figure 27-3 Similar technique performed with a short 1.5 cm active tip using the Decompression Catheter (Smith & Nephew), where the most active heating occurs within 2 mm of the outer annulus on the opposite side of the disc (**A** axial view, **B** anterior view).

the electrode inevitably ends up in the outer annular fibers. Although clinicians may attempt multiple catheter placements and even bend the outer catheter to achieve the ideal position 5 mm from the outer annulus, this goal is seldom achieved. Furthermore, repeated insertion and removal of the catheter may increase the risk of infection, and often results in permanent damage to a costly medical device. The catheter should not be placed outside of the annulus of the disc. Before heating, catheter position should be confirmed and documented with both anterior-posterior and lateral views.

Heating Protocol

The original 5-cm active heating element catheter introduced by Oratec placed the temperature sensor electrode deep within the catheter and reported temperatures that were on average 13° C higher than those administered to tissue at the tip of the catheter. The empirically derived heating protocol recommended beginning at 65° C, with incremental increases of 1° C every 30 seconds to achieve a final temperature of 80° C to 90° C that should be maintained for 5 minutes; the total treatment time was approximately 15 minutes.[10] Although some clinicians advocated using higher temperatures, there was no standard method for determining the actual final temperature delivered to targeted tissues.

Derby and colleagues were not able to demonstrate a correlation between higher final temperatures and improved

Figure 27-4 The introducer needle is directed into the outer posterior lateral annulus, rather than nucleus, and the active electrode (discTRODE RF catheter; Radionics Burlington, MA) is advanced across the posterior annulus (**A** axial view, **B** anterior view). Utilizing radiofrequency energy, the temperature is incrementally elevated beginning at 65° C, and is maintained for 4 minutes. The final temperature is determined by measuring contralateral outer annulus using a temperature monitoring needle that can be placed into the outer posterior annulus. (**A** from Finch PM, Price LM, Drummond PD. Radiofrequency heating of painful annular disruptions: one-year outcomes. J Spinal Disord Tech, Volume 18, Number 1, February 2005, pp 6-13. Courtesy Professor JA Taylor.)

outcomes with IDET after 8 or 16 months.[11] In fact, when catheter positions were less than 5 mm from the outer annulus, higher temperatures were associated with longer postprocedure increased pain. Based on these results, it was proposed that temperatures should be incrementally increased to 80° C but that the final temperature and total duration of the intervention should be based on the patient's pain response. In this scenario, incremental increases in temperature would be stopped when the patient reported pain rated higher than 6 to 8 out of 10. This temperature would then be maintained for up to 4 minutes as long as pain remained less than 8 out of 10.

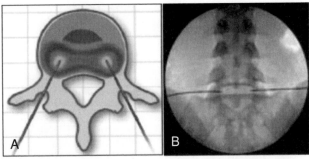

Figure 27-5 Two water-cooled straight radiofrequency electrodes (Baylis Medical, Inc., Montreal, Canada) with a 6 mm active tip placed on the posterolateral sides of the intervertebral annulus fibrosus (**A** axial view, **B** anterior view). Bipolar heating with tissue ablation occurs utilizing radiofrequency energy, up to 55° C maintained for 4 minutes for total of 15 minutes of treatment time. (Courtesy of Baylis Medical Company, Inc. Images found at www.baylismedical.com/images/PDF%20pain/PM1007_TD.pdf.)

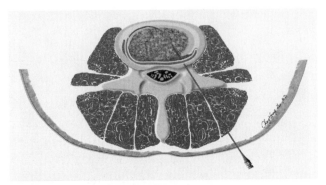

Figure 27-6 A SpineCATH Intradiscal Catheter (Smith & Newphew) is place circumferentially in the outer posterior annulus.

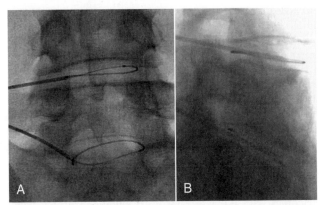

Figure 27-7 Fluoroscopic image of the IDET procedures. The Intradiscal Electrothermal Catheter electrode (SpineCATH Intradiscal Catheter, Smith & Newphew) is place within the L4/5 and L5/S1 discs (**A** anterior view, **B** lateral view).

The newer IDET catheter (Decompression Catheter, Smith & Nephew) used a shorter 1.5-cm heating element, which was thought to help limit destruction of normal annulus tissue (Figures 27-8 and 27-9). Because the temperature sensor was placed on the outside of the catheter, measurements were more likely to reflect those of adjacent tissues. The heating

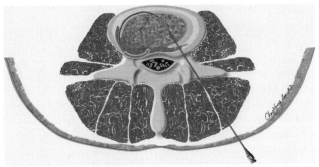

Figure 27-8 Using a standard posterolateral discogram technique, a Decompression Catheter (Smith & Nephew) with a 1.5 cm active electrothermal tip is inserted through a 17-gauge introducer needle and advanced circumferentially to the posterior annulus. Most of the active heating tip remains in the outer annulus on the opposite side. The very outer part of the catheter is usually within 2 mm of the outer annulus.

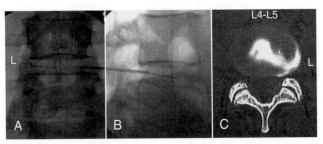

Figure 27-9 Fluoroscopic image of the IDET procedure. The shorter 1.5 cm electrothermal wire (Decompression Catheter, Smith & Nephew) has been positioned within the torn outer posterior annulus of the L4/5 disc (**A** anterior view, **B** lateral view, **C** axial view).

protocol using the newer IDET catheter also called for beginning at 65° C, incrementally increasing temperatures 1° C every 30 seconds up to 90° C, which was to be maintained for 6 minutes. Because the newer catheter was shorter than the original, the total dose of heat delivered with this protocol was probably less. Anecdotally, some practitioners reported improved outcomes with shorter post-procedure pain and greater tolerance of increased temperature before patients complained of excessive pain when using the newer catheter.

Post-Procedure Care

Following the IDET procedure, the patient is typically monitored in a recovery room for 1 to 3 hours before discharge.[8] Patients are warned to expect a significant increase in pain, and are told that this may last 2 to 7 days, although infrequently this may be permanent. Patients typically wear a lumbar brace for weeks to months after the procedure while healing of the outer annulus occurs to minimize the risk of reinjury from excessive disc loading during this period. Activities such as walking and pool exercises are encouraged, but aggressive physical therapy is usually not begun until 1 to 2 months after the procedure.[12] Most patients have reached maximal improvement by 3 months but a minority may take up to 3 to 6 months.[9,12-14]

Intradiscal Radiofrequency Treatment

This approach is similar to IDET but rather than passing the introducer needle into the nucleus, the needle tip is placed directly into the outer posterior lateral annulus, and the active electrode is advanced across the posterior annulus (Figure 27-10). The device used for the procedure, the DiscTRODE radiofrequency catheter, is manufactured by Radionics (Burlington, Massachusetts) and includes a sensor that measures tissue resistance, detecting the higher resistance of the disc annulus with both sound and digital readings. By passing the needle tip slightly more posteriorly and medially in the annulus, an asymmetric opening in the needle tip helps direct the active electrode across the posterior disc annulus. The device also includes a temperature monitoring needle that can be placed into the outer posterior annulus to monitor the increase as the electrode is heated. A graduated temperature protocol beginning at 65° C is used, but the final temperature is determined by measuring that of the contralateral outer annulus. Although this is thought to represent a more accurate method of determining final temperature, the distance of the measuring electrode from the radiofrequency electrode varies. When using this device, the temperature is incrementally elevated to 65° C, which is maintained for 4 minutes. Similar post-procedure care is followed.

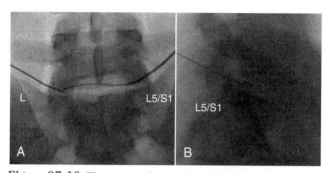

Figure 27-10 Fluoroscopy image of the IDRT procedure. The needle tip is directed into the outer posterior lateral annulus and the active tip is advanced across the posterior annulus. The temperature sensing electrode is shown on the left of the AP image (**A** anterior view, **B** lateral view).

Intradiscal Biacuplasty

The IDB procedure is somewhat similar to the IDET procedure described above. However, the probes are heated to 45° C for 15 minutes (approximately 60° C to 65° C tissue temperature) while water is continuously circulated around the probes. The heating is typically less painful than heating using the IDET catheters. Disc IDB is a method of heating the outer annulus that uses a bipolar cooled radiofrequency system (TransDiscal System, Baylis Medical, Montreal, Quebec, Canada). The lesion is created between two water-cooled radiofrequency probes placed into the right and left outer disc annuli. Using a standard posterior lateral approach to the lumbar IVD, introducer needles are passed into the outer disc annulus from the right and left side. The stylettes are removed and radiofrequency probes are passed through the introducer needle to lie within the middle and inner annular fibers (Figure 27-11). By placing two electrodes in a disc in a bipolar arrangement, radiofrequency current is concentrated in the disc and creates a larger size lesion compared to standard radiofrequency electrodes.[15] Water circulating in the electrodes cools the electrode surfaces, which allows for greater power delivery while at the same time not overheating tissue local to the electrodes. This allows a three-dimensional lesion to develop between the electrodes, which theoretically would be able to seal radial and circumferential fissures throughout the posterior annulus.

An animal study of the histologic effects and thermal distribution of disc IDB in an in vivo porcine model has shown that the IDB procedure achieves suitable temperatures for neural ablation in the disc (44° C to 55° C) while showing no evidence of damage to adjacent nerve roots.[16] Pauza assessed temperature profiles created by IDB in human cadaver discs, showing safe temperatures below 45° C in the anterior disc and posterior longitudinal ligament, while posterior annulus fibrosus outer and inner two-thirds reached 54° C to 60° C, respectively.[17] A cadaver study by Kapural and colleagues reported that measured temperatures across the posterior annulus using the IDB technique were sufficient to ablate nerves in the disc while maintaining safe temperatures in the epidural space and neural foramina.[18]

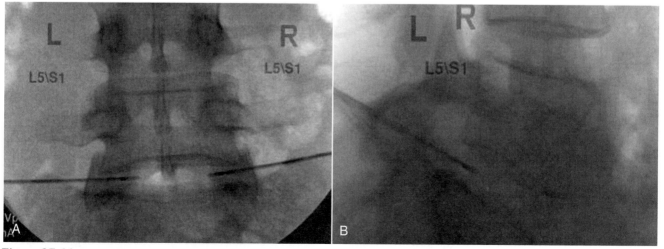

Figure 27-11 Fluoroscopy image of the biacuplasty procedure. Two water-cooled radiofrequency electrodes (Baylis Medical, Inc., Montreal, Canada) are placed on the posterolateral side of the annulus at the L5-S1 disc (**A** anterior view, **B** lateral view).

The possible advantages of this technique over previously available procedures include the following: (1) relative ease of placement of bipolar electrodes, eliminating the need to thread a long, flexible IDET catheter; (2) concentration of the heating energy primarily at the posterior wall of the disc; and (3) a greater volume of tissue heated, while sparing adjacent tissue with the use of cooling electrodes; and (4) better tolerability of the procedure by patients due to lower peak temperatures within the disc compared to IDET.

Regulatory Status

The FDA gave clearance to the medical device used during IDET, the SpineCATH intradiscal catheter, in March 1998, for the coagulation and decompression of contained herniated discs in patients with low back pain (LBP). Obtaining approval as a class II medical device mainly requires that the manufacturer submits evidence that the new device is substantially equivalent to a currently approved similar device. The IDB system was approved for use by the FDA in 2006, when initial spinal temperature measurements and histologic studies reported an appropriate safety profile.[18]

THEORY

Mechanism of Action

Despite many in vivo and in vitro studies using human and animal models, the precise mechanism of action through which IDET can help patients with chronic low back pain (CLBP) is unclear. Various changes have been reported with electron microscopy of IVDs obtained from cadavers following IDET, including extensive collagen disorganization, decreased quantity of collagen, collagen fibril shrinkage, and chondrocyte damage when compared with controls.[19] Numerous theoretical explanations for these observations have been offered, such as changes in disc biomechanics, annular contraction, thermally induced healing response, sealing of annular tears, annular denervation, and decreased intradiscal pressure; each is briefly summarized here.

Changes in Disc Biomechanics

Although changes in the biomechanical properties of discs (e.g., compliance) could alter the function of a vertebral segment, studies have not provided clear evidence that this occurs. Studies in human cadaver discs after following IDET at 65° C to 90° C over 17 minutes with a 6-cm active tip thermal-resistive coil resulted in decreased disc compliance and increased motion in all planes, although this was greatest in lateral bending.[20] The amount of increased motion did not, however, approach clinical significance and the authors concluded that IDET did not adversely affect segmental stability.

Similarly, Wang and colleagues heated bovine disc core samples consisting of the vertebrae and disc nucleus in a water bath and found no difference in either stiffness or failure strength.[21] Failures occurred only in the midsubstance of the specimen. In contrast, Kleinstueck and colleagues, in a larger series of discs, found that heating cadaver IVDs with IDET placed 10 to 15 mm from the outer annulus resulted in a significant (6% to 12%) decrease in stiffness, though temperatures greater than 65° C were seen only within a 2-mm radius of the catheter.[22] To achieve a more uniform heating, Bass and colleagues heated their human cadaver segments in a water bath to 75° C and found that the annulus was more compliant at higher applied stresses.[23]

Annular Contraction

A decrease in the size of disc herniations secondary to contraction of collagen in the annulus could potentially lead to decreased discogenic pain. Indeed, when bovine annular tissue was placed in a tube and heated, Schaufele and colleagues measured a 2% decrease in mass, 15% decrease in volume, and 3% decrease in diameter.[24] In addition, there were two cases in which magnetic resonance imaging (MRI) showed a reduction in herniation size after clinical application of heat using a thermal-resistive coil. However, a retrospective case series by Cohen and colleagues reported new disc herniation in 2 of 79 (2.5%) patients following IDET.[25] He postulated that the slow recovery post-IDET and observed results were more consistent with collagen modulation rather than reduced nociception. Additionally, Bass showed that the annulus will only shrink 8% after heating to 85° C, compared with 60% to 80% in the shoulder capsule. Further shrinkage is likely prevented by the attachment of the annulus to the vertebral end plates.

Thermally Induced Healing Response

Heating is thought to first disrupt the weaker intramolecular bonds unraveling and denaturing the triple helix. The stronger nonreducible intermolecular cross-links remain intact and thus the amount of collagen is unchanged. This "melting" into an amorphous state causes the observed "tissue shrinkage" and is a phase transition from a highly ordered crystalline structure to a random coil state. The effect plateaus at temperatures above 75°C, but higher temperatures eventually cause tissue destruction. Because temperatures above 45° C cause necrosis, cells are assumed to be destroyed after treatment. By 2 weeks, animal experiments show an enhanced healing response with the proliferation of cells and capillary sprouting. However, the treated ligaments were two to three times more susceptible to cyclic and static creep strains and in one study, two in eight treated ligaments experienced partial failure during creep testing.[26]

Although there is a loss of cell viability staining following IDET, discs maintained in cell culture conditions have demonstrated the ability to recover within 2 to 4 weeks.[27] Studies have demonstrated thermal modification of collagen after IDET treatment, with changes in both histologic and scanning electron microscopy collagen morphology, consistent with other studies showing that shoulder capsular tissues regain biomechanical integrity after thermal treatment. In contrast, an in vitro ovine study by Freeman and colleagues found that IDET did not modulate the healing response in any way at various time intervals up to 12 weeks.[28] Both treated and untreated discs showed similar degrees of degeneration, and the sheep discs in which an annular incision was made showed the most pronounced degenerative changes. At 12 weeks, there was pronounced granulation tissue accompanied by small nerves up to the outer three layers.

Bass and colleagues confirmed these findings by heating bovine cervical discs and harvesting up to 3 months after the procedure.[29] There was no evidence that thermal treatment lead to increased stability, and no indication that high temperatures delivered to large regions of the disc had any discernable therapeutic benefit. Similarly, Derby and colleagues found that in clinical practice, higher temperatures and larger total heating doses during IDET with catheters placed in the outer annulus increased the duration of subsequent pain and led to less favorable outcomes after 8 months, though long-term outcomes at 16 months were unaffected by these differences in heating protocols.[11]

Sealing of Annular Tears

Although several authors have postulated that IDET might "seal" annular tears, thereby leading to decreased pain, there are no clinical data to support this hypothesis. In fact, Narvani and colleagues reported that in 6 of the 10 patients with discogenic pain, MRI confirmed that high-intensity zones in the outer posterior annulus were unchanged 6 months after IDET.[30]

Annular Denervation

Studies using a heating element placed in close proximity to the outer annulus and heated according to protocol will most likely achieve temperatures greater than 45° C within 5 to 9 mm from the catheter.[10,29,31] Because most current techniques involve catheters placed in the outer annulus, denervation is theoretically possible. Bono and colleagues showed that a zone of potential denervation occurred at distances 12 to 14 mm from the catheter.[32] Using an IDET catheter placed close to the area of pathology, Wright and Gatchel measured mean outer annular temperatures of 43.9° C ± 2.3° C and concluded that these temperatures were sufficient to coagulate nociceptors.[31] Although a catheter placed within 5 mm of the outer annulus will achieve temperatures toxic to nociceptors within outer and middle annular fibers, it is unclear if this mechanism correlates with clinical recovery after IDET.[32] Of particular interest is the duration of subsequent pain, which may last from several days to a week because of tissue trauma, followed by clinical improvement. However, few studies have reported the frequency and duration of post-IDET pain. Derby and colleagues[8] showed that in a series of 32 patients, subsequent pain lasted an average of 5 days. If patients having no or only minimal (<1 week) subsequent pain achieved a significantly better outcome, these data would be consistent with the theory that intradiscal heating reduces pain by destroying nociceptor input.

Decreased Intradiscal Pressure

Using a recently introduced shorter electrothermal IDET catheter (SpineCATH intradiscal catheter, Smith & Nephew), the controlled intradiscal application of thermal energy on bovine disc material resulted in a 15% decrease in volume, 2% decrease in mass, and a 3% decrease in disc diameter.[33] The authors postulated that this mechanism might provide an explanation for observed improvements in radicular symptoms in patients with lumbar herniated nucleus pulposus. In a similar study, Podhajsky and Belous found pressure reductions approximating 30% to 50% in sheep nucleus pulposus after IDET treatment using a 1.5-cm electrothermal device (decompression catheter, Smith & Nephew).[33] The authors also found that the hydrophilic property of nucleus pulposus is temperature-dependent and that increasing treatment temperature resulted in a decreasing ability for the nucleus to absorb water. Such pressure reduction might account for a more substantial reduction in referred leg symptoms than LBP after IDET procedure in one retrospective study.[34]

Indication

The following indications have been proposed for IDET[35]:
1. Axial CLBP with or without leg pain that persists for more than 6 months
2. MRI findings of high intensity zones with greater than 50% normal disc height
3. MRI or computed tomography (CT) findings of posterior annulus disruption
4. Normal lower extremity neurologic examination
5. Symptoms consistent with CLBP related to discogenic involvement (e.g., pain with motion, difficulty with prolonged sitting)
6. Symptoms reproduced by discography with pressure less than 50 PSI
7. Unresponsive to at least 6 weeks of appropriate conservative care

Assessment

Before receiving IDET, patients should first be assessed for LBP using an evidence-based and goal-oriented approach focused on the patient history and neurologic examination, as discussed in Chapter 3. Clinicians should also inquire about medication history to note prior hypersensitivity/allergy or adverse events (AEs) with drugs similar to those which may be used during the IDET procedure, and evaluate contraindications for these types of drugs. Advanced imaging such as MRI or CT is required to help guide the spine specialist to target the appropriate spinal levels involved in a patient's CLBP.[36] Findings on advanced imaging that may be of interest for IDET include loss of disc height and decreased T2-weighted signal, which may be predictive of outer annular disc tears.[37] Similarly, high intensity zone lesions marked by a localized peripheral area of increased T2-weighted signal may indicate symptomatic annular disruption.[37-39] Advanced imaging may also need to be repeated following the IDET procedure.[40]

Interventional diagnostic testing is also frequently used prior to recommending or performing IDET, especially in cases of symptoms that persist for more than 6 months and prove recalcitrant to exhaustive conservative treatment measures. The use of provocative discography for CLBP remains controversial, but is used by some clinicians to identify painful annular defects that may subsequently be targeted with other interventions. When interpreting provocative discography, extension of isotopic dye into or beyond the outer annulus has been suggested as a strong predictor of concordant pain.[41] Findings of concordantly painful outer annular disruption on discography would indicate to the clinician which disc may be targeted with IDET to achieve maximum impact. However, such a strategy has not been critically evaluated.

EFFICACY

Evidence supporting the efficacy of these interventions for CLBP was summarized from recent clinical practice guidelines (CPGs), systematic reviews (SRs), and randomized controlled trials (RCTs). Observational studies (OBSs) were also summarized where appropriate. Findings are summarized by study design for each intervention.

Clinical Practice Guidelines

IDET

Four of the recent national CPGs on the management of CLBP have assessed and summarized the evidence to make specific recommendations about the efficacy of IDET.

The CPG from Belgium in 2006 found low-quality and conflicting evidence to support the efficacy of IDET in the management of CLBP.[42]

The CPG from Europe in 2004 found conflicting evidence that IDET is more effective than sham interventions in the management of CLBP with discogenic pain.[43] That CPG also found limited evidence to support the efficacy of IDET with respect to short-term improvements in pain for CLBP. That CPG did not recommend IDET in the management of CLBP.

The CPG from the United Kingdom in 2009 found no evidence to support the efficacy of IDET for the management of CLBP.[44] That CPG did not recommend IDET for CLBP.

The CPG from the United States in 2009 found insufficient evidence to make a recommendation about the use of IDET for the management of CLBP.[45]

Other

The CPG from the American Society of Interventional Pain Physicians (ASIPP) assessed the evidence supporting IDET as limited (level II-2) based on United States Preventive Services Task Force (USPSTF) criteria.[46]

Intradiscal Radiofrequency Thermocoagulation

Four of the recent national CPGs on the management of CLBP have assessed and summarized the evidence to make specific recommendations about the efficacy of IRFT.

The CPG from Belgium in 2006 found conflicting evidence to support the efficacy of IRFT in the management of CLBP.[42]

The CPG from Europe in 2004 found conflicting evidence that IRFT is more effective than sham interventions in the management of CLBP with discogenic pain.[43] That CPG also found limited evidence to support the efficacy of IRFT with respect to short-term improvements in pain for CLBP. That CPG did not recommend IRFT in the management of CLBP.

The CPG from the United Kingdom in 2009 found no evidence to support the efficacy of IRFT for the management of CLBP.[44] That CPG did not recommend IRFT for CLBP.

TABLE 27-2	Clinical Practice Guideline Recommendations on Intradiscal Electrothermal Therapy for Chronic Low Back Pain	
Reference	Country	Conclusion
IDET		
42	Belgium	Low-quality and conflicting evidence to support efficacy
43	Europe	Not recommended
44	United Kingdom	Not recommended
45	United States	Insufficient evidence to make a recommendation
46	United States (ISIS)	Limited evidence to support efficacy (level II-2)
IRFT		
42	Belgium	Conflicting evidence to support efficacy
43	Europe	Not recommended
44	United Kingdom	Not recommended
45	United States	Insufficient evidence to make a recommendation
IDB		
46	United States (ISIS)	Limited evidence to support efficacy (level III)

IDB, intradiscal biacuplasty; IDET, intradiscal electrothermal therapy; IRFT, intradiscal radiofrequency thermocoagulation.

The CPG from the United States in 2009 found insufficient evidence to make a recommendation about the use of IRFT for the management of CLBP.[45]

Intradiscal Biacuplasty

The CPG from ASIPP reported that the evidence supporting IDB was very limited (level III) based on USPSTF criteria.[46]

Findings from the above CPGs are summarized in Table 27-2.

Systematic Reviews

Cochrane Collaboration

An SR was conducted in 2005 by the Cochrane Collaboration on surgical procedures including IDET for LBP and/or associated leg symptoms secondary to degenerative lumbar spondylosis.[47] A total of 31 RCTs were identified, including 3 RCTs related to IDET for patients with chronic discogenic pain or CLBP.[36,48,49] One trial reported significantly greater improvement in pain and disability for IDET versus placebo, while the other two trials found no significant differences between IDET and placebo for all outcomes.[36,48,49] This review concluded that there is conflicting evidence supporting IDET for chronic discogenic pain and CLBP and recommended that future RCTs be conducted to examine the effectiveness of IDET.[47]

American Pain Society and American College of Physicians

The American Pain Society and American College of Physicians CPG committee on nonsurgical therapies conducted an SR in 2008 for acute and chronic LBP.[50] That review identified four SRs related to IDET including the Cochrane Collaboration review mentioned earlier.[47,51-53] Two other SRs concluded that there was inconsistent evidence supporting IDET, whereas two SRs concluded that IDET is effective.[47,51-53] These SRs included two RCTs, both of which were also included in the Cochrane review described above.[36,49] No new trials were identified in this review. This SR was unable to make any definitive conclusions about the effectiveness of IDET for CLBP because of the conflicting results found in the RCTs.[50] The SR recommended that more RCTs be conducted to assess the effects of IDET of CLBP.

Other

Appleby and colleagues recently published a meta-analysis of 17 IDET studies with follow-up of 6 to 24 months and validated outcome measures related to pain or function.[52] The pooled analysis from these studies found a mean decrease in visual analog scale (VAS) of 2.9 (95% confidence interval [CI] 2.5 to 3.4), a mean decrease in short-form 36 (SF-36) physical function of 21.1 (95% CI 13.4 to 28.8), a mean decrease in SF-36 bodily pain of 18 (95% CI 11.9 to 24.1), and a mean decrease in Oswestry Disability Index (ODI) of 7.0 (95% CI 2.0 to 11.9), all of which were statistically significant. This study was funded by Smith & Nephew, the manufacturer of equipment used in IDET, and concluded that there was compelling evidence supporting the relative efficacy and safety of this procedure.[52]

A review by Andersson and colleagues compared validated outcome measurements of 18 IDET studies with the same outcome measurements reported by 33 studies of fusion for degenerative disc disease (DDD).[51] Pain severity was measured by VAS or numerical pain scores, functional improvement measured by ODI, and quality of life measured by the physical function (PF) or physical component summary (PCS) of the SF-36. Outcomes were summarized by percentage improvement according to study design: RCTs, non-RCTs before-and-after cohorts, and case series. The overall median decrease in pain reported after IDET was very similar to that reported after spinal fusion. For example, eight before and after studies had a 61% mean decrease in VAS score for surgery, compared with 50% for IDET. Function, as measured by the ODI, showed a median 40% drop in eight RCTs of spinal fusion, compared with 20% in two RCTs of IDET. Improvements in quality of life was two to three times greater for surgery than IDET.

A meta-analysis by Freeman reviewed the same studies as the review by Appleby and colleagues but reached different conclusions.[6] This review reported a mean improvement in VAS scores of 3.4 (compared with 2.9 for Appleby), and only slightly lower mean ODI improvement of 5.2 (compared with 7.0 for Appleby). In addition, only 13% to 23% of the patients treated with IDET subsequently required surgery. Despite these seemingly positive findings, Freeman concluded that the evidence supporting the efficacy of IDET remains weak. Six IDET studies contained enough data to calculate the percentage of patients obtaining 50% or more pain relief as measured by the VAS or a numerical pain score. The studies included one RCT and five OBSs.[9,12-14,40,54-56] Between 38% and 94% (average 71%) of patients reported greater than 50% pain relief 6 to 24 months after IDET.

A critical review with strict interpretation of the procedure followed by RCTs in interventional spine procedures for spine disorders concluded that IDET is modestly effective in the treatment of lumbosacral discogenic pain in carefully selected patients.[57]

A recent SR of IDET procedures by Helm and colleagues in 2009 identified 2 RCTs and 16 OBSs with an indicated evidence of level II-2 according to USPSTF criteria.[58] The review of radiofrequency annuloplasty identified no RCTs but found two OBSs with uncertain evidence rated as level II-3. This review identified one OBS pilot study for intradiscal IDB, with very limited level III evidence. The authors cited limitations including the paucity of the literature and lack of evidence with internal validity and generalizability and concluded that IDET offers functionally significant relief in approximately one half of appropriately chosen patients with discogenic CLBP. This review also concluded that there was minimal evidence supporting the use of radiofrequency annuloplasty and IDB.

Findings from the above SRs are summarized in Table 27-3.

TABLE 27-3	Systematic Review Findings on Intradiscal Electrothermal Therapy for Chronic Low Back Pain		
Reference	# RCTs in SR	# RCTs for CLBP	Conclusion
44	31	3	Conflicting evidence supporting IDET for CLBP
50	4 SRs		Unable to make any definitive conclusions about effectiveness for CLBP because of conflicting results in RCTs
52	17	NR	Compelling evidence supporting relative efficacy
51	33	NR	Pain decrease similar to that reported with spinal fusion
6	Same studies as Ref. 52	NR	Weak evidence supporting efficacy of IDET
57	2	2	Modestly effective in carefully selected patients
58	2	2	Limited evidence supporting IDET (level II-2) Minimal evidence supporting use of IDRT Very limited evidence IDB due to current paucity of published studies (level III)

CLBP, chronic low back pain; IDB, intradiscal biacuplasty; IDET, intradiscal electrothermal therapy; NR, not reported; RCT, randomized controlled trial; SR, systematic review.

TABLE 27-4	Randomized Controlled Trials of Intradiscal Electrothermal Therapy for Chronic Low Back Pain		
Reference	Indication	Intervention	Control
49	DDD, discrete annular tear, LBP with or without neurologic involvement, symptoms >3 months	IDET via SpineCATH Surgeon 1 session Cointervention: rehabilitation program including Pilates n = 38	Sham placebo group Surgeon 1 session Cointervention: rehabilitation program including Pilates n = 55
36	IDD, posterior annular tear only, LBP without neurologic involvement, symptoms >6 months	IDET via SpineCATH 2 clinicians 1 session Cointervention: rehabilitation program including corset and exercise, acetaminophen for postprocedural pain n = 32	Sham placebo group 2 clinicians 1 session Cointervention: rehabilitation program including corset and exercise, acetaminophen for postprocedural pain n = 24
48	CLBP without neurologic involvement, symptoms >1 year	IDET via PIRFT Clinicians 1 session Cointervention: NR n = 13	Sham placebo group Clinicians 1 session Cointervention: NR n = 15
59	Disc disruption, duration of LBP NR, with or without neurologic involvement NR	IDET Provider type NR # sessions NR Cointervention: NR n = 11	Sham placebo group Provider type NR # sessions NR Cointervention: NR n = 6

CLBP, chronic low back pain; DDD, degenerative disc disease; IDD, internal disc disruption; IDET, intradiscal electrothermal therapy; LBP, low back pain; NR, not reported; PIRFT, percutaneous intradiscal radiofrequency thermocoagulation.

Randomized Controlled Trials

Four RCTs were identified.[36,48,49,59] Their methods are summarized in Table 27-4. Their results are briefly described here.

Freeman and colleagues[49] performed an RCT in which patients were selected on the basis of one- or two-level symptomatic disc degeneration with posterior or posterolateral annular tears as determined by provocative CT discography. To be included, participants had to have degenerative disc derangement symptoms lasting longer than 3 months; those with greater than 50% loss of disc height or previous back surgery were excluded. One session of IDET was delivered via the SpineCATH equipment by a surgeon while individuals in the sham placebo group experienced the same session without activating the electrical current. After 6 months, the sham group experienced a statistically significant increase in bodily pain from baseline. No other statistically significant differences in pain or function were observed for either group compared with baseline and no differences were noted between groups for pain or function at any time.

Pauza and colleagues[36] performed an RCT in patients with painful disc disruption identified by pressure-controlled lumbar discography. In order to be included, participants had to have LBP lasting longer than 6 months. Those with neurologic involvement, litigation, previous back surgery or worker's compensation issues were excluded. One session of IDET was delivered via the SpineCATH equipment by two clinicians; individuals in the sham placebo group experienced the same session without the activation of the electrical current. After 6 months, more people in the IDET group experienced pain relief than those in the sham placebo group (statistical significance not reported). The IDET group experienced statistically significant improvements in pain on one score (VAS) but not on another (SF-36 Bodily Pain) versus the sham placebo group. Similarly, the IDET group experienced statistically significant improvements in function on one score (ODI) but not on another (SF-36 Physical Function) versus the sham placebo group.

Barendse and colleagues[48] performed an RCT in patients with CLBP. To be included, participants had to have LBP lasting longer than 1 year. Those with a VAS score less than 5 and comorbidities (e.g., spinal stenosis) were excluded. One session of IDET was delivered via PIRFT by clinicians and individuals in the sham placebo group experienced the same session without the activation of the electrical current. Differences occurring within the IDET and sham placebo groups from baseline were not reported. After 8 weeks, no statistically significant differences were observed between the IDET and sham placebo groups regarding pain and function.

Lau and colleagues[59] presented their RCT at the 2004 ISIS Annual Scientific Meeting. Patients with single-level painful disc disruption were identified by a positive discogram using ISIS criteria. The study included 11 patients randomized to the IDET group and 6 patients randomized to the control sham group. After 12 months, more patients in the IDET group experienced more pain relief (statistical significance not reported), yet no statistically significant differences in pain were observed between the IDET and sham control groups. The RCT was stopped early because it was deemed that too large a number of patients would be required to show statistically significant differences between groups.

Observational Studies

As with many other newly introduced CLBP treatments, early IDET OBSs reported optimistic results (Tables 27-5 and 27-6). The initial prospective case series by Saal and colleagues, the cofounders of Oratec Interventions (later

TABLE 27-5 | **Design of Observational Studies of Intradiscal Electrothermal Therapy for Chronic Low Back Pain**

Reference	Sample Size (Final)	Follow-Up Period	Equipment Used	Indication	Pain Duration	Provocative Discography	Performed By	Secondary Gain*
IDET								
13	IDET: 36 CM: 17	24 months	SpineCATH	IDD	30 months 32 months	yes	INT	17/35 WC 3/17 WC
9	IDET: 36 CM: 17	12 months 3 months	SpineCATH	IDD	32 months 30 months	yes	INT	NR
64	25	12 months	SpineCATH	CLBP	2 years	yes	SURG	WC excluded
55	34 (33)	15 months	SpineCATH	CLBP	46 months	yes	SURG	15/34 WC Or no-fault cases
56	62 (41)	2 y (up to 4 years)	SpineCATH	CLBP, IDD	46 months	yes	SURG	20/61 WC
83	27	12 months	SpineCATH	DDD	38 months	yes	SURG	19/27 WC
14	58	24 months	SpineCATH	CLBP	60.7 months	yes	INT	20/58 WC
60	20 (19)	6 months	SpineCATH	DDD (with leg pain 50%)	44.2 months	yes	SURG	NR
40	NR	6 months	NR	NR	NR	NR	NR	NR
8	32	>6 months	SpineCATH	IDD (Discrete and global annular fissures, DDD)	NR	yes	INT	4/32 WC
12	62 (58)	12 months	SpineCATH	CLBP	60 months	yes	INT	23/62 WC
84	25	>6 months	SpineCATH	CLBP	58.5 months	yes	INT	5/25 WC
85	21	1 to 6 months	SpineCATH	IDD	91.9 months	yes	INT	3/21 WC
86	100	24 months	SpineCATH	CLBP	38.5 months	NR	INT	NR
87	75	12 months	NR	CLBP	NR	yes	NR	NR
88	IDET: 74 IRI: 35	15.5 months 7.7 months	SpineCATH	DDD, IDD	NR	yes	INT	NR
34	99	18 months	SpineCATH	IDD RLB	41.2 months	yes	INT	NR
61	60 (44)	20.4 months	SpineCATH	IDD with annular fissures Contained Disc herniation Discogenic Pain	>6 months	yes	SURG	WC excluded
62	142	22 months	SpineCATH	CLBP (68% not meeting the criteria)	26.4 months	yes (78% performed)	SURG and INT	All WC cases, 45% litigation involved

Continued

TABLE 27-5 | **Design of Observational Studies of Intradiscal Electrothermal Therapy for Chronic Low Back Pain—cont'd**

Reference	Sample Size (Final)	Follow-Up Period	Equipment Used	Indication	Pain Duration	Provocative Discography	Performed By	Secondary Gain*
25	79	6 months	SpineCATH	CLBP	5.7 years	yes	INT	NR
89	36 (31)	24 months	SpineCATH	CLBP	>6 months	yes	INT	NR
90	54	12 to 108 weeks	SpineCATH	70% discogenic pain, 24% DDD, 6% LBP	>9 months	yes	INT	NR
67	15	1, 3, 6 months	TransDiscal	DDD	>6 months	yes	NR	WC, litigation excluded
68	34	2 weeks; 2, 3, 6, 9, 12 months	NR	DDD	1.6 years	yes	INT	NR
91	34 (32)	12 months	SpineCATH	CLBP	1.1 years	yes	INT	10/34 WC, 19/34 PI
68	DDD: 17 MDDD: 17	12 months	SpineCATH	DDD	1.6 years	yes	NR	NR
92	21	1 to 6 months	SpineCATH	IDD	91.9 months	yes	INT	3/21 WC
93	86 (NR)	24 months	SpineCATH	CLBP	>6 months	yes	INT	NR
70	56	24 months	SpineCATH	CLBPIDD Contained disc herniation	38.8 months	yes	NR	9/56 WC
69	53	72 months	NR	CLBPIDD	NR	yes	NR	All WC cases
94	39	18 months	NR	Chronic Discogenic LBP DDD without nerve root compression	32 months	yes	NR	NR
IDRT								
65	IDRT: 31 CM: 15	12 months	Disctrode	CLBP	>6 months	yes	NR	65% WC 60% WC
63	IDET: 21 RFA: 21	12 months	SpineCATH and RFA	CLBP No disc herniation	3.2 years	yes	NR	WC, litigation excluded
IDB								
71	1	6 months	Baylis Medical Inc	Chronic axial LBP	2.5 years	yes	INT	NR
67	15 (13)	6 months	Baylis Medical Inc	CLBP > leg pain	>6 months	yes	INT	WC excluded
72	15 (13)	12 months	Baylis Medical Inc	CLBP > leg pain	>6 months	yes	INT	WC excluded
73	1	12 months	Baylis Medical Inc	DDD post-discectomy	>4 years	yes	INT	WC excluded
74	8	6 months	Baylis Medical Inc	CLBP	NR	-	INT	WC excluded

CLBP, chronic low back pain; CM, conservative management; DDD, degenerative disc disease; IDB, intradiscal biacuplasty; IDD, internal disc disruption; INT, interventionalist; IRI, intradiscal restorative injection; LBP, low back pain; MDDD, multilevel degenerative disc disease; NR, not reported; PI, personal injury; RFA, radiofrequency posterior annuloplasty; RLB, referred leg and back pain; SpineCATH, SpineCATH by Oratec International; SURG, surgeon; WC, worker's compensation.

*Includes worker's compensation, claims, or litigation.

TABLE 27-6	Outcomes of Observational Studies of Intradiscal Electrothermal Therapy for Chronic Low Back Pain			
Reference	Outcomes	Initial (Mean ± SD)	Follow-Up (Mean, SD)	% Improvement
IDET				
91	VAS	WC: 7.44 ± 1.5	WC: 4.33 ± 2.5	78
		Non-WC: 8.0 ± 1.6	Non-WC: 1.77 ± 1.8	53
		Overall: 8.0	Overall: 2.3	71
	Return to work		WC: 40%	
			Non-WC: 82%	
68	VAS	DDD: 7.7 ± 2	DDD: 2.5 ± 2.4	68
		MDDD: 7.4 ± 1.8	MDDD: 4.9 ± 2.9	34
	PDI (MDDD-DDD)		Change 13.6	
92	VAS-current	6.2	3.9	37
	VAS-best	3.5	2.0	
	VAS-worst	8.4	5.7	
	Opioid use	81%	29%	
	Improvement VAS >50%		67%	
	Improvement VAS >75%		57%	
93	"Current day" pain VAS	Male: 5.5, Female: 7	Changed −1.5 ± 2.9 (all patients)	
	"Last week" pain VAS	Male: 7.0, Female: 7.1	Changed −2.4 ± 3.2 (all patients)	
	RMDQ	Male: 75, Female: 75	Changed −26.7 ± 36 (all patients)	
70	VAS	6.1 ± 1.8	2.4 ± 2.6	61
	Sitting	40.9 ± 40.6	84.5 ± 54.4	107
	Standing	46.8 ± 42.9	84.4 ± 54.2	80
	Walking	39.2 ± 39.6	77.9 ± 50.8	99
	SF-36 General Health	96% of the norm	97% of the norm	
	SF-36 Physical function	61% of the norm	90% of the norm	
	SF-36 Role Physical	44% of the norm	79% of the norm	
	SF-36 Bodily Pain	61% of the norm	93% of the norm	
	SF-36 Vitality	82% of the norm	103% of the norm	
	SF-36 Social Functioning	64% of the norm	93% of the norm	
	SF-36 Role Emotional	64% of the norm	96% of the norm	
	SF-36 Mental Health	87% of the norm	103% of the norm	
69	VAS (0-100)	63.77	19.43	62.6
	ODI	24.83	5.15	69.3
	Economic productivity	5.3%	47.2%	
	Narcotic use	51%	13.2%	
94	ODI	45.7	24.8	21.0
	– 6 months		23.0	22.7
	– 12 months		21.5	24.3
	– 18 months			
13	VAS	IDET: 8.0 (7.0-9.0)	IDET: 3.0 (1.0-7.0)	IDET: 63
		CM: 8.0 (5.0-8.0)	CM: 7.5 (4.0-8.0)	CM: 6
	Any improvement VAS		80%	
	>50% improvement VAS		IDET: 57%	
			CM: 12%	
	Complete pain relief		20%	
9	VAS	IDET: 8.0 (7.0-9.0)	IDET: 3.0 (1.0-7.0)	IDET: 63
		CM: 8.0 (5.0-8.0)	CM: 8.0 (7.0-8.0)	CM: 0
	>50% improvement VAS		IDET: 60% (12 months)	
			CM: 6% (3 months)	
	Any improvement VAS		94%	
64	VAS	7.3	4.9	32
	Any improvement VAS		56%	
	SAT		8	
55	VAS-Back Pain	7.5	3.9	52
	VAS-Lower Extremity	5.7	2.0	65
	RMDQ	13.9	6.6	53
	NASS		77	
	Improvement VAS >3		69.6%	
	No pain		24%	

Continued

TABLE 27-6	Outcomes of Observational Studies of Intradiscal Electrothermal Therapy for Chronic Low Back Pain—cont'd			
Reference	Outcomes	Initial (Mean ± SD)	Follow-Up (Mean, SD)	% Improvement
56	VAS-LB	7.9 ± 1.3	4.7 ± 3.0	41
	VAS-LE	5.0 ± 3.6	2.7 ± 3.2	46
	RMDQ	15.4 ± 5.3	8.8 ± 7.5	43
	NASS		63%	
	Improvement VAS >2		53%	
	Decreased medication use		68%	
83	ODI	34	30	12
	SF-36 Physical Function	32	47	47
	SF-36 Bodily Pain	27	38	41
	Improved symptoms		75%	
14	VAS	6.6 ± 1.9	3.4 ± 2.0	48
	SF-36 Physical Function	40.5 ± 25.0	71.8 ± 22.9	77
	SF-36 Bodily Pain	29.8 ± 16.0	51.7 ± 22.6	72
	Sitting time	32.6 ± 47.5	85.3 ± 61.2	62
	Improvement VAS >2		72%	
	Improvement VAS >4		50%	
	Return to work		PP: 97%	
			WC: 83%	
60	VAS	65.4 ± 14.89	50.6 ± 26.5	22
	ODI	43.1 ± 7.35	36.7 ± 21.1	14
	SF-36 Physical Function	46	56	22
	SF-36 Bodily Pain	32	42	31
40	Improvement VAS >4		94%	
	SF-Physical Function		75	
8	VAS		Decreased 1.84 ± 2.38	
	RMDQ		Decreased 4.03 ± 4.82	
	Overall activity—better or much better		53.1%	
	Overall favorable outcome		62.5%	
12	VAS	6.6 ± 1.8	3.5 ± 2.4	46
	SF-36 Physical Function	39.7 ± 25.5	59.9 ± 22.7	51.3
	SF-36 Bodily Pain	29.5 ± 16.6	46.4 ± 19.2	59.3
	Any improvement VAS		71%	
	Improvement VAS >60%		50%	
	Return to work		PP: 97%	
			WC: 83%	
			NW: 95%	
84	VAS	7.3	3.6	51
	SF-36 Physical Function	40.1 ± 5.4	55.2 ± 5.4	38
	SF-36 Bodily Pain	28.5 ± 3.3	42.2 ± 3.6	45
	Sitting	23.6	47.2	50
	Any improvement VAS		80%	
	Improvement VAS >2		Single level: 85%	
			Multilevel: 75%	
85	VAS-current	6.2	3.9	37
	VAS-best	3.5	2.0	
	VAS-worst	8.4	5.7	
	Opioid use	81%	29%	
	Improvement VAS >50%		67%	
	Improvement VAS >75%		57%	

TABLE 27-6	Outcomes of Observational Studies of Intradiscal Electrothermal Therapy for Chronic Low Back Pain—cont'd			
Reference	Outcomes	Initial (Mean ± SD)	Follow-Up (Mean, SD)	% Improvement
86	VAS	6.7 ± 1.7	3.6 ± 2.9	46
	SF-36 Physical Function	36.6 ± 23.1	62.1 ± 28.4	9
	SF-36 Bodily Pain	26.1 ± 16.0	49.2 ± 30.0	97
	Sitting	34.6 ± 35.6	77.3 ± 52.8	120
	Standing	31.9 ± 36.7	54.8 ± 47.2	73
	Walking	32.3 ± 27.6	65.2 ± 52.1	101
	Any improvement VAS		81%	
	Reduced medication use		60%	
87	VAS	6.0	3.6	40
	Any improvement VAS		85.3%	
88	VAS		IDET: changed 1.27	
			IRI: changed 2.24	
	Any improvement VAS		IDET: 47.8%	
			IRI: 65.6%	
34	VAS-back dominant		Changed 1.13 ± 3.13	
	VAS-leg and back		Changed 2.28 ± 2.49	
	VAS-leg dominant		Changed 2.64 ± 3.41	
	NASS-back dominant	3.37 ± 0.82	2.59 ± 1.08	23
	NASS leg dominant		1.79 ± 1.35	
	Any improvement VAS	2.36 ± 1.25	63.90%	24
61	Satisfied with outcome		37%	
	Less pain		39%	
	Return to work		29%	
	Reduced opioid use		45%	
62	Return to work		37%	
	Opioid use		66%	
	– 3 months		70%	
	– 6 months			
	Significant postintervention pain		>67%	
	Required surgery		n = 3	
	Required injections		n = 7	
25	VAS	Positive outcome group: 5.9 ± 1.8	Positive outcome group: 5.9 ± 1.8	
	Any improvement VAS	Negative outcome group: 6.2 ± 1.9	Negative outcome group: 6.2 ± 1.9	
	Improvement VAS >50%		48%	
	Improvement VAS >90%		10%	
89	VAS		Changed 2.5 ± 1	
	VAS-improved		29%	
	VAS-improved, returned to same		23%	
	VAS-stayed the same		29%	
	VAS-worsened		19%	
	Any improvement VAS		65%	
	Improvement VAS >2		52%	
	Improvement VAS >50%		16%	
	Return to work		61%	
	Opioid use	n = 7	n = 2	

Continued

TABLE 27-6	Outcomes of Observational Studies of Intradiscal Electrothermal Therapy for Chronic Low Back Pain—cont'd			
Reference	Outcomes	Initial (Mean ± SD)	Follow-Up (Mean, SD)	% Improvement
90	VAS		Changed 2.49 (median 2)	
	Any improvement VAS		77%	
	Sitting-car		60.4	
	Sitting-firm surface		41.3	
	Improvement VAS >2		65%	
	Improvement VAS >3		52%	
	Walking		50.0 months	
	Return to work		66%	
IDRT				
63	VAS	IDRT: 7.4 ± 1.9	IDRT: 1.4 ± 1.9	IDRT: 81
		RFA: 6.6 ± 2.0	RFA: 4.4 ± 2.4	RFA: 84
	PDI	IDRT: 55	IDRT: 9	IDRT: 83
		RFA: 48	RFA: 31	RFA: 35
	>30% improvement PDI		86%	
	>60% improvement PDI		81%	
65	VAS	IDET: 7.2 ± 1.3	IDET: 4.5 ± 2.5	IDET: 37
		CM: 6.2 ± 1.2	CM: 6.3 ± 1.5	CM: 3
	ODI	IDET: 48.1 ± 11.5	IDET: 35.5 ± 16.6	IDET: 25
		CM: 46.1 ± 15.0	CM: 46.0 ± 14.0	CM: 7
	MQS	IDET: 16.8 ± 10.5	IDET: 13.5 ± 11.8	IDET: 0
		CM: 15.9 ± 14.9	CM: 19.3 ± 13.6	CM: 0
IDB				
72	VAS	7	4	50%
	ODI	23.3	17.5	
	SF-36 Physical Function	51	67	
	SF-36 Bodily Pain	38	57	
	Opioid use	40 mg (95% CI)	0 mg (95% CI)	
73	VAS	5	3	
	ODI	52	14	
	SF-36 Physical Function	55	95	
74	Median pain	69	35 (P < .05) at 1 month	4 patients (50%)
			41 (P < .14) at 3, 6 months	achieved >50%
	ODI	69		By 11 points at 3 months
				By 10 at 6 months
	SF-36 Physical Function			By 15 points at 3 months
				By 5 at 6 months
67	VAS	7.2 ± 1.9	1 month: 3.3 ± 2.1	
			3 months: 3.8 ± 1.9	
			6 months: 3.4 ± 1.9	
	ODI	23.3 ± 7.0	1 month: 16.5 ± 6.8	
			3 months: 16.9 ± 7.1	
			6 months: 17.1 ± 8.1	
	SF-36 Physical Function	50.8 ± 17.5	1 month: 59.4 ± 6.8	
			3 months: 65.7 ± 7.1	
			6 months: 69.9 ± 8.1	
	SF-36 Bodily Pain	37.5 ± 15.0	1 month: 49.7 ± 19.3	
			3 months: 51.2 ± 16.8	
			6 months: 53.8 ± 22.7	
	Opioid use (morphine sulphate equivalent dose)	73.5 ± 59.7	1 month: 56.5 ± 62.6	
			3 months: 45.0 ± 59.2	
			6 months: 38.8 ± 61.6	

TABLE 27-6	Outcomes of Observational Studies of Intradiscal Electrothermal Therapy for Chronic Low Back Pain—cont'd			
Reference	Outcomes	Initial (Mean ± SD)	Follow-Up (Mean, SD)	% Improvement
71	VAS	5	1	
	ODI	14	6	
	SF-36 Physical Function	67	82	
	SF-36 General Health	80	90	
	SF-36 Role Physical	75	88	
	SF-36 Bodily Pain	68	80	
	SF-36 Vitality	70	75	
	SF-36 Social Functioning	75	88	
	SF-36 Role Emotional	100	100	
	SF-36 Mental Health	60	80	

1,2DDD, 1 or 2 level degenerative disc disease; BP, bodily pain; CM, conservative management; DDD, degenerative disc disease; IDB, intradiscal biacuplasty; IDET, intradiscal electrothermal therapy; IDRT, intradiscal radiofrequency treatment; LB, low back; LE, lower extremity; MDDD, multilevel degenerative disc disease; MQS, medication quantification score; NASS, North American Spine Society Low Back Pain questionnaire; ODI, Oswestry Disability Index; PDI, pain disability index; PP, private pay patients; RFA, radiofrequency posterior annuloplasty; RMDQ, Roland Morris Disability Questionnaire; SAT, satisfaction score; SD, standard deviation; SF, short form; SF-BP, Short form-36, Bodily Pain score; SF-PF, short form-36, Physical Function score; VAS, visual analog scale; WC, worker's compensation.

purchased by Smith & Nephew), reported a positive response rate in 80% of participants.[12,14] A study by Derby and colleagues reported positive response rates of 73% when the catheter position was optimal, but only 16.5% in patients with a catheter placement described as only fair.[8] Saal and colleagues also reported decreases in the SF-36 bodily pain of 59% to 78% and average decreases in VAS of 62% to 72%.[12,14] Despite early published results similar to the Saal and colleagues study, Derby's study reported that approximately one-third of his patients treated with IDET were much better, one-third were slightly better, and one-third were the same or worse. In addition, his patients had on average only a 1.84/10 (18%) decrease in VAS. Since then, prospective and retrospective OBS case series have reported a dichotomy of results as described below.[8]

Three studies reported overall poor results with an average decrease in VAS of about 20%.[60-62] The worst results are reported by Davis, whose retrospective OBS was conducted by surgeons who had not performed the IDET procedure. They reported that 29% had more pain than before the procedure, 39% had less pain, and 29% had the same amount of pain. While 37% of patients reported being satisfied with the procedure, 50% were dissatisfied with IDET.[61] The other retrospective study conducted by the Liberty Mutual Center reported on narcotic use, spine surgery, and epidural steroid injections after IDET was performed on 142 patients in 23 states.[62] They found that 68% of the cases did not meet Medicare's published criteria for medical necessity, 37% had at least one epidural steroid injection post-IDET, 55% had at least two narcotic prescriptions, 23% had spinal surgery, and only 20% returned to work.

On the other hand, the mean decrease in VAS was approximately 50% in the five published case series with different population groups, only one of which was approved by an institutional review board.[25,34,55,63,64] The best reported outcome scores were from a recent study by Kapural and

colleagues,[63] who compared the results in 42 patients randomized to IDET or IDRT. From months 3 to 12, the IDET group had significantly lower mean pain scores than the IDRT group. VAS pain scores decreased from 6.6 ± 2.0 (mean ± standard deviation) at baseline to 4.4 ± 2.4 at 1 year after IDRT ($P = .001$), whereas in the IDET group the average VAS pain score decreased from 7.4 ± 1.9 at baseline IDET to 1.4 ± 1.9 at the 1-year follow-up. Similarly, ODI scores in the IDET group had a significantly larger improvement from baseline than the IDRT group.

Two prospective case series used a convenience control group of patients who were offered IDET but could either not afford the procedure or failed to obtain prior authorization from their insurance companies.[9,13,65] Although the results were criticized because the denial of care introduced a potential selection bias and probably immediate patient dissatisfaction in the control population, one could argue that they had greater external validity than RCTs performed under artificial conditions because they represented the patients who would normally have received this intervention.[66]

Karasek and Bogduk[9] studied a group of 17 patients who were denied insurance authorization and were reported to have continued a conservative treatment protocol identical to 36 patients receiving IDET. Only patients with well-hydrated discs in whom annular disruption was limited to two quadrants or less were selected. At one year, only 1 patient in the control group had significant relief of pain. In the IDET group, VAS was decreased by 63% and 60% of the patients had greater than 50% pain relief, with 23% obtaining complete relief of pain. All 18 patients working before IDET returned to work, and 8 of 15 not working returned to work after IDET. At the 2-year follow-up, 54% of the patients continued to have greater than 50% reduction in pain.[13]

In a more recent but similar study, Finch and colleagues[65] performed IDRT on the posterior annulus using a flexible radiofrequency electrode (DiscTRODE) in 46 patients with single-level painful discs and compared outcomes with 17 patients who were unable to obtain funding for the procedure. The VAS decreased 37% in treated patients at the 12-month follow-up, compared with an increase of 3% in control subjects.

Kapural and colleagues[68] performed a study examining the effects of IDTA among patients with chronic DDD. Seventeen patients with multiple-level DDD were matched with 17 patients with one- or two-level DDD and all received IDTA. After 12 months of follow-up, patients with one- or two-level DDD experienced statistically significant improvement in pain ($P < .00273$) and disability versus those with multiple-level DDD. The authors concluded that IDTA is an effective treatment for DDD and that the number of affected discs is an important factor to consider for this treatment.

Nunley and colleagues in 2008 prospectively studied 53 consecutive worker's compensation patients undergoing IDET for CLBP.[69] At a mean follow-up of 53 months the authors reported a mean reduction ($P < .001$) of 62.6% in the VAS and 69.3% in the ODI. The patient's initial VAS and ODI scores ($P < .05$) significantly affected the final outcomes. In addition, approximately 47.2% of the patients had resumed some degree of economic productivity (e.g., employment), while only 7 (initial 26) continued to consume opioid analgesics.

Using a single-arm prospective clinical trial, Maurer and colleagues in 2008 reported outcomes of 56 patients undergoing IDET for CLBP selected by MRI scan and pressure-controlled discography at an average follow-up of 20 months.[70] The mean pain severity scores (VAS) improved from 6.1 ± 1.8 before treatment to 2.4 ± 2.6 at final follow-up ($P = .0001$). The mean tolerance times (minutes) improved from 40.9 ± 40.6 to 84.5 ± 54.4, 46.8 ± 42.9 to 84.4 ± 54.2, and 39.2 ± 39.6 to 77.9 ± 50.8 between baseline and final follow-up for sitting, standing, and walking, respectively ($P = .0001$ for all comparisons). Seven of eight quality-of-life domains from the SF-36 showed significant ($P = .0001$ for all comparisons) improvement over baseline. Forty-two patients (75%) were classified as a treatment success by virtue of at least a 2-point improvement in pain severity or at least a 10-point improvement in either the physical function or bodily pain domain of the SF-36.

Intradiscal Biacuplasty

Kapural and Mekhail reported the first clinical case of IDB done for a patient with severe chronic axial LBP on a single-level painful disc confirmed by provocative discography.[71] VAS decreased from 5 before the procedure to 2 at 1 month, and down to 1 at 6 months after the procedure. ODI improved from 14 to 6 points (from moderate to minimal disability) and physical function score of the SF-36 improved from 67 to 82 with patient satisfaction reported as "absolute."

Kapural and colleagues conducted an observational study on patients with CLBP (>6 months) who were not responsive to nonoperative care.[67] All patients had one- or two-level DDD without evidence of additional degenerative changes. After confirmation by provocative discography, the patients

underwent a one- or two-level biacuplasty procedure of their painful discs. Thirteen of 15 patients (86.7%) completed the study. At 6 months, pain was significantly improved, with a decrease in mean VAS scores of 53% compared with baseline. Disability was also significantly improved at 6 months, with a decrease in ODI of 27% compared with baseline. There were also statistically significant improvements in the SF-36 scores for physical function and bodily pain. Opioid use did not significantly change from baseline, but showed a trend to decline. More than half of patients had more than 50% improvement in their pain scores when followed up over a 6-month period.

Kapural reported 12-month follow-up results of the aforementioned study with the same 13 patients.[72] VAS remained reduced from 7 to 4 at 12 months (3 at 6 months); ODI remained improved 17.5 points at 12 months (16.6 at 6 months). The SF-36 scores for physical function and bodily pain remained similarly reduced. The difference was noted in the daily opioid use at 12 months: 0 mg (95% CI 0 to 20) of morphine equivalent compared to 5 mg (95% CI 0 to 40) at 6 months after the procedure and 40 mg (95% CI 40 to 120) before the procedure. More than half of patients maintained greater than 50% pain relief.

Kapural and colleagues reported a case study of IDB done on a single disc level for a woman who had an open discectomy procedure 4 years earlier.[73] She had axial LBP aggravated by sitting, single-level DDD with greater than 50% disc height confirmed by MRI, and concordant pain on provocative discography with two negative control levels. Twelve months after the procedure, the patient's VAS score improved from 5 to 3. ODI showed functional improvement from severe disability (52%) to minimal (14%). The SF-36 score for physical function improved from 55 to 95.

Bogduk and colleagues reported the results of a prospective OBS in eight patients with CLBP due to internal disc disruption who received IDB.[74] Median pain score improved from 69 to 35 at 1 month ($P < .05$), but deteriorated at 3 months to 41, and remained at that level at 6 months, after which the charge from the baseline was no longer statistically significant ($P < .14$). Scores for disability and physical function improved (to 50 and 50), but this did not achieve statistical significance.[33,54] ODI decreased by 11 points at 3 months and by 10 points at 6 months, with increase in physical function on the SF-36 by 15 points at 3 months and 5 points at 6 months. Overall, four of eight patients (50%) achieved greater than 50% decrease in pain at 6 months.

Summary of Evidence by Category and Subcategory

Although the various methods of applying intradiscal thermal therapies are based on somewhat similar principles, their application is not necessarily equal with respect to demonstrated efficacy. Each method must therefore stand or fall on the evidence that the particular method achieves its primary goal which is to reduce discogenic pain and thereby improve function. The original intradiscal heating that delivered heat only to the nucleus was never widely used and was for the most part abandoned after an RCT showed an effect no larger than placebo. An overview of the

TABLE 27-7	Summary Outcomes by Category and Subcategory of Intradiscal Thermal Therapy for Chronic Low Back Pain				
Type	Reference	Study Type	Pain Improvement	Functional Improvement	Overall Outcome
Intranuclear	48	RCT	Approximately 6	Approximately 3 (ODI)	Negative
	95	OBS	Approximately 20	38 (ODI)	Negative
Intra-annular (IDET)	74	RCT	25	NR	Inconclusive
	36	RCT	24	11 (ODI)	Positive
	49	RCT	3 (SF-BP)	13 (ODI)	Negative
	9, 13	OBS	50	NR	Positive
	88	OBS	13	NR	Positive
	68	OBS	42	Significantly better (PDI)	Positive
	63	OBS	60	60 (PDI)	Positive
	92	OBS	Approximately 23	Better (tolerance)	Positive
	12	OBS	30	20 (SF-PF)	Positive
	14	OBS	32	31 (SF-PF)	Positive
	84	OBS	51	38 (SF-PF)	Positive
	60	OBS	14	6 (ODI)	Negative
	83	OBS	41 (SF-BP)	12 (ODI)	Positive
	55	OBS	39	30 (RMDQ)	Positive
	56	OBS	32	28 (RMDQ)	Positive
	91	OBS	66	75 (ADL)	Positive
	64	OBS	24	NR	Negative
	93	OBS	20	27 (RMDQ)	Positive
	70	OBS	61	95 (Tolerance)	Positive
	69	OBS	63	69 (ODI)	Positive
	94	OBS	NR	24 (ODI)	Positive
	25	OBS	Approximately 20	NR	Positive
	89	OBS	NA	NA	Positive
	61	OBS	NA	NA	Negative
	34	OBS	Approximately 8	NR	Positive
Intra-annular (IDRT)	65	OBS	37	25 (ODI)	Positive
	63	OBS	22	14 (PDI)	Negative
Intra-annular (IDB)	71	OBS	40	8 (ODI)	Positive
	67	OBS	40	7 (ODI)	Positive
	72	OBS	30	6 (ODI)	Positive
	73	OBS	20	38 (ODI)	Positive
	74	OBS	29	4 (ODI)	Positive

Pain improvement: mean % change in VAS or SF-36 bodily pain (BP).
Functional improvement: mean % change in ODI, PDI, SF-36 physical function (SF), RMDQ, or ADL.
IDB, intradiscal biacuplasty; IDRT, intradiscal radiofrequency treatment; short form; NA, not applicable; NR, not reported; OBS, observational study; ODI, Oswestry Disability Index; PDI, pain disability index; RCT, randomized controlled trial; RMDQ: Roland Morris Disability Questionnaire; SF-BP, SF-36 bodily pain score; SF-PF, SF-36 physical function score; VAS, visual analog scale.

evidence supporting efficacy for the various categories and subcategories of intradiscal thermal therapies is presented in Table 27-7.

SAFETY

Contraindications

The following contraindications have been proposed for the spinal level targeted by IDET: >50% disc height loss, extruded or sequestered herniation, major psychological impairment, moderate to severe spinal stenosis, moderate to severe spondylosis, nerve root compression with motor deficit, obesity, pregnancy, previous IDET in past 6 months, previous lumbar surgery, and spondylolisthesis with instability.[6,35]

Adverse Events

CPGs on the management of LBP have reported that AEs associated with IDET include burning sensations in the legs, radicular pain, disc herniation, numbness, and paresis.[43] A retrospective study of 1675 IDET procedures and 35,000

SpineCATH intradiscal catheters reported a total of 40 serious AEs.[75] Nineteen cases of catheter breakage were reported, which was associated with repeated catheter manipulation during positioning; the broken catheter was left uneventfully within the disc in 16 cases. Eight cases of superficial skin burn at the needle puncture site were reported. Six nerve root injuries were reported, five of which occurred when inserting the introducer needle; these cases resolved completely. Six disc herniations were reported 2 to 12 months after IDET, of which four resolved with nonoperative care and two required surgical excision. One case of bladder dysfunction was reported following IDET.

Other AEs have also been reported, including disc infections and nerve injury.[76] When the catheter is placed in the outer periphery of the disc and lies within a few millimeters of the spinal nerve root, the spinal nerve roots and dorsal root ganglions may be vulnerable.[77] The catheter can be inadvertently introduced into the epidural space, but this can be easily identified on a lateral fluoroscopic image. When this occurs, withdrawing the catheter and reorienting it into the disc should prevent injury. If a misplaced catheter remains unnoticed and is heated, the patient will likely complain of immediate onset radicular leg pain. However, this can only be communicated by patients who are not heavily sedated or anesthetized. Although transient increases in leg pain are not uncommon after IDET, these may be related to the reappearance of previous leg pain rather than a new onset related to the procedure.

Temperatures greater than 45° C applied for an extended period of time might also result in transient or prolonged leg pain. One case of cauda equina syndrome was reported following IDET at the L4-5 level, possibly from direct injury by the introducer needle or catheter rather than heat transfer through the disc.[66,78] End-plate heat injury is another possible AE. Although cadaver studies have not demonstrated significantly elevated end-plate temperatures, it is difficult to determine the proximity of the catheter to the end plates with fluoroscopy and in some instances a portion of the catheter may contact an adjoining end plate.[79] There has been one case report of possible end-plate necrosis following an IDET procedure.[80] Accelerated disc degeneration may occur after IDET, though there seems to be little change in MRI findings after 12 months.[81]

COSTS

Fees and Third-Party Reimbursement

In the United States, IDET for CLBP can be reported by physicians using CPT code 22526 (single level, including fluoroscopic guidance) or 22527 (additional levels, including fluoroscopic guidance). These are new category 1 CPT codes added on January 1, 2007. Codes 0062T and 0063T have now been deleted. These codes can only be reported for electrothermal annuloplasty. For percutaneous intradiscal annuloplasty using a method other than electrothermal, CPT code 22899 (unlisted procedure of the spine) should be used, along with a description of the procedure. The disposable catheter

itself can be charged using Healthcare Common Procedure Coding System code C1754. Additional fees also apply for any other disposable medical equipment (e.g., needles, syringes), as well as any medications injected. The outpatient surgical center in which the procedure takes place will also charge facility fees for use of their operating room, recovery room, other disposable medical equipment, nurses, radiology, and other services. Because of these ancillary fees, the total cost of an IDET procedure can reach $8000 or more, although there is wide variation in fees.

These procedures are not currently reimbursed by Medicare and are considered experimental and investigational.[82] If the Medicare patient is expected to pay for this service out of pocket, an Advanced Beneficiary Notice should be executed before the service. The procedures may be covered by other third-party payers such as health insurers and worker's compensation insurance. Preauthorization may be required to obtain reimbursement from third-party payers, which generally indicates that patients and physicians must adhere to specific criteria in order to deem the procedure medically necessary.

Cost Effectiveness

No cost effectiveness analyses or cost utility analyses were identified that evaluated the cost effectiveness of IDET as an intervention for LBP.

The CPG from Europe in 2004 indicated that the cost effectiveness of IDET for CLBP (>3 months) is unknown.[43]

The CPG from Belgium in 2006 indicated that the cost effectiveness of IRFT for CLBP (>3 months) is unknown.[42]

The CPG from Europe in 2004 indicated that the cost effectiveness of IRFT in the treatment of CLBP (>3 months) is unknown.[43]

SUMMARY

Description

Intradiscal thermal therapies use a number of devices that deliver heat energy to IVDs for the purpose of contracting tissue, lowering pressure, destroying nociceptors, and creating a seal to limit expression of matrix components. The original method of heating the nucleus with a radiofrequency probe has largely been abandoned and now other devices target the outer annulus. IDET uses a catheter inserted into the nucleus and circumferentially navigated to the outer annulus and is heated using either electrothermal energy or RFE. IDRT heats the outer annulus using RFE delivered through an electrode passed across the posterior annulus through an introducer needle. The latest method uses two water-cooled radiofrequency probes inserted into the outer annulus from both sides and may have the advantage of providing a more uniform distribution of heat across the outer posterior annulus. Nonsurgical or surgical spine specialists in secondary care settings typically perform these procedures in facilities in which fluoroscopy is available, such as specialty spine clinics, pain management clinics, and hospitals.

Theory

The precise mechanism of action through which intradiscal heating can help patients with CLBP is unclear and numerous theoretical explanations for these observations have been offered, such as changes in disc biomechanics, annular contraction, thermally-induced healing response, sealing of annular tears, annular denervation, and decreased intradiscal pressure. Indications for intradiscal heating include axial CLBP with or without leg pain that persists for more than 6 months, greater than 50% normal disc height, MRI or CT findings of posterior annulus disruption, symptoms consistent with CLBP related to discogenic involvement (e.g., pain with motion, difficulty with prolonged sitting), a positive discography that reproduces concordant pain at 7/10 intensity at a pressure less than 50 PSI (preferably at less than 15 PSI) above opening, and unresponsiveness to at least 12 weeks of appropriate conservative care. CT discography is typically performed prior to the procedure to help guide the spine specialist to target the appropriate spinal levels involved in a patient's CLBP and to assess the location and magnitude of annular disruption. Greater than 50% relief of pain following injection of local anesthetic into an IVD may theoretically offer a better method of predicting outcome.

Efficacy

Two CPGs found conflicting evidence, two CPGs found insufficient evidence, and one other CPG found level II-2 evidence based on USPSTF criteria supporting IDET. Similarly for IDRT, two CPGs found conflicting evidence, one CPG found no evidence, and another CPG found insufficient evidence of effectiveness. Two SRs did not recommend IDET due to inconsistent evidence; one review indicated limited effectiveness, while two SRs concluded that IDET is effective. Four published RCTs have assessed intradiscal heating and generally reported mixed result. Some studies found statistically significant improvement in pain scores or other indices of physical function for IDET compared to sham control, while others found no change over baseline, or no significant difference in improvement when compared to a sham procedure.

Safety

Contraindications of IDET include greater than 50% disc height loss, extruded or sequestered herniation, major psychological impairment, moderate to severe spinal stenosis, moderate to severe spondylosis, nerve root compression with motor deficit, obesity, pregnancy, previous IDET in past 6 months, previous lumbar surgery, and spondylolisthesis with instability. AEs include burning sensations in the legs, radicular pain, disc herniation, numbness, paresis, disc infections, and nerve injury.

Costs

The cost of IDET, IDRT, and IDB varies, but can be as high as $8000. The cost effectiveness of intradiscal heating is unknown.

Comments

Our review finds no evidence that intranuclear heating is effective. Likewise there is little evidence to support the IDRT method based on one controlled study showed no significant effect and one study comparing IDET and IDRT that showed IDET was clearly more effective. However, the evidence for IDET, while conflicting, weakly supports the method of heating the outer annulus using the catheter technique in well-selected patients. In particular, almost all retrospective and prospective OBSs report positive results. A controlled but non-randomized study clearly showed superiority of IDET over continued conservative care. There are mixed results in published RCTs evaluating the IDET procedure, some showing a difference, albeit small, and some showing no difference from control. The negative RCT is often used to dissuade many reviewing organizations from endorsing IDET for LBP. Although this study should not be discounted, the negative findings do not outweigh all the other positive results reported in OBS studies since the highly unusual finding of no placebo response and the reported 0% success rate are inconsistent with all other observational IDET studies. Finally, with only one OBS and several case reports, there is not enough information available to adequately evaluate the efficacy of IDB.

The reviewed CPGs, SRs, and OBSs report conflicting evidence regarding the effectiveness of intradiscal heating, although available studies weakly support IDET method for CLBP. However, it should be considered that intradiscal heating is significantly less invasive than conventional decompression surgery and may therefore be beneficial for a small subset of patients who fail to improve after conservative therapy and are not appropriate candidates for surgery. This subgroup of patients is currently difficult to define, but may include those with CLBP who have less functional impairment, relatively well-maintained disc heights, and discogenic pain caused by annular tears or protrusions less than 3 to 4 mm. Patients interested in trying IDET should be advised about the potential AEs associated with this intervention.

CHAPTER REVIEW QUESTIONS

Answers are located on page 452.

1. At which tissue is the heat used in IDET targeted?
   a. tendon
   b. cartilage
   c. collagen
   d. iliolumbar ligaments
2. What attribute gives type I collagen the ability to resist tensile forces?
   a. triple-helical configuration
   b. fibrous protein
   c. gelatinous properties
   d. high solubility

3. What is the tissue temperature above which necrosis can occur?

   a. 45° C

   b. 55° C

   c. 65° C

   d. 75° C

4. Which of the following is most often used to produce the energy used in intradiscal thermal therapies?

   a. laser

   b. thermal cautery

   c. electrocautery

   d. radiofrequency energy

5. What is an advantage of the shorter heating element catheter over the longer catheter?

   a. allows collagen tissue to shrink quickly

   b. helps limit destruction of normal disc annulus

   c. allows the disc annulus to heal quicker

   d. is more precise

6. What type of probes are often used for RFE?

   a. depressed probes

   b. bipolar probes

   c. copper probes

   d. stainless steel probes

7. True or false: CPGs generally recommend IDET and IRFT due to strong evidence of effectiveness.

8. Why do some physicians use provocative discography prior to IDET?

   a. to detect disc herniations

   b. to rule out the need for decompression surgery

   c. to identify annular defects

   d. to examine if there is a fracture

REFERENCES

1. Chou LH, Lew HL, Coelho PC, et al. Intradiscal electrothermal annuloplasty. Am J Phys Med Rehabil 2005;84:538-549.
2. Biyani A, Andersson GB, Chaudhary H, et al. Intradiscal electrothermal therapy: a treatment option in patients with internal disc disruption. Spine 2003;28:8-14.
3. Hecht P, Hayashi K, Lu Y, et al. Monopolar radiofrequency energy effects on joint capsular tissue: potential treatment for joint instability. An in vivo mechanical, morphological, and biochemical study using an ovine model. Am J Sports Med 1999;27:761-771.
4. Hayashi K, Massa KL, Thabit G III, et al. Histologic evaluation of the glenohumeral joint capsule after the laser-assisted capsular shift procedure for glenohumeral instability. Am J Sports Med 1999;27:162-167.
5. Hayashi K, Thabit G III, Massa KL, et al. The effect of thermal heating on the length and histologic properties of the glenohumeral joint capsule. Am J Sports Med 1997;25:107-112.
6. Freeman BJ. IDET: a critical appraisal of the evidence. Eur Spine J 2006;15:S448-S457.
7. Saal JA, Saal JS. Intradiscal electrothermal therapy for the treatment of chronic discogenic low back pain. Clin Sports Med 2002;21:167-187.
8. Derby R, Eek B, Chen Y, et al. Intradiscal electrothermal annuloplasty (IDET): a novel approach for treating chronic discogenic back pain. Neuromodulation 2000;3:82-88.
9. Karasek M, Bogduk N. Twelve-month follow-up of a controlled trial of intradiscal thermal anuloplasty for back pain due to internal disc disruption. Spine 2000;25:2601-2607.
10. Kleinstueck FS, Diederich CJ, Nau WH, et al. Temperature and thermal dose distributions during intradiscal electrothermal therapy in the cadaveric lumbar spine. Spine 2003;28:1700-1708.
11. Derby R, Seo KS, Kazala K, et al. A factor analysis of lumbar intradiscal electrothermal annuloplasty outcomes. Spine J 2005;5:256-261.
12. Saal JA, Saal JS. Intradiscal electrothermal treatment for chronic discogenic low back pain: a prospective outcome study with minimum 1-year follow-up. Spine 2000;25:2622-2627.
13. Bogduk N, Karasek M. Two-year follow-up of a controlled trial of intradiscal electrothermal anuloplasty for chronic low back pain resulting from internal disc disruption. Spine J 2002;2:343-350.
14. Saal JA, Saal JS. Intradiscal electrothermal treatment for chronic discogenic low back pain: prospective outcome study with a minimum 2-year follow-up. Spine 2002;27:966-973.
15. Pilcher TA, Sanford AL, Saul JP, et al. Convective cooling effect on cooled-tip catheter compared to large-tip catheter radiofrequency ablation. Pacing Clin Electrophysiol 2006;29:1368-1374.
16. Petersohn JD, Conquergood LR, Leung M. Acute histologic effects and thermal distribution profile of disc Biacuplasty using a novel water-cooled bipolar electrode system in an in vivo porcine model. Pain Med 2008;9:26-32.
17. Pauza K. Cadaveric intervertebral disc temperature mapping during disc Biacuplasty. Pain Physician 2008;11:669-676.
18. Kapural L, Mekhail N, Hicks D, et al. Histological changes and temperature distribution studies of a novel bipolar radiofrequency heating system in degenerated and nondegenerated human cadaver lumbar discs. Pain Med 2008;9:68-75.
19. Shah RV, Lutz GE, Lee J, et al. Intradiskal electrothermal therapy: a preliminary histologic study. Arch Phys Med Rehabil 2001;82:1230-1237.
20. Lee J, Lutz GE, Campbell D, et al. Stability of the lumbar spine after intradiscal electrothermal therapy. Arch Phys Med Rehabil 2001;82:120-122.
21. Wang JC, Kabo JM, Tsou PM, et al. The effect of uniform heating on the biomechanical properties of the intervertebral disc in a porcine model. Spine J 2005;5:64-70.
22. Kleinstueck FS, Diederich CJ, Nau WH, et al. Acute biomechanical and histological effects of intradiscal electrothermal therapy on human lumbar discs. Spine 2001;26:2198-2207.
23. Bass EC, Wistrom EV, Diederich CJ, et al. Heat-induced changes in porcine annulus fibrosus biomechanics. J Biomech 2004;37:233-240.
24. Schaufele M, Andrews N, Huckle J. Volumetric reduction of bovine intervertebral discs with the use of an intradiscal decompression catheter. Presentation at ISIS 12th annual scientific meeting, Maui, HI: 2004.
25. Cohen SP, Larkin T, Abdi S, et al. Risk factors for failure and complications of intradiscal electrothermal therapy: a pilot study. Spine 2003;28:1142-1147.
26. Wallace AL, Hollinshead RM, Frank CB. Creep behavior of a rabbit model of ligament laxity after electrothermal shrinkage in vivo. Am J Sports Med 2002;30:98-102.
27. Andersson G, Andrews N, Huckle J. Alteration of the collagen and cell viability within the disc following intradiscal electrothermal therapy. Presentation at ISIS 12th annual scientific meeting, Maui, HI: 2004.

28. Freeman BJ, Walters RM, Moore RJ, et al. Does intradiscal electrothermal therapy denervate and repair experimentally induced posterolateral annular tears in an animal model? Spine 2003;28:2602-2608.

29. Bass EC, Nau WH, Diederich CJ, et al. Intradiscal thermal therapy does not stimulate biologic remodeling in an in vivo sheep model. Spine 2006;31:139-145.

30. Narvani AA, Tsiridis E, Wilson LF. High-intensity zone, intradiscal electrothermal therapy, and magnetic resonance imaging. J Spinal Disord Tech 2003;16:130-136.

31. Wright AR, Gatchel RJ. Occupational musculoskeletal pain and disability. In: Turk DC, Gatchel RJ, editors. Psychological approaches to pain management: a practitioner's handbook, 2nd ed. New York: Guilford; 2002. p. 349-364.

32. Bono CM, Iki K, Jalota A, et al. Temperatures within the lumbar disc and endplates during intradiscal electrothermal therapy: formulation of a predictive temperature map in relation to distance from the catheter. Spine 2004;29:1124-1129.

33. Podhajsky R., Belous A. The effects of temperature on nucleus pulposus: pressure and hydrokinetics. Presentation at ISIS 12th annual scientific meeting, Maui, HI: 2004.

34. Derby R, Lee SH, Seo KS, et al. Efficacy of IDET for relief of leg pain associated with discogenic low back pain. Pain Pract 2004;4:281-285.

35. Kloth DS, Fenton DS, Andersson GB, et al. Intradiscal electrothermal therapy (IDET) for the treatment of discogenic low back pain: patient selection and indications for use. Pain Physician 2008;11:659-668.

36. Pauza KJ, Howell S, Dreyfuss P, et al. A randomized, placebo-controlled trial of intradiscal electrothermal therapy for the treatment of discogenic low back pain. Spine J 2004;4:27-35.

37. Milette PC, Fontaine S, Lepanto L, et al. Differentiating lumbar disc protrusions, disc bulges, and discs with normal contour but abnormal signal intensity. Magnetic resonance imaging with discographic correlations. Spine 1999;24:44-53.

38. Aprill C, Bogduk N. High-intensity zone: a diagnostic sign of painful lumbar disc on magnetic resonance imaging. Br J Radiol 1992;65:361-369.

39. Schellhas KP, Pollei SR, Gundry CR, et al. Lumbar disc high-intensity zone. Correlation of magnetic resonance imaging and discography. Spine 1996;21:79-86.

40. Maurer P, Squillante D, Dawson K. Is IDET effective treatment for discogenic low back pain? A prospective cohort outcome study (1-2 year follow-up). Identifying successful patient selection criteria. Proceedings of the 16 Annual Meeting of the North American Spine Society, Seattle, WA: 2001.

41. Moneta GB, Videman T, Kaivanto K, et al. Reported pain during lumbar discography as a function of anular ruptures and disc degeneration. A re-analysis of 833 discograms. Spine 1994;19:1968-1974.

42. Nielens H, van Zundert J, Mairiaux P, et al. Chronic low back pain. Brussels, 2006, Report No.: KCE reports Vol 48C.

43. Airaksinen O, Brox JI, Cedraschi C, et al. European guidelines for the management of chronic nonspecific low back pain. Eur Spine J 2006;15(Suppl 2):192-300.

44. National Institute for Health and Clinical Excellence (NICE). Low back pain: early management of persistent non-specific low back pain. London: National Institute of Health and Clinical Excellence; 2009. Report No.: NICE Clinical Guideline 88.

45. Chou R, Loeser JD, Owens DK, et al. Interventional therapies, surgery, and interdisciplinary rehabilitation for low back pain: an evidence-based clinical practice guideline from the American Pain Society. Spine 2009;34:1066-1077.

46. Manchikanti L, Boswell MV, Singh V, et al. Comprehensive evidence-based guidelines for interventional techniques in the management of chronic spinal pain. Pain Physician 2009;12:699-802.

47. Gibson JN, Waddell G. Surgery for degenerative lumbar spondylosis. Cochrane Database Syst Rev 2005;(4):CD001352.

48. Barendse GA, van Den Berg SG, Kessels AH, et al. Randomized controlled trial of percutaneous intradiscal radiofrequency thermocoagulation for chronic discogenic back pain: lack of effect from a 90-second 70 C lesion. Spine 2001;26:287-292.

49. Freeman BJ, Fraser RD, Cain CM, et al. A randomized, double-blind, controlled trial: intradiscal electrothermal therapy versus placebo for the treatment of chronic discogenic low back pain. Spine 2005;30:2369-2377.

50. Chou R, Atlas SJ, Stanos SP, et al. Nonsurgical interventional therapies for low back pain: a review of the evidence for an American Pain Society clinical practice guideline. Spine 2009;34:1078-1093.

51. Andersson GB, Mekhail NA, Block JE. Treatment of intractable discogenic low back pain. A systematic review of spinal fusion and intradiscal electrothermal therapy (IDET). Pain Physician 2006;9:237-248.

52. Appleby D, Andersson G, Totta M. Meta-analysis of the efficacy and safety of intradiscal electrothermal therapy (IDET). Pain Med 2006;7:308-316.

53. Urrutia G, Kovacs F, Nishishinya MB, et al. Percutaneous thermocoagulation intradiscal techniques for discogenic low back pain. Spine 2007;32:1146-1154.

54. Bogduk N, Long DM. The anatomy of the so-called "articular nerves" and their relationship to facet denervation in the treatment of low-back pain. J Neurosurg 1979;51:172-177.

55. Lutz C, Lutz GE, Cooke PM. Treatment of chronic lumbar diskogenic pain with intradiskal electrothermal therapy: a prospective outcome study. Arch Phys Med Rehabil 2003;84:23-28.

56. Lee MS, Cooper G, Lutz GE, et al. Intradiscal electrothermal therapy (IDET) for treatment of chronic lumbar discogenic pain: a minimum 2-year clinical outcome study. Pain Physician 2003;6:443-448.

57. Levin JH. Prospective, double-blind, randomized placebo-controlled trials in interventional spine: what the highest quality literature tells us. Spine J 2009;9:690-703.

58. Helm S, Hayek SM, Benyamin RM, et al. Systematic review of the effectiveness of thermal annular procedures in treating discogenic low back pain. Pain Physician 2009;12:207-232.

59. Lau P, Mercer S, Govind J, et al. The surgical anatomy of lumbar medial branch neurotomy (facet denervation). Pain Med 2004;5:289-298.

60. Spruit M, Jacobs WC. Pain and function after intradiscal electrothermal treatment (IDET) for symptomatic lumbar disc degeneration. Eur Spine J 2002;11:589-593.

61. Davis TT, Delamarter RB, Sra P, et al. The IDET procedure for chronic discogenic low back pain. Spine 2004;29:752-756.

62. Webster BS, Verma S, Pransky GS. Outcomes of workers' compensation claimants with low back pain undergoing intradiscal electrothermal therapy. Spine 2004;29:435-441.

63. Kapural L, Hayek S, Malak O, et al. Intradiscal thermal annuloplasty versus intradiscal radiofrequency ablation for the treatment of discogenic pain: a prospective matched control trial. Pain Med 2005;6:425-431.

64. Park SY, Moon SH, Park MS, et al. Intradiscal electrothermal treatment for chronic lower back pain patients with internal disc disruption. Yonsei Med J 2005;46:539-545.

65. Finch PM, Price LM, Drummond PD. Radiofrequency heating of painful annular disruptions: one-year outcomes. J Spinal Disord Tech 2005;18:6-13.

66. Hsia AW, Isaac K, Katz JS. Cauda equina syndrome from intradiscal electrothermal therapy. Neurology 2000;55:320.

67. Kapural L, Ng A, Dalton J, et al. Intervertebral disc Biacuplasty for the treatment of lumbar discogenic pain: results of a six-month follow-up. Pain Med 2008;9:60-67.

68. Kapural L, Mekhail N, Korunda Z, et al. Intradiscal thermal annuloplasty for the treatment of lumbar discogenic pain in patients with multilevel degenerative disc disease. Anesth Analg 2004;99:472-476.

69. Nunley PD, Jawahar A, Brandao SM, et al. Intradiscal electrothermal therapy (IDET) for low back pain in worker's compensation patients: can it provide a potential answer? Long-term results. J Spin Disord Techn 2008;21:11-18.

70. Maurer P, Block JE, Squillante D. Intradiscal electrothermal therapy (IDET) provides effective symptom relief in patients with discogenic low back pain. J Spinal Disord Tech 2008; 21:55-62.

71. Kapural L, Mekhail N. Novel intradiscal biacuplasty (IDB) for the treatment of lumbar discogenic pain. Pain Pract 2007;7: 130-134.

72. Kapural L. Intervertebral disk cooled bipolar radiofrequency (intradiskal biacuplasty) for the treatment of lumbar diskogenic pain: a 12-month follow-up of the pilot study. Pain Med 2008;9:407-408.

73. Kapural L, Cata JP, Narouze S. Successful treatment of lumbar discogenic pain using intradiscal biacuplasty in previously discectomized disc. Pain Pract 2009;9:130-134.

74. Bogduk N, Lau P, Gowaily K, et al. A pilot audit of radiofrequency biacuplasty for back pain due to internal disc disruption. 16th annual scientific meeting of the ISIS, Las Vegas, NV 2008.

75. Saal JA, Saal JS, Wetzel FT, et al. IDET related complications: a multi-center study of 1675 treated patients with a review of the FDA MDR data base. Proceedings of the 16th Annual Meeting of the North American Spine Society, Seattle, Washington, 2001.

76. Thomas PS. Image-guided pain management. Philadelphia: Lippincott-Raven, 1997.

77. Konno S, Olmarker K, Byrod G, et al. The European Spine Society AcroMed Prize 1994. Acute thermal nerve root injury. Eur Spine J 1994;3:299-302.

78. Wetzel FT. Cauda equina syndrome from intradiscal electrothermal therapy. Neurology 2001;56:1607.

79. Yetkinler DN, Nau WH, Brandt LL. Disc temperature measurements during nucleoplasty and IDET procedures. Paper presented at 6th International Congress on Spinal Surgery, September 4-7, 2002; Ankara, Turkey.

80. Scholl BM, Theiss SM, Lopez-Ben R, et al. Vertebral osteonecrosis related to intradiscal electrothermal therapy: a case report. Spine 2003;28:E161-E164.

81. Ho C, Kaiser J, Saal J, et al. Does IDET cause advancement of disc degeneration? A one year MRI follow-up study of 72 patients. Proceedings of the 16th Annual Meeting of the North American Spine Society. Seattle, WA: 2001.

82. Centers for Medicare and Medicaid Services. Medicare claims processing manual. 2008. Report No.: 100-104, transmittal 1646.

83. Gerszten PC, Welch WC, McGrath PM, et al. A prospective outcomes study of patients undergoing intradiscal electrothermy (IDET) for chronic low back pain. Pain Physician 2002;5:360-364.

84. Saal JS, Saal JA. Management of chronic discogenic low back pain with a thermal intradiscal catheter. A preliminary report. Spine 2000;25:382-388.

85. Singh V. Percutaneous disc decompression for the treatment of chronic atypical cervical discogenic pain. Pain Physician 2004;7:115-118.

86. Thompson K, Eckel T. Two-year results from the Intradiscal electrothermal therapy nationwide registry. Spine J 2002;2(2 Suppl 1).

87. Wetzel FT, Andersson G, Peloza J. Intradiscal electrothermal therapy (IDET) to treat discogenic low back pain: preliminary results of a multicenter prospective cohort study. Proceedings of the 15th Annual Meeting of the North American Spine Society. New Orleans, LA: 2000.

88. Derby R, Eek B, Lee SH, et al. Comparison of intradiscal restorative injections and intradiscal electrothermal treatment (IDET) in the treatment of low back pain. Pain Physician 2004;7:63-66.

89. Freedman BA, Cohen SP, Kuklo TR, et al. Intradiscal electrothermal therapy (IDET) for chronic low back pain in active-duty soldiers: 2-year follow-up. Spine J 2003;3:502-509.

90. Endres SM, Fiedler GA, Larson KL. Effectiveness of intradiscal electrothermal therapy in increasing function and reducing chronic low back pain in selected patients. Wisconsin Medical Journal 2002;101:31-34.

91. Mekhail N, Kapural L. Intradiscal thermal annuloplasty for discogenic pain: an outcome study. Pain Pract 2004;4: 84-90.

92. Singh V. Intradiscal electrothermal therapy: a preliminary report. Pain Physician 2000;3:367-373.

93. Bryce DA, Nelson J, Glurich I, et al. Intradiscal electrothermal annuloplasty therapy: a case series study leading to new considerations. Wisconsin Medical Journal 2005;104:39-46.

94. Ergun R, Sekerci Z, Bulut H, et al. Intradiscal electrothermal treatment for chronic discogenic low back pain: a prospective outcome study of 39 patients with the Oswestry disability index at 18 month follow-up. Neurol Res 2008;30:411-416.

95. Ercelen O, Bulutcu E, Oktenoglu T, et al. Radiofrequency lesioning using two different time modalities for the treatment of lumbar discogenic pain: a randomized trial. Spine 2003; 28:1922-1927.

RICHARD DERBY
RAY M. BAKER
CHANG-HYUNG LEE

CHAPTER 28

Nucleoplasty

DESCRIPTION

Terminology and Subtypes

Nucleoplasty, also termed *minimally invasive nuclear decompression*, refers to an intervention in which a probe is inserted through a catheter and into the nucleus of an injured intervertebral disc (IVD) thought to be responsible for symptoms of chronic low back pain (CLBP), and energy is targeted at a portion of the nucleus in order to eliminate it.[1] This procedure can be considered minimally invasive when it is compared with traditional surgical discectomy because it does not require direct visualization of the structures and it can be delivered through a very small skin incision. The type of energy used during nucleoplasty is a form of radiofrequency termed *coblation*, which involves disrupting molecular bonds in the surrounding plasma with only minimal production of heat.[1] The terminology surrounding nucleoplasty is not standardized, and various names have emerged emphasizing one or more of its characteristics. Nucleoplasty has also been referred to (sometimes incorrectly) as *minimally invasive disc decompression, percutaneous disc decompression, percutaneous disc decompression using coblation therapy, percutaneous nucleotomy, percutaneous radiofrequency thermomodulation, percutaneous plasma discectomy,* or *coblation nucleoplasty*.

History and Frequency of Use

The IVD was first proposed as a potential source of CLBP when the concept of disc herniations was proposed by Mixter and Barr in 1934.[2] Since that discovery was made, numerous surgical interventions have been devised to address and correct perceived injuries to the IVD. Traditional operative disc decompression has long been accepted as the standard treatment for large disc herniations resulting in progressive or severe neurologic deficits or unbearable lower extremity symptoms. Although advances are continually made in traditional disc decompression in an attempt to increase its efficacy and safety, it remains a surgical procedure that involves substantial disruption to surrounding tissues in order to expose the targeted IVD. Clinicians and scientists have relentlessly pursued progressively less invasive approaches to disc decompression to increase the accessibility and use of this procedure in selected patients.[3,4] Some of the

innovative interventions that have been offered as percutaneous alternatives to traditional decompression include automated percutaneous lumbar discectomy (APLD), laser disc decompression, hydrodiscectomy (e.g., SpineJet MicroResector), and intradiscal electrothermal therapy (IDET); the latter is discussed in Chapter 27 of this text.

During percutaneous endoscopic discectomy, surgeons have often noted an inflamed outer annulus adjacent to the disc protrusion.[5] Removing the herniated disc within the protrusion was commonly thought to remove the source of inflammation and decrease pressure on the innervated outer annulus and adjacent posterior longitudinal ligament and nerve roots. However, percutaneous techniques using medium and smaller diameter cannulae were not designed to remove nucleus material directly behind the protrusion. Unlike larger 3- to 5-mm outer diameter cannulae used for "surgical" percutaneous disc decompression, those performed though smaller 2.5- to 3-mm cannulae used in APLD, laser disc decompression, or hydrodiscectomy are designed to allow easy access only to the disc nucleus and not to herniated nucleus material located within posterior annular fissures or protrusions. These techniques primarily eliminate injured tissue by cutting, aspirating, or vaporizing the nucleus within the center of the disc, and do not necessarily remove nuclear material within the protrusion unless the protrusion is located along its access path.

One of the newer approaches developed as an alternative to both traditional and percutaneous disc decompression is nuclear decompression using a bipolar radiofrequency device, which was introduced in the United States in 1999. The technique, commonly named *nucleoplasty*, was patterned after existing devices for knee debridement and marketed as a percutaneous technique to ablate nuclear tissue by creating channels within the nucleus. Nucleoplasty was thought to offer advantages over IDET because it did not involve the use of heat, which can damage adjacent tissues.

Practitioner, Setting, and Availability

Nucleoplasty is typically performed in secondary care settings by nonsurgical or surgical spine specialists, including physiatrists, anesthesiologists, orthopedic surgeons, or interventional pain management specialists. Because this intervention must be conducted under fluoroscopy, it is typically limited to specialty spine or pain management clinics in outpatient centers or hospitals. Nucleoplasty is available throughout the United States, but mostly in larger cities.

Procedure

Nucleoplasty uses the Perc-D SpineWand bipolar radiofrequency device manufactured by ArthroCare (Sunnyvale, CA). The procedure begins with the patient wearing a medical gown and lying prone on a treatment table (Figure 28-1A). The area to be treated is typically cleaned with sequential alcohol or betadine wipes. The procedure can be performed under conscious sedation to minimize patient discomfort or anxiety. Nucleoplasty is performed under image guidance using fluoroscopy. A 17 gauge (G) introducer needle is first inserted through the skin, subcutaneous tissue, and muscle, and advanced to the annulus-nucleus junction using standard posterolateral access techniques; catheter position is critical to a successful nucleoplasty procedure.

Once the needle is in place, the nucleoplasty "wand" is introduced through the needle placed into the annular-nuclear junction. The nuclear tissue is then ablated using a high-voltage (typically 100 to 300 V) electrical current produced by bipolar radiofrequency energy and delivered at a frequency of 120 KHz. In hydrated-tissue conductive medium containing normal saline, this current creates a plasma field approximately 75 mm thick that is composed of highly ionized particles with sufficient energy to break organic molecular bonds and thus vaporize tissue. By advancing the wand in ablation mode and retracting the probe while delivering a bipolar radiofrequency coagulation, 1 mm channels are created in the nucleus (see Figures 28-1B and 28-1C).

Following nucleoplasty, the patient is typically monitored in a recovery room for 1 to 3 hours before discharge. Patients may wear lumbar supports for a few weeks following the procedure to minimize the risk of reinjury from excessive disc loading during this healing period. Activities like walking and pool exercises are encouraged, but aggressive physical therapy is usually not begun until a few weeks after the procedure.

Regulatory Status

The Perc-D SpineWand bipolar radiofrequency device manufactured by ArthroCare that is used during nucleoplasty was approved by the US Food and Drug Administration in 2005 for the ablation, coagulation, and decompression disc material for patients with symptomatic, contained disc herniations. Obtaining approval as a class II medical device mainly requires that the manufacturer submits evidence that the new device is substantially equivalent to a currently approved similar device.

THEORY

Mechanism of Action

The precise mechanism of action through which nucleoplasty can help patients with CLBP is unclear, but is thought

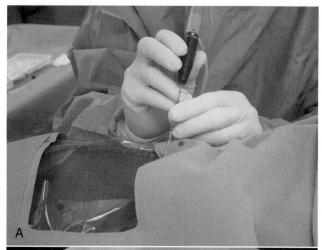
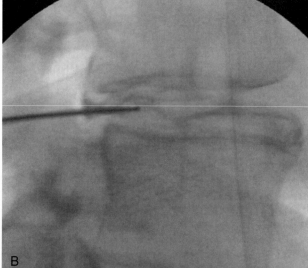
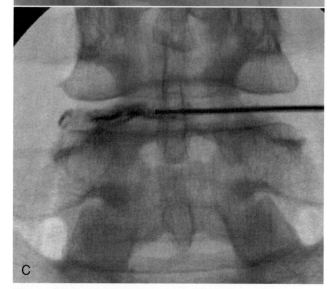

Figure 28-1 Lumbar nucleoplasty. **A,** Procedure view. **B,** Lateral view with needle placed posteriorly to achieve decompression behind the central disc protrusion. **C,** anterior view.

to involve decreased pressure in the nucleus, thereby reducing nerve root tension and allowing a protrusion to implode inward, reducing any contact pressure between the protruding disc and spinal nerve root. Although pressure on a nerve root is considered a primary cause of radicular low back pain (LBP), few studies have validated this mechanism. Takahashi and colleagues measured the contact pressure between the nerve and annulus in patients under general anesthesia in a prone position before and after removing a herniated disc.[6] Pressure ranged from 7 mm Hg to 256 mm Hg (mean 54.2) before discectomy and decreased to 0 mm following the procedure, and was directly correlated with the amount of trunk list and degree of neurologic deficit before the operation.

Because nerve edema can be induced by pressure of only 50 mm Hg sustained for only 2 minutes, this study suggests that nerve not compression could in fact contribute to radicular CLBP.[7] One might logically conclude that removing a herniated disc would relieve pressure on an affected spinal nerve root. However, the effect of lowering nuclear pressure by removing a small amount of nucleus from the center of the disc is conceptually harder to understand, especially if the desired effect is to lower annular tension for the purpose of decreasing axial CLBP. This mechanism was confirmed by histologic examination after channel "coblation" (coagulation ablation) in harvested sheep discs in which there was no evidence of collateral tissue or cell destruction.[8] The main explanations that have been offered for the effects of nucleoplasty are the pressure theory, implosion theory, and chemical theory; each is briefly summarized here.

Pressure Theory

The concept of lowering pressure was postulated by surgeons to justify nuclear decompression using laser heat ablation. Case and colleagues measured a rapid rise in the pressure of cadaver discs while slowly infusing normal saline into the disc nucleus.[9] These findings were consistent with the concept that the nucleus, surrounded by a relatively inelastic annulus and solid vertebral end plates, acts like a tight hydraulic space where large pressure rises occur with a small increase in volume. On the basis of these findings, it was suggested that small decreases in volume must lead to large decreases in intradiscal pressure.[9]

In a follow-up study using a 1000-J Nd:YAG 1.32-micron laser delivered through a quartz fiber, the mean intradiscal pressure in cadaver discs was decreased by 43%.[10,11] Likewise, using a 350 Nd:YAG laser, Yonezawa and colleagues vaporized central nuclear tissue in rabbit discs, creating a hole in the nucleus that, over an 8-week period, gradually filled with fibrous tissue and lowered the vertically measured disc pressure by approximately 50%.[12] Removing even less nuclear material by creating six channels in the nucleus of cadaver discs, Chen and colleagues showed a 100% drop in pressure in normal discs from young cadavers, but only a negligible drop in pressure in degenerated discs.[13]

In addition to direct pressure measurements in animal models, Hellinger and colleagues indirectly studied disc pressure changes in 21 patients by comparing the disc densities in computed tomography (CT) scans before and after nonendoscopic Nd:YAG laser nuclear ablation.[14] Density within disc protrusions showed a statistical difference of 66.3 Houndsfield units, corresponding to a 20% postoperative density reduction. Therapeutic results were attributed to improved flow of venous and cerebrospinal fluid. Although these studies suggest that pressure is lowered within the nucleus immediately after ablation, little is known about the effect on tensional forces in the outer annulus or the duration of decreased pressure. Because injecting the disc with fluid will increase outer annular pressure when radial annular tears extend to the outer annulus, one might reasonably conclude that lowering the fluid pressure would decrease annular tension.[15]

Several studies suggest that it may be preferable to remove a smaller amount of nuclear material through ablation. Mochida and colleagues performed percutaneous discectomy on 47 young (average age 27 years) patients with herniations causing radicular pain.[16] They compared results of 25 cases in which an average of 3.8 g of tissue was removed from the central nucleus to 22 cases in which an average of only 1 g was removed from the posterior protrusion. Although 2-year outcomes were comparable at about 70% in both groups, 10-year results were favorable in 71% for the group that had less tissue removed compared with only 36% in those having more tissue removed. More importantly, disc space collapse greater than 30% was observed in 57% of the group with more tissue removed, compared with 20% of the group with less tissue removed. A decrease in disc herniation size did not correlate with outcome.

Further supporting these findings, another study showed that in elite athletes a more extensive arthroscopic removal of tissue was associated with an acute worsening of symptoms and a delayed return to sports activity.[17] Similarly, Carragee and colleagues had better outcomes after open surgical removal of herniated discs when less nuclear material was removed.[18] The study compared removal of all the free fragments through an annulotomy incision to a more limited removal of the herniated mass alone. Although recurrent herniation rate was higher in the group with limited disc material removal, clinical outcomes measured by satisfaction, pain, and function were superior to the group with more removed disc material.

Although removing nuclear tissue will decrease disc pressure in the inner and middle annular fibers, little effect is seen on the outer and more commonly innervated collagenous layers.[19] In addition, during creep loading the reduced nuclear tension allows the inner layers to bulge inward, reducing height and compressive strength, and potentially leading to lateral segmental instability.[20] Reduced nuclear pressure shifts load to the relatively thin outer annulus causing high, irregular stress concentrations that may cause pain.[20-24] In addition, the lowered pressure in the nucleus and the elevated pressures in the annulus will suppress chondrocyte metabolism leading to further disc dehydration and reduction of osmotic forces.[25,26]

Wognum and colleagues showed that decreased osmotic pressure exposes the tips of annular tears to increased stress concentrations, causing cracks to open, potentially increasing the risk of herniation.[27] In addition, a drop in nuclear pressure will cause disc space narrowing and disc bulging. In hydrated cadaver discs, Brinckmann and colleagues[28] showed a significant drop of pressure when up to 3 g of nuclear material was removed. For every gram of tissue removed from the nucleus, disc height collapsed by an average of 0.8 mm and the disc bulged by 0.02 mm. Similarly, Castro and colleagues showed that removal of 4.6 g of nuclear material by APLD narrowed the disc space by 1.42 mm and increased the disc bulge by 0.45 mm.[29]

Interpreting findings of decreased IVD pressure is challenging, because the majority of discs selected for this procedure may already have lowered nuclear pressures from end-plate injury or disc herniations. With the nucleus already decompressed, the benefits of further decompression may be questionable, but removing less disc material would perhaps cause less harm in such cases. Interestingly, studies have suggested that elevating nuclear pressures may be theoretically beneficial in those cases where an annular tear alone is present in an otherwise healthy hydrated nucleus.[19] Although elevated pressure will increase the risk of disruption, decreased chondrocyte metabolism should eventually relieve the pressure.[30] Furthermore, nuclear decompression typically occurs after injuries such as an end-plate fracture, annular tear with herniation, outer rim lesion, or concentric annular tears.[31,32] One could postulate that minimal nuclear decompression might initiate, assist, or hasten this response. Further studies, however, are required to understand the effects of nucleoplasty on disc pressure and the potential role for this phenomenon to explain clinical outcomes in CLBP.

Implosion Theory

Another goal of central nuclear decompression is to allow room for the herniated fragment to implode inward and reduce the tension on the nerve root and annulus. There is little evidence to support this theory. In fact, Delamarter and colleagues reviewed the magnetic resonance imaging (MRI) scans of 33 patients with radicular pain as the result of a disc herniation before and after APLD and saw no measurable changes at 6 weeks.[33] At the L4-5 level and above, a more lateral approach will facilitate posterior needle placement and targeted tissue removal.[34]

Chemical Theory

The application of heat through nucleoplasty may also enhance the chemical environment within the disc. Coblation in cultured disc cells increased inflammatory mediators in normal nuclear and annular cells, but decreased inflammatory mediators in abnormal nuclear cells.[35]

Indication

The following indications have been proposed for nucleoplasty and primarily radicular CLBP[36]:
- Leg pain greater than back pain
- MRI evidence of contained disc protrusion
- Positive discography (if indicated)
- Failure of 6 weeks of conservative therapy

The following indications have been proposed for nucleoplasty and primarily axial CLBP[36]:

- MRI evidence of contained disc protrusion
- Positive discography
- Failure of 12 weeks of conservative therapy

Assessment

Prior to receiving nucleoplasty, patients should first be assessed for LBP using an evidence-based and goal-oriented approach focused on the patient history and neurologic examination, as discussed in Chapter 3. Clinicians should also inquire about medication history to note prior hypersensitivity/allergy or adverse events (AEs) with drugs similar to those being considered, and evaluate contraindications for these types of drugs. Advanced imaging such as MRI or CT is required to help guide the spine specialist to target the appropriate spinal levels involved in a patient's CLBP.[37] Findings on advanced imaging that may be of interest to nucleoplasty include MRI or CT findings of substantial disc herniations concordant with patient symptoms. Interventional diagnostic testing may also be used prior to recommending or performing nucleoplasty, especially in cases of symptoms that persist for more than 6 months and prove recalcitrant to exhaustive conservative treatment measures. The use of provocative discography for CLBP remains controversial, but is used by some clinicians to identify painful disc herniations that may subsequently be targeted with other interventions, including nucleoplasty.

EFFICACY

Evidence supporting the efficacy of this intervention for CLBP was summarized from recent clinical practice guidelines (CPGs), systematic reviews (SRs), and randomized controlled trials (RCTs). Observational studies (OBSs) were also summarized where appropriate. Findings are summarized by study design.

Clinical Practice Guidelines

Two of the recent national CPGs on the management of CLBP have assessed and summarized the evidence to make specific recommendations about the efficacy of nucleoplasty.

The CPG from Belgium in 2006 found insufficient evidence to support the efficacy nucleoplasty in the management of CLBP.[38]

The CPG from the United States in 2009 found insufficient evidence to make a recommendation about the use of coblation nucleoplasty for the management of CLBP with or without radicular pain.[39]

Findings from the CPGs are summarized in Table 28-1.

Systematic Reviews

Cochrane Collaboration

A Cochrane review of surgical interventions for lumbar disc prolapse was conducted in 2007.[40] That review stated that until better scientific evidence is available, coblation therapy should be regarded as an investigational technique.

American Pain Society and American College of Physicians

An SR was conducted in 2008 by the American Pain Society and American College of Physicians CPG committee on non-surgical therapies for acute and chronic LBP.[41] That review identified one SR related to nucleoplasty, which concluded that there was insufficient evidence on nucleoplasty.[42] However, no RCTs on nucleoplasty were identified in that review. As such, this SR was unable to make any definitive conclusions about the effectiveness of nucleoplasty.[41] The SR concluded that RCTs are required to assess the effectiveness of nucleoplasty for CLBP.

Other

Another SR was conducted in 2009 on the effectiveness of percutaneous mechanical disc decompression with nucleoplasty for patients with disc protrusions.[43] That review included five OBSs.[44-48] The SR concluded that there is no evidence for nucleoplasty among patients with axial LBP. Based on OBSs, the SR concluded that there is low-quality evidence supporting nucleoplasty for patients presenting with LBP and lower extremity pain from disc herniation.

The National Institute for Clinical Excellence (NICE) in the United Kingdom published an Interventional Procedure Guidance report in May 2006 related to nucleoplasty for LBP.[49] The report stated that although there are no major safety concerns associated with percutaneous disc decompression using coblation for LBP, and there is some evidence of short-term efficacy, this is not sufficient to support its use without special arrangements for consent, audit, or research. The guidance stated that the lack of data makes it difficult to

draw conclusions regarding the efficacy of the procedure. The lack of long-term and comparative data also makes it difficult to distinguish between the treatment effect and the natural history of the disease, or to determine whether the benefits (if any) are sustained beyond 12 months.

The American Society for Interventional Pain Physicians (ASIPP) published Practice Guidelines for the Management of Chronic Spinal Pain in 2007.[50] That report stated that the evidence supporting the efficacy of coblation nucleoplasty was limited for both short- and long-term relief of LBP.[50]

The American College of Occupational and Environmental Medicine (ACOEM) published evidence-based practice guidelines on LBP in 2007.[51] That report stated that there was no high-quality evidence supporting the efficacy of coblation therapy as an effective treatment for LBP with or without radiculopathy.

Findings from some of the above SRs are summarized in Table 28-2.

Randomized Controlled Trials

Based on the SRs summarized above, no RCTs were identified examining the efficacy of nucleoplasty for CLBP. A literature search conducted in MEDLINE and the Cochrane Library in November 2009 also did not uncover any RCTs for this intervention.

Observational Studies

In 2001, Sharps and colleagues reported outcomes after nucleoplasty in 49 patients after 1 month, 41 patients after 3 months, 24 patients after 6 months, and 13 patients after 12 months.[36] Participants had CLBP (mean duration 38 months) with or without leg pain, and protrusions greater than one-third the sagittal canal diameter were excluded. The procedure was performed as recommended by the device manufacturer. The 1- through 12-month outcomes based on visual analog scale (VAS) pain score showed a relatively consistent drop in VAS pain score of between 4.3 (54%) and 3.6 (45%) from a preoperative average of 7.9. Despite the reported near 50% drop in VAS pain score, mean postprocedural patient satisfaction (0 = unsatisfactory, 4 = excellent) was only 2.14. Nonetheless, authors reported a 79% success rate based on patient satisfaction change of greater than 1 in a group of patients with relatively severe pain secondary to small disc protrusions.

In the following year, Singh and colleagues reported results on a group of 67 patients with CLBP and leg pain of

TABLE 28-1	Clinical Practice Guideline Recommendations on Minimally Invasive Nuclear Decompression for Chronic Low Back Pain	
Reference	Country	Conclusion
38	Belgium	Insufficient evidence to support efficacy
39	United States	Insufficient evidence to make a recommendation

TABLE 28-2	Systematic Review Findings on Minimally Invasive Nuclear Decompression for Chronic Low Back Pain		
Reference	# RCTs in SR	# RCTs for CLBP	Conclusion
41	1 SR	0	Insufficient evidence on nucleoplasty
43	0 (5 observational studies only)	0	Low-quality evidence for lower extremity pain from disc herniation

CLBP, chronic low back pain; NR, not reported; RCT, randomized controlled trial; SR, systematic review.

long duration (5.4 to 5.6 years).[45] Outcomes were available in 61 patients at 6 months and 41 patients at 12 months. The average decrease in numerical pain rating (NPRS) score was 38%, from a preoperative average score of 6.80. NPRS decreased by more than 50% in 59% of participants at 6 months and 56% of participants at 12 months. The authors also presented improvements in self-reported sitting and standing tolerance.

The same group extended their study, and in 2003 published results of a consecutive series of 84 patients with LBP with or without leg pain.[46] The study is presumably included the 67 participants from the previous study, but this was unclear. Although not specifically stated in their first published report, the second study excluded any patient with "secondary gain issues" and therefore left open to the authors' discretion which patients would be enrolled in the study. At 12 months, there was a 34% decrease in the NPRS; only 15% of the patients who were unemployed before receiving nucleoplasty returned to work after the study intervention.

In 2005, Reddy and colleagues reported on 67 patients undergoing nucleoplasty for LBP and leg pain.[52] Follow-up data were available for 16 patients at 3 months, 22 patients at 6 months, and 11 patients at 12 months. Small but statistically significant improvements were reported in a 5-point impairment score for work and leisure activities, with 56%, 64%, and 45% of patients achieving greater than 50% pain relief at 3, 6, and 12 months, respectively. However, there was only a 15% (7.1 to 5.2) decrease in NPRS reported by the 11 patients who were followed up to 12 months, consistent with 5 responders having greater than 50% relief and 6 nonresponders having no relief.

Cohen and colleagues reported on 16 active duty soldiers with CLBP and leg pain (average duration 5.6 years).[53] Seven had nucleoplasty alone and nine had IDET followed by nucleoplasty at the same level. The average decrease in VAS pain score was 16%, and only one patient reported greater than 50% relief of pain. There was no significant difference in outcome between the two groups.

Derby compared 67 patients undergoing IDET with 92 patients undergoing nucleoplasty.[54,55] Both groups had similar eligibility criteria and included a large percentage of patients with worker's compensation or litigation claims. Axial LBP was worse than leg pain in 60% to 70% of patients. At an average 1-year follow-up, NPRS had decreased 17% (7.60 to 6.06) in the IDET group and 32% (7.45 to 5.02) in the nucleoplasty group. An index rating improvement in axial LBP and leg pain showed approximately equal improvement in the nucleoplasty group. Patient satisfaction based on a standard questionnaire was 44% in the IDET group and 68% in the nucleoplasty group.

Marin[44] performed a cohort study in which patients with LBP were selected on the basis of having a contained disc herniation with or without leg pain. To be included, participants had to have symptoms lasting longer than 3 months. One group received one session of nucleoplasty that was delivered using coblation technology via Perc-DLE equipment while another group received coblation-assisted microdiscectomy administered by a surgeon. After 12 months,

improvements in pain were observed compared with baseline scores in both groups but statistical difference between groups was not reported.

Alexandre and colleagues[56] performed a cohort study in which patients were selected on the basis of having CLBP with a contained disc herniation. To be included, participants had to have symptoms lasting longer than 3 months. One session of nucleoplasty was delivered using coblation technology to each participant. After 12 months, improvements in pain were observed compared with baseline scores but the statistical significance of this improvement was not reported.

Sharps and Isaac[36] performed a controlled before-after study in which patients were selected on the basis of having LBP of mixed duration without neurologic involvement due to a contained disc herniation. To be included, participants had to have failed conservative therapy; those with large disc herniations (occupying more than one-third of the spinal canal) and neurologic deficits were excluded. One session of nucleoplasty was delivered by a surgeon to each participant. After 12 months, statistically significant improvements in pain were observed compared with baseline scores.

In 2008, Al-Zain and colleagues[47] reported on a prospective case series of 96 patients treated with nucleoplasty. Patients had LBP and/or radiating pain to the lower extremities from a contained disc herniation, and were not responsive to at least 6 weeks of conservative treatment. One session of nucleoplasty was delivered to each participant. After 1 year, mean pain scores (VAS) were significantly improved compared with baseline. Disability in activities of daily living also improved significantly during this period.

Calisaneller and colleagues[57] reported on a prospective case series of 29 patients treated with nucleoplasty. Patients had LBP and/or leg pain due to disc bulging and/or protrusion less than or equal to 5 mm at one or two levels, and were not responsive to at least 6 weeks of conservative treatment. One session of nucleoplasty was delivered to each participant. After 6 months, mean pain scores (VAS) were not significantly different compared with those measured before the procedure.

Mirzai and colleagues[48] reported on a prospective case series of 52 patients treated with nucleoplasty. Patients had radicular pain due to one- or two-level, small- and medium-sized contained lumbar disc herniations, and were not responsive to at least 3 months of conservative treatment. One session of nucleoplasty was delivered by a surgeon to each participant. After 1 year, there was an improvement in mean pain scores (VAS) by 72% (P values not reported) compared with baseline. There was also an improvement in mean disability scores (ODI) by 51% (P values not reported).

Yakovlev and colleagues[58] reported on a retrospective case series of 22 patients treated with nucleoplasty. Patients had LBP with or without radicular pain due to contained disc herniation, and were not responsive to conservative treatment. One session of nucleoplasty was delivered to each participant. After 1 year, mean pain scores (VAS) decreased significantly compared with before the procedure, with 73% of patients reporting an improvement. There was also a statistically significant improvement in functional status, as measured by physical therapy assessment and activities of daily living, with 81.8% of patients reporting an improvement.

Masala and colleagues[59] reported on a prospective case series of 72 patients treated with nucleoplasty. Patients had LBP and/or radicular pain due to contained disc herniation, and were not responsive to 6 weeks of conservative treatment. One session of nucleoplasty was delivered to each participant. At 1-year follow-up, mean pain scores (VAS) decreased by 50% (P values not reported).

The OBSs discussed above are summarized in Tables 28-3 and 28-4.

SAFETY

Contraindications

Contraindications for nucleoplasty include severe disc degeneration with greater than 33% loss of disc height, disc herniation that is larger than one-third the sagittal diameter of the spinal canal at that level, disc extrusion or sequestration, moderate to severe spinal stenosis, tumor, infection, and fracture.[36]

Adverse Events

AEs associated with nucleoplasty include increased symptoms, infection, nerve injury, end-plate damage, and disc injury. An OBS reported short-term AEs in 53 participants following nucleoplasty.[60,61] The most common AE was soreness at the needle insertion site (76%), followed by new onset of numbness and tingling (26%), increased intensity of LBP (15%), and new areas of LBP (15%). These symptoms generally resolved within 2 weeks, but some participants continued to experience numbness, tingling, and increased LBP beyond that period.

As with other interventional and surgical procedures targeting the IVD, nucleoplasty may occasionally result in

TABLE 28-3	Design of Observational Studies on Minimally Invasive Nuclear Decompression for Chronic Low Back Pain			
Reference	Study Design	Indication	Intervention	Control
36	Prospective cohort without an unexposed group	LBP with or without neurologic involvement, symptoms >6 weeks	Nucleoplasty via SpineWand (ArthroCare, Sunnyvale, CA) Surgeon 1 session Cointervention: limited physical activity n = 49	NA
45	Controlled before-after study	Contained, discogenic, LBP with or without neurologic involvement, symptoms >3 months	Nucleoplasty via Perc-DLE SpineWand Clinician 1 session Cointervention: exercise with physical therapist n = 67	NA
46	Controlled before-after study	Discogenic, LBP with or without neurologic involvement, symptoms >3 months	Nucleoplasty via Perc-DLE SpineWand Clinician 1 session Cointervention: home exercise program n = 69	NA
52	Retrospective cohort without an unexposed group	Lumbar herniated disc, leg pain with or without LBP, symptoms >6 months	Nucleoplasty via Perc-DLE SpineWand plus IDET Administrator: NR Cointervention: NR n = 9	Nucleoplasty via Perc-DLE SpineWand Administrator: NR Cointervention: NR n = 7
53	Retrospective cohort	Lumbar herniated disc, leg pain with or without LBP, symptoms >6 months	Nucleoplasty via Perc-DLE SpineWand plus IDET Administrator: NR Cointervention: NR n = 49	NA

Continued

TABLE 28-3	Design of Observational Studies on Minimally Invasive Nuclear Decompression for Chronic Low Back Pain—cont'd			
Reference	**Study Design**	**Indication**	**Intervention**	**Control**
54, 55	Cohort study	Discogenic, with or without leg pain	Nucleoplasty Clinician Cointervention: NR n = 92	IDET Clinician Cointervention: NR n = 63
44	Cohort study	Contained discogenic, LBP with or without neurologic involvement, symptoms >3 months	Nucleoplasty via Perc-DLE SpineWand Surgeon 1 session Cointervention: NR n = 60	Coblation-assisted microdiscectomy Surgeon 1 session Cointervention: NR n = 13
56	Cohort study	Discogenic, LBP with neurologic involvement, symptoms >3 months	Nucleoplasty Administrator: NR 1 session Cointervention: NR n = 64	NA
36	Controlled before-after study	LBP with or without neurologic involvement, contained, discogenic, duration of symptoms >6 weeks	Nucleoplasty via Perc-DLE SpineWand Administrator: NR 1 session Cointervention: home exercise and physical therapy n = 49	NA
47	Prospective case series	LBP with or without neurologic involvement, disc herniation, duration of symptoms >1 month	Nucleoplasty via Perc-DLE SpineWand Administrator: NR 1 session Cointervention: NR n = 96	NA
57	Prospective case series	LBP and/or leg pain, contained, discogenic, duration of symptoms >6 months	Nucleoplasty via SpineWand Administrator: NR 1 session Cointervention: NR n = 29	NA
48	Prospective case series	Lumbar disc herniation, leg pain with or without LBP, duration of symptoms NR	Nucleoplasty via Perc-DLR SpineWand Surgeon 1 session Cointervention: NR n = 52	NA
58	Retrospective case series	LBP with or without neurologic involvement, contained, discogenic, duration of symptoms >6 months	Nucleoplasty via SpineWand Administrator: NR 1 session Cointervention: NR n = 22	
59	Prospective case series	Lumbar disc herniation, LBP and/or radicular pain, contained, duration of symptoms >6 weeks	Nucleoplasty via Perc-DLE SpineWand Administrator NR 1 session Cointervention: NR n = 72	

IDET, intradiscal electrothermal therapy; LBP, low back pain; NR, not reported; NA, not applicable.

TABLE 28-4	**Outcomes of Observational Studies on Minimally Invasive Nuclear Decompression for Chronic Low Back Pain**			
Reference	Outcomes	Initial (Mean ± SD)	Follow-Up (Mean, SD)	% Improvement
44	VAS – any improvement			78%
	Improvement – walking, standing, sitting			N: >75%
54, 55	VAS	N: 7.45 ± 1.44	N: 5.02 ± 2.21	33
		I: 7.60 ± 1.78	I: 6.06 ± 2.08	20
	Improvement VAS >10%			N: 80.4%
				I: 55.5%
	Improvement VAS >50%		N: 27.59	
			I: 7.62	
	BPI			68.20%
	SAT			44.40%
36	VAS-back	6.74	4.27	37%
	VAS-right leg	5.14	3.59	30%
	VAS-left leg	6.63	4.01	40%
	VAS	7.9 ± 1.3	4.3 ± 2.8	46%
	VAS – any improvement			OP: 67%
				Non-OP: 82%
				Overall: 79%
	Improvement VAS >50%			56%
56	JOA-excellent			55.80%
	JOA-good			24.90%
	JOA-scanty			12.40%
	JOA-none			6.90%
	Overall excellent outcome			51.50%
	Overall good outcome			31.50%
46	VAS	6.8	4.2 (6 months)	34%
			4.5 (12 months)	38%
	VAS – any improvement			75%
	Improvement VAS >50%			54%
	Improvement – sitting			54%
	Improvement – standing			44%
	Improvement – walking			49%
45	VAS	6.8 ± 1.1	4.1 ± 2.5	40%
	VAS – any improvement			80%
	Improvement VAS >50%			56%
	Improvement – sitting			62%
	Improvement – standing			59%
	Improvement – walking			60%
53	VAS	N: 6.0 ± 2.0	N: 4.8 ± 1.8	20%
		N + I: 7.2 ± 0.8	N + I: 6.3 ± 1.0	13%
	Improvement VAS >50%	N: 86%	N: 20%	
		N + I: 34%	N + I: 0%	
	Return to work		N: 83%	
			N + I: 86%	
	Medication use		N: 71%	
			N + I: 34%	
52	VAS	Overall: 8.08	Overall: 4.41	45%
		<6 months: 8.1	<6 months: 4.5	56.4%
		6-12 months: 8.0	6-12 months: 3.9	64.6%
		>1 year: 7.1	>1 year: 5.4	45%
	SAT		<6 months: 75%	
			6-12 months: 73%	
			>1 year: 91%	
	Work impairment	<6 months: 3.9	<6 months: 2.7	
		6-12 months: 3.7	6-12 months: 2.2	
		>1 year: 4.2	>1 year: 3.0	
	Medication use	<6 months: 3.8	<6 months: 2.7	
		6-12 months: 3.2	6-12 months: 2.0	
		>1 year: 3.7	>1 year: 2.4	

Continued

TABLE 28-4	Outcomes of Observational Studies on Minimally Invasive Nuclear Decompression for Chronic Low Back Pain—cont'd			
Reference	**Outcomes**	**Initial (Mean ± SD)**	**Follow-Up (Mean, SD)**	**% Improvement**
47	VAS back pain	6.59	3.36 (1 year)	49%
	VAS radicular pain	5.68	2.50	56%
	Improvement VAS >50% (back)			59%
	Improvement VAS >50% (radicular)			58%
	Analgesics consumption			NR
	Disability in daily living			NR
	Inability to work			NR
57	VAS – 6 months	6.95 ± 1.87	4.53 ± 3.60	35%
	Improvement VAS >50%			51.72%
48	VAS	7.5 ± 1.3	2.1 ± 1.6 (1 year)	72%
	ODI	42.2 ± 5.5	20.5 ± 8.9	51%
	Satisfied patients (%)			88%
	Stopped or reduced analgesic use (% patients)			94%
58	VAS	7.6	3.6 (1 year)	53%
	Improvement VAS (mean)		3.98	
	Improvement VAS >50%			68.2%
	Improvement in functional status (% patients)			81.8%
	Return to work (% patients)			63.6%
	Stopped or reduced opioid intake (% patients)			72.7%
59	VAS	8.2	4.1 (1 year)	50%
	Improvement VAS >4 units (% patients)			79%
	Patient satisfaction good or very good (%)			79%

BPI, brief pain inventory; CAM, coblation-assisted microdiscectomy; CM, conservative management; I, IDET procedure; JOA, Japanese Orthopaedic Association scale; N, nucleoplasty; Non-OP, no previous surgical intervention; NR, not reported; ODI, Oswestry disability index; OP, previous surgery; SAT, satisfaction score; VAS, visual analog scale.

infection or spinal nerve root injury. The use of both intradiscal and intravenous antibiotics prior to and during the procedure is thought to reduce the incidence of infection. Because the introducer needle is only 17G and the patient is awake throughout the procedure, the potential for prolonged nerve root injury should be minimized. If the wand is introduced outside of the disc, injury could also occur to neural structures.

Common to any procedure that uses heat within the IVD, there is the risk of end-plate damage. A study in human cadaver discs reported transient peak temperatures of 80° C to 90° C along the channel paths created by nucleoplasty, temperatures greater than 65° C at radial distances of 3 to 4 mm from the channels, and exposure to heat exceeding 250 minutes up to 6 mm from the probes.[62] Because operators cannot guarantee the exact placement of the advancing wand in relation to its transient proximity to the end plate, end-plate damage is possible with nucleoplasty.

Nucleoplasty may also result in disc injury if the wand is placed outside the targeted area within the nucleus and activated. This could inadvertently destroy normal annulus tissue. This is typically minimized by the advancing wand encountering tactile resistance and not penetrating normal annulus tissue. If one is trying to achieve a more posterior placement closer to the protrusion, there would be a risk that one would create channels in normal annulus on either side of the annular tear because the probe will be advanced roughly perpendicular to the annular tear.

COSTS

Fees and Third-Party Reimbursement

Before 2010, nucleoplasty for CLBP could be reported by physicians using category III CPT code 0062T (intradiscal annuloplasty, except electrothermal; single level, including fluoroscopic guidance), or 0063T (intradiscal annuloplasty, except electrothermal; additional levels, including fluoroscopic guidance). However, those codes were deleted in 2010. The most recent CPT guidelines, effective January 1, 2010, recommend reporting CPT code 22899 (unlisted procedure, spine) for percutaneous intradiscal annuloplasty (any method other than electrothermal), or 62287 (aspiration or decompression procedure, nucleus pulposus, single or multiple levels). If imaging guidance is used, CPT code 77003 (fluoroscopic imaging) can be reported. When reporting unlisted procedures such as (22899), the initial submission of the claim will often be denied and additional information will be requested to describe the service, substantiate medical necessity, and support the effectiveness of the procedure. The claim will then be manually reviewed and if it is determined that payment can be made, the examiner will also determine the reimbursement amount based on the data provided. Disposable medical equipment, needles, and syringes used in conjunction with these procedures are included in the practice expense for the procedure. Additional fees will apply for any medications injected. The outpatient surgical center in which the procedure takes place will also charge facility fees for use of the operating room, recovery room, other disposable medical equipment, nurses, radiology, and other services. Because of these ancillary fees, the total cost of a nucleoplasty procedure can reach $8000 or more, though there is wide variation in fees.

These procedures may be covered by other third-party payers such as health insurers and worker's compensation insurance, however, it is recommended that payment policies be verified prior to submitting claims. Although some payers continue to base their reimbursements on usual, customary, and reasonable payment methodology, the majority have developed reimbursement tables based on the Resource Based Relative Value Scale used by Medicare. Reimbursement by other third-party payers is generally higher than Medicare. Preauthorization may be required to obtain reimbursement from third-party payers, which generally indicates that patients and physicians must adhere to specific criteria in order to deem the procedure medically necessary.

Typical fees reimbursed by Medicare in New York and California for these services are summarized in Table 28-5.

Cost Effectiveness

No cost effectiveness analyses or cost utility analyses were identified which evaluated the cost effectiveness of

TABLE 28-5	Medicare Fee Schedule for Related Services	
CPT Code	New York	California
22899	*	*
62287	$539	$574
77003	$61	$6

2010 Participating, nonfacility amount.
*When reporting unlisted procedures such as (22899), the initial submission of the claim will often be denied and additional information will be requested to describe the service, substantiate medical necessity, and support the effectiveness of the procedure. The claim will then be manually reviewed and if it is determined that payment can be made, the examiner will also determine the reimbursement amount based on the data provided.

minimally invasive nuclear decompression as an intervention for CLBP.

SUMMARY

Description

Minimally invasive nuclear decompression (or nucleoplasty) is a procedure in which a probe is inserted through a catheter into the nucleus of an injured IVD and a form of radiofrequency termed *coblation* is targeted at a portion of the nucleus to eliminate it. It is typically performed by nonsurgical or surgical spine specialists in secondary care settings where fluoroscopy is available, such as specialty spine clinics, pain management clinics, and hospitals.

Theory

The exact mechanism of action through which nucleoplasty improves LBP is unclear, but is thought to involve decreased pressure in the nucleus, allowing a disc protrusion to implode inward, reducing any contact pressure between the protruding disc and spinal nerve root. The indications for nucleoplasty for LBP with neurologic involvement include leg pain greater than back pain, MRI-verified contained disc protrusion, positive discography, and failure of at least 6 weeks of conservative therapy. For LBP without neurologic involvement, the indications include MRI-verified contained disc protrusion, positive discography, and failure of at least 6 weeks of conservative therapy. Advanced imaging such as MRI or CT is usually performed prior to the procedure to help guide the spine specialist to target the appropriate spinal levels involved in a patient's CLBP. The use of provocative discography for CLBP remains controversial, but is used by some clinicians to identify painful disc herniations that may subsequently be targeted with other interventions.

Efficacy

Two CPGs and two SRs found insufficient evidence supporting nucleoplasty due to a lack of RCTs. One SR found low-quality evidence supporting nucleoplasty, but this conclusion was based on OBSs. RCTs examining the efficacy of nucleoplasty for LBP were not identified in our search.

Safety

Contraindications for nucleoplasty include severe disc degeneration with more than 33% loss of disc height, disc herniation that is larger than one-third the sagittal diameter of the spinal canal at that level, disc extrusion or sequestration, moderate to severe spinal stenosis, tumor, infection, and fracture. AEs associated with nucleoplasty include increased symptoms, infection, nerve injury, end-plate damage, and disc injury.

Costs

The cost of nucleoplasty varies, but can be as high as $8000 due to ancillary fees. The cost effectiveness of nucleoplasty is unknown.

Comments

There are many OBSs supporting the use of nucleoplasty as an intervention for radicular pain and a few studies supporting its use for CLBP. However, few CPGs and SRs endorse the technique for radicular pain and none endorse the technique for CLBP. On the other hand, nuclear decompression is relatively less invasive than conventional surgical decompression approaches and may therefore represent an option for a subset of patients with CLBP coexisting with significant radicular pain who fail to improve after conservative therapy and who are not appropriate candidates for traditional decompression surgery. This subgroup of patients may include those with referred lower extremity pain, protrusions less than 4 mm to 6 mm (preferably foraminal disc protrusions), minimal stenosis, and relatively well-maintained disc heights. If patients with CLBP are considering nucleoplasty, they should be advised about the potential AEs associated with this intervention. Future studies on nucleoplasty should enhance our current understanding of protrusions and incorporate enhanced methods to safely remove herniated nuclear material without compromising other disc tissue integrity or damaging adjacent tissues.

Minimally invasive interventions in the future target tissue restoration rather than removal. Noncommercial options may include injectable solutions like hypertonic saline and dextrose that transiently lower disc pressure, and may be used alone or combined with inexpensive chemicals that may either promote regeneration or otherwise favorably affect the chemical environment in the disc.[15,63-65] Future products could include injectable solutions that may be combined with growth factors, cultured chondrocytes, or gene vectors to stimulate disc repair. Various collagen fillers have already been used clinically and are under patent and investigation.[66,67] These substances could be used to fill annular tears with the hope that the injected fillers will provide scaffolding on which healthy tissue can grow, with the potential to accelerate both the healing and regeneration processes.[68]

CHAPTER REVIEW QUESTIONS

Answers are located on page 452.
1. What form of radiofrequency is used for nucleoplasty?
   a. ablation
   b. neurotomy
   c. lesioning
   d. coblation
2. True or false: Nucleoplasty has been shown to be cost effective.
3. True or false: CPGs have found insufficient evidence supporting nucleoplasty.
4. Which of the following is a proposed mechanism of action for nucleoplasty?
   a. the protrusion theory
   b. the pressure theory
   c. explosion therapy
   d. neurologic theory
5. What type of electrical current is generally used in nucleoplasty?
   a. low-voltage electrical current (0-50 V)
   b. medium-voltage electrical current (50-100 V)
   c. high-voltage electrical current (100-300 V)
   d. none of the above
6. At which frequency is bipolar radiofrequency energy delivered in nucleoplasty?
   a. 120 KHz
   b. 110 KHz
   c. 100 KHz
   d. 90 KHz
7. What diagnostic test is required prior to nucleoplasty?
   a. EMG or NCV
   b. MRI or CT
   c. diagnostic medial branch blocks
   d. x-rays
8. True or false: It is not recommended that fluoroscopy be used to guide the nucleoplasty procedure.

REFERENCES

1. Chen YC, Lee SH, Chen D. Intradiscal pressure study of percutaneous disc decompression with nucleoplasty in human cadavers. Spine (Phila Pa 1976) 2003;28:661-665.
2. Mixter WJ, Barr JS. Rupture of the intervertebral disc with involvement of the spinal canal. N Engl J Med 1934;211: 210-215.
3. Benz RJ, Garfin SR. Current techniques of decompression of the lumbar spine. Clin Orthop Relat Res 2001;(384):75-81.
4. Singh V, Derby R. Percutaneous lumbar disc decompression. Pain Physician 2006;9:139-146.
5. Yeung AT, Tsou PM. Posterolateral endoscopic excision for lumbar disc herniation: surgical technique, outcome, and complications in 307 consecutive cases. Spine 2002;27:722-731.
6. Takahashi K, Shima I, Porter RW. Nerve root pressure in lumbar disc herniation. Spine 1999;24:2003-2006.
7. Olmarker K, Rydevik B, Holm S, et al. Effects of experimental graded compression on blood flow in spinal nerve roots. A vital microscopic study on the porcine cauda equina. J Orthop Res 1989;7:817-823.

8. Lee MS, Cooper G, Lutz GE, et al. Histologic characterization of coblation nucleoplasty performed on sheep intervertebral discs. Pain Physician 2003;6:439-442.

9. Case RB, Choy DS, Altman P. Change of intradisc pressure versus volume change. J Clin Laser Med Surg 1995;13: 143-147.

10. Choy DS, Diwan S. In vitro and in vivo fall of intradiscal pressure with laser disc decompression. J Clin Laser Med Surg 1992;10:435-437.

11. Maroon JC. Current concepts in minimally invasive discectomy. Neurosurgery 2002;51(Suppl 5):137-145.

12. Yonezawa T, Onomura T, Kosaka R, et al. The system and procedures of percutaneous intradiscal laser nucleotomy. Spine 1990;15:1175-1185.

13. Chen YC, Lee SH, Saenz Y, et al. Histologic findings of disc, end plate and neural elements after coblation of nucleus pulposus: an experimental nucleoplasty study. Spine J 2003;3: 466-470.

14. Hellinger J, Linke R, Heller H. A biophysical explanation for Nd:YAG percutaneous laser disc decompression success. J Clin Laser Med Surg 2001;19:235-238.

15. Derby R, Eek B, Lee SH, et al. Comparison of intradiscal restorative injections and intradiscal electrothermal treatment (IDET) in the treatment of low back pain. Pain Physician 2004;7:63-66.

16. Mochida J, Toh E, Nomura T, et al. The risks and benefits of percutaneous nucleotomy for lumbar disc herniation. A 10-year longitudinal study. J Bone Joint Surg Br 2001;83:501-505.

17. Mochida J, Nishimura K, Okuma M, et al. Percutaneous nucleotomy in elite athletes. J Spinal Disord 2001;14:159-164.

18. Carragee EJ, Han MY, Suen PW, et al. Clinical outcomes after lumbar discectomy for sciatica: the effects of fragment type and anular competence. J Bone Joint Surg Am 2003; 85:102-108.

19. Martinez JB, Oloyede VO, Broom ND. Biomechanics of load-bearing of the intervertebral disc: an experimental and finite element model. Med Eng Phys 1997;19:145-156.

20. Adams MA, McMillan DW, Green TP, et al. Sustained loading generates stress concentrations in lumbar intervertebral discs. Spine 1996;21:434-438.

21. Adams MA, McNally DS, Dolan P. "Stress" distributions inside intervertebral discs. The effects of age and degeneration. J Bone Joint Surg Br 1996;78:965-972.

22. Edwards WT, Ordway NR, Zheng Y, et al. Peak stresses observed in the posterior lateral anulus. Spine 2001;26: 1753-1759.

23. McNally DS, Shackleford IM, Goodship AE, Mulholland RC. In vivo stress measurement can predict pain on discography. Spine 1996;21:2580-2587.

24. McNally DS, Adams MA. Internal intervertebral disc mechanics as revealed by stress profilometry. Spine 1992;17: 66-73.

25. Hutton WC, Elmer WA, Boden SD, et al. The effect of hydrostatic pressure on intervertebral disc metabolism. Spine 1999; 24:1507-1515.

26. Hutton WC, Elmer WA, Bryce LM, et al. Do the intervertebral disc cells respond to different levels of hydrostatic pressure? Clin Biomech (Bristol, Avon) 2001;16:728-734.

27. Wognum S, Huyghe JM, Baaijens FP. Influence of osmotic pressure changes on the opening of existing cracks in 2 intervertebral disc models. Spine 2006;31:1783-1788.

28. Brinckmann P, Grootenboer H. Change of disc height, radial disc bulge, and intradiscal pressure from disctomy. An in vitro investigation on human lumbar discs. Spine 1991 Jun;16(6): 641-646.

29. Castro WH, Halm H, Rondhuis J. The influence of automated percutaneous lumbar discectomy (APLD) on the biomechanics of the lumbar intervertebral disc. An experimental study. Acta Orthop Belg 1992;58:400-405.

30. Simunic DI, Robertson PA, Broom ND. Mechanically induced disruption of the healthy bovine intervertebral disc. Spine 2004;29:972-978.

31. Osti OL, Vernon-Roberts B, Moore R, et al. Annular tears and disc degeneration in the lumbar spine. A post-mortem study of 135 discs. J Bone Joint Surg Br 1992;74:678-682.

32. Osti OL, Vernon-Roberts B, Fraser RD. 1990 Volvo Award in experimental studies. Anulus tears and intervertebral disc degeneration. An experimental study using an animal model. Spine 1990;15:762-767.

33. Delamarter RB, Howard MW, Goldstein T, et al. Percutaneous lumbar discectomy. Preoperative and postoperative magnetic resonance imaging. J Bone Joint Surg Am 1995;77:578-584.

34. Derby R. Percutaneous disc decompression. 13th Annual Scientific Meeting of the International Spine Intervention Society. New York, NY, July 15-17, 2005.

35. O'Neill CW, Liu JJ, Leibenberg E, et al. Percutaneous plasma decompression alters cytokine expression in injured porcine intervertebral discs. Spine J 2004;4:88-98.

36. Sharps LS, Isaac Z. Percutaneous disc decompression using nucleoplasty. Pain Physician 2002;5:121-126.

37. Pauza KJ, Howell S, Dreyfuss P, et al. A randomized, placebo-controlled trial of intradiscal electrothermal therapy for the treatment of discogenic low back pain. Spine J 2004; 4:27-35.

38. Nielens H, van Zundert J, Mairiaux P, et al. Chronic low back pain. Brussels, 2006, Report No.: KCE reports Vol 48C.

39. Chou R, Loeser JD, Owens DK, et al. Interventional therapies, surgery, and interdisciplinary rehabilitation for low back pain: an evidence-based clinical practice guideline from the American Pain Society. Spine 2009;34:1066-1077.

40. Gibson JN, Waddell G. Surgical interventions for lumbar disc prolapse. Cochrane Database Syst Rev 2007;(2):CD001350.

41. Chou R, Atlas SJ, Stanos SP, et al. Nonsurgical interventional therapies for low back pain: a review of the evidence for an American Pain Society clinical practice guideline. Spine 2009;34:1078-1093.

42. Urrutia G, Kovacs F, Nishishinya MB, et al. Percutaneous thermocoagulation intradiscal techniques for discogenic low back pain. Spine 2007;32:1146-1154.

43. Manchikanti L, Derby R, Benyamin RM, et al. A systematic review of mechanical lumbar disc decompression with nucleoplasty. Pain Physician 2009;12:561-572.

44. Marin FZ. CAM versus nucleoplasty. Acta Neurochir Suppl 2005;92:111-114.

45. Singh V, Piryani C, Liao K, et al. Percutaneous disc decompression using coblation (nucleoplasty TM) in the treatment of chronic discogenic pain. Pain Physician 2002;5:250-259.

46. Singh V, Piryani C, Liao K. Evaluation of percutaneous disc decompression using coblation in chronic back pain with or without leg pain. Pain Physician 2003;6:273-280.

47. Al-Zain F, Lemcke J, Killeen T, et al. Minimally invasive spinal surgery using nucleoplasty: a 1-year follow-up study. Acta Neurochir (Wien) 2008;150:1257-1262.

48. Mirzai H, Tekin I, Yaman O, et al. The results of nucleoplasty in patients with lumbar herniated disc: a prospective clinical study of 52 consecutive patients. Spine J 2007;7:88-92.

49. National Institute for Health and Clinical Excellence (NICE). Percutaneous disc decompression using coblation for lower back pain. London, 2006, Report No.: Interventional procedure guidance 173.

50. Boswell MV, Trescot AM, Datta S, et al. Interventional techniques: evidence-based practice guidelines in the management of chronic spinal pain. Pain Physician 2007;10:7-111.

51. American College of Occupational and Environmental Medicine. Low back disorders. In: Glass LS, editor. Occupational medicine practice guidelines: evaluation and management of common health problems and functional recovery in workers, 2nd ed. Elk Grove Village, IL: American College of Occupational and Environmental Medicine (ACOEM); 2007. p. 366.

52. Reddy AS, Loh S, Cutts J, et al. New approach to the management of acute disc herniation. Pain Physician 2005;8: 385-390.

53. Cohen SP, Williams S, Kurihara C, et al. Nucleoplasty with or without intradiscal electrothermal therapy (IDET) as a treatment for lumbar herniated disc. J Spinal Disord Tech 2005;18(Suppl):119-124.

54. Derby R. Outcome comparison between IDET, combined IDET nucleoplasty and biochemical injection treatment. International Spine Intervention Society, 10th Annual Scientific Meeting, Austin, Texas. September, 2002.

55. Derby R. Comparison between IDET and nucleoplasty outcome in patients with discogenic pain. International Spine Intervention Society, 14th Annual Scientific Meeting. Salt Lake City, Utah. July, 2006.

56. Alexandre A, Coro L, Azuelos A, et al. Percutaneous nucleoplasty for discoradicular conflict. Acta Neurochir Suppl 2005;92:83-86.

57. Calisaneller T, Ozdemir O, Karadeli E, et al. Six months postoperative clinical and 24 hour post-operative MRI examinations after nucleoplasty with radiofrequency energy. Acta Neurochir (Wien) 2007;149:495-500.

58. Yakovlev A, Tamimi MA, Liang H, et al. Outcomes of percutaneous disc decompression utilizing nucleoplasty for the treatment of chronic discogenic pain. Pain Physician 2007;10: 319-328.

59. Masala S, Massari F, Fabiano S, et al. Nucleoplasty in the treatment of lumbar diskogenic back pain: one year follow-up. Cardiovasc Intervent Radiol 2007;30:426-432.

60. Bhagia SM, Slipman CW, Nirschl M, et al. Side effects and complications after percutaneous disc decompression using coblation technology. Am J Phys Med Rehabil 2006;85: 6-13.

61. Slipman CW. Nucleoplasty procedure for cervical radicular pain-initial case series. International Spine Intervention Society, 11th Annual Scientific Meeting. Orlando, FL, 2003.

62. Nau WH, Diederich CJ. Evaluation of temperature distributions in cadaveric lumbar spine during nucleoplasty. Phys Med Biol 2004;49:1583-1594.

63. Miller MR, Mathews RS, Reeves KD. Treatment of painful advanced internal lumbar disc derangement with intradiscal injection of hypertonic dextrose. Pain Physician 2006;9: 115-121.

64. Klein RG, Eek BC, O'Neill CW, et al. Biochemical injection treatment for discogenic low back pain: a pilot study. Spine J 2003;3:220-226.

65. Kim JH. In vivo safety study of intradiscal restorative injection. Interventional Spine 2006;5:60-67.

66. Derby R, Kim BJ. Effect of intradiscal electrothermal treatment with a short heating catheter and fibrin on discogenic low back pain. Am J Phys Med Rehabil 2005;84:560-561.

67. Derby R. Injection of fibrin sealant into discs following IDET and nucleoplasty early outcome in six cases. Interventional Spine 2005;5:12-19.

68. Taylor W. Biologic collagen PMMA injection (Artefill) repairs mid-annular concentric defects in the ovine model. Spine J 2006;6(5S):48-49 (Abstract no. 4:3499).

EUGENE K. WAI
DARREN M. ROFFEY
ANDREA C. TRICCO
SIMON DAGENAIS

CHAPTER **29**

Decompression Surgery

DESCRIPTION

Terminology and Subtypes

Decompression surgery refers to the various forms of lumbar surgery whose primary goal is to remove structures in the neural canal that are thought to cause neural impingement.[1,2] *Neural impingement* is a term used to describe both sensory (e.g., pain, numbness, tingling, burning) and motor (e.g., reduced strength, muscle atrophy) changes that may result from a compression of structures within the neural canal. In the cervical and thoracic spine, the neural canal contains the spinal cord, from which anterior and dorsal roots emerge to form spinal nerve roots (Figure 29-1). In the lumbar spine, the neural canal contains the cauda equina, composed of lumbar and sacral spinal nerve roots (Figure 29-2). The borders of the neural canal include the vertebral body, intervertebral disc, pedicles, lamina, and zygapophysial joints (also called facet joints), as well as the longitudinal ligament and the ligamentum flavum. The lateral recess is defined by the medial border of the superior facet and the medial border of the pedicle (Figure 29-3). This area, also called the subarticular space, is a common location for nerve root impingement within the neural canal (Figure 29-4). The term *degenerative cascade* is used to describe changes in the discs, facet joints, and ligamentum flavum that may eventually lead to neural impingement.[3] Disc herniations are often described according to the direction in which the bulge occurs, that is, posterolateral, central, or far lateral. *Spinal stenosis* refers to the narrowing of the neural canal, which often results from advanced degenerative changes in surrounding structures.[4]

Symptoms associated with neural canal impingement in the lumbosacral region may include radiculopathy and neurogenic claudication.[2] *Radiculopathy* is a general term used to describe symptoms involving a spinal nerve root, both sensory and motor. *Sciatica* is the term given to radiculopathy of the sciatic nerve. *Claudication* refers to intermittent pain in the legs that is often worse after activities such as walking or standing and is relieved only by sitting or leaning forward. Neurogenic claudication describes claudication from neural canal impingement, usually from spinal stenosis. Cauda equina syndrome represents a medical emergency in which severe neural impingement affects multiple lumbar or sacral spinal nerve roots. Signs and symptoms of cauda equina syndrome may include bowel and bladder dysfunction (e.g., incontinence, inability to urinate), saddle anesthesia, or progressive leg weakness.

There are many types of decompression surgery, which are usually named according to the structure that is surgically removed. The two main types of decompression surgery are discectomy and laminectomy. Discectomy implies surgical excision of an intervertebral disc, whereas laminectomy involves removal of the lamina. Either procedure may involve partial or complete removal of the targeted structures. There are several variants of decompression surgery procedures according to the surgical technique used. Standard, traditional, or open decompression usually describes a procedure in which the skin incision made is large enough to completely visualize the targeted structures. Microscopic decompression is a loosely defined term in which the skin incision made is typically smaller and different surgical instruments are used to improve visualization of the targeted structures with less tissue disruption (Figure 29-5). An endoscope or arthroscope may be used in microscopic decompression to improve visualization of deeper structures. The procedures and techniques used in decompression surgery are often combined to name a particular approach (e.g., microscopic discectomy, microdiscectomy, or endoscopic discectomy). Multiple decompression procedures may also be combined (e.g., discectomy with or without laminectomy).

History and Frequency of Use

The earliest evidence of spinal pathology can be traced back to the preserved remnants of Egyptian mummies approximately 5000 years ago.[5] The first written account of spinal pathology originated in 1600-1700 BC in a surgical textbook from Egypt that was later transcribed as the Edwin Smith Papyrus.[6,7] In more modern times, Andreas Vesalius was one of the first to raise awareness about the intervertebral disc in

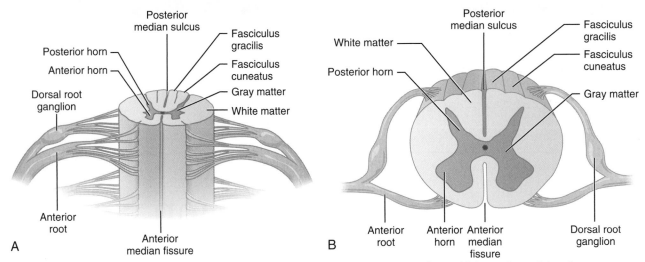

Figure 29-1 The neural canal in the cervical and thoracic spine contains the spinal cord, from which anterior and dorsal roots emerge to form spinal nerve roots (**A** anterior view, **B** axial view). (**B** modified from Swartz MH. Textbook of physical diagnosis: history and examination, ed. 5. St. Louis, 2006, Saunders.)

his publication *De Humani Corporis Fabrica*.[8] However, it was only in the past two centuries that decompression surgery was attempted to address specific spinal pathology.

In 1829, Smith reported performing a lumbar laminectomy in the United States for the treatment of progressive paresis attributed to a vertebral fracture.[9] Lumbar laminectomy for the treatment of spinal stenosis followed several decades later when the procedure was performed by Lane in 1893.[10] One of the earliest accounts of discectomy is attributed to Oppenheim and Krause, who performed a laminectomy followed by transdural disc resection in 1909.[11,12] In 1910, a unilateral laminectomy was performed in cadavers by Taylor.[12] Shortly thereafter, there were published accounts of a herniated disc.[13,14] The term *neurogenic claudication* was also coined around that time by Dejerine, although the link with lumbar spinal stenosis was not made until 1954 by Verbiest.[15,16]

In 1929, Dandy operated on two individuals presenting with compression of the cauda equina following traumatic disc herniation.[17] The now seminal report by Mixter and Barr in 1934 was the first to correlate sciatica with a herniated lumbar disc and elaborate on its operative management with a laminectomy and discectomy.[18] The procedure for decompression surgery remained largely unchanged until microsurgical techniques were developed in the early 1970s to improve outcomes and minimize adverse events (AEs).[19-21] In 1978, Williams reported on 532 patients who received lumbar microdiscectomy through an intralaminar window.[22] A decade later, Young and colleagues described a unilateral approach for bilateral spinal canal decompression.[23] In the 1990s, development of tubular retractor systems and low-profile automatic instrumentation revolutionized decompression surgery through smaller incisions, less operative blood loss, increased visualization of pathology, decreased hospitalization, shorter postoperative recovery, and earlier return to activities.

The United States has the highest rate of spine surgery in the world.[24-28] Lumbar discectomy is the most common

surgical procedure performed in the United States for patients presenting with chronic low back pain (CLBP) and radiculopathy due to neural impingement.[29-31] Spinal stenosis is the most common indication for lumbar spine decompression surgery in patients older than 65 years of age.[32,33] Between 1979 and 1992, surgical treatment for spinal stenosis increased in the United States by almost 700%, from 8 to 61 procedures per 100,000 persons.[34] Between 1992 and 2003, the rate of lumbar discectomy and laminectomy in the United States increased from 1.7 to 2.1 per 1000 Medicare enrollees, resulting in nearly 300,000 procedures annually in that population.[29,35,36]

Practitioner, Setting, and Availability

Decompression surgery is usually performed by orthopedic spine surgeons or neurologic spine surgeons. In the United States, spine surgeons (orthopedic or neurologic) typically complete 4 years of undergraduate education, 4 years of medical school, and 5 to 7 years of surgical residency. Many spine surgeons also complete 1 or 2 years of optional subspecialty fellowship training to further develop clinical skills in spine surgery. Spine surgery fellowship training programs have been accredited by the Accreditation Council for Graduate Medical Education (ACGME) since 1991 and by the American College of Spine Surgery (ACSS) since 1998. After completion of residency/fellowship training, orthopedic and neurologic surgeons are eligible for board certification by the American Board of Orthopaedic Surgery (ABOS) and the American Board of Neurological Surgery (ABNS), which were founded in 1934 and 1940, respectively. Obtaining certification means the surgeon has met the specified educational, evaluation, and examination requirements of the respective board.

According to the American Academy of Orthopaedic Surgeons (AAOS), there were 17,673 orthopedic surgeons and 4605 residents practicing in the United States as of January 2010.[37] Corresponding figures from the American

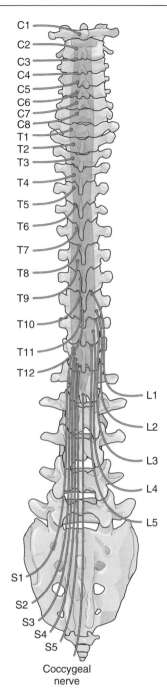

Figure 29-2 The neural canal in the lumbar spine contains the cauda equina, composed of lumbar and sacral spinal nerve roots. (Modified from Swartz MH. Textbook of physical diagnosis: history and examination, ed. 5. St. Louis, 2006, Saunders.)

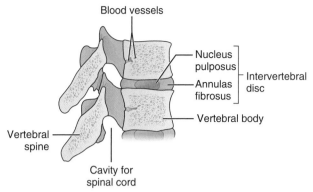

Figure 29-3 The lateral recess is defined by the medial border of the superior facet and the medial border of the pedicle. (Modified from Patton KT, Thibodeau GA. Anatomy & physiology, ed. 7. St. Louis, 2010, Elsevier.)

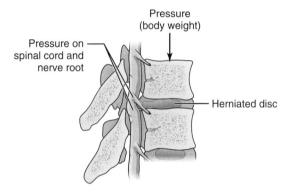

Figure 29-4 The lateral recess is a common location for spinal nerve root impingement secondary to disc herniations. (Modified from Patton KT, Thibodeau GA. Anatomy & physiology, ed. 7. St. Louis, 2010, Elsevier.)

Association of Neurological Surgeons (AANS) were 3519 neurologic surgeons and 1663 residents/fellows as of December 2009.[38] The number of orthopedic and neurologic surgeons with subspecialty training in spine surgery is difficult to estimate because board certification in spine surgery is optional in the United States. The American Board of Spine Surgery (ABSS) was approved as a specialty certification board by the Medical Board of California in 2002 and reported 180 board-certified spine surgeons in the United States as of January 2010 (personal communication, Eckert M. Executive administrator, American Board of Spine Surgery, 2010).

Decompression surgery is generally performed in hospitals because it requires general anesthesia and postoperative care. Some procedures may also be performed on an outpatient basis in ambulatory surgical centers. Decompression surgery for CLBP is widely available throughout the United States.

Procedure

Preoperative

Conventional decompression surgery usually begins with an anesthesiologist performing a preoperative examination and history, followed by induction of general anesthesia. An endotracheal tube is inserted and the patient breathes with the assistance of a ventilator during the surgery. Microscopic decompression surgery, on the other hand, can be performed under local anesthesia with minimal or no sedation. Preoperative intravenous antibiotics are often given to minimize postoperative infection. Depending upon the surgical approach used, patients are positioned in a prone (common) or supine

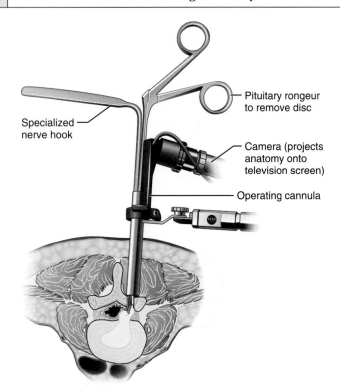

Specialized nerve hook

Pituitary rongeur to remove disc

Camera (projects anatomy onto television screen)

Operating cannula

Figure 29-5 Microscopic decompression surgery uses smaller incisions and instruments to improve visualization of the targeted structures. (From MED surgical technique booklet, Memphis, Tenn, 1997, Medtronic Sofamor Danek.)

(rare) position using a flexible operating table with padding and supports. The skin in the lumbosacral region is cleaned repeatedly using antimicrobial cleaning solutions. Sterile drapes are then placed around the area of the operation, and the surgical team wears sterile surgical attire to maintain a bacteria-free environment throughout the procedure.

General Surgical Approach

A skin incision is then made by the surgeon above the area to be operated on. The length of the incision varies according to the surgical approach (e.g., conventional vs. microscopic). The incision is then made gradually deeper by cutting through subcutaneous tissues, using retractors to maximize visualization. Conventional decompression surgery requires stripping the muscles from the posterior vertebral structures. This approach allows for excellent exposure of the posterior midline structures, including the lamina, central and posterolateral disc, and medial facet joint. A paramedian approach (also called a *Wiltse approach*) also involves exposing the lateral aspect of the facet joint and foramen through the intermuscular plane between the erector spinae and multifidus. Although anterior approaches to decompression surgery are possible, they are generally used to facilitate reconstruction of structural abnormalities rather than to perform simple discectomy or laminectomy procedures.

Posterior Elements

Once the targeted vertebra is exposed, the structures contributing to the neural impingement are then removed. Laminectomy requires removal of the lamina, usually along with the

associated spinous process. Alternatively, a laminotomy involves partial removal of the lamina but preserves the posterior aspect (e.g., spinous process). Laminoplasty involves cutting only one side of the lamina to allow the other side to swing posteriorly as if on a hinge, thereby relieving some neural impingement without removing any bone. Flavectomy involves removal of the ligamentum flavum to expose the cauda equina and spinal nerve roots. Medial facetectomy involves removing any hypertrophy of the facet joint capsule and surrounding osteophytes. Foraminotomy involves removing the portion of the superior facet in the foraminal space to relieve stenosis that may be present in the intervertebral foramen. As neural impingement is often associated with all of the above structures, the term laminectomy has been used to denote surgical removal of all of the surrounding structures. Posterior decompression surgery is another term used to represent the global resection of all structures contributing to neural impingement.

Intervertebral Disc

Patients with sciatica related to large disc herniations usually require surgical removal of the prolapsed portion of the disc. This can be accomplished through a unilateral approach with only minimal resection of the posterior elements as described above to identify the spinal nerve root. Once exposed, the spinal nerve root is then mobilized and protected prior to exposing the prolapsed section of the disc to be removed. The amount of intervertebral disc removal varies considerably, and debate continues over removal of disc fragments contained within the annulus (Figure 29-6).

Microscopic Surgery

The basic steps involved in the microscopic approach to decompression surgery are generally similar to the steps described for conventional decompression. However, microscopic decompression surgery usually involves a smaller skin incision, use of tube retractors rather than surgical musculature removal, greater illumination of the surgical field with more powerful lighting, and magnification of targeted structures through surgical microscopes. An endoscope may also be used to facilitate visualization of targeted structures.

Regulatory Status

Equipment and instruments used during decompression surgery are regulated by the US Food and Drug Administration (FDA) as class I or class II medical devices. Class I medical devices present a negligible potential for harm and are subject only to general controls that provide reasonable assurance of the safety and effectiveness of the device. Surgical devices in this category include rongeurs (bone pliers), rotary burrs (bone drill bits), retractors, and other nonpowered hand-held surgical instruments. Class II medical devices are subjected to general controls and additional special controls to provide reasonable assurance that they will perform as indicated and will not cause harm or injury to the patient and/or surgeon. Obtaining approval to market a class II medical device requires a 510(k) premarket submission to the FDA with evidence from the manufacturer that the new device is substantially equivalent to a currently approved and

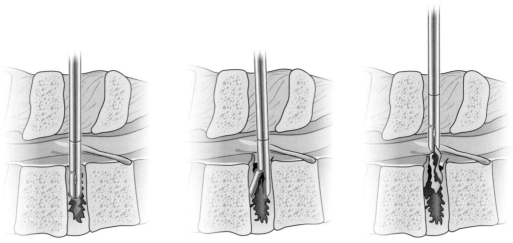

Figure 29-6 Decompression surgery with discectomy requires removal of herniated disc material while preserving the structural integrity of the remaining disc. (Modified from Kirkaldy-Willis WH, editor. Managing low back pain, ed. 2, New York, 1988, Churchill Livingstone.)

legally marketed similar device. Devices in this category include surgical drapes, suture materials, electrically powered arthroscopes, and digital fluoroscopic equipment.

In reaction to the increasing frequency with which decompression surgery is being performed, the FDA has approved a raft of new medical devices designed to streamline certain procedures. In 2000, the Medtronic METRx system was approved as a class II medical device, and it is indicated for use in the visualization of the surgical area to allow for herniated disc repair, circumferential decompression of nerve roots, and the search and removal of nucleus material. Similarly, in 2009, the FDA approved the Tiger Discectomy Device as a class II medical device for use in endoscopic and nonendoscopic spinal procedures to assist in the removal of fibrous disc material between the T12 to S1 spinal segments.

As a function of the continual development of new decompression surgery technologies, a trend has emerged toward the manufacturing of sterile, single-use, single-level, disposable medical devices. In 2003, the FDA approved a class II medical device called the Stryker Dekompressor Percutaneous Discectomy Probe, which is indicated for use in the aspiration of disc material during minimally invasive percutaneous discectomy procedures. The FDA approved another class II medical device called the Clarus Model 21200 Nucleotome Discectomy Probe in 2004, which is also indicated for use in the aspiration of disc material during minimally invasive percutaneous discectomy procedures. In 2009, the FDA approved and regulated a class II medical device called the Laurimed Discectomy System, which is indicated for use in the cutting and aspiration of nucleus material from discs during open discectomy procedures.

THEORY

Mechanism of Action

Decompression surgery may be used for a variety of indications, including spinal trauma, spinal tumor, spinal infection, or cauda equina syndrome. The outcomes of decompression surgery for each of those indications may be attributed to specific mechanisms of action such as removal of diseased tissue, or prevention of disease progression. In the context of CLBP, decompression surgery is generally thought to alleviate signs and symptoms of neural impingement associated with structures that are compressing the spinal canal secondary to advanced degeneration.

Kirkaldy-Willis and colleagues described a degenerative cascade involving the intervertebral discs, facet joints, and ligamentum flavum that could eventually lead to neural impingement if severe.[3] This degenerative cascade initially involves dehydration of the disc and loss of disc height that naturally occurs with aging. These changes in disc composition and morphology may then lead to posterior bulging, which exerts pressure on the ligamentum flavum and pushes it toward the neural canal. Further degeneration or injury to a degenerated disc may then lead to tears in the annulus, resulting in prolapse of the nucleus pulposus into the neural canal.

Degenerative changes in the disc may then affect the biomechanical properties of the motion segment, leading to mild instability that increases the mechanical load on surrounding structures. In response to this increased load, the facet joints may undergo degenerative changes including growth of osteophytes as well as facet joint capsule and ligament hypertrophy, which may grow into the neural canal. Continued degeneration of the facet joints may eventually lead to segmental instability and contribute to degenerative spondylolisthesis or lateral listhesis, resulting in narrowing of the neural canal or intervertebral foramen, leading to further impingement of the neural canal.

Impingement of the neural canal may result in neurologic dysfunction from direct or indirect causes. Spinal nerve root function may be disrupted due to direct mechanical compression, though the amount of pressure required to do this remains a matter of continued research. An alternative mechanism that has been proposed is that spinal nerve root function may be affected indirectly by chemical mediators of the acute inflammatory cascade (e.g., cytokines).[39] Claudication may result from direct mechanical compression of spinal nerve roots or from focal ischemia.[39]

Decompression surgery is therefore thought to alleviate neurologic dysfunction by removing one or more of the structures with degenerative changes that may be causing or contributing to impingement of the neural canal. Removal of these structures may also temporarily decrease acute inflammatory changes, reducing the role of chemical mediators and related neural irritation. A careful balance must be achieved when performing decompression surgery to remove an amount of tissue that is sufficient to alleviate neural impingement but will not exacerbate segmental stability in the lumbar spine that may require subsequent fusion surgery.

Indication

As described above, the primary goal of decompression surgery is to remove structures that may be contributing to neural impingement and any resulting neurologic dysfunction from the spinal nerve roots.[2] The indication for decompression surgery in the context of CLBP is persistent and disabling pain or neurological dysfunction associated with impingement of the neural canal. Radicular and claudicant leg pain are the typical pain syndromes associated with impingement of the neural canal. Specific diagnoses that may cause impingement of the neural canal include spinal stenosis, lateral foramen impingement, and large disc herniations. Because of the potential harms involved with decompression surgery, it should only be considered when patients have failed to achieve meaningful improvement of their CLBP and neurologic dysfunction following appropriate nonoperative management, since many patients will improve without treatment given sufficient time.[40,41]

The precise nature and duration of the ideal nonoperative management regime that should be attempted prior to considering decompression surgery remains difficult to define. However, it appears reasonable to include at least a few months of education, analgesics, therapeutic exercise, lifestyle improvements, epidural steroid injections, manual therapy, behavioral, and/or other more conservative interventions described elsewhere in this text. Trial and error will be unavoidable, and failure to improve following a limited attempt at one form of nonoperative care should not be construed as an absolute need for decompression surgery for patients who do not have progressive neurologic deficits or intractable pain preventing them from engaging in most activities of daily living. Once it has been determined that decompression surgery may be warranted for a particular patient, there should be a full discussion of the potential short- and long-term harms associated with this procedure prior to the patient and their health care team deciding to proceed with surgical management.

Assessment

Before undergoing decompression surgery, patients should first be assessed for LBP using an evidence-based and goal-oriented approach focused on the patient history and neurologic examination, as discussed in Chapter 3. Clinicians should also inquire about medication history to note prior hypersensitivity/allergy or AEs with drugs similar to those being considered, and evaluate contraindications for these types of drugs. Advanced imaging such as magnetic resonance imaging (MRI), computed tomography (CT), or CT myelography is required to help guide the spine specialist to target the appropriate spinal levels involved in a patient's CLBP and related neurologic dysfunction.

Findings on advanced imaging that may be of particular interest when considering decompression surgery include large disc herniations or advanced degenerative changes in the facet joints resulting in impingement of intervertebral foramen or neural canal, or spinal stenosis. However, the mere presence of these findings on advanced imaging is not sufficient to justify proceeding with decompression surgery. It is of the utmost importance that any findings on advanced imaging be correlated with findings made independently from the medical history, symptoms, physical examination, and neurologic examination.

For patients in whom there is uncertainty about the significance of findings present on advanced imaging, electrodiagnostic testing may be used. Electromyography and nerve conduction velocity may provide objective evidence of neurologic dysfunction. These tests may not always clearly identify the spinal nerve root involved since muscle groups in the lower extremities are jointly innervated. Nevertheless, electrodiagnostic testing may be helpful in distinguishing neurogenic claudication from vascular claudication, as well as spinal nerve root impairment from peripheral neuropathy.

Another aspect that should be considered for the assessment of patients with CLBP who may be candidates for decompression surgery is to clearly identify the location of predominant pain symptoms. It has been suggested that decompression surgery is most beneficial for patients whose CLBP is associated with predominant leg pain rather than predominant axial LBP. Because symptom severity is expected to fluctuate over time and the wording of a question may influence its answer, establishing the location of the predominant pain may require a validated instrument. Responses to a three-item questionnaire developed for this purpose was as useful as assessment by a pain management physician or advanced imaging findings in determining the likelihood that patients presenting with CLBP were deemed appropriate candidates for decompression surgery by a spine surgeon.[42]

Other differential diagnoses to consider before proceeding with decompression surgery for CLBP and neurologic dysfunction include fibromyalgia, myofascial pain syndromes, spinal cord or central nervous system pathology, peripheral neuropathy, peripheral nerve entrapment, vascular claudication, arthropathy, and other pathologies affecting the lower extremities. Additional screening may be required to identify spinal instability associated with pars defects, spondylolisthesis, lateral listhesis, or scoliosis, which may require surgical fusion in addition to decompression surgery. This screening may usually be performed using standing and flexion-extension lumbar spine x-rays.

EFFICACY

Evidence supporting the efficacy of these interventions for CLBP was summarized from recent clinical practice guidelines (CPGs), systematic reviews (SRs), and randomized controlled trials (RCTs).

TABLE 29-1	Clinical Practice Guideline Recommendations on Decompression Surgery for Chronic Low Back Pain

Reference	Country	Conclusion
43	Belgium	Not recommended for disc prolapse without neurologic involvement
		Low-quality evidence for discoradicular conflict with neurologic involvement
45	Europe	Not recommended
131	Italy	Recommended for LBP with neurologic involvement

LBP, low back pain.

Clinical Practice Guidelines

Discectomy

Two of the recent national CPGs on the management of CLBP have assessed and summarized the evidence to make specific recommendations about the efficacy of discectomy, while one CPG made recommendations related to the efficacy of decompression surgery in general.

The CPG from Belgium in 2006 found no evidence supporting discectomy among patients with disc prolapse without neurologic involvement.[43] That CPG also reported low-quality evidence supporting discectomy among patients with discoradicular conflict and neurologic involvement.

The CPG from Italy in 2006 recommended discectomy for LBP with neurologic involvement.[44]

The CPG from Europe in 2006 did not recommend decompression surgery in general for CLBP.[45]

Laminectomy

None of the recent national CPGs on the management of CLBP have assessed and summarized the evidence to make specific recommendations about the efficacy of laminectomy.

Findings from the above CPGs are summarized in Table 29-1.

Systematic Reviews

Discectomy

Cochrane Collaboration. The Cochrane Collaboration conducted an SR in 2007 on surgery for degenerative lumbar disc prolapse.[46] A total of 42 RCTs were identified, of which 22 involved some form of discectomy. Sixteen of these RCTs examined disc herniation,[47-62] one examined nerve root compromise,[63] one examined root lesion,[64] two examined nerve root pain with or without LBP,[65,66] one examined disc prolapse,[67] and one examined a mixture of patients without specifying the duration of LBP or condition.[68]

One RCT found that discectomy was superior to conservative treatment after 1 year yet statistically significant differences were not observed after 4 and 10 years of follow-up. Another RCT observed similar findings for microdiscectomy

versus physical therapy.[51] A meta-analysis of two RCTs showed no statistically significant differences between discectomy and chymopapain injection for subjective outcomes, which was consistent with another meta-analysis of three RCTs reporting on the surgeon's rating of patient improvement.[49,55,59]

However, another meta-analysis showed that discectomy was superior to chymopapain injection regarding the need for a second procedure within 1 to 2 years.[49,50,59,65] Yet another meta-analysis of two RCTs indicated that chymopapain injection was superior to automated percutaneous discectomy regarding the need for a second procedure within 1 year.[53,57] RCTs of microdiscectomy versus open discectomy did not show any differences.[54,58] Two RCTs did not observe differences between percutaneous endoscopic discectomy and microdiscectomy, yet a meta-analysis found microdiscectomy superior regarding repeat surgery within 6 months.[48,56,60]

This review concluded that discectomy provides faster relief from an acute attack of LBP versus conservative management among patients with LBP and neurologic involvement.[46] This review also concluded that comparable results are expected for microdiscectomy and open discectomy, yet there is insufficient evidence supporting other types of discectomy (e.g., percutaneous).[46]

American Pain Society and American College of Physicians. An SR was conducted in 2008 by the American Pain Society and American College of Physicians CPG committee on surgical interventions for acute and chronic LBP.[69] That review identified two SRs related to discectomy for radiculopathy with herniated lumbar disc, one of which was the Cochrane Collaboration review mentioned above.[46,70] The other SR concluded that there is insufficient evidence regarding the comparative effectiveness of the different types of discectomy.[70] Collectively, these SRs summarized data from 30 RCTs, which were also described in the Cochrane review.[71]

In addition, five other RCTs were identified, two examining disc prolapse and three examining disc herniation.[72-76] One RCT did not find any differences between microdiscectomy and open discectomy.[75] Another RCT found that microdiscectomy was superior to nonsurgical treatment, and another observed no statistically significant differences in pain relief for microdiscectomy versus nonsurgical treatment after 1 to 2 years of follow-up.[72,73] Results of the other RCTs were not reported.

This SR concluded that there is good quality evidence that discectomy or microdiscectomy leads to moderate net benefit among patients with lumbar disc prolapse and radiculopathy.[68] However, these benefits may decrease after only 3 months of follow-up. This SR also concluded that there is insufficient evidence supporting the superiority of microdiscectomy over open discectomy (and vice versa), as well as the efficacy of other types of discectomy, such as percutaneous, laser-assisted, and endoscopic discectomy.[69]

Laminectomy

Cochrane Collaboration. The Cochrane Collaboration conducted an SR in 2005 on surgery for degenerative lumbar spondylosis.[71] A total of 31 RCTs were identified, of which 6 examined the effects of laminectomy. Of these RCTs, four

TABLE 29-2	Systematic Review Findings on Decompression Surgery for Chronic Low Back Pain		
Reference	# RCTs in SR	# RCTs for CLBP	Conclusion
Discectomy			
46	22	NR	Discectomy provides faster relief from an acute attack of LBP versus conservative management among patients with LBP and neurologic involvement Comparable results are expected for microdiscectomy and open discectomy Insufficient evidence supporting the other types of discectomy
69	30	NR	Good-quality evidence that discectomy or microdiscectomy leads to moderate net benefit among patients with lumbar disc prolapse and radiculopathy Insufficient evidence supporting the superiority of microdiscectomy over open discectomy Insufficient evidence supporting percutaneous, laser-assisted, and endoscopic discectomy
Laminectomy			
71	6	NR	Insufficient evidence to identify the most effective technique of decompression surgery for spinal stenosis Decompression surgery combined with fusion surgery might be beneficial for degenerative spondylolisthesis
69	18	NR	Good evidence that laminectomy with or without fusion leads to moderate net benefit among patients with spinal stenosis with or without degenerative spondylolisthesis Additive benefit of fusion surgery combined with laminectomy is unclear

CLBP, chronic low back pain; LBP, low back pain; NR, not reported; RCT, randomized controlled trial; SR, systematic review.

examined spinal stenosis, one examined spondylolisthesis, one examined isthmic spondylolisthesis, and one examined a mixture of patients without specifying the duration of LBP or condition.[77-82]

One RCT did not find any statistically significant effects between decompression and conservative therapy after 10 years of follow-up and another RCT did not observe any statistically significant differences between laminectomy and laminotomy.[77,78] Three RCTs examined laminectomy alone versus laminectomy plus fusion and their pooled results via meta-analysis did not find any statistically significant differences.[79-81] In addition, another RCT did not find any differences between fusion alone versus fusion plus laminectomy and decompression for patients with isthmic spondylolisthesis.[82]

This review concluded that there is insufficient evidence to identify the most effective technique of decompression surgery for spinal stenosis.[71] This review also concluded that fusion plus decompression might be beneficial for degenerative spondylolisthesis but that fusion alone is as effective as fusion plus decompression for isthmic spondylolisthesis without significant neurologic involvement.

American Pain Society and American College of Physicians. The American Pain Society and American College of Physicians CPG committee on surgical interventions conducted an SR in 2008 for acute and chronic LBP.[69] That review identified two SRs related to laminectomy for symptomatic spinal stenosis with or without degenerative spondylolisthesis, one of which was the Cochrane Collaboration review mentioned earlier. The other SR concluded that there is insufficient evidence regarding the comparative effectiveness of laminectomy plus fusion versus laminectomy alone.[83] Collectively, these SRs summarized data from 18 RCTs. In

addition, three other RCTs were identified, one examining chronic spinal stenosis and two examining patients with spinal stenosis and degenerative spondylolisthesis.[84-86] One of these RCTs observed superiority of laminectomy with or without fusion versus nonsurgical therapy, whereas two RCTs did not observe these differences after 2 years of follow-up.[84-86]

This SR concluded that there is good quality evidence that laminectomy with or without fusion leads to moderate net benefits among patients with spinal stenosis with or without degenerative spondylolisthesis.[69] This SR also concluded that these benefits might still be observed after 1 to 2 years of follow-up. However, this SR concluded that the additive benefit of fusion to laminectomy alone is unclear.[69]

Findings from the SRs are summarized in Table 29-2.

Randomized Controlled Trials

A total of 36 RCTs were identified, 16 of which were published after the year 2000.[47-68,72-82,84-86] The methods for the most recent RCTs are summarized in Tables 29-3 and 29-4, and their results are briefly described below.

Discectomy

Buttermann[47] performed a prospective study to compare discectomy to epidural steroid injections in patients with LBP and lumbar disc herniation (>25% cross section of spinal canal) who had symptoms lasting longer than 3 months.[87,88] A third group of patients in which epidural steroid injection treatment failed and were subsequently given a discectomy constituted the crossover group. After 3 years of follow-up, there was significant improvement in pain (visual analog scale [VAS]) and disability (Oswestry Disability Index

TABLE 29-3	Randomized Controlled Trials Examining Discectomy for Radiculopathy with Herniated Lumbar Disc			
Reference	Indication	Intervention	Control (C1)	Control (C2)
47	Lumbar disc herniation, with neurologic involvement, symptoms >3 months	Open discectomy Orthopedic surgeon n = 50	Epidural steroid injection 10-15 mg betamethasone up to 3× Radiologist or anesthesiologist n = 50	Epidural steroid injection followed by discectomy (cross-over) 10-15 mg betamethasone up to 3× Radiologist or anesthesiologist, orthopedic surgeon n = 27
51	Lumbar disc herniation, with neurologic involvement, symptom duration NR	Microdiscectomy Orthopedic surgeon n = 44	Physical therapy exercises + education Frequency NR Practitioner NR n = 44	NA
53	Lumbar disc herniation, with neurologic involvement, symptom duration average 3 years	Automated percutaneous discectomy Orthopedic surgeon n = 10	Chemonucleolysis 4000 IU chymopapain Practitioner NR n = 12	NA
60	Lumbar disc herniation with neurologic involvement, symptom duration NR	Automated percutaneous discectomy Orthopedic surgeon n = 21	Open discectomy Orthopedic surgeon n = 13	NA
61	Lumbar disc herniation, with neurologic involvement, symptom duration NR	Microdiscectomy Orthopedic surgeon n = 10	Open discectomy Orthopedic surgeon n = 12	NA
62	Lumbar disc herniation, with neurologic involvement, acute symptoms >2 months	Microdiscectomy Orthopedic surgeon n = 42	Sequestrectomy Orthopedic surgeon n = 42	NA
66	Lumbar disc herniation with nerve root irritation, with neurologic involvement, symptom duration NR	Open discectomy Orthopedic surgeon n = 245	Usual care with nonoperative treatments (physical therapy + education/ counseling with home exercise instruction + NSAIDs + other individualized treatments) GP n = 256	NA
72	Lumbar disc herniation, with neurologic involvement, symptoms of radicular pain 6-12 weeks	Microdiscectomy + physical therapy instructions Orthopedic surgeon n = 28	Physical therapy instructions + isometric exercises Frequency NR Practitioner NR n = 28	NA
73	Lumbar disc herniation, with neurologic involvement, symptoms of sciatica 6-12 weeks	Open discectomy and microdiscectomy Orthopedic surgeon n = 141	Conservative treatment followed by microdiscectomy if indicated 6 months GP n = 142	NA

Continued

TABLE 29-3	Randomized Controlled Trials Examining Discectomy for Radiculopathy with Herniated Lumbar Disc—cont'd			
Reference	Indication	Intervention	Control (C1)	Control (C2)
75	Lumbar disc herniation, with neurologic involvement, symptom duration NR	Open discectomy Orthopedic surgeon n = 62	Microdiscectomy Orthopedic surgeon n = 57	NA
74	Lumbar disc herniation, with neurologic involvement, symptom duration NR	Microdiscectomy Orthopedic surgeon n = 142	Microdiscectomy + chemonucleolysis 1000 IU intradiscal chymopapain Orthopedic surgeon n = 138	NA
76	Lumbar disc herniation, with neurologic involvement, symptom duration average 82 days	Full-endoscopic microdiscectomy via interlaminar and transforaminal technique Orthopedic surgeon n = 91	Conventional microdiscectomy Orthopedic surgeon n = 87	NA

GP, general practitioner; NA, not applicable; NR, not reported; NSAID, nonsteroidal anti-inflammatory drug.

TABLE 29-4	Randomized Controlled Trials Examining Laminectomy for Symptomatic Spinal Stenosis with or without Degenerative Spondylolisthesis		
Reference	Indication	Intervention	Control
77	Lumbar spinal stenosis, with neurologic involvement, symptom duration NR	Decompression (partial or total laminectomy, medial facetectomy, discectomy, and/or removal of osteophytes from vertebral margins or facet joints) Surgeons Cointervention: lumbar support, back school, advice to remain active n = 13	Conservative treatment (lumbar support, 1 month of back school, advice to remain active) Clinician, physical therapist Cointervention: n = 18
84	Lumbar spinal stenosis, with neurologic involvement, symptoms >6 months	Decompression and an undercutting facetectomy Surgeons Cointervention: education, exercise, ergonomics, fusion surgery (n = 10 participants) n = 50	Nonsurgical group (NSAIDs, PT, education) Physical therapist, physiatrist PT 1-3 times in total n = 44
85	Spinal stenosis with degenerative spondylolisthesis, with neurologic involvement, symptoms >3 months	Laminectomy with or without bilateral single-level fusion Surgeons Cointervention: NSAIDs, epidural steroid injection, opioids n = 159	Nonsurgical group (PT, education, home exercise, NSAIDs) Physical therapist Cointervention: epidural steroid injection, opioids n = 145
86	Spinal stenosis, with neurologic involvement, symptoms >3 months	Laminectomy Surgeons Cointervention: injections, gabapentin n = 138	Nonsurgical group (PT, education, home exercise, NSAIDs) Physical therapist Cointervention: injections, gabapentin n = 151

NR, not reported; NSAID, nonsteroidal anti-inflammatory drug; PT, physical therapy.

[ODI]) in all groups compared with baseline. The differences in pain and disability between the groups were not statistically significant at 3 years.

Greenfield and colleagues[51] performed an RCT to compare microdiscectomy to physical therapy exercises in patients with LBP and small or moderate lumbar disc herniation and sciatica. At the end of 24 months, there were significant improvements in disability (ODI) in both groups compared to baseline. However, disability scores between the two groups were not statistically significant. There were also no significant differences in pain (VAS) between the two groups at 24 months.

Krugluger and Knahr[53] performed an RCT to compare automated percutaneous discectomy (APD) to chemonucleolysis in patients with LBP and disc herniation and neurologic deficit. Patients had symptoms for an average of 3 years. After 24 months, there was no significant change in pain or disability (ODI) in the chemonucleolysis group. In the APD group, recurrence of pain occurred in half the patients, and there was a significant deterioration of disability scores compared with baseline. Disability in the APD group at 24 months was significantly worse than that of the chemonucleolysis group.

Haines and colleagues[60] conducted an RCT to compare APD with conventional discectomy in patients with lumbar disc herniation and leg pain. After 12 months, there were improvements in disability (SF-36 physical function, modified RMDQ) in both groups, but there were no significant differences between the groups. Pain was measured in the study but these results were not reported separately.

Huang and colleagues[61] conducted an RCT to compare microdiscectomy to conventional discectomy in patients with lumbar disc herniation who did not respond to conservative treatment after 3 months or had acute attacks of intractable LBP and leg pain that did not improve with 1 to 2 weeks of bed rest. The patients were followed up for an average of 18.9 months. Although involved leg pain was measured in this study, LBP and disability were not measured.

Thome and colleagues[62] conducted an RCT to compare microdiscectomy to sequestrectomy in patients with LBP and free, subligamentary, or transannular herniated lumbar discs for which conservative treatment failed. After 18 months of follow-up, patients in both groups experienced an improvement in pain (VAS) compared with baseline, but this improvement was not statistically significant. There were no significant differences in pain between the two groups at baseline or at 18-months. There was a significant improvement in disability (SF-36 physical function) in both groups, but no significant differences between groups.

An RCT conducted by Weinstein and colleagues[66] compared open discectomy to nonoperative treatment in patients with LBP and lumbar disc herniation with radicular pain and nerve root irritation for which non-operative treatment of at least 6 weeks failed. Nonoperative treatment included active physical therapy, education/counseling with home exercise instruction, and NSAIDs, if tolerated, and any other treatment individualized to the patient. Nonadherence in the study

was high, with patients crossing over to the other treatment arm. After 2 years, there were significant improvements in pain (SF-36 bodily pain) and disability (ODI) in both groups compared with baseline. There were no significant differences in pain or disability between the two groups after 2 years.

An RCT conducted by Osterman and colleagues[72] compared microdiscectomy with conservative treatment consisting of physical therapy instruction and isometric exercises in patients with LBP and lumbar disc herniation with radicular pain (symptoms lasting 6 to 12 weeks) and nerve root compression. Among the control patients, 11 of 28 crossed over to the surgery group. After 2 years, there were improvements in pain (VAS) and disability (ODI) in both groups (P values not reported). However, no significant differences were observed between the groups.

An RCT conducted by Peul and colleagues[73] compared early surgery to conservative treatment for 6 months in patients with LBP and lumbar disc herniation with sciatica (symptoms lasting 6 to 12 weeks) and nerve root compression. Patients in the conservative treatment groups were assigned to have a microdiscectomy if indicated. After 2 years of follow-up, there were significant improvements in pain (VAS) and disability (ODI) in both groups. However, no significant differences were observed between the groups.

An RCT conducted by Katayama and colleagues[75] compared open discectomy with microdiscectomy in patients with LBP and lumbar disc herniation and sciatica. Postoperatively, mean pain scores (VAS) improved in both groups compared with preoperative scores (P values not reported). Pain scores in the microdiscectomy group were significantly better than those in the open discectomy group both before and after the operation.

An RCT conducted by Hoogland and colleagues[74] compared microdiscectomy to microdiscectomy with chemonucleolysis in patients with LBP and lumbar disc herniation with radicular pain and nerve root compression for which conservative treatment failed. After 2 years of follow-up, pain (VAS) improved in both groups (P values not reported). Mean pain scores in the two groups were similar preoperatively and after 2 years (P values not reported).

An RCT conducted by Ruetten and colleagues[76] compared conventional microdiscectomy to full endoscopic (FE) discectomy using transforaminal or intralaminar technique in patients with LBP and lumbar disc herniation and radicular pain who previously had a discectomy. Patients had symptoms lasting an average of 82 days. After 24 months of follow-up, there was an improvement in pain (VAS) in the FE group but not in the conventional microdiscectomy group compared with preoperative measurements (P values not reported). Mean pain scores in the conventional group were higher than those in the FE group (P values not reported). A significantly greater number of patients in the conventional group had postsurgical than in the FE group. There were also large improvements in disability (ODI) in both groups (P values not reported). Disability scores were slightly higher than those in the FE group (P values not reported).

Laminectomy

Amundsen and colleagues[77] performed an RCT to compare partial or total laminectomy, medial facetectomy, discectomy, and/or removal of osteophytes from vertebral margins or facet joints to conservative treatment in patients with LBP and lumbar spinal stenosis. Conservative treatment consisted of lumbar support, 1 month of back school, and advice to remain active. After 10 years of follow-up, there was no significant change in pain between the groups.

Malmivaara and colleagues[84] performed an RCT to compare surgery with nonsurgical treatment among patients with chronic LBP and lumbar spinal stenosis. Individuals in the surgery group received segmental decompression and an undercutting facetectomy with or without fusion. The nonsurgical group received nonsteroidal anti-inflammatory drugs (NSAIDs), physical therapy, and education. They had one to three sessions with the physical therapist during the intervention period. After 2 years of follow-up, individuals in the decompression group experienced statistically significant improvement in disability (ODI) versus those in the nonsurgical group. However, there was no significant change in pain between the groups after 2 years of follow-up.

Weinstein and colleagues[85] performed an RCT to compare surgery with nonsurgical treatment among patients with chronic LBP and spinal stenosis with degenerative spondylolisthesis. Individuals in the surgery group received laminectomy with or without fusion. The nonsurgical group received standard care, including physical therapy, education, home exercise, and NSAIDs. The number of physical therapy sessions was not reported. After 2 years of follow-up, no statistically significant differences were observed between the laminectomy and nonsurgical groups regarding improvement in pain and disability.

Weinstein and colleagues[86] performed another RCT to compare surgery with nonsurgical treatment among patients with chronic LBP and spinal stenosis. Individuals in the surgery group received laminectomy, while the nonsurgical group received standard care, including physical therapy, education, home exercise, and NSAIDs. The number of physical therapy sessions was not reported. After 2 years of follow-up, individuals in the surgery group experienced statistically significant improvement in pain versus the nonsurgical treatment group. However, no statistically significant differences were observed between the laminectomy and nonsurgical groups regarding improvement in disability.

SAFETY

Many contraindications to decompression surgery are nonspecific and can include medical considerations of cardiac, pulmonary, and metabolic reserves, prohibitive anesthetic risk, tumor, pregnancy, active infection, severe physical deconditioning, significant psychosocial comorbidities, and patients unable to comprehend the intentions and limitations of surgery.[51,68,72,74,75] A number of factors have been shown to predict a poor outcome with decompression surgery for CLBP, including smoking, patients with high fear avoidance of pain, psychological distress, compensation claims, personal injury litigation, and job dissatisfaction.[88-92] Such risk factors are much more common in patients without specific pathology or destructive processes to explain the etiology of their LBP.[93,94]

Decompression surgery should not be considered unless there is an appropriate correlation between the patient's symptoms, clinical examination and radiographic findings supporting pain and/or dysfunction mediated by a specific neurologic compression. Because CLBP with or without radicular or claudicant leg pain is often mediated by pathology other than neurologic compression, decompression surgery alone would not address the LBP. As such, back-dominant pain should be considered a relative contraindication for decompression surgery alone. Contraindications specific to decompression surgery used to treat certain CLBP conditions are summarized below.

Spinal Stenosis

The major contraindications for laminectomy include kyphotic misalignment, lumbar segmental instability related to a pars defect, associated fracture, and neoplastic involvement of the vertebrae.[2,33,61,70,74] Fusion procedures should be considered in addition to laminectomy for patients with degenerative lumbar instability as manifested by degenerative spondylolisthesis or scoliosis.[95]

Intervertebral Disc Herniation

The most common contraindications for open discectomy are spinal stenosis, calcified disc herniation, and severe degenerative facet disease.[96,97] Additional contraindications for microdiscectomy include multilevel herniation and pain originating from structures other than contained herniated discs.[98,99] In these situations, more extensive decompressive procedures would be required.

In regard to minimally invasive percutaneous, arthroscopic and endoscopic microdiscectomy, the main contraindications common to all three procedures are free or extruded disc fragments, which would not be accessible via the provided surgical corridor.[100,101] Although minimally invasive surgical techniques have evolved to allow for broader indications, open decompression surgery should be considered with certain indications. These include disc herniations that occupy more than 30% of the spinal canal, severe bony stenosis, severely degenerative discs, extruded/sequestered disc herniation, bone spur impingement on the nerve root, previous surgery with scar tissue nerve entrapment, spondylolisthesis, disc herniation between L5-S1, and the calcification of longitudinal ligaments, interspaces, and discs associated with a higher degree of technical difficulty.

Adverse Events

Many AEs resulting from decompression surgery are nonspecific and can include reactions to anesthesia, myocardial infarction, infection, hematoma, pneumonia, stroke, wound dehiscence, delayed healing, and pain or discomfort at the operative site. Although death resulting from decompression surgery is a possible AE, randomized trials and large observational studies of open discectomy or microdiscectomy for disc herniation have shown no operative deaths in more than 1400 patients who underwent surgery.[31,99,107-111]

Results from the SPORT studies[31,109] also showed there were no complications in 95% of open discectomies. Similarly, no operative deaths were recorded in four RCTs of decompressive surgery for spinal stenosis, while Benz and colleagues found serious complications that could affect quality of life occurred in only 12% of patients who underwent a lumbar laminectomy.[112-116] Despite these findings, both minor and serious AEs can and do occur during and following decompression surgery procedures used to treat a number of conditions related to CLBP.

Randomized trials and large observational studies indicate that dural tears (1% to 4%) and reoperations (3% to 10%) were the most common complications associated with surgery for lumbar disc herniation.[31,108-111,113] Likewise, dural tears (7% to 11%) and reoperation (8% to 15%) were the most common complications associated with surgery for lumbar spinal stenosis.[107,112-115,117]

National registry data suggests that the rate of reoperation following spinal decompression surgery varies between 10% and 15%.[118] However, this may be mediated by the degenerative nature of the spine that led to the original operation and as such, it is uncertain what the rate of surgery would be if no operation was originally performed. Additional AEs specific to decompression surgery used to treat certain CLBP conditions are summarized below.

Spinal Stenosis

As well as dural tears and reoperation, the AEs which may occur in relation to a laminotomy and laminectomy procedure include epidural hematoma, neural injury, thromboembolic events, instability following wide decompression, nonunion or hardware failure following fusion (if performed along with decompression), adjacent segment degeneration, recurrent stenosis, and scarring of the epidural space.[61,69,86,117,119,120]

Intervertebral Disc Herniation

In addition to dural tears and reoperation, AEs resulting from open discectomy surgery can include neural injury, intraoperative bleeding, and recurrent disc herniation.[36,69,121,122] Neurovascular trauma and discitis are also possible AEs associated with microdiscectomy.[123,124]

Although long-term follow-up data are scarce, AEs occurring during or after minimally invasive percutaneous, arthroscopic, or endoscopic microdiscectomy may include discitis, device malfunction, and a requirement for open decompression surgery reoperation.[69,125-127]

COSTS

Fees and Third-Party Reimbursement

In the United States, decompression surgery procedures for CLBP are reported by orthopedic surgeons and neurosurgeons using a variety of specific CPT codes appropriate to the procedure performed, which may include 62287

(decompression procedure, percutaneous, of nucleus pulposus of intervertebral disc, any method, single or multiple levels, lumbar [e.g., manual or automated percutaneous discectomy, percutaneous laser discectomy]), 63005 (laminectomy with exploration and/or decompression of spinal cord and/or cauda equina, without facetectomy, foraminotomy, or discectomy [e.g., spinal stenosis]), one or two vertebral segments; lumbar, except for spondylolisthesis), 63012 (laminectomy with removal of abnormal facets and/or pars interarticularis with decompression of cauda equina and nerve roots for spondylolisthesis, lumbar [Gill type procedure]), 63017 (laminectomy with exploration and/or decompression of spinal cord and/or cauda equina, without facetectomy, foraminotomy, or discectomy [e.g., spinal stenosis], more than two vertebral segments; lumbar), 63030 (laminotomy [hemilaminectomy], with decompression of nerve roots, including partial facetectomy, foraminotomy and/or excision of herniated intervertebral disc, including open and endoscopically assisted approaches; one interspace; lumbar), 63042 (laminotomy [hemilaminectomy], with decompression of nerve roots, including partial facetectomy, foraminotomy and/or excision of herniated intervertebral disc, reexploration, single interspace; lumbar), 63047 (laminectomy, facetectomy, and foraminotomy [unilateral or bilateral with decompression of spinal cord, cauda equina, and/or nerve roots] such as spinal or lateral recess stenosis, single vertebral segment; lumbar), or 63055 (transpedicular approach with decompression of spinal cord, cauda equina, and/or nerve roots [e.g., herniated intervertebral disc], single segment; lumbar). Other related procedures may also be reported, such as fluoroscopic imaging guidance or the use of surgical microscopes, other instruments, or surgical devices.

In addition to the professional surgical fees, hospital charges also apply. Hospital charges for decompression surgery may be reported using ICD-9 procedural codes, including 80.50 (excision or destruction, intervertebral disc, unspecified), 80.51 (excision, intervertebral disc), or 80.59 (destruction, other intervertebral disc). Alternatively, hospital charges may report a diagnostic related group (DRG), which is a system used to classify hospital stays by combining diagnostic and procedural ICD-9 codes. The DRGs that may be reported for decompression surgery include 499 (back and neck procedures except spinal fusion with complications), or 500 (back and neck procedures except spinal fusion without complications).

These procedures are typically covered by most third-party payers such as health insurers and worker's compensation insurance. Although some payers continue to base their reimbursements on usual, customary, and reasonable payment methodology, the majority have developed reimbursement tables based on the Resource Based Relative Value Scale used by Medicare. Reimbursement by other third-party payers is generally higher than Medicare. Preauthorization may be required to obtain reimbursement from third-party payers.

Typical fees reimbursed by Medicare in New York and California for these services are summarized in Table 29-5. Hospital charges for these services are summarized in Table 29-6.

Cost Effectiveness

Evidence supporting the cost effectiveness of treatment protocols that compared these interventions, often in combination with one or more cointerventions, with control groups who received one or more other interventions, for either acute or chronic LBP, was identified from two SRs on this topic and is summarized here.[128,129] Although many of these study designs are unable to clearly identify the individual contribution of any intervention, their results provide some insight as to the clinical and economic outcomes associated with these approaches.

An RCT in the United States compared spinal cord stimulation (SCS) versus reoperation for patients with neurologic involvement with or without LBP after one or more lumbar spine surgeries.[130] To ensure that surgery was indicated, a series of diagnostic tests were conducted, such as x-rays and MRI. Patients randomized to reoperation received laminectomy and/or foraminotomy and/or discectomy with or without fusion. The SCS group experienced statistically significant improvement in pain versus the reoperation group after an average of 2.9 years of follow-up. However, no statistically significant differences were observed regarding improvement in disability. After 3.1 years of follow-up, 62% of the patients randomized to SCS crossed over to receive reoperation and 26% of the patients randomized to reoperation crossed over to receive SCS. The average cost per success was $117,901 for individuals who crossed over to SCS and no successes were observed for those who crossed over to reoperation (per-patient expenditure of $260,584). For the intention-to-treat analysis, the average costs per patient were $31,530 for SCS and $38,160 for reoperation. The cost-utility analysis indicated that SCS resulted in better effectiveness, less costs, and greater quality-adjusted life-year gains versus reoperation (Table 29-7).

Other

Conservative estimates suggest that up to $306 million is spent on inpatient decompression surgery (without fusion) each year in the United States.[35]

Findings from the aforementioned cost effectiveness analysis are summarized in Table 29-7.

SUMMARY

Description

Decompression surgery has been performed for CLBP for nearly 200 years and involves complete or partial removal of anatomic structures in the lumbar spine that are thought to be causing neural impingement. The main types of decompression surgery include discectomy and laminectomy, which are often performed together. Procedures for decompression surgery include open, conventional, and microscopic approaches. Orthopedic and neurologic spine surgeons typically offer this procedure, which is widely available throughout the US.

Theory

The primary indication for decompression surgery is CLBP with signs or symptoms of neurologic dysfunction associated with impingement of the neural canal. Common indications for decompression surgery include large disc herniations and spinal stenosis. Decompression surgery is thought to alleviate neural impingement by removing mechanical pressure on

TABLE 29-5	Medicare Fee Schedule for Related Services	
CPT Code	New York	California
62287	$539	$574
63005	$1123	$1193
63012	$1136	$1206
63017	$1185	$1258
63030	$921	$981
63042	$1248	$1326
63047	$1052	$1119
63055	$1553	$1645

2010 Participating, nonfacility amount.

TABLE 29-6	Hospital Charges for Related Services
Code	Charges
ICD-9 procedure	
80.50	$24,281
80.51	$24,639
80.59	$29,534
DRG	
499	$33,033
500	$22,936

Source: http://hcupnet.ahrq.gov/HCUPnet.jsp (HCUP Nationwide Inpatient Sample).

TABLE 29-7	Cost Effectiveness and Cost Utility Analyses of Decompressions Surgery for Chronic Low Back Pain					
Ref Country Follow-Up	Group	Direct Medical Costs	Indirect Productivity Costs	Total Costs	Conclusion
130 United States 3.1 years (mean)	1. Reoperation using laminectomy, foraminotomy, discectomy, with or without fusion 2. Spinal cord stimulation	1. $31,530 2. $38,160	NR	NR	SCS was cost effective over reoperation

NR, not reported; SCS, spinal cord stimulation.

elements inside the neural canal from abutting structures that may occur following advanced degenerative changes or trauma. Improvement may also be attributed to removal of structures contributing to an acute inflammatory cascade that releases chemical mediators which may indirectly irritate spinal nerve roots.

Efficacy

Discectomy

Two recent CPGs provided recommendations related to discectomy and another CPG provided recommendations on decompression surgery in general. The first CPG reported no evidence for discectomy among patients with disc prolapse without neurologic involvement, yet reported low-quality evidence supporting discectomy among patients with disco-radicular conflict and neurologic involvement. The second CPG recommended discectomy for LBP with neurologic involvement and the third CPG did not recommend decompression surgery in general for CLBP. Two SRs concluded that discectomy is effective for patients with LBP and neurologic involvement or disc prolapse and radiculopathy. These SRs also concluded that microdiscectomy is comparable to open discectomy, yet there is insufficient evidence supporting the other types of discectomy. At least 12 RCTs examined the efficacy of discectomy, the majority finding no statistically significant benefits for this type of surgery versus various surgical or nonsurgical comparators.

Laminectomy

None of the recent CPGs made specific recommendations about the efficacy of laminectomy for CLBP. One SR concluded that there is insufficient evidence supporting the most effective technique of decompression surgery for spinal stenosis, while another SR concluded that laminectomy with or without fusion leads to moderate net benefit among patients with spinal stenosis with or without degenerative spondylolisthesis. At least four RCTs examined the efficacy of laminectomy; two examined the effects of laminectomy plus other types of decompression surgery and two examined the effects of laminectomy plus fusion. Two of these RCTs did not find any statistically significant differences between decompression surgery and other comparators, while the other two studies reported statistically significant improvement in disability or pain compared to nonsurgical care.

Safety

Contraindications to decompression surgery include poor general health with comorbidities that may preclude general anesthesia, as well as risk factors associated with poor outcomes. Predictors of negative outcomes with decompression surgery include physical deconditioning, psychosocial or emotional distress, unrealistic expectations, smoking, fear avoidance behavior, litigation, and job dissatisfaction. Other contraindications to decompression surgery include inadequate correlation between symptoms and findings on physical examination, neurologic examination, imaging, or other diagnostic testing. CLBP alone without predominant leg symptoms may also be considered a relative contraindication for decompression surgery.

AEs associated with decompression surgery include those related to general anesthesia and surgery such as cardiopulmonary AEs, infection, vascular trauma, thromboembolism, or death. Other AEs related to operating on the lumbar spine include dural tears, spinal nerve root injury, spinal cord injury, adjacent segment degeneration, surgical instability, scarring, delayed healing, lower extremity pain, lower extremity neurologic findings, increased LBP, and disc infection. Approximately 10% to 15% of patients who receive decompression surgery will require a subsequent operation.

Costs

The cost of decompression surgery is estimated at $30,000 to $40,000 per procedure for professional and hospital fees, excluding any diagnostic testing or rehabilitation required before or after the procedure. At least one study examined the cost effectiveness of decompression surgery (including discectomy and/or laminectomy) with or without fusion versus SCS. The cost-utility analysis indicated that SCS resulted in better effectiveness, less costs, and greater quality-adjusted life-year gains versus reoperation.

CHAPTER REVIEW QUESTIONS

Answers are located on page 452.
1. Which of the following is not an appropriate indication for decompression surgery?
   a. neurogenic claudication
   b. progressive motor deficits in the lower extremities
   c. cauda equina syndrome
   d. instability
2. Which of the following is not a symptom associated with cauda equina syndrome?
   a. inability to urinate
   b. pain on urination
   c. incontinence
   d. loss of bowel control
3. Which is one of the earliest reported accounts of decompression surgery?
   a. Dr. Smith in the United States in 1829
   b. Dr. Johnson in the United Kingdom in 1867
   c. Dr. Smith in the United States in 1929
   d. Dr. Johnson in the United Kingdom in 1827
4. Which of the following structures are generally not removed during laminectomy?
   a. spinous process
   b. ligamentum flavum
   c. pedicle
   d. facet joint capsule hypertrophy
5. True or false: Evidence generally favors laminectomy over discectomy when performing decompression surgery for LBP.
6. True or false: The superiority of microdiscectomy over conventional open discectomy has been clearly established in RCTs.

7. Which of the following is not a predictor of poor outcomes with decompression surgery?
   a. high fear avoidance
   b. psychological distress
   c. poor job dissatisfaction
   d. none of the above

REFERENCES

1. Allen RT, Rihn JA, Glassman SD, et al. An evidence-based approach to spine surgery. Am J Med Qual 2009;24: 15S-24S.
2. Siebert E, Pruss H, Klingebiel R, et al. Lumbar spinal stenosis: syndrome, diagnostics and treatment. Nat Rev Neurol 2009;5:392-403.
3. Kirkaldy-Willis WH, Wedge JH, Yong-Hing K, et al. Pathology and pathogenesis of lumbar spondylosis and stenosis. Spine 1978;3:319-328.
4. Joaquim AF, Sansur CA, Hamilton DK, et al. Degenerative lumbar stenosis: update. Arq Neuropsiquiatr 2009;67: 553-558.
5. Feldtkeller E, Lemmel EM, Russell AS. Ankylosing spondylitis in the pharaohs of ancient Egypt. Rheumatol Int 2003; 23:1-5.
6. Atta HM. Edwin Smith Surgical Papyrus: the oldest known surgical treatise. Am Surg 1999;65:1190-1192.
7. Hughes JT. The Edwin Smith Surgical Papyrus: an analysis of the first case reports of spinal cord injuries. Paraplegia 1988;26:71-82.
8. Robinson JS. Sciatica and the lumbar disk syndrome: a historic perspective. South Med J 1983;76:232-238.
9. Keller T, Holland MC. Some notable American spine surgeons of the 19th century. Spine 1997;22:1413-1417.
10. Lane WA. Case of spondylolisthesis associated with progressive paraplegia; laminectomy. Lancet 1893;141:991-992.
11. Holdsworth FW, Hardy A. Early treatment of paraplegia from fractures of the thoraco-lumbar spine. J Bone Joint Surg Br 1953;35:540-550.
12. Patwardhan RV, Hadley MN. History of surgery for ruptured disk. Neurosurg Clin N Am 2001;12:173-179.
13. Goldthwait JE. The lumbosacral articulation: an explanation of many cases of lumbago, sciatica, and paraplegia. Boston Med Surg J 1911;164:365-372.
14. Middleton GS, Treacher JH. Injury to the spinal cord due to rupture of an intervertebral disc during muscular effort. Glasgow Med J 1911;76:1-6.
15. Verbiest H. A radicular syndrome from developmental narrowing of the lumbar vertebral canal. J Bone Joint Surg Br 1954;36:230-237.
16. Dejerine J. Intermittent claudication of the spinal cord [French]. Presse Med 1911;19:981-984.
17. Dandy WE. Loose cartilage from intervertebral disk simulating tumor of the spinal cord. Arch Surg 1929;19:660-672.
18. Mixter WJ, Barr JS. Rupture of the intervertebral disc with involvement of the spinal canal. N Engl J Med 1934;211: 210-215.
19. Yasargil MG, Krayenbuhl H. The use of the binocular microscope in neurosurgery. Bibl Ophthalmol 1970;81:62-65.
20. Yasargil MG. Microsurgical operations for herniated lumbar disc. Adv Neurosurg 1977;4:81-82.
21. Caspar W. A new surgical procedure for lumbar disc herniation causing less tissue damage through a microsurgical approach. Adv Neurosurg 1977;4:74-80.
22. Williams RW. Microlumbar discectomy: a conservative surgical approach to the virgin herniated lumbar disc. Spine 1978;3:175-182.
23. Young S, Veerapen R, O'Laoire SA. Relief of lumbar canal stenosis using multilevel subarticular fenestrations as an alternative to wide laminectomy: preliminary report. Neurosurgery 1988;23:628-633.
24. Ehrlich GE. Low back pain. Bull World Health Org 2003; 81:671-676.
25. Cherkin DC, Deyo RA, Loeser JD, et al. An international comparison of back surgery rates. Spine 1994;19:1201-1206.
26. Taylor VM, Deyo RA, Cherkin DC, et al. Low back pain hospitalization. Recent United States trends and regional variations. Spine 1994;19:1207-1212.
27. Deyo RA, Gray DT, Kreuter W, et al. United States trends in lumbar fusion surgery for degenerative conditions. Spine 2005;30:1441-1445.
28. Irwin ZN, Hilibrand A, Gustavel M, et al. Variation in surgical decision making for degenerative spinal disorders. Part I: lumbar spine. Spine 2005;30:2208-2213.
29. Bruske-Hohlfeld I, Merritt JL, Onofrio BM, et al. Incidence of lumbar disc surgery. A population-based study in Olmsted County, Minnesota, 1950-1979. Spine 1990;15:31-35.
30. Deyo RA, Weinstein JN. Low back pain. N Engl J Med 2001;344:363-370.
31. Weinstein JN, Tosteson TD, Lurie JD, et al. Surgical vs nonoperative treatment for lumbar disk herniation: the Spine Patient Outcomes Research Trial (SPORT): a randomized trial. JAMA 2006;296:2441-2450.
32. Lurie JD, Birkmeyer NJ, Weinstein JN. Rates of advanced spinal imaging and spine surgery. Spine 2003;28:616-620.
33. Atlas SJ, Delitto A. Spinal stenosis: surgical versus nonsurgical treatment. Clin Orthop Relat Res 2006;443: 198-207.
34. Ciol MA, Deyo RA, Howell E, et al. An assessment of surgery for spinal stenosis: time trends, geographic variations, complications, and reoperations. J Am Geriatr Soc 1996;44: 285-290.
35. Weinstein JN, Lurie JD, Olson PR, et al. United States' trends and regional variations in lumbar spine surgery: 1992-2003. Spine 2006;31:2707-2714.
36. Ambrossi GL, McGirt MJ, Sciubba DM, et al. Recurrent lumbar disc herniation after single-level lumbar discectomy: incidence and health care cost analysis. Neurosurgery 2009;65:574-578.
37. American Academy of Orthopaedic Surgeons. Membership Growth. American Academy of Orthopaedic Surgeons, 2010 [cited 2010 Feb 7]. Available at: http://www.aaos.org/about/memchart.asp.
38. American Association of Neurological Surgeons. Membership as of December 2009. American Association of Neurological Surgeons, 2010 [cited 2010 Feb 7]. Available at: http://www.aans.org/membership/.
39. Garfin SR, Rydevik BJ, Lipson SJ, Herkowitz HH. Pathophysiology of pain in spinal stenosis. In: Herkowitz HH, Garfin SR, Balderston RA, Eismont FJ, Bell GR, Wisel SW, editors. The Spine. 4th ed. Philadelphia: WB Saunders; 1999.
40. Vroomen PC, de Krom MC, Slofstra PD, et al. Conservative treatment of sciatica: a systematic review. J Spinal Disord 2000;13:463-469.
41. Johnsson KE, Rosen I, Uden A. The natural course of lumbar spinal stenosis. Clin Orthop Relat Res 1992;(279): 82-86.

42. Simon D, Coyle M, Dagenais S, et al. Potential triaging of referrals for lumbar spinal surgery consultation: a comparison of referral accuracy from pain specialists, findings from advanced imaging and a 3-item questionnaire. Can J Surg 2010;52:473-480.

43. Nielens H, van Zundert J, Mairiaux P, et al. Chronic low back pain. Brussels, 2006, Report No.: KCE reports Vol 48C.

44. Negrini S, Giovannoni S, Minozzi S, et al. Diagnostic therapeutic flow-charts for low back pain patients: the Italian clinical guidelines. Eura Medicophys 2006;42:151-170.

45. Airaksinen O, Brox JI, Cedraschi C, et al. European guidelines for the management of chronic nonspecific low back pain. Eur Spine J 2006;15(Suppl 2):192-300.

46. Gibson JN, Waddell G. Surgical interventions for lumbar disc prolapse. Cochrane Database Syst Rev 2007;(2):CD001350.

47. Buttermann GR. The effect of spinal steroid injections for degenerative disc disease. Spine J 2004;4:495-505.

48. Chatterjee S, Foy PM, Findlay GF. Report of a controlled clinical trial comparing automated percutaneous lumbar discectomy and microdiscectomy in the treatment of contained lumbar disc herniation. Spine 1995;20:734-738.

49. Crawshaw C, Frazer AM, Merriam WF, et al. A comparison of surgery and chemonucleolysis in the treatment of sciatica. A prospective randomized trial. Spine 1984;9:195-198.

50. Ejeskar A, Nachemson A, Herberts P, et al. Surgery versus chemonucleolysis for herniated lumbar discs. A prospective study with random assignment. Clin Orthop Relat Res 1983;(174):236-242.

51. Greenfield K, Nelson RJ, Findlay GD, et al. Microdiscectomy and conservative treatment for lumbar disc herniation with back pain and sciatica: a randomised clinical trial. Proceedings of the 30th meeting of the International Society for the Study of the Lumbar Spine, Vancouver, 2003:254. www.issls.org.

52. Hermantin FU, Peters T, Quartararo L, et al. A prospective, randomized study comparing the results of open discectomy with those of video-assisted arthroscopic microdiscectomy. J Bone Joint Surg Am 1999;81:958-965.

53. Krugluger J, Knahr K. Chemonucleolysis and automated percutaneous discectomy—a prospective randomized comparison. Int Orthop 2000;24:167-169.

54. Lagarrigue J, Chaynes P. [Comparative study of disk surgery with or without microscopy. A prospective study of 80 cases.] Neurochirurgie 1994;40:116-120.

55. Lavignolle B, Vital JM, Baulny D, et al. [Comparative study of surgery and chemonucleolysis in the treatment of sciatica caused by a herniated disk.] Acta Orthop Belg 1987;53:244-249.

56. Mayer HM, Brock M. Percutaneous endoscopic discectomy: surgical technique and preliminary results compared to microsurgical discectomy. J Neurosurg 1993;78:216-225.

57. Revel M, Payan C, Vallee C, et al. Automated percutaneous lumbar discectomy versus chemonucleolysis in the treatment of sciatica. A randomized multicenter trial. Spine 1993;18:1-7.

58. Tullberg T, Isacson J, Weidenhielm L. Does microscopic removal of lumbar disc herniation lead to better results than the standard procedure? Results of a one-year randomized study. Spine 1993;18:24-27.

59. van Alphen HA, Braakman R, Bezemer PD, et al. Chemonucleolysis versus discectomy: a randomized multicenter trial. J Neurosurg 1989;70:869-875.

60. Haines SJ, Jordan N, Boen JR, et al. Discectomy strategies for lumbar disc herniation: results of the LAPDOG trial. J Clin Neurosci 2002;9:411-417.

61. Huang TJ, Hsu RW, Li YY, et al. Less systemic cytokine response in patients following microendoscopic versus open lumbar discectomy. J Orthop Res 2005;23:406-411.

62. Thome C, Barth M, Scharf J, et al. Outcome after lumbar sequestrectomy compared with microdiscectomy: a prospective randomized study. J Neurosurg Spine 2005;2:271-278.

63. Henriksen L, Schmidt K, Eskesen V, et al. A controlled study of microsurgical versus standard lumbar discectomy. Br J Neurosurg 1996;10:289-293.

64. Weber H. Lumbar disc herniation. A controlled, prospective study with ten years of observation. Spine 1983;8:131-140.

65. Muralikuttan KP, Hamilton A, Kernohan WG, et al. A prospective randomized trial of chemonucleolysis and conventional disc surgery in single level lumbar disc herniation. Spine 1992;17:381-387.

66. Weinstein JN, Tosteson TD, Lurie JD, et al. Surgical vs nonoperative treatment for lumbar disk herniation: the Spine Patient Outcomes Research Trial (SPORT): a randomized trial. JAMA 2006;296:2441-2450.

67. Jensen TT, Asmussen K, Berg-Hansen EM, et al. First-time operation for lumbar disc herniation with or without free fat transplantation. Prospective triple-blind randomized study with reference to clinical factors and enhanced computed tomographic scan 1 year after operation. Spine 1996;21:1072-1076.

68. Steffen R, Luetke A, Wittenberg RH, et al. A prospective comparative study of chemonucleolysis and laser discectomy. Orthop Trans 1996;20:388.

69. Chou R, Baisden J, Carragee EJ, et al. Surgery for low back pain: a review of the evidence for an American Pain Society Clinical Practice Guideline. Spine 2009;34:1094-1109.

70. Boult M, Fraser RD, Jones N, et al. Percutaneous endoscopic laser discectomy. Aust N Z J Surg 2000;70:475-479.

71. Gibson JN, Waddell G. Surgery for degenerative lumbar spondylosis. Cochrane Database Syst Rev 2005;(4):CD001352.

72. Osterman H, Seitsalo S, Karppinen J, et al. Effectiveness of microdiscectomy for lumbar disc herniation: a randomized controlled trial with 2 years of follow-up. Spine 2006;31:2409-2414.

73. Peul WC, van den Hout WB, Brand R, et al. Prolonged conservative care versus early surgery in patients with sciatica caused by lumbar disc herniation: two year results of a randomised controlled trial. BMJ 2008;336:1355-1358.

74. Hoogland T, Schubert M, Miklitz B, et al. Transforaminal posterolateral endoscopic discectomy with or without the combination of a low-dose chymopapain: a prospective randomized study in 280 consecutive cases. Spine 2006;31:E890-E897.

75. Katayama Y, Matsuyama Y, Yoshihara H, et al. Comparison of surgical outcomes between macro discectomy and micro discectomy for lumbar disc herniation: a prospective randomized study with surgery performed by the same spine surgeon. J Spinal Disord Tech 2006;19:344-347.

76. Ruetten S, Komp M, Merk H, et al. Full-endoscopic interlaminar and transforaminal lumbar discectomy versus conventional microsurgical technique: a prospective, randomized, controlled study. Spine 2008;33:931-939.

77. Amundsen T, Weber H, Nordal HJ, et al. Lumbar spinal stenosis: conservative or surgical management? A prospective 10-year study. Spine 2000;25:1424-1435.

78. Postacchini F, Cinotti G, Perugia D, et al. The surgical treatment of central lumbar stenosis. Multiple laminotomy compared with total laminectomy. J Bone Joint Surg Br 1993;75:386-392.

79. Grob D, Humke T, Dvorak J. Degenerative lumbar spinal stenosis. Decompression with and without arthrodesis. J Bone Joint Surg Am 1995;77:1036-1041.

80. Bridwell KH, Sedgewick TA, O'Brien MF, et al. The role of fusion and instrumentation in the treatment of degenerative spondylolisthesis with spinal stenosis. J Spinal Disord 1993; 6:461-472.

81. Herkowitz HN, Kurz LT. Degenerative lumbar spondylolisthesis with spinal stenosis. A prospective study comparing decompression with decompression and intertransverse process arthrodesis. J Bone Joint Surg Am 1991;73:802-808.

82. Carragee EJ. Single-level posterolateral arthrodesis, with or without posterior decompression, for the treatment of isthmic spondylolisthesis in adults. A prospective, randomized study. J Bone Joint Surg Am 1997;79:1175-1180.

83. Ibrahim T, Tleyjeh IM, Gabbar O. Surgical versus non-surgical treatment of chronic low back pain: a meta-analysis of randomised trials. Int Orthop 2008;32:107-113.

84. Malmivaara A, Slatis P, Heliovaara M, et al. Surgical or nonoperative treatment for lumbar spinal stenosis? A randomized controlled trial. Spine 2007;32:1-8.

85. Weinstein JN, Lurie JD, Tosteson TD, et al. Surgical versus nonsurgical treatment for lumbar degenerative spondylolisthesis. N Engl J Med 2007;356:2257-2270.

86. Weinstein JN, Tosteson TD, Lurie JD, et al. Surgical versus nonsurgical therapy for lumbar spinal stenosis. N Engl J Med 2008;358:794-810.

87. Jamison RN, Raymond SA, Slawsby EA, et al. Opioid therapy for chronic noncancer back pain. A randomized prospective study. Spine 1998;23:2591-2600.

88. Carragee EJ, Alamin TF, Miller JL, et al. Discographic, MRI and psychosocial determinants of low back pain disability and remission: a prospective study in subjects with benign persistent back pain. Spine J 2005;5:24-35.

89. Burton AK, Tillotson KM, Main CJ, et al. Psychosocial predictors of outcome in acute and subchronic low back trouble. Spine 1995;20:722-728.

90. Boos N, Semmer N, Elfering A, et al. Natural history of individuals with asymptomatic disc abnormalities in magnetic resonance imaging: predictors of low back pain-related medical consultation and work incapacity. Spine 2000;25: 1484-1492.

91. Hurwitz EL, Morgenstern H, Yu F. Cross-sectional and longitudinal associations of low-back pain and related disability with psychological distress among patients enrolled in the UCLA Low-Back Pain Study. J Clin Epidemiol 2003;56: 463-471.

92. Cassidy JD, Carroll L, Cote P, et al. Low back pain after traffic collisions: a population-based cohort study. Spine 2003;28: 1002-1009.

93. Cairns MC, Foster NE, Wright CC, et al. Level of distress in a recurrent low back pain population referred for physical therapy. Spine 2003;28:953-959.

94. Carragee EJ. Psychological and functional profiles in select subjects with low back pain. Spine J 2001;1:198-204.

95. Resnick DK, Choudhri TF, Dailey AT, et al. Guidelines for the performance of fusion procedures for degenerative disease of the lumbar spine. Part 9: fusion in patients with stenosis and spondylolisthesis. J Neurosurg Spine 2005;2:679-685.

96. Hurme M, Alaranta H. Factors predicting the result of surgery for lumbar intervertebral disc herniation. Spine 1987;12: 933-938.

97. Katz JN, Stucki G, Lipson SJ, et al. Predictors of surgical outcome in degenerative lumbar spinal stenosis. Spine 1999; 24:2229-2233.

98. Riesenburger RI, David CA. Lumbar microdiscectomy and microendoscopic discectomy. Minim Invasive Ther Allied Technol 2006;15:267-270.

99. Osterman H, Seitsalo S, Karppinen J, et al. Effectiveness of microdiscectomy for lumbar disc herniation: a randomized controlled trial with 2 years of follow-up. Spine 2006;31: 2409-2414.

100. Deen HG, Fenton DS, Lamer TJ. Minimally invasive procedures for disorders of the lumbar spine. Mayo Clin Proc 2003;78:1249-1256.

101. Mathews HH, Long BH. Minimally invasive techniques for the treatment of intervertebral disk herniation. J Am Acad Orthop Surg 2002;10:80-85.

102. Hirsch JA, Singh V, Falco FJ, et al. Automated percutaneous lumbar discectomy for the contained herniated lumbar disc: a systematic assessment of evidence. Pain Physician 2009;12: 601-620.

103. Hirsch JA, Singh V, Falco FJ, et al. Automated percutaneous lumbar discectomy for the contained herniated lumbar disc: a systematic assessment of evidence. Pain Physician 2009;12: 601-620.

104. Armin SS, Holly LT, Khoo LT. Minimally invasive decompression for lumbar stenosis and disc herniation. Neurosurg Focus 2008;25:E11.

105. Ruetten S, Komp M, Merk H, et al. Use of newly developed instruments and endoscopes: full-endoscopic resection of lumbar disc herniations via the interlaminar and lateral transforaminal approach. J Neurosurg Spine 2007;6: 521-530.

106. Kambin P. Arthroscopic microdiscectomy. Spine J 2003;3: 60-64.

107. Weinstein JN, Lurie JD, Tosteson TD, et al. Surgical compared with nonoperative treatment for lumbar degenerative spondylolisthesis. Four-year results in the Spine Patient Outcomes Research Trial (SPORT) randomized and observational cohorts. J Bone Joint Surg Am 2009;91:1295-1304.

108. Peul WC, van Houwelingen HC, van den Hout WB, et al. Surgery versus prolonged conservative treatment for sciatica. N Engl J Med 2007;356:2245-2256.

109. Weinstein JN, Lurie JD, Tosteson TD, et al. Surgical vs nonoperative treatment for lumbar disk herniation: the Spine Patient Outcomes Research Trial (SPORT) observational cohort. JAMA 2006;296:2451-2459.

110. Atlas SJ, Deyo RA, Keller RB, et al. The Maine Lumbar Spine Study, Part II. 1-year outcomes of surgical and nonsurgical management of sciatica. Spine 1996;21:1777-1786.

111. Weinstein JN, Lurie JD, Tosteson TD, et al. Surgical versus nonoperative treatment for lumbar disc herniation: four-year results for the Spine Patient Outcomes Research Trial (SPORT). Spine 2008;33:2789-2800.

112. Malmivaara A, Slatis P, Heliovaara M, et al. Surgical or nonoperative treatment for lumbar spinal stenosis? A randomized controlled trial. Spine 2007;32:1-8.

113. Weinstein JN, Lurie JD, Tosteson TD, et al. Surgical versus nonsurgical treatment for lumbar degenerative spondylolisthesis. N Engl J Med 2007;356:2257-2270.

114. Weinstein JN, Tosteson TD, Lurie JD, et al. Surgical versus nonsurgical therapy for lumbar spinal stenosis. N Engl J Med 2008;358:794-810.

115. Amundsen T, Weber H, Nordal HJ, et al. Lumbar spinal stenosis: conservative or surgical management? A prospective 10-year study. Spine 2000;25:1424-1435.

116. Benz RJ, Ibrahim ZG, Afshar P, et al. Predicting complications in elderly patients undergoing lumbar decompression. Clin Orthop Relat Res 2001;384:116-121.

117. Ruetten S, Komp M, Merk H, et al. Surgical treatment for lumbar lateral recess stenosis with the full-endoscopic interlaminar approach versus conventional microsurgical technique: a prospective, randomized, controlled study. J Neurosurg Spine 2009;10:476-485.

118. Osterman H, Sund R, Seitsalo S, et al. Risk of multiple reoperations after lumbar discectomy: a population-based study. Spine 2003;28:621-627.

119. Yuan PS, Booth RE Jr, Albert TJ. Nonsurgical and surgical management of lumbar spinal stenosis. Instr Course Lect 2005;54:303-312.

120. Castro-Menendez M, Bravo-Ricoy JA, Casal-Moro R, et al. Midterm outcome after microendoscopic decompressive laminotomy for lumbar spinal stenosis: 4-year prospective study. Neurosurgery 2009;65:100-110.

121. Harrington JF, French P. Open versus minimally invasive lumbar microdiscectomy: comparison of operative times, length of hospital stay, narcotic use and complications. Minim Invasive Neurosurg 2008;51:30-35.

122. Peul WC, van den Hout WB, Brand R, et al. Prolonged conservative care versus early surgery in patients with sciatica caused by lumbar disc herniation: two year results of a randomised controlled trial. BMJ 2008;336:1355-1358.

123. Kraemer R, Wild A, Haak H, et al. Classification and management of early complications in open lumbar microdiscectomy. Eur Spine J 2003;12:239-246.

124. Schoeggl A, Reddy M, Matula C. Functional and economic outcome following microdiscectomy for lumbar disc herniation in 672 patients. J Spinal Disord Tech 2003;16:150-155.

125. Singh V, Benyamin RM, Datta S, et al. Systematic review of percutaneous lumbar mechanical disc decompression utilizing Dekompressor. Pain Physician 2009;12:589-599.

126. Yeung AT, Tsou PM. Posterolateral endoscopic excision for lumbar disc herniation: surgical technique, outcome, and complications in 307 consecutive cases. Spine 2002;27:722-731.

127. Wu X, Zhuang S, Mao Z, et al. Microendoscopic discectomy for lumbar disc herniation: surgical technique and outcome in 873 consecutive cases. Spine 2006;31:2689-2694.

128. Dagenais S, Roffey DM, Wai EK, et al. Can cost utility evaluations inform decision making about interventions for low back pain? Spine J 2009;9:944-957.

129. van der Roer N, Goossens MEJB, Evers SMAA, et al. What is the most cost-effective treatment for patients with low back pain? A systematic review. Best Pract Res Clin Rheumatol 2005;19:671-684.

130. North RB, Kidd D, Shipley J, et al. Spinal cord stimulation versus reoperation for failed back surgery syndrome: a cost effectiveness and cost utility analysis based on a randomized, controlled trial. Neurosurgery 2007;61:361-368.

131. Negrini S, Giovannoni S, Minozzi S, et al. Diagnostic therapeutic flow-charts for low back pain patients: the Italian clinical guidelines. Eura Medicophys 2006;42:151-170.

EUGENE K. WAI
DARREN M. ROFFEY
ANDREA C. TRICCO
ANGUS SHANE DON
SIMON DAGENAIS

CHAPTER 30

Fusion Surgery and Disc Arthroplasty

DESCRIPTION

Terminology and Subtypes

In the context of chronic low back pain (CLBP) and degenerative disc disease (DDD), *fusion surgery* is a broad term used to indicate various forms of lumbar surgery whose primary goal is to join bony anatomic structures in the lumbar spine that are thought to have excessive movement or otherwise contribute to presenting symptoms. Fusion surgery is also known as *arthrodesis*. The main types of fusion surgery are named according to the surgical approach taken (i.e., where the incision is made and the direction from which the spine is operated on) and include posterior approaches (Figure 30-1), anterior approaches, and combined anterior and posterior approaches, which are also known as circumferential or 360-degree approaches (Figure 30-2). Posterior approaches to fusion surgery include posterior lateral intertransverse fusion surgery (PLF), posterior lumbar interbody fusion surgery (PLIF), and transforaminal lumbar interbody fusion surgery (TLIF) (Figure 30-3). The main anterior approach to fusion surgery is known as anterior lumbar interbody fusion surgery (ALIF).

Fusion surgery may also be categorized according to the use of surgical hardware such as plates, screws, hooks, cables, and cages, which are collectively termed instrumentation. Although surgical instrumentation was traditionally made of metal, it is now composed of a wide range of materials, such as titanium mesh, carbon fiber, and polyetheretherketone (PEEK). Noninstrumentation fusion surgery involves the use of bone grafts to fuse adjacent vertebrae. Autograft fusion surgery involves taking small bone chips from the patient's own body such as the iliac crest, whereas allograft fusion surgery uses bone chips harvested from another person (i.e. bone bank). Autograft bone is also known as autologous or autogenous bone. Bone morphogenic protein (BMP) is a substance used to enhance the body's natural bone growth processes and is occasionally (incorrectly) termed artificial or synthetic bone. It is also termed recombinant human bone morphogenetic protein (rhBMP).

Arthroplasty is a generic term indicating that a targeted structure is surgically removed and replaced. Disc arthroplasty describes a surgical procedure in which an intervertebral disc is removed through decompression surgery and replaced with a device intended to function as a disc replacement. Disc arthroplasty is also known as total disc replacement or artificial disc replacement. The artificial disc device normally consists of two metal plates between which a polyethylene core glides.

History and Frequency of Use

In 1891, the first spinal instrumentation procedure was performed by Hadra, who used wires to repair a spinous process fracture.[1] Bone augmentation and arthrodesis for the treatment of lumbar DDD initially occurred in 1911, with successful noninstrumented fusion surgery using tibial grafts between spinal processes to stabilize the spine.[2] Another technique "feathered" the lamina, decorticated the facet joints, and then added morsalized bone derived from the spinous processes, representing the first documented example of flexible stabilization utilizing autologous bone for reconstructive purposes.[3] Kleinberg then pioneered the concept of using bone graft for fusion surgery in 1922.[4] In 1933, the ALIF procedure was first documented by Burns.[5] Internal fixation as an adjuvant to fusion surgery using bone graft was described shortly thereafter by Venable and Stuck in 1939.[6] With an increased understanding of spinal fusion surgery, the PLIF procedure was developed and first performed in 1944 by Briggs and Milligan, who used bone chips collected during the laminectomy procedure in the disc space as an interbody autograft.[7] In 1946, Jaslow modified the PLIF procedure by positioning an excised portion of the spinous process within the intervertebral space.[8]

Instrumentation advances were also occurring in the middle of the 20th century, with the original pedicle fixation procedure described in 1949.[9] In 1953, Cloward described a PLIF technique that used impacted blocks of iliac crest autograft, after which the popularity of this approach increased.[10] Holdsworth and Hardy were the first to report on internal

422

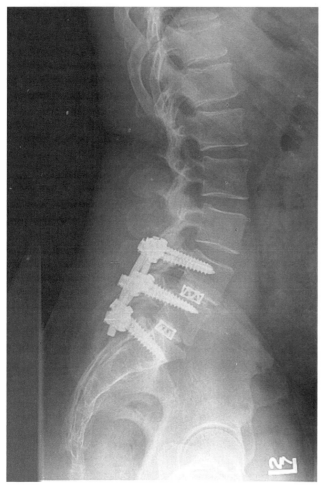

Figure 30-1 Lumbar fusion surgery: posterior approach. (From Paz, JC. Acute care handbook for physical therapists, 3rd Edition. St. Louis, 2009, Saunders.)

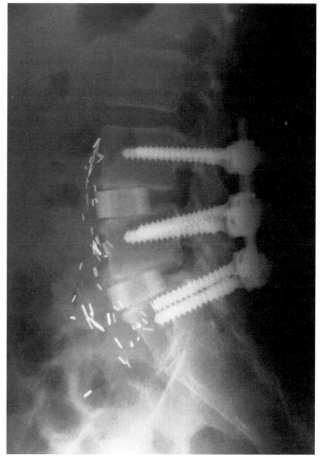

Figure 30-2 Lumbar fusion surgery: circumferential approach. (From Maxey L, Magnusson J. Rehabilitation for the postsurgical orthopedic patient, ed. 2. St. Louis, 2007, Mosby.)

fixation of the spine in patients with fracture dislocations of the thoracolumbar spine in 1953.[11] The use of rigid interbody instrumentation to promote fusion surgery was originally reported in horses by DeBowes and colleagues[12] and Wagner and colleagues.[13] Boucher was the first to use transpedicular screws for spinal fusion surgeries in 1959.[14] Harrington published his results for fusion surgery with instrumentation for scoliosis in 1962.[15] Luque developed the segmental stabilization system in the late 1970s, in which two flexible L-shaped rods were wired to each of the vertebrae to correct the curve and achieve a more stable, stronger fixation.[16] Bagby followed up this research using a slightly oversized, extensively perforated stainless steel cylinder (the "Bagby Basket") filled with local bone autograft to restore the intervertebral disc space.[17] Butts and colleagues furthered this concept using two parallel implants interposed between the lumbar vertebral bodies and reported achieving immediate stabilization; this technology would eventually become known as the Bagby and Kuslich (BAK) vertebral interbody cage.[18]

TLIF was introduced by Harms and Rolinger in 1982, enabling placement of the bone graft within the anterior or middle of the disc space to restore lumbar lordosis.[19] This procedure preserved the contralateral laminae and spinous

processes, making additional surface area available to help achieve a posterior fusion surgery. The first percutaneous screw placement technique was reported by Magerl in 1982 and involved the use of external fixators.[20] The Cotrel-Dubousset system for spine surgery was introduced in 1984, followed by the Texas Scottish Rite system in 1991, the Moss Miami system in 1994, the Xia spine system in 1999, and the Expedium system in 2008. Although a large number of these surgical instrumentations, techniques, and devices were originally designed for scoliosis, many were later used to treat patients with DDD and CLBP. The initial discovery of rhBMP was made in 1965 by Urist and colleagues.[21] Since then, at least 14 different types have been isolated and analyzed.[22]

Disc arthroplasty devices were first proposed in the early 1950s.[23] Nachemson was the first to begin implanting a silicon testicular prosthesis into the disc space, although this procedure was later abandoned when the implants disintegrated.[23] Fernstrom reported his experience with implanting a steel ball in the disc space in 1966, but this also met with poor results.[23,24] Since that time, there has been a plethora of failed artificial disc designs including inelastic and elastic devices, silicon spacers, plastic spacers, silicon or plastic spacers with metal end plates, and various end plate designs including screws, pins, keels, cones, and suction caps.[25,26] Various hygroscopic agents have also been used, followed by elastic beads, springs,

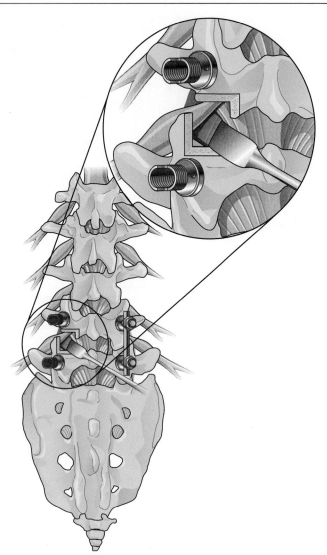

Figure 30-3 Lumbar fusion surgery: transforaminal lumbar interbody approach. (Adapted from Kim DH, Henn J, Vaccaro AR, Dickman CA (eds). Surgical Anatomy & Techniques to the Spine. Philadelphia, 2006, Saunders.)

oils, and expandable gels.[25] The first such arthroplasty device approved for use in the United States was the Charite artificial disc, which was developed in the mid-1980s at the Charite University Hospital in Berlin, Germany.

Practitioner, Setting, and Availability

Fusion surgery and disc arthroplasty are usually performed by orthopedic spine surgeons or neurologic spine surgeons. In the United States, spine surgeons (orthopedic or neurologic) typically complete 4 years of undergraduate education, 4 years of medical school, and 5 to 7 years of surgical residency. Many spine surgeons also complete 1 or 2 years of optional subspecialty fellowship training to further develop clinical skills in spine surgery. Spine surgery fellowship training programs have been accredited by the Accreditation Council for Graduate Medical Education (ACGME) since 1991 and by the American College of Spine Surgery (ACSS) since 1998. After completion of residency/fellowship training, orthopedic and neurologic surgeons are eligible for board certification by the American Board of Orthopaedic Surgery (ABOS) and the American Board of Neurological Surgery (ABNS), which were founded in 1934 and 1940, respectively. Obtaining certification means the surgeon has met the specified educational, evaluation, and examination requirements of the respective board.

According to the American Academy of Orthopaedic Surgeons (AAOS), there were 17,673 orthopedic surgeons and 4605 residents practicing in the United States as of January 2010.[27] Corresponding figures from the American Association of Neurological Surgeons (AANS) were 3519 neurologic surgeons and 1663 residents/fellows as of December 2009.[28] The number of orthopedic and neurologic surgeons with subspecialty training in spine surgery is difficult to estimate because board certification in spine surgery is optional in the United States. The American Board of Spine Surgery (ABSS) was approved as a specialty certification board by the Medical Board of California in 2002 and reported 180 board-certified spine surgeons in the United States as of January 2010 (personal communication, Eckert M. Executive administrator, American Board of Spine Surgery, 2010).

Fusion surgery and disc arthroplasty are inpatient procedures performed in hospitals because they require general anesthesia and may require extensive postoperative care. Fusion surgery and disc arthroplasty procedures are both widely available throughout the United States.

Procedure

Preoperative

Fusion surgery and disc arthroplasty usually begin with an anesthesiologist performing a preoperative examination and history, followed by induction of general anesthesia. An endotracheal tube is inserted and the patient breathes with the assistance of a ventilator during the surgery. Preoperative intravenous antibiotics are often given to minimize the risk of postoperative infection. Depending upon the surgical approach used, patients are positioned in a prone or supine position using a flexible operating table with padding and supports. The skin in the lumbosacral region is then cleaned repeatedly using antimicrobial cleaning solutions. Sterile drapes are then placed around the area of the operation, and the surgical team wears sterile surgical attire to maintain a bacteria-free environment throughout the procedure.

General Surgical Approach

A skin incision is made by the surgeon above the area to be operated on. The length of the incision varies according to the surgical approach. The incision is then made gradually deeper by cutting through subcutaneous tissues and muscular planes, using retractors to maximize visualization (Figure 30-4). Decompression surgery is often performed before fusion surgery or disc arthroplasty to remove disc tissue and bone; that procedure is described in Chapter 29 of this text.

Fusion Surgery

Once the intervertebral disc has been removed, fusion surgery is performed according to the particular approach selected by

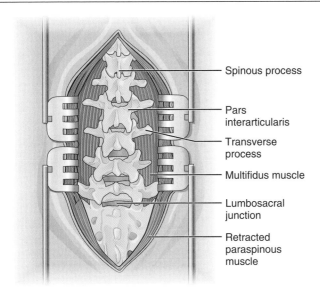

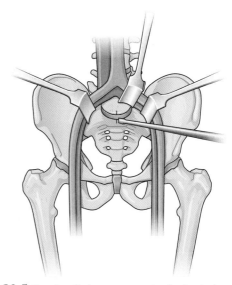

Figure 30-4 Lumbar fusion surgery: complete dissection to maximize visualization of operative field. (In Shen FH, Shaffrey C: Arthritis and arthroplasty: the spine. Philadelphia, 2010, Saunders. Adapted from Kim DH, Henn J, Vaccaro AR, Dickman CA (eds). Surgical Anatomy & Techniques to the Spine. Philadelphia, 2006, Saunders.)

Figure 30-5 Lumbar fusion surgery: standard anterior approach retracting major vessels to expose intervertebral disc. (Modified from Yue JJ, Bertagnoli R, McAfee PC, An HS. Motion preservation surgery of the spine. Philadelphia, 2008, Saunders.)

the surgeon. Although a detailed discussion of surgical technique is beyond the scope of this chapter, each approach will briefly be described. Noninstrumented fusion surgery requires bone chips. If these could not be obtained from the bone removed during the decompression surgery procedure, the surgeon will harvest additional bone chips from the posterior iliac crest (autograft) or obtain them from a bone bank (allograft). Bone chips will then be placed in the intervertebral disc space while applying axial distraction (ALIF, TLIF, or FLIF), or along the transverse processes (PLF). BMP may also be used with, or instead of, bone chips, depending on availability and the surgeon's preference. Instrumented fusion surgery may use a variety of devices to fix adjacent vertebrae, such as metal rods held in place by screws placed through the pedicles and drilled into the vertebral bodies. Intervertebral body cages may also be placed in the intervertebral disc space while applying axial distraction; serrated edges on the cages help keep them in place, as does gravity using the weight of the upper body.

Disc Arthroplasty

To perform disc arthroplasty, a standard anterior approach to the lumbar discs is used, with the patient lying in a supine position (Figure 30-5). After the intervertebral disc has been removed, the artificial disc device will be placed in the intervertebral disc space while held under axial distraction. Positioning of the device should be verified extensively using fluoroscopic guidance in an attempt to preserve alignment with adjacent vertebral bodies and maximize lumbosacral motion. The device remains fixed to the adjacent end plates with small keels.

Regulatory Status

Equipment and instruments used during fusion surgery or disc arthroplasty are regulated by the US Food and Drug

Administration (FDA) as class I or class II medical devices. Class I medical devices present a negligible potential for harm and are subject only to general controls which provide reasonable assurance of the safety and effectiveness of the device. Surgical devices in this category include rongeurs (bone pliers), rotary burrs (bone drill bits), retractors, and other nonpowered hand-held surgical instruments. Class II medical devices are subjected to general controls and additional special controls to provide reasonable assurance that they will perform as indicated and will not cause harm or injury to the patient and/or surgeon. Obtaining approval to market a class II medical device requires a 510(k) premarket submission to the FDA with evidence from the manufacturer that the new device is substantially equivalent to a currently approved and legally marketed similar device. Devices in this category include surgical drapes, suture materials, electrically powered arthroscopes, and digital fluoroscopic equipment.

Many of the developmental trends in spine surgery over the past 20 years have been driven by the challenge of achieving arthrodesis in the lumbar spine. Because of this, the FDA has seen a dramatic increase in the number of applications for bone graft substitutes and disc arthroplasty technologies. Currently, there are two genetically engineered rhBMP bone graft substitutes available in the United States. In 2002, rhBMP-2 (Infuse Bone Graft, Medtronic) was approved by the FDA for use in ALIF cage (LT-Cage, Medtronic) procedures, with results subsequently indicating fusion surgery rates superior to those associated with autograft.[29] In 2006, rhBMP-7 (Osteogenic Protein-1 [OP-1] Putty, Stryker) was approved by the FDA for revision posterolateral (intertransverse) lumbar spinal fusion surgery.[30]

Currently, there are four intervertebral disc arthroplasty devices available in the United States: Charité (Depuy) (Figure 30-6), ProDisc-L (Synthes) (Figure 30-7), Maverick (Medtronic), and Flexicore (Stryker). The Charité and ProDisc-L received FDA approval in 2004 and 2006

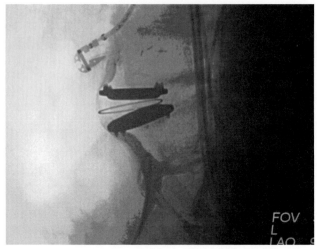

Figure 30-6 Total disc arthroplasty device: Charité (Depuy). (From Yue JJ, Bertagnoli R, McAfee PC, An HS. Motion preservation surgery of the spine. Philadelphia, 2008, Saunders.)

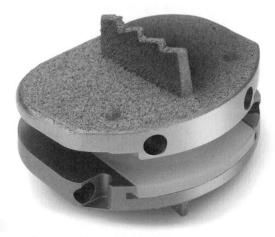

Figure 30-7 Total disc arthroplasty device: ProDisc-L (Synthes). (© Synthes, Inc. or its affiliates. All rights reserved.)

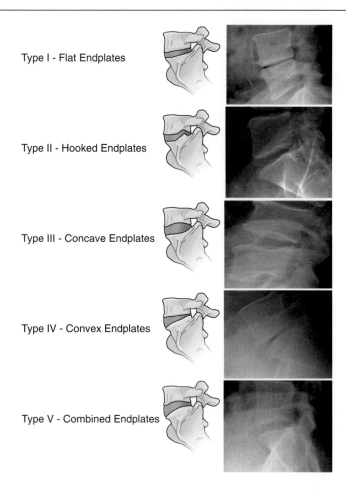

Type I - Flat Endplates

Type II - Hooked Endplates

Type III - Concave Endplates

Type IV - Convex Endplates

Type V - Combined Endplates

Figure 30-8 Lack of end plate structural integrity may represent a contraindication to total disc arthroplasty. (From Yue JJ, Bertagnoli R, McAfee PC, An HS. Motion preservation surgery of the spine. Philadelphia, 2008, Saunders.)

respectively, while Maverick and Flexicore multicenter trials have completed enrollment in their RCTs and are currently operating in continued access, nonrandomized modes. Spinal-Motion (Mountain View, California), developer of the Kineflex lumbar artificial disc implant, submitted their premarketing approval application to the FDA in 2009. One of the potential barriers to using any of the disc arthroplasty devices instead of traditional fusion surgery for CLBP with advanced DDD is lack of end plate structural integrity (Figure 30-8).

THEORY

Mechanism of Action

Fusion Surgery

Kirkaldy-Willis and colleagues described a degenerative cascade involving the intervertebral discs, facet joints, and ligamentum flavum that could eventually lead to neural impingement if sufficiently severe.[31] This degenerative cascade initially involves dehydration of the disc and loss of disc height that naturally occurs with aging. These changes in disc composition and morphology may lead to posterior bulging, which exerts pressure on the ligamentum flavum and pushes it toward the neural canal. Further degeneration or injury to a degenerated disc may then lead to tears in the annulus, resulting in posterior prolapse of the nucleus pulposus into the neural canal.

Degenerative changes in the disc may affect the biomechanical properties of the motion segment, leading to mild instability that increases the mechanical load on surrounding structures. In response to this increased load, the facet joints may undergo degenerative changes including growth of osteophytes as well as facet joint capsule and ligament hypertrophy, which may eventually grow into the neural canal. Continued degeneration of the facet joints may eventually lead to segmental instability and contribute to degenerative spondylolisthesis or lateral listhesis, resulting in narrowing of the neural canal or intervertebral foramen, leading to further impingement of the neural structures.

Impingement of the neural canal may result in neurologic dysfunction from direct or indirect causes. Spinal nerve root function may be disrupted due to direct mechanical compression, although the amount of pressure required to do this remains a matter of continued research. An alternative mechanism that has been proposed is that spinal nerve root function may be indirectly affected by chemical mediators of the acute inflammatory cascade (e.g., cytokines).[32] Claudication may result from direct mechanical compression of spinal nerve roots or from focal ischemia.[33]

Whereas decompression surgery may alleviate neurologic dysfunction by removing one or more of the structures with degenerative changes that may be causing or contributing to impingement of the neural canal, decompression alone may not be sufficient to address an underlying etiology related to severe degeneration. Because the elimination of motion after solid arthrodesis has been effective for pain relief in other arthritic joints within the body (e.g., ankle, wrist, hip), it is no surprise that fusion surgery to eliminate excessive motion leading to segmental instability has been used to treat CLBP. However, it should be acknowledged that the precise mechanism of action by which fusion surgery may alleviate symptoms of CLBP is not completely understood. The complexity of the multiple spinal articulations and uncertainty in determining whether these joints are in fact related to the etiology of CLBP underlines the inherent challenge presented by fusion surgery when compared to arthrodesis in smaller joints with less complex movement. Some authors have previously reported that clinical outcomes obtained following fusion surgery did not correlate with the presence of a radiographically solid arthrodesis.[34-36]

Disc Arthroplasty

The premise for disc arthroplasty stems from the assumption that CLBP is due to an abnormal and painful spinal motion segment, and that the artificial disc would function as a painless and physiologic replacement for the degenerated disc. This premise is buoyed by the success in treating arthritic hips and knees with arthroplasty, where replacements are now expected to last 15 to 20 years in an elderly population with generally favorable outcomes. Proponents of disc arthroplasty often argue that this approach is superior to the unsatisfactory results observed with fusion surgery because it avoids the morbidity associated with pseudarthrosis, prolonged healing required for fusion surgery, bone graft donor site pain, increased adjacent segment strain, and risk of accelerated DDD. Disc arthroplasty purports to reproduce the natural load transmission properties of the intervertebral disc and maintain spinal motion segment characteristics, theoretically avoiding some of the above problems related to fusion surgery and the associated adjacent level strain this may cause. It should be acknowledged that these assertions have not been conclusively demonstrated and may represent an oversimplification of a complex phenomenon.

Indication

Fusion Surgery

Fusion surgery is often used for a variety of indications. Given its primary objective, fusion surgery is most commonly used for CLBP with persistent, severe symptoms that may be due to underlying surgical instability secondary to degenerative spondylolisthesis, DDD, isthmic spondylolisthesis, spondylolysis, or failed back surgery syndrome. However, defining patients with CLBP who may be appropriate candidates for fusion surgery remains challenging because findings from the physical and neurologic examination, as well as advanced imaging or other diagnostic testing, have generally failed to identify a clear pathoanatomic cause for CLBP. This lack of consensus regarding appropriate indications has led to large geographic variations in the rate of lumbar spine surgery across the United States that cannot be explained by demographics alone.[37] This uncertainty may perhaps best be illustrated by contrasting the two main schools of thought with respect to CLBP in the absence of serious spinal pathology, which are briefly discussed here.

Pain Generator Approach. The pain generator approach to CLBP generally focuses on attempting to identify a specific anatomic structure that is the root "pain generator" responsible for the symptoms observed in patients with CLBP. Following this approach requires several assumptions. First, this approach assumes that a specific pathoanatomic cause exists for CLBP, independently of any psychological, social, economical, neurophysiologic, or other contributing factors. Second, this approach assumes that one or more diagnostic tests are able to identify that specific pathoanatomic cause with certainty. Third, this approach assumes that one or more interventions may be recommended based on the underlying pathoanatomic cause. In an ideal world, this approach would be expected to be highly effective in eliminating symptoms of CLBP after instituting appropriate interventions aimed at correcting abnormal findings identified through diagnostic testing.

Biopsychosocial Approach. The biopsychosocial approach to CLBP is founded on findings from many epidemiologic, scientific, and clinical studies, which generally suggest that no specific pathoanatomic cause or structure can be identified to explain symptoms of CLBP in the vast majority of patients. This approach acknowledges the consistently poor long-term outcomes reported in many clinical trials of interventions directed at specific anatomic structures thought to contribute to CLBP. This approach also acknowledges that although subgroups with specific, correctable pathology may exist in the large number of patients with CLBP, the ability to identify those subgroups and institute interventions to improve their long-term prognosis is generally limited. The biopsychosocial approach accepts that pathoanatomic findings alone cannot fully explain the clinical course of CLBP, and other factors must be involved in its genesis, chronicity, and prognosis. Although these other factors are not completely understood, they likely include psychological, social, economic, occupational, and behavioral factors influencing a person's response to experiencing CLBP. Rather than targeting interventions at specific pathoanatomic structures, this approach is generally aimed at restoring normal physical and mental function through education, behavioral therapy, activity modification, and multidisciplinary physical rehabilitation.

Combined Approach. The combined approach to CLBP attempts to integrate the best elements of both approaches described above. For fusion surgery, this combined approach would first attempt to identify patients with CLBP in whom there is a high degree of certainty that instability may be responsible for their symptoms and offer them a surgical intervention. For other patients where the likelihood of long-term benefit from fusion surgery is uncertain, the combined approach would likely promote the use of multidisciplinary rehabilitation combining educational, behavioral, and exercise approaches (described elsewhere in this text) rather than recommend fusion surgery. An important consideration in this combined approach is the timing of any proposed surgical intervention. Generally, fusion surgery should not be considered for CLBP unless the patient has suffered substantial functional disability and unremitting pain for a prolonged period despite receiving appropriate conservative interventions. Although the specific definition of appropriate conservative interventions remains elusive and depends on the clinical scenario, it may be appropriate to at least consider fusion surgery for severe CLBP of more than 6 months duration if no clinically meaningful improvement is noted following a coordinated approach with analgesics, supervised therapeutic exercise, manual therapy, education, and behavioral therapy.[38]

Disc Arthroplasty

The indications for disc arthroplasty are generally the same as those described above for fusion surgery. Because the goal of disc arthroplasty is to preserve some degree of motion at the targeted vertebral segment, this approach is generally recommended for younger patients with CLBP in whom preserving the maximal possible range of motion while restoring stability is desired. Because disc arthroplasty is predicated on preserving normal motion in the lumbosacral region, it is generally indicated in patients with CLBP who are thought to have degenerative or other changes that are isolated to one particular motion segment rather than widespread DDD. Those patients are thought to benefit the most from a motion preserving approach, while those with broader, multilevel degenerative changes may not be appropriate candidates for disc arthroplasty.

Assessment

Before receiving fusion surgery or disc arthroplasty, patients should first be assessed for LBP using an evidence-based and goal-oriented approach focused on the patient history and neurologic examination, as discussed in Chapter 3. Clinicians should also inquire about medication history to note prior hypersensitivity/allergy or adverse events (AEs) with drugs similar to those being considered, and evaluate contraindications for these types of drugs. Advanced imaging such as magnetic resonance imaging (MRI), computed tomography (CT), or CT myelography is required to help guide the spine specialist to target the appropriate spinal levels involved in a patient's CLBP and related neurologic dysfunction. Findings on advanced imaging that may be of particular interest when considering fusion surgery include advanced degenerative changes. However, the presence of these findings on advanced imaging is not sufficient to justify proceeding with spinal surgery. It is of the utmost importance that any findings on advanced imaging be correlated with findings made independently from the medical history, symptoms, physical examination, and neurologic examination. Screening for

biopsychosocial risk factors associated with poor outcomes should also be conducted before considering fusion surgery or disc arthroplasty.

EFFICACY

Evidence supporting the efficacy of these interventions for CLBP was summarized from recent clinical practice guidelines (CPGs), systematic reviews (SRs), and randomized controlled trials (RCTs).

Clinical Practice Guidelines

Fusion Surgery

Five of the recent national CPGs on the management of CLBP have assessed and summarized the evidence to make specific recommendations about the efficacy of fusion surgery.

The CPG from Belgium in 2006 found low-quality evidence against fusion surgery for LBP without neurologic involvement.[39]

The CPG from Europe in 2004 could not recommend fusion surgery for CLBP because multidisciplinary rehabilitation was shown to be as effective as fusion surgery. However, fusion surgery could be used if all other conservative treatments were unsuccessful and combined behavioral and exercise interventions are not available in the patient's geographic area.[40]

Similarly, the CPG from Italy in 2007 only recommended fusion surgery if 2 years of all other conservative therapy failed and psychological prognostic factors were absent.[41]

The CPG from the United Kingdom in 2009 recommended fusion surgery only if the patient was in severe enough pain to consider surgery an option and all other treatments had failed including combined physical and psychological interventions.[42]

The CPG from the United States in 2009 found fair evidence of a moderate net benefit for fusion surgery versus standard nonsurgical therapy and fair evidence of no benefit versus intensive rehabilitation for managing CLBP without neurologic involvement.[43]

Disc Arthroplasty

One of the recent national CPGs on the management of CLBP has assessed and summarized the evidence to make specific recommendations about the efficacy of disc arthroplasty.

For DDD without neurologic involvement, the CPG from the United States in 2009 found fair evidence of no difference for disc arthroplasty versus fusion surgery for up to 2 years of follow-up and insufficient evidence for longer-term outcomes.[43]

Findings from the above CPGs are summarized in Table 30-1.

Systematic Reviews

Fusion Surgery

Cochrane Collaboration. The Cochrane Collaboration conducted an SR in 2005 on various forms of lumbar surgery for

TABLE 30-1	Clinical Practice Guideline Recommendations of Fusion Surgery and Disc Arthroplasty for Chronic Low Back Pain	
Reference	Country	Conclusion
Fusion Surgery		
39	Belgium	Not recommended
40	Europe	Not recommended
41	Italy	Recommended
42	United Kingdom	Recommended
43	United States	Recommended
Disc Arthroplasty		
43	United States	Insufficient evidence

degenerative lumbar spondylosis.[45] A total of 31 RCTs were identified, of which 19 examined the effects of fusion surgery. Of the 19 RCTs identified for fusion surgery, 4 examined CLBP, 2 examined chronic DDD, 3 examined DDD without specifying the duration of symptoms, 5 examined spondylolisthesis, 2 included a mixture of spondylolisthesis and spinal stenosis, 1 included spinal stenosis, 1 included a mixture of failed back surgery syndrome, DDD, degenerative spondylolisthesis, and isthmic spondylolisthesis, and 1 included a mixture of patients without specifying the duration of LBP or condition.[35,45-61]

Three RCTs examined decompression surgery alone versus decompression surgery combined with fusion surgery, and their pooled results via meta-analysis did not find any statistically significant differences between the two approaches.[34,58,59] In addition, another RCT did not find any differences between fusion surgery alone versus fusion surgery combined with decompression surgery for patients with isthmic spondylolisthesis.[57] One RCT observed a statistically significant improvement in pain and disability for fusion surgery versus an intensive exercise program after 2 years of follow-up for patients with isthmic spondylolisthesis.[54] One RCT randomized patients to three different forms of fusion surgery or to physical therapy and observed statistically significant improvements in pain and disability after 2 years of follow-up among the groups who received fusion surgery.[46] Another RCT examined the effects of fusion surgery versus a multidisciplinary rehabilitation program (including a cognitive behavioral component) and observed no statistically significant differences in pain and function.[46] Two RCTs compared fusion surgery versus disc arthroplasty and observed no statistically significant differences at the end of follow-up.[49,50] Eight RCTs were pooled via meta-analysis to show that fusion surgery with instrumentation improved the radiologic fusion surgery rate, while four RCTs provided inconsistent evidence about the relative superiority of different techniques for fusion surgery (i.e., anterior, posterior, circumferential).

This review concluded that there is conflicting evidence regarding the effectiveness of fusion surgery versus other interventions for degenerative lumbar spondylosis. The review also concluded that instrumented fusion surgery may produce a higher radiologic fusion surgery rate but is also associated with higher complication rates.[44] In addition, this review concluded that the evidence was insufficient regarding the relative effectiveness of the different procedures involved with fusion surgery (i.e., anterior, posterior, circumferential).

American Pain Society and American College of Physicians. The American Pain Society and American College of Physicians CPG committee on surgical interventions conducted an SR in 2008 on acute and chronic LBP.[62] That review identified five SRs related to fusion surgery, one of which was the Cochrane Collaboration review mentioned earlier.[44,63-66] Two of the SRs concluded there was inconsistent evidence for fusion surgery versus no surgery,[44,63] one SR did not find any significant differences between fusion surgery and nonsurgical therapy,[64] and two SRs pooled data from observational studies and observed a 67% to 79% success rate for fusion surgery.[65,66]

These SRs summarized data from 20 RCTs, which were the same as those described in the Cochrane review above.[44] No additional RCTs were identified. This SR concluded that there is fair-quality evidence that fusion surgery does not lead to improved pain or function versus intensive rehabilitation with a cognitive behavioral component but is superior to nonsurgical therapy for CLBP without neurologic involvement and common degenerative changes.[62] This SR also concluded that there was insufficient evidence supporting one type of fusion surgery procedure over another, and that instrumented and noninstrumented fusion surgery showed similar results after older, lower quality RCTs were excluded.[62]

Disc Arthroplasty

Cochrane Collaboration. The Cochrane Collaboration conducted an SR in 2005 on surgery for degenerative lumbar spondylosis.[44] A total of 31 RCTs were identified, of which 2 examined the effects of disc arthroplasty for chronic DDD.[49,50] Both RCTs compared disc arthroplasty to fusion surgery and observed no statistically significant differences at the end of the study.[49,50] This review reported that no definitive conclusions could be made regarding disc arthroplasty for lumbar DDD.[44]

American Pain Society and American College of Physicians. The American Pain Society and American College of Physicians CPG committee on surgical interventions conducted an SR in 2008 on acute and chronic LBP.[62] That review identified no SRs related to disc arthroplasty and two RCTs related to disc arthroplasty, which were both included in the Cochrane review mentioned earlier.[44] This SR concluded that disc arthroplasty provides similar results to fusion surgery and that insufficient data exists regarding the long-term safety and efficacy of this procedure.[62]

Findings from the above SRs are summarized in Table 30-2.

Randomized Controlled Trials

A total of 19 RCTs were identified related to fusion surgery for CLBP, of which 10 were published after the year 2000.[34,35,45-61,67-82] The methods of these more recent RCTs are summarized in Table 30-3, and their results are briefly described here.

TABLE 30-2	Systematic Review Findings on Fusion Surgery and Disc Arthroplasty for Chronic Low Back Pain		
Reference	# RCTs in SR	# RCTs for CLBP	Conclusion
Fusion Surgery			
44	19	19	Conflicting evidence for effectiveness of fusion surgery versus other interventions for degenerative lumbar spondylosis Instrumented fusion surgery may produce a higher fusion surgery rate but has more complications Insufficient evidence regarding the relative effectiveness of the different forms of fusion surgery
62	20	20	Fair-quality evidence that fusion surgery is not superior to intensive rehabilitation with a cognitive behavioral component Fusion surgery is superior to nonsurgical therapy for CLBP without neurologic involvement and common degenerative changes Insufficient evidence to determine superiority of one fusion surgery procedure over another
Arthroplasty			
44	2	2	No definitive conclusions supporting disc arthroplasty for degenerative lumbar spondylosis
62	2	2	Disc arthroplasty results appear similar to those of fusion surgery Insufficient data exists regarding long-term safety and efficacy of disc arthroplasty

CLBP, chronic low back pain; RCT, randomized controlled trial; SR, systematic review.

Fusion Surgery

Brox and colleagues[45] conducted an RCT including patients with CLBP without neurologic involvement. Only those experiencing symptoms for more than 12 months were eligible for inclusion. Participants were randomized to fusion surgery or behavioral therapy plus exercise. Physical therapists administered behavioral therapy and therapeutic exercise for an average of 25 hours a week over 4 weeks. After 12 months of follow-up, both groups experienced statistically significant improvement in pain and disability compared to baseline scores. However, no statistically significant differences were observed between the groups.

Fritzell and colleagues[46] conducted an RCT including patients with CLBP with or without neurologic involvement. Only those experiencing symptoms for more than 24 months were eligible for inclusion. Participants were randomized to fusion surgery or a physical therapy program, which could include education, transcutaneous electrical nerve stimulation, acupuncture, injections, cognitive behavioral therapy, and functional training. After 24 months of follow-up, participants in the fusion surgery group experienced statistically significant improvement in pain compared with both baseline scores and the control group. Furthermore, individuals in the fusion surgery group experienced statistically greater improvement in disability versus those in the control group.

Christensen and colleagues[47] conducted an RCT including patients with CLBP with or without neurologic involvement. The duration of symptoms was not reported. Participants were randomized to posterior lateral fusion surgery or circumferential fusion surgery. After 24 months of follow-up, participants in both groups experienced statistically significant improvement in disability compared with baseline scores. No statistically significant differences were observed between groups for disability outcomes after 24 months of follow-up.

Similarly, no statistically significant differences in pain were observed between groups after 24 months of follow-up.

Sasso and colleagues[51] conducted an RCT including patients with DDD with or without neurologic involvement. The duration of symptoms was not reported. Participants were randomized to fusion surgery with the INTER FIX threaded fusion surgery device or fusion surgery with femoral ring allograft. After 24 months of follow-up, both groups experienced statistically significant improvement in pain compared to baseline scores. However, no statistically significant differences were observed between the two groups after 24 months of follow-up.

Madan and Boeree[52] conducted an RCT including patients with DDD with or without neurologic involvement. The duration of symptoms was not reported. Participants were randomized to anterior lumbar interbody fusion surgery with the Hartshill horseshoe cage or Graf ligamentoplasty. After an average of 2.7 years of follow-up, participants in both groups experienced statistically significant improvement in pain and disability compared to baseline scores. The authors reported that the Graf ligamentoplasty group had superior outcomes to the anterior lumbar interbody fusion surgery group, but did not specify which outcomes were affected.

Moller and Hedlund[54] conducted an RCT of patients with isthmic spondylolisthesis with or without neurologic involvement; the duration of symptoms was not reported. Participants were randomized to receive fusion surgery or exercise therapy. A physical therapist supervised the exercise therapy, which occurred during 3 weekly 45-minute sessions for the first 6 months and 2 weekly 45-minute sessions for the final 6 months. After 24 months of follow-up, participants in the fusion surgery group experienced statistically significant improvement in pain and disability compared with baseline

TABLE 30-3	Randomized Controlled Trials of Fusion Surgery for Chronic Low Back Pain		
Reference	**Indication**	**Intervention**	**Control**
45	CLBP without neurologic involvement, symptoms >12 months	Fusion surgery Orthopedic surgeon Cointervention: pain medication n = 34	Behavioral therapy + exercise Physical therapist 25 hours/wk × 4 weeks Cointervention: pain medication, education n = 26
46	CLBP with or without neurologic involvement, symptoms >24 months	Fusion surgery Surgeon Cointervention: NR n = 219	Physical therapy supplemented with education, TENS, acupuncture, injections, cognitive and functional training Administrator: NR Schedule: NR Cointervention: NR n = 70
47	CLBP with or without neurologic involvement, symptom duration NR	Posterolateral fusion surgery Surgeon Cointervention: reoperation n = 73	Circumferential fusion surgery Surgeon Cointervention: reoperation n = 73
51	DDD with or without neurologic involvement, symptom duration NR	Fusion surgery with the INTER FIX threaded device Surgeon Cointervention: NR n = 78	Fusion surgery with femoral ring allograft Surgeon Cointervention: NR n = 62
52	DDD with or without neurologic involvement, symptom duration NR	Anterior lumbar interbody fusion surgery with Hartshill horseshoe cage Surgeon Cointervention: NR n = 27	Graf ligamentoplasty Surgeon Cointervention: NR n = 28
54	Isthmic spondylolisthesis with or without neurologic involvement, symptom duration NR	Fusion surgery Surgeon Cointervention: NR n = 77	Exercise (strength, postural) Physical therapist 12 exercises, 8 could be done at home 45-minute sessions 3×/wk × 6 months then 2×/wk × 12 months Cointervention: NR n = 34
61	Unspecified indications, neurologic involvement NR, symptom duration NR	360-degree fusion surgery Vascular surgeon Cointervention: NR n = 26	270-degree fusion surgery Cointervention: NR n = 22
56	Degenerative spondylolisthesis, neurologic involvement NR, symptom duration NR	Interbody + posterolateral fusion surgery Surgeon Cointervention: NR n = 30	Posterolateral fusion surgery only Surgeon Cointervention: NR n = 32
50	DDD with or without neurologic involvement, symptoms >6 months	BAK fusion surgery General or vascular surgeon Cointervention: back brace, progressive activity n = 99	Disc arthroplasty with Charité General or vascular surgeon Cointervention: progressive activity n = 205
49	DDD with or without neurologic involvement, symptoms >6 months	Fusion surgery Surgeon Cointervention: narcotic medication n = 18	Disc arthroplasty with ProDisc-L Surgeon Cointervention: narcotic medication n = 35

CLBP, chronic low back pain; DDD, degenerative disc disease; NR, not reported; TENS, transcutaneous electrical nerve stimulation.

TABLE 30-4	Randomized Controlled Trials of Disc Arthroplasty for Chronic Low Back Pain		
Reference	Indication	Intervention	Control
50	DDD with or without neurologic involvement, symptoms >6 months	Disc arthroplasty with Charité General or vascular surgeon Cointervention: progressive activity n = 205	BAK fusion surgery General or vascular surgeon Cointervention: back brace, progressive activity n = 99
49	DDD with or without neurologic involvement, symptoms >6 months	Disc arthroplasty with ProDisc Surgeon Cointervention: narcotic medication n = 35	Fusion surgery Surgeon Cointervention: narcotic medication n = 18

DDD, Degenerative disc disease.

scores. Participants in the exercise group did not experience statistically significant improvement in pain or disability when post-intervention scores were compared with baseline scores. Participants in the fusion surgery group experienced statistically significant improvement in pain and disability versus those in the exercise group after 24 months of follow-up.

Schofferman and colleagues[61] conducted an RCT including patients with unspecified indications amenable to fusion surgery. Neurologic involvement and symptom duration were not reported. Participants were randomized to 360-degree fusion surgery or 270-degree fusion surgery. After an average of 34.5 months of follow-up, both groups experienced statistically significant improvement in pain and disability compared with baseline values. However, no statistically significant differences were observed between the two groups at this follow-up.

Kitchel and Matteri[56] conducted an RCT including patients with degenerative spondylolisthesis. Neurologic involvement and symptom duration were not reported. Participants were randomized to interbody fusion surgery plus posterior lateral fusion surgery or posterior lateral fusion surgery only. Results for pain or disability were not reported.

Zigler and colleagues[49] conducted an RCT including patients with DDD with or without neurologic involvement. To be included, participants had to experience symptoms for at least 6 months. Participants were randomized to receive fusion surgery or disc arthroplasty with ProDisc-L. After 24 months of follow-up, both groups experienced statistically significant improvement in pain relief and disability compared to baseline values. However, no statistically significant differences were observed between the two groups after 24 months of follow-up in either pain or disability.

Blumenthal and colleagues[50] conducted an RCT including patients with DDD with or without neurologic involvement. To be included, participants had to experience symptoms for at least 6 months. Participants were randomized to receive the BAK interbody fusion surgery or disc arthroplasty with Charité. After 24 months of follow-up, both groups experienced statistically significant improvement in pain and disability compared with baseline scores. No statistically significant differences in pain or disability were observed between groups after 24 months of follow-up.

Disc Arthroplasty

A total of two RCTs were identified related to disc arthroplasty for CLBP.[50,51] Their methods are summarized in Table 30-4. Their results are briefly described below.

Zigler and colleagues[49] conducted an RCT including patients with DDD with or without neurologic involvement. To be included, participants had to experience symptoms for at least 6 months. Participants were randomized to receive fusion surgery or disc arthroplasty with the ProDisc-L device. After 24 months of follow-up, both groups experienced statistically significant improvement in pain relief and disability compared to baseline values. However, no statistically significant differences were observed between the two groups after 24 months of follow-up in either pain or disability.

Blumenthal and colleagues[50] conducted an RCT including patients with DDD with or without neurologic involvement. To be included, participants had to experience symptoms for at least 6 months. Participants were randomized to receive the BAK interbody fusion surgery or disc arthroplasty with Charité. After 24 months of follow-up, both groups experienced statistically significant improvement in pain and disability compared with baseline scores. However, no statistically significant differences in pain or disability were observed between groups after 24 months of follow-up.

Fusion Surgery vs. Disc Arthroplasty. For the treatment of nonspecific CLBP, the clinical results comparing disc arthroplasty with fusion surgery have been mostly inconclusive. Results of these trials have reported minimal differences in functional outcomes, pain intensity, medication intake, or occupational disability.[50,83,84] Approximately 50% of the subjects who participated in clinical trials of disc arthroplasty in the United Kingdom and United States, despite rigorous study eligibility criteria intended to maximize the likelihood of success, were reported to in fact be clinical failures.[50,83] The study conducted to support the investigational device exemption of the ProDisc-L was an exception to this observation and demonstrated marginally superior results using the visual analog scale, Oswestry Disability Index, and employment status when compared with circumferential fusion surgery.[49] According to criteria established by the FDA, successful outcomes reported in 53% with disc arthroplasty were compared with 41% for fusion surgery.[49]

It should also be noted that these efficacy results are in many ways an optimistic estimate of the effectiveness of fusion surgery and disc arthroplasty for CLBP because study eligibility criteria excluded subjects with multiple segment disease, serious psychological distress, compensation claims, osteoporosis, metabolic diseases, and other risk factors associated with poor outcomes. Furthermore, follow-up in these trials was generally limited to short-term results, and long-term outcomes are required to determine the longevity of these implants given the higher physical demands that will likely be placed on them by younger patients than those previously studied. Possible wear changes, debris disease, implant settling, and other complications are difficult to predict without long-term data. Furthermore, a study with a 17-year follow-up conducted in Europe with Charité disc arthroplasty reported that preservation of spinal motion may not result in any clinically beneficial improvement in pain intensity.[85]

SAFETY

Contraindications

Many contraindications to fusion surgery and disc arthroplasty are nonspecific and include general medical considerations of cardiac, pulmonary, and metabolic reserves, prohibitive anesthetic risk, and patients unable to comprehend the intentions and limitations of surgery. Although there is no absolute contraindication specifically related to the spine, there are certainly factors that have been shown to predict a poor outcome to surgical intervention for CLBP. Patients with high fear avoidance of pain, psychological distress, compensation claims, personal injury litigation, and job dissatisfaction generally have poorer outcomes than those without these risk factors.[86-90] Such risk factors are much more common in patients without any definite pathology or destructive processes related to their CLBP.[91,92]

Fusion Surgery

Contraindications for fusion surgery may include unilateral compression of a lumbar spinal nerve root or single-level disc disease causing radicular pain without symptoms of mechanical CLBP or instability (which should likely be managed with decompression surgery), severe physical deconditioning (i.e., obesity), smoking, multilevel (greater than three levels) disc disease without lumbar spinal deformities, and severe osteoporosis.[93-97] Infuse Bone Graft (Medtronic) is contraindicated for use during posterior fusion surgery in patients with a known hypersensitivity to rhBMP-2 or type I bovine bone collagen, in pregnant women, in patients with an active infection at the site of the surgical incision, in patients who have had a tumor removed from the area of the implantation site or currently have a tumour in that area, or in patients who are skeletally immature (i.e., younger than 18 years of age or no radiographic evidence of epiphyseal closure).[98] OP-1 Putty (Stryker Biotech) should not be applied at or near the vicinity of a resected tumor or in patients with a history of malignancy, and is contraindicated for use as an alternative to autograft during revision fusion surgery in patients with a known hypersensitivity to rhBMP-7 (also known as

Osteogenic Protein 1 or OP-1) or type I bovine bone collagen, in patients who are skeletally immature (younger than 18 years of age or no radiographic evidence of closure of epiphyses), and in pregnant women.[99]

Disc Arthroplasty

There are many more contraindications to disc arthroplasty than to fusion surgery. When strictly enforced, these contraindications should severely limit the number of patients with CLBP who are considered appropriate candidates for disc arthroplasty. In a study of 100 patients undergoing fusion surgery, it was reported that 95% had at least one contraindication to disc arthroplasty and would therefore not be considered appropriate candidates for that alternative procedure.[99]

The most common contraindications for disc arthroplasty are facet arthrosis, prior resection of facets through decompression surgery, central spinal stenosis, lateral recess spinal stenosis, fixed deformity, allergy to implant material, spondylolysis, spondylolisthesis, herniated nucleus pulposus with radiculopathy, facet cyst, scoliosis, osteoporosis, active systemic infection or infection localized to site of implantation, deficiency of end plate structural integrity, severe sagittal or coronal plane misalignment, severe obesity, and insufficient bone quality (e.g., osteoporosis, osteopenia).[100-103]

Adverse Events

Many AEs resulting from fusion surgery and disc arthroplasty are nonspecific and can include reactions to anesthesia such as cardiovascular events, infection, hematoma, pneumonia, stroke, wound dehiscence, clinically significant blood loss requiring transfusion surgery, delayed healing, thrombosis, pulmonary edema, pain or discomfort at the operative site, and peripheral nerve injury or blindness to awkward operative positioning or ischemia.

Fusion Surgery

Adverse events that may occur as a result of fusion surgery include permanent or transient lumbar or sacral root injury, pain, paresis or weakness, iliac vein laceration, reoperation (i.e., instrumentation removal, laminectomy, pedicle screw exploration), nonunion, new sensation of nerve root pain, incorrect pedicle screw placement (Figure 30-9), pain, fracture or hematoma at the iliac crest donor site, dural tear and cerebrospinal fluid leak, wound infection, hardware loosening (Figure 30-10), and adjacent level degeneration or fracture.[45,46,54,104-107] Anterior fusion surgery is associated with approach-related AEs including abdominal wall hematoma, retrograde ejaculation, sympathetic chain injury, deep venous thrombosis, iliac vein laceration, incisional hernias, major artery/venous injury, ileus, viscous injury, and incision hernia.

One large RCT evaluating three different types of fusion surgery technique found that the rate of AEs after 2 years was 12% with noninstrumented posterior lateral fusion surgery, 22% with instrumented posterior lateral fusion surgery, and 40% with circumferential fusion surgery.[108] A study using administered data from the Nationwide Inpatient Sample

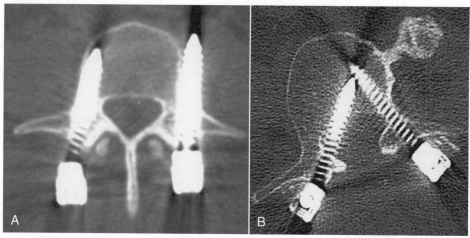

Figure 30-9 Incorrect pedicle screw placement: laterally (30-9A) and medially (30-9B). (From Shen FH, Shaffrey, C. Arthritis and Arthroplasty: The Spine. Philadelphia, 2010, Saunders.)

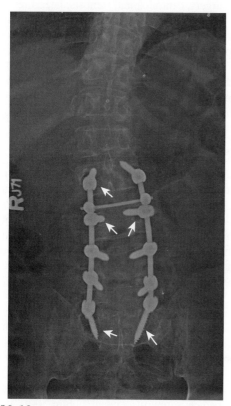

Figure 30-10 Pedicle screw loosening. (Modified from Shen FH, Shaffrey, C. Arthritis and Arthroplasty: The Spine. Philadelphia, 2010, Saunders.)

database from 1993 to 2002 in the United States reported that the rate of AEs for 66,601 patients undergoing posterior lumbar fusion surgery for degenerative spondylolisthesis was 13 per 100 operations.[109]

AEs associated with the Infuse Bone Graft (Medtronic) may include allergic reaction to the implant materials, bone fracture or failure to fuse, bone formation that is abnormal, excessive, or in an unintended location, damage to nearby tissues, fetal development complications, infection, paralysis or other neurologic problems, postoperative changes in spinal curvature, loss of correction or disc height, scar tissue formation or other problems with the surgical incision, and spinal cord or nerve damage.[110,111]

AEs associated with the OP-1 Putty (Stryker Biotech) may include gastrointestinal disorders, general disorders and administration site condition, infections and infestations, injury, poisoning and procedural complications, musculoskeletal and connective tissue disorders (i.e., joint inflammation, pseudarthrosis), nervous system disorders (i.e., transient ischemic attach), skin and subcutaneous tissue disorders (i.e., wound infection).[112]

Although a large body of evidence suggests that pedicle screws promote fusion surgery and decrease pseudarthrosis, there is little evidence to support their clinical benefits. After almost 100 years of use, several authors have demonstrated the safety and efficacy of iliac crest autograft in fusion surgery.[116-119] However, while iliac crest autograft is an excellent material to promote fusion surgery, harvest site morbidity is reported in a significant percentage of patients.[120-122]

Although death resulting from fusion surgery is a rare but possible serious AE, four large RCTs have reported no operative deaths in more than 400 patients with at least 1 year of follow-up.[45,46,106,107,123-125] In general, because of the differences in techniques, study populations, and methodologic shortcomings, AEs following fusion surgery have been shown to vary widely and are difficult to interpret.[65,126] However, it is worth mentioning that a recent retrospective population-based cohort study of 2378 lumbar fusion surgery subjects found that harms associated with analgesics were responsible for more deaths and more potential life lost among young and middle-aged workers than any other cause.[123]

Disc Arthroplasty

The AEs resulting from disc arthroplasty can include anterior subluxation of the prosthesis, subsidence of the prosthesis, polyethylene wear, surgical approach-related complications (as described earlier), disc degeneration at adjacent levels, facet joint arthrosis at the same or other levels, vertebral body fracture, transient or permanent radicular injury, pain, paresis or weakness, implant malposition, device failures necessitating reoperation (i.e., artificial disc removal or subsequent fusion surgery), and anterior dislocation of the polyethylene inlay.[49,50,84,85,127-132]

There were no serious AEs in the ProDisc-L trial, and in the Charité trial there were no differences between disc arthroplasty and fusion surgery in terms of overall or serious AEs (i.e., 1% of patients in both groups).[50,133] Long-term data following disc arthroplasty are limited, but a recent 5-year follow-up study of disc arthroplasy using the Charité disc arthroplasty reported no mortality in 90 patients, and noninferiority versus both ALIF with BAK and iliac crest autograft.[134]

Only one death was reported in 366 patients randomized to undergo disc arthroplasy using the Charité disc arthroplasty or ProDisc-L disc arthroplasty.[50,133]

COSTS

Fees and Third-Party Reimbursement

Fusion Surgery

In the United States, fusion surgery procedures for CLBP are reported by orthopedic surgeons and neurosurgeons using a variety of specific CPT codes appropriate to the procedure performed, which may include 22533 (arthrodesis, lateral extracavitary technique, including minimal discectomy to prepare interspace [other than for decompression]; lumbar), 22558 (arthrodesis, anterior interbody technique, including minimal discectomy to prepare interspace [other than for decompression]; lumbar), 22612 (arthrodesis, posterior or posterolateral technique, single level; lumbar [with or without lateral transverse technique]), 22630 (arthrodesis, posterior interbody technique, including laminectomy and/or discectomy to prepare interspace [other than for decompression], single interspace; lumbar), 22842 (posterior segmental instrumentation [e.g., pedicle fixation, dual rods with multiple hooks and sublaminar wires]; three to six vertebral segments), 22845 (anterior instrumentation; two to three vertebral segments), or 22851 (application of intervertebral biomechanical devices [e.g., synthetic cages, threaded bone dowels, methylmethacrylate] to vertebral defect or interspace). Other related procedures may also be reported, such as fluoroscopic imaging guidance, use of surgical microscopes or other instruments, or surgical devices.

In addition to the professional surgical fees, hospital charges also apply. Hospital charges for fusion surgery may be reported using ICD-9 procedural codes, including 81.06 (fusion surgery, anterior, lumbar/lumbosacral), 81.07 (fusion surgery, lateral, lumbar/lumbosacral), or 81.08 (fusion surgery, posterior, lumbar/lumbosacral). Alternatively, hospital charges may report a diagnostic related group (DRG), which is a system used to classify hospital stays by combining diagnostic and procedural ICD-9 codes. The DRGs that may be reported for fusion surgery include 496 (combined anterior/posterior spinal fusion surgery), 497 (spinal fusion surgery except cervical, with complications), or 498 (spinal fusion surgery except cervical, without complications).

Fusion surgery is typically covered by most third-party payers such as health insurers and worker's compensation insurance. Although some payers continue to base their reimbursements on usual, customary, and reasonable payment methodology, the majority have developed reimbursement tables based on the Resource Based Relative Value Scale used by Medicare. Reimbursement by other third-party payers is generally higher than Medicare. Preauthorization may be required to obtain reimbursement from third-party payers.

Disc Arthroplasty

In the United States, disc arthroplasty procedures for CLBP are reported by orthopedic surgeons and neurosurgeons using a variety of specific CPT codes appropriate to the procedure performed, which may include 22857 (total disc arthroplasty [artificial disc], anterior approach, including discectomy to prepare interspace [other than for decompression], lumbar, single interspace) or 22862 (revision including replacement of total disc arthroplasty [artificial disc] anterior approach, lumbar, single interspace).

Hospital charges for disc arthroplasty surgery may be reported using ICD-9 procedural code 84.65 (insertion of total spinal disc prosthesis, lumbosacral). The DRGs that may be reported for disc arthroplasty include 499 (back and neck procedures except spinal fusion surgery with complications), or 500 (back and neck procedures except spinal fusion surgery without complications).

Disc arthroplasty may or may not be covered by third-party payers such as health insurers based on their individual medical policies.

Typical fees reimbursed by Medicare in New York and California for these services are summarized in Table 30-5. Hospital charges for these services are summarized in Table 30-6.

Cost Effectiveness

Evidence supporting the cost effectiveness of treatment protocols that compared these interventions, often in combination with one or more cointerventions, with control groups

TABLE 30-5	Medicare Fee Schedule for Related Services	
CPT Code	New York	California
Fusion Surgery		
22533	$1616	$1717
22612	$1537	$1632
22630	$1478	$1571
22842	$754	$796
22845	$722	$761
22851	$402	$424
Disc Arthroplasty		
22857	$1658	$1757
22862	$1892	$1998

2010 Participating, nonfacility amount.

TABLE 30-6	Hospital Charges for Related Services
Code	Charges
Fusion Surgery	
ICD-9 Procedure	
81.06	$104,608
81.07	$78,607
81.08	$81,890
DRG	
496	$145,085
497	$89,022
498	$74,316
Disc Arthroplasty	
ICD-9 Procedure	
84.65	$61,826
DRG	
499	$33,033
500	$22,936

From: http://hcupnet.ahrq.gov/HCUPnet.jsp (HCUP Nationwide Inpatient Sample [NIS]).

who received one or more other interventions, for either acute or chronic LBP, was identified from two SRs on this topic and is summarized below.[135,136] Although many of these study designs are unable to clearly identify the individual contribution of any intervention, their results provide some insight as to the clinical and economic outcomes associated with these approaches.

An RCT in Denmark compared two types of fusion surgery for patients with severe CLBP with or without neurologic involvement.[137] To ensure that lumbar fusion surgery was indicated, patient history was augmented with a series of diagnostic tests, such as x-rays, CT with myelography, or MRI. The patients were randomized to posterior lateral or circumferential fusion surgery. The circumferential group experienced statistically significant improvement in clinical outcomes after 2 years, including improved function, fusion rate, and number of reoperations compared with the posterior lateral group. The total direct (medication, appointments, surgery) and indirect (family time, paid help) costs were estimated at $68,567 for the posterior lateral group and $55,624 for the circumferential group. The results indicated that circumferential surgery dominated posterior lateral surgery. The cost utility analysis indicated that circumferential fusion surgery had incremental savings of $49,306 for each quality-adjusted life-year (QALY) gained.

An RCT in the United Kingdom compared two types of circumferential fusion surgery for patients with CLBP with or without neurologic involvement.[138] To ensure that fusion surgery was indicated, a series of diagnostic tests were conducted, such as x-rays, MRI, and discography. The patients were randomized to circumferential fusion surgery via femoral ring allograft (FRA) or titanium cage (TC). The FRA group experienced statistically significant improvement in function and pain on one pain score versus the TC group after 2 years. The direct medical costs were $17,732 in the TC group and $13,912 in the FRA group. The indirect costs were

$12,519 in the TC group and $0 in the FRA group. The total costs were therefore $30,251 in the TC group vs. $13,912 in the FRA group. The results indicate that not only is FRA more efficacious, it has a lower cost. The cost utility analysis indicated that fusion surgery with FRA resulted in greater QALY gains versus fusion surgery with TC.

An RCT in the United States compared spinal cord stimulation (SCS) versus reoperation for patients with neurologic involvement with or without LBP after one or more lumbar spine surgeries.[139] To ensure that fusion surgery was indicated, a series of diagnostic tests were conducted, such as x-rays and MRI. Patients randomized to reoperation received decompression surgery with or without fusion surgery as determined by the surgeon. The SCS group experienced statistically significant improvement in pain versus the reoperation group after an average of 2.9 years of follow-up. However, no statistically significant differences were observed regarding improvement in disability. After 3.1 years of follow-up, 62% of the patients randomized to SCS crossed over to receive reoperation and 26% of the patients randomized to reoperation crossed over to receive SCS. The average cost per success was $117,901 for individuals who crossed over to SCS and no successes were observed for those who crossed over to reoperation (per-patient expenditure of $260,584). For the intention-to-treat analysis, the average costs per patient were $31,530 for SCS and $38,160 for reoperation. The cost utility analysis indicated that SCS resulted in better effectiveness, less costs, and greater QALY gains versus reoperation.

Other. Conservative estimates suggest that up to $482 million is spent on lumbar fusion surgery each year in the United States (Table 30-7).[37]

SUMMARY

Description

The main approaches used for fusion surgery are anterior, posterior, or circumferential. Fusion surgery is also categorized as instrumented or noninstrumented according to its use of surgical hardware to achieve fusion. Autograft fusion surgery uses bone chips from the patient to promote fusion, while allograft fusion surgery uses bone from another person; BMP is a substance used to promote bone growth. Disc arthroplasty involves removing an intervertebral disc and replacing it with a device intended to act as an artificial disc. Fusion surgery has been used for over a century and has seen many technological and procedural advances since its inception. Disc arthroplasty was proposed in the 1950s but only approved by the FDA in the 2000s.

Theory

Because the main objective for fusion surgery is to join adjacent vertebrae, its primary indication is severe CLBP with instability that may be due to advanced degenerative changes in the lumbar spine. Fusion surgery is thought to alleviate symptoms that may be related to excessive movement in a

TABLE 30-7	Cost Effectiveness and Cost Utility Analyses of Fusion Surgery or Disc Arthroplasty for Chronic Low Back Pain				
Ref Country Follow-Up	Group	Direct Medical Costs	Indirect Productivity Costs	Total Costs	Conclusion
138 United Kingdom 2 years	1. Fusion surgery with TC 2. Fusion surgery with FRA	1. $17,732 2. $13,912	1. $12,519 2. $0	1. $30,251 2. $13,912	Fusion surgery with FRA dominated TC
137 Denmark 3 years	1. Posterior lateral fusion surgery 2. Circumferential fusion surgery	1. $64,994 2. $51,151	1. $3363 2. $4473	1. $68,357 2. $55,624	Circumferential fusion surgery dominated posterior lateral fusion surgery
139 United States 3.1 years (mean)	1. Reoperation using laminectomy, foraminotomy, discectomy, with or without fusion surgery 2. Spinal cord stimulation	1. $31,530 2. $38,160	NR	NR	SCS was more cost effective than reoperation

FRA, femoral ring allograft; NR, not reported; SCS, spinal cord stimulation; TC, titanium cage.

vertebral motion segment. Given the inherent risks to fusion surgery and uncertain outcomes, fusion surgery should only be considered in patients with CLBP who have failed a prolonged period of appropriate conservative care. The indications for disc arthroplasty are degenerative changes that are isolated to one vertebral motion segment. Because it intends to preserve motion in the lumbosacral spine when compared to fusion surgery, disc arthroplasty is perhaps most appropriate for younger or more active patients in whom this possibility is necessary.

Efficacy

Fusion Surgery

Five recent CPGs provided recommendations related to fusion surgery for CLBP. One CPG reported low-quality evidence against fusion surgery for LBP without neurologic involvement. Three CPGs recommended fusion surgery for CLBP only if all other conservative treatment fails (including combined exercise and behavioral interventions) if psychosocial factors are absent, and if the pain is severe. One CPG found fair evidence of a moderate net benefit for fusion surgery versus standard nonsurgical therapy and fair evidence of no benefit versus intensive rehabilitation for managing CLBP. Two SRs concluded that there is inconsistent evidence supporting fusion surgery; one found no significant differences between fusion surgery and nonsurgical therapy, and another concluded that there is fair-quality evidence that fusion surgery does not lead to improved pain or function versus intensive rehabilitation with a cognitive behavioral component but is superior to nonsurgical therapy for CLBP without neurologic involvement and common degenerative changes. One SR also concluded that there was insufficient evidence supporting one type of fusion surgery procedure over another.

Disc Arthroplasty

One recent CPG provided recommendations related to disc arthroplasty for CLBP. For DDD without neurologic involvement, this CPG found fair evidence of no difference for disc arthroplasty versus fusion surgery for up to 2 years of follow-up and insufficient evidence for longer-term outcomes. One SR reported that no definitive conclusions could be made supporting disc arthroplasty for degenerative lumbar spondylosis and another SR concluded that disc arthroplasty provides similar results to fusion surgery and that insufficient data exist regarding the long-term safety and efficacy of the procedure.

Safety

The contraindications to fusion surgery and disc arthroplasty include poor health representing a risk for general anesthesia, severe physical deconditioning, obesity, smoking, and allergy or hypersensitivity to drugs, materials, or devices used. Patients with psychosocial risk factors may experience poor outcomes with fusion surgery. Contraindications to disc arthroplasty include facet arthrosis, central stenosis, deformity, multilevel DDD, and insufficient bone quality of the end plates. General AEs associated with fusion surgery and disc arthroplasty include reactions to anesthesia, infection, hematoma, stroke, myocardial infarction, blood loss, pulmonary edema, blindness, and death. Additional AEs associated with fusion surgery include spinal nerve root injury, nonunion, incorrect surgical hardware placement requiring revision, dural tears, increased axial or radicular CLBP, and donor site pain. AEs related to disc arthroplasty include subluxation of the device requiring revision surgery, adjacent level degeneration, increased axial or radicular CLBP, and device failure.

Costs

The costs associated with fusion surgery and disc arthroplasty are substantial. Professional fees for the surgeon are likely to approach several thousand dollars, while hospital fees for the operating room, monitoring, equipment, and postsurgical recovery are in the tens of thousands of dollars.

Additional fees are also associated with presurgical diagnostic testing and postsurgical rehabilitation. When various forms of fusion surgery were compared in cost effectiveness analyses or cost utility analyses, it was reported that fusion surgery using FRA dominated fusion surgery with TC, circumferential fusion surgery dominated posterior lateral fusion surgery, and SCS was more cost-effective than decompression surgery with or without fusion surgery. However, the cost effectiveness of fusion surgery or disc arthroplasty over intensive rehabilitation has not yet been evaluated.

Comments

The use of surgery for CLBP in the absence of serious structural disease is a complex issue in which decisions about the type of procedure used should be secondary to evaluating the underlying cause of pain and establishing that a particular individual is in fact an appropriate surgical candidate. Although there are multiple surgical options for the treatment of CLBP, there is currently insufficient evidence on which to draw any firm conclusions as to their effectiveness on clinical outcomes. Lumbar fusion surgery for common degenerative changes appears to offer limited relative benefits, if any, over intensive nonoperative rehabilitation. Emerging technologies for surgical treatment of CLBP may include biologic modification of disc metabolism, alteration of disc genetic expression to change mechanical properties, synthetic nuclear augmentation devices, and combined facet and disc mechanical replacements. Before adopting these techniques, high-quality RCTs comparing them with placebo, nonoperative treatment, or natural history, will be required. Ultimately, the central question that remains unanswered and is critical to the appropriate use of surgery is establishing the precise cause of CLBP. At present, the poor correlation between apparent degenerative changes and clinical presentation of CLBP argues against the expectation that modifying the degenerative process surgically will be highly effective in modifying pain and disability.

CHAPTER REVIEW QUESTIONS

Answers are located on page 452.
1. Which of the following is not an approach used in fusion surgery?
   a. anterior
   b. posterior
   c. coronal
   d. circumferential
2. How many weeks of conservative treatment should be attempted before proceeding with fusion surgery for a patient with CLBP?
   a. 4 weeks
   b. 8 weeks
   c. 12 weeks
   d. 24 weeks

3. Which of the following is not a technique used in fusion surgery?
   a. allograft
   b. autograft
   c. BMP
   d. xenograft
4. When was disc arthroplasty first proposed?
   a. 1950s
   b. 1960s
   c. 1970s
   d. 1980s
5. True or false: Decompression surgery procedures are often performed in conjunction with fusion surgery for CLBP with neurologic involvement.
6. True or false: Scientific evidence has clearly demonstrated that the long-term outcomes of modern fusion surgery with instrumentation are superior to those of traditional autograft fusion surgery.
7. True or false: Disc arthroplasty is more effective than traditional fusion surgery.

REFERENCES

1. Hadra BE. Wiring the spinous process in Pott's disease. Trans Am Orthop Assoc 1891;4:206-208.
2. Albee FH. Transplantation of a portion of the tibia into the spine for Pott's disease. A preliminary report. JAMA 1911; 57:885-886.
3. Hibbs RA. An operation for progressive spinal deformities: a preliminary report of three cases from the service of the orthopaedic hospital. 1911. Clin Orthop Relat Res 2007;460: 17-20.
4. Kleinberg S. The operative treatment of scoliosis. Arch Surg 1922;5:631-645.
5. Burns BH. An operation for spondylolisthesis. Lancet 1933;1:12-33.
6. Venable CS, Stuck WG. Electrolysis controlling factor in the use of metals in treating fractures. JAMA 1939;3:349.
7. Briggs H, Milligan P. Chip fusion of the low back following exploration of the spinal canal. J Bone Joint Surg 1944; 26:125-130.
8. Jaslow I. Intracorporeal bone graft in spinal fusion after disc removal. Surg Gynecol Obstet 1946;82:215-222.
9. Albert TJ, Jones AM, Balderston RA. Spinal instrumentation. In: Rothman RH, Simeone FA, editors. The spine, 3rd ed. Philadelphia: WB Saunders; 1992. p. 1777-1796.
10. Cloward RB. The treatment of ruptured lumbar intervertebral discs by vertebral body fusion. I. Indications, operative technique, after care. J Neurosurg 1953;10:154-168.
11. Holdsworth FW, Hardy A. Early treatment of paraplegia from fractures of the thoraco-lumbar spine. J Bone Joint Surg Br 1953;35:540-550.
12. DeBowes RM, Grant BD, Bagby GW, et al. Cervical vertebral interbody fusion in the horse: a comparative study of bovine xenografts and autografts supported by stainless steel baskets. Am J Vet Res 1984;45:191-199.
13. Wagner P, Grant B, Bagby G. Evaluation of cervical spinal fusion as a treatment in the equine "wobbler" syndrome. Vet Surg 1979;8:84-89.
14. Boucher HH. A method of spinal fusion. J Bone Joint Surg Br 1959;41:248-259.

15. Harrington PR. Treatment of scoliosis. Correction and internal fixation by spine instrumentation. J Bone Joint Surg Am 1962;44:591-643.

16. Luque ER. Segmental spinal instrumentation of the lumbar spine. Clin Orthop Relat Res 1986;(203):126-134.

17. Bagby GW. Arthrodesis by the distraction-compression method using a stainless steel implant. Orthopedics 1988; 11:931-934.

18. Butts M, Kuslick S, Bechtold J. Biomechanical analysis of a new method for spinal interbody fusion. Boston, MA: American Society of Mechanical Engineers; 1987.

19. Harms J, Rolinger H. [A one-stager procedure in operative treatment of spondylolistheses: dorsal traction-reposition and anterior fusion (author's transl).] Z Orthop Ihre Grenzgeb 1982;120:343-347.

20. Magerl F. External skeletal fixation of the lower thoracic and lumbar spine. In: Uhthoff HK, Stahl E, editors. Current concepts of external fixation of fractures. New York: Springer-Verlag; 1982. p. 353-366.

21. Urist MR, Huo YK, Brownell AG, et al. Purification of bovine bone morphogenetic protein by hydroxyapatite chromatography. Proc Natl Acad Sci U S A 1984;81:371-375.

22. Cheng H, Jiang W, Phillips FM, et al. Osteogenic activity of the fourteen types of human bone morphogenetic proteins (BMPs). J Bone Joint Surg Am 2003;85:1544-1552.

23. Szpalski M, Gunzburg R, Mayer M. Spine arthroplasty: a historical review. Eur Spine J 2002;11(Suppl 2):S65-S84.

24. Fernstrom U. Arthroplasty with intercorporal endoprothesis in herniated disc and in painful disc. Acta Chir Scand Suppl 1966;357:154-159.

25. Frelinghuysen P, Huang RC, Girardi FP, et al. Lumbar total disc replacement part I: rationale, biomechanics, and implant types. Orthop Clin North Am 2005;36:293-299.

26. Bono CM, Garfin SR. History evolution of disc replacement. Spine J 2004;4(6 Suppl):S145-S150.

27. American Academy of Orthopaedic Surgeons. Membership Growth. American Academy of Orthopaedic Surgeons, 2010 [cited 2010 Feb 7]. Available at: http://www.aaos.org/about/memchart.asp.

28. American Association of Neurological Surgeons. Membership as of December 2009. American Association of Neurological Surgeons, 2010 [cited 2010 Feb 7]. Available at: http://www.aans.org/membership/.

29. Burkus JK, Heim SE, Gornet MF, et al. Is INFUSE bone graft superior to autograft bone? An integrated analysis of clinical trials using the LT-CAGE lumbar tapered fusion device. J Spinal Disord Tech 2003;16:113-122.

30. Brown A, Stock G, Patel AA, et al. Osteogenic protein-1: a review of its utility in spinal applications. BioDrugs 2006;20:243-251.

31. Kirkaldy-Willis WH, Wedge JH, Yong-Hing K, et al. Pathology and pathogenesis of lumbar spondylosis and stenosis. Spine 1978;3:319-328.

32. Wiseneski RJ, Garfin SR, Rothman RH, et al. Radicular pain. In: Herkowitz HH, Garfin SR, Balderston RA, et al, editors. The spine, 4th ed. Philadelphia: WB Saunders; 1999.

33. Garfin SR, Rydevik BJ, Lipson SJ, et al. Pathophysiology of pain in spinal stenosis. In: Herkowitz HH, Garfin SR, Balderston RA, et al, editors. The spine, 4th ed. Philadelphia: WB Saunders; 1999.

34. Herkowitz HN, Kurz LT. Degenerative lumbar spondylolisthesis with spinal stenosis. A prospective study comparing decompression with decompression and intertransverse process arthrodesis. J Bone Joint Surg Am 1991;73:802-808.

35. Fischgrund JS, Mackay M, Herkowitz HN, et al. 1997 Volvo Award winner in clinical studies. Degenerative lumbar spondylolisthesis with spinal stenosis: a prospective, randomized study comparing decompressive laminectomy and arthrodesis with and without spinal instrumentation. Spine 1997;22: 2807-2812.

36. Axelsson P, Johnsson R, Stromqvist B, et al. Posterolateral lumbar fusion. Outcome of 71 consecutive operations after 4 (2-7) years. Acta Orthop Scand 1994;65:309-314.

37. Weinstein JN, Lurie JD, Olson PR, et al. United States' trends and regional variations in lumbar spine surgery: 1992-2003. Spine 2006;31:2707-2714.

38. van Tulder MW, Koes BW, Bouter LM. Conservative treatment of acute and chronic nonspecific low back pain. A systematic review of randomized controlled trials of the most common interventions. Spine 1997;22:2128-2156.

39. Nielens H, van Zundert J, Mairiaux P, et al. Chronic low back pain. Brussels, 2006, Report No.: KCE reports Vol 48C.

40. Airaksinen O, Brox JI, Cedraschi C, et al. European guidelines for the management of chronic nonspecific low back pain. Eur Spine J 2006;15(Suppl 2):192-300.

41. Negrini S, Giovannoni S, Minozzi S, et al. Diagnostic therapeutic flow-charts for low back pain patients: the Italian clinical guidelines. Eura Medicophys 2006;42:151-170.

42. National Institute for Health and Clinical Excellence (NICE). Low back pain: early management of persistent nonspecific low back pain . London, 2009, National Institute of Health and Clinical Excellence. Report No.: NICE clinical guideline 88.

43. Chou R, Loeser JD, Owens DK, et al. Interventional therapies, surgery, and interdisciplinary rehabilitation for low back pain: an evidence-based clinical practice guideline from the American Pain Society. Spine 2009;34:1066-1077.

44. Gibson JN, Waddell G. Surgery for degenerative lumbar spondylosis. Cochrane Database Syst Rev 2005;(4): CD001352.

45. Brox JI, Sorensen R, Friis A, et al. Randomized clinical trial of lumbar instrumented fusion and cognitive intervention and exercises in patients with chronic low back pain and disc degeneration. Spine 2003;28:1913-1921.

46. Fritzell P, Hagg O, Wessberg P, et al. Swedish Lumbar Spine Study Group. 2001 Volvo Award Winner in Clinical Studies: Lumbar fusion versus nonsurgical treatment for chronic low back pain: a multicenter randomized controlled trial from the Swedish Lumbar Spine Study Group. Spine 2001;26: 2521-2532.

47. Christensen FB, Hansen ES, Eiskjaer SP, et al. Circumferential lumbar spinal fusion with Brantigan cage versus posterolateral fusion with titanium Cotrel-Dubousset instrumentation: a prospective, randomized clinical study of 146 patients. Spine 2002;27:2674-2683.

48. Thomsen K, Christensen FB, Eiskjaer SP, et al. 1997 Volvo Award winner in clinical studies. The effect of pedicle screw instrumentation on functional outcome and fusion rates in posterolateral lumbar spinal fusion: a prospective, randomized clinical study. Spine 1997;22:2813-2822.

49. Zigler J, Delamarter R, Spivak JM, et al. Results of the prospective, randomized, multicenter Food and Drug Administration investigational device exemption study of the ProDisc-L total disc replacement versus circumferential fusion for the treatment of 1-level degenerative disc disease. Spine 2007;32:1155-1162.

50. Blumenthal S, McAfee PC, Guyer RD, et al. A prospective, randomized, multicenter Food and Drug Administration investigational device exemptions study of lumbar total disc replacement with the CHARITE artificial disc versus lumbar fusion: part I: evaluation of clinical outcomes. Spine 2005;30:1565-1575.

51. Sasso RC, Kitchel SH, Dawson EG. A prospective, randomized controlled clinical trial of anterior lumbar interbody fusion using a titanium cylindrical threaded fusion device. Spine 2004;29:113-122.

52. Madan S, Boeree NR. Outcome of the Graf ligamentoplasty procedure compared with anterior lumbar interbody fusion with the Hartshill horseshoe cage. Eur Spine J 2003;12:361-368.

53. Zdeblick TA. A prospective, randomized study of lumbar fusion. Preliminary results. Spine 1993;18:983-991.

54. Moller H, Hedlund R. Surgery versus conservative management in adult isthmic spondylolisthesis—a prospective randomized study: part 1. Spine 2000;25:1711-1715.

55. McGuire RA, Amundson GM. The use of primary internal fixation in spondylolisthesis. Spine 1993;18:1662-1672.

56. Kitchel S, Matteri RE. Prospective randomized evaluation of PLIF in degenerative spondylolisthesis patients over 60 years old. Spine J 2002;2(Suppl 2):21.

57. Carragee EJ. Single-level posterolateral arthrodesis, with or without posterior decompression, for the treatment of isthmic spondylolisthesis in adults. A prospective, randomized study. J Bone Joint Surg Am 1997;79:1175-1180.

58. Bridwell KH, Sedgewick TA, O'Brien MF, et al. The role of fusion and instrumentation in the treatment of degenerative spondylolisthesis with spinal stenosis. J Spinal Disord 1993;6:461-472.

59. Grob D, Humke T, Dvorak J. Degenerative lumbar spinal stenosis. Decompression with and without arthrodesis. J Bone Joint Surg Am 1995;77:1036-1041.

60. France JC, Yaszemski MJ, Lauerman WC, et al. A randomized prospective study of posterolateral lumbar fusion. Outcomes with and without pedicle screw instrumentation. Spine 1999;24:553-560.

61. Schofferman J, Slosar P, Reynolds J, et al. A prospective randomized comparison of 270 degrees fusions to 360 degrees fusions (circumferential fusions). Spine 2001;26:E207-E212.

62. Chou R, Baisden J, Carragee EJ, et al. Surgery for low back pain: a review of the evidence for an American Pain Society Clinical Practice Guideline. Spine 2009;34:1094-1109.

63. Mirza SK, Deyo RA. Systematic review of randomized trials comparing lumbar fusion surgery to nonoperative care for treatment of chronic back pain. Spine 2007;32:816-823.

64. Ibrahim T, Tleyjeh IM, Gabbar O. Surgical versus non-surgical treatment of chronic low back pain: a meta-analysis of randomised trials. Int Orthop 2008;32:107-113.

65. Andersson GB, Mekhail NA, Block JE. Treatment of intractable discogenic low back pain. A systematic review of spinal fusion and intradiscal electrothermal therapy (IDET). Pain Physician 2006;9:237-248.

66. Bono CM, Lee CK. Critical analysis of trends in fusion for degenerative disc disease over the past 20 years: influence of technique on fusion rate and clinical outcome. Spine 2004;29:455-463.

67. Buttermann GR. The effect of spinal steroid injections for degenerative disc disease. Spine J 2004;4:495-505.

68. Amundsen T, Weber H, Nordal HJ, et al. Lumbar spinal stenosis: conservative or surgical management? A prospective 10-year study. Spine 2000;25:1424-1435.

69. Greenfield K, Nelson RJ, Findlay GD, et al. Microdiscectomy and conservative treatment for lumbar disc herniation with back pain and sciatica: a randomised clinical trial. Proceedings of the 30th meeting of the International Society for the Study of the Lumbar Spine, Vancouver, 2003:254. www.issls.org.

70. Krugluger J, Knahr K. Chemonucleolysis and automated percutaneous discectomy—a prospective randomized comparison. Int Orthop 2000;24:167-169.

71. Weinstein JN, Tosteson TD, Lurie JD, et al. Surgical vs nonoperative treatment for lumbar disk herniation: the Spine Patient Outcomes Research Trial (SPORT): a randomized trial. JAMA 2006;296:2441-2450.

72. Haines SJ, Jordan N, Boen JR, et al. Discectomy strategies for lumbar disc herniation: results of the LAPDOG trial. J Clin Neurosci 2002;9:411-417.

73. Huang TJ, Hsu RW, Li YY, et al. Less systemic cytokine response in patients following microendoscopic versus open lumbar discectomy. J Orthop Res 2005;23:406-411.

74. Thome C, Barth M, Scharf J, et al. Outcome after lumbar sequestrectomy compared with microdiscectomy: a prospective randomized study. J Neurosurg Spine 2005;2:271-278.

75. Osterman H, Seitsalo S, Karppinen J, et al. Effectiveness of microdiscectomy for lumbar disc herniation: a randomized controlled trial with 2 years of follow-up. Spine 2006;31:2409-2414.

76. Peul WC, van den Hout WB, Brand R, et al. Prolonged conservative care versus early surgery in patients with sciatica caused by lumbar disc herniation: two year results of a randomised controlled trial. BMJ 2008;336(7657):1355-1358.

77. Malmivaara A, Slatis P, Heliovaara M, et al. Surgical or nonoperative treatment for lumbar spinal stenosis? A randomized controlled trial. Spine 2007;32:1-8.

78. Weinstein JN, Lurie JD, Tosteson TD, et al. Surgical versus nonsurgical treatment for lumbar degenerative spondylolisthesis. N Engl J Med 2007;356:2257-2270.

79. Weinstein JN, Tosteson TD, Lurie JD, et al. Surgical versus nonsurgical therapy for lumbar spinal stenosis. N Engl J Med 2008;358:794-810.

80. Katayama Y, Matsuyama Y, Yoshihara H, et al. Comparison of surgical outcomes between macro discectomy and micro discectomy for lumbar disc herniation: a prospective randomized study with surgery performed by the same spine surgeon. J Spinal Disord Tech 2006;19:344-347.

81. Hoogland T, Schubert M, Miklitz B, et al. Transforaminal posterolateral endoscopic discectomy with or without the combination of a low-dose chymopapain: a prospective randomized study in 280 consecutive cases. Spine 2006;31:E890-E897.

82. Ruetten S, Komp M, Merk H, et al. Full-endoscopic interlaminar and transforaminal lumbar discectomy versus conventional microsurgical technique: a prospective, randomized, controlled study. Spine 2008;33:931-939.

83. Freeman BJ, Davenport J. Total disc replacement in the lumbar spine: a systematic review of the literature. Eur Spine J 2006;15:439-447.

84. Delamarter RB, Bae HW, Pradhan BB. Clinical results of ProDisc-II lumbar total disc replacement: report from the United States clinical trial. Orthop Clin North Am 2005;36:301-313.

85. Putzier M, Funk JF, Schneider SV, et al. Charite total disc replacement—clinical and radiographical results after an average follow-up of 17 years. Eur Spine J 2006;15:183-195.

86. Carragee EJ, Alamin TF, Miller JL, et al. Discographic, MRI and psychosocial determinants of low back pain disability and remission: a prospective study in subjects with benign persistent back pain. Spine J 2005;5:24-35.

87. Burton AK, Tillotson KM, Main CJ, et al. Psychosocial predictors of outcome in acute and subchronic low back trouble. Spine 1995;20:722-728.

88. Boos N, Semmer N, Elfering A, et al. Natural history of individuals with asymptomatic disc abnormalities in magnetic resonance imaging: predictors of low back pain-related medical consultation and work incapacity. Spine 2000;25:1484-1492.

89. Hurwitz EL, Morgenstern H, Yu F. Cross-sectional and longitudinal associations of low-back pain and related disability with psychological distress among patients enrolled in the UCLA Low-Back Pain Study. J Clin Epidemiol 2003;56:463-471.

90. Cassidy JD, Carroll L, Cote P, et al. Low back pain after traffic collisions: a population-based cohort study. Spine 2003;28:1002-1009.

91. Cairns MC, Foster NE, Wright CC, et al. Level of distress in a recurrent low back pain population referred for physical therapy. Spine 2003;28:953-959.

92. Carragee EJ. Psychological and functional profiles in select subjects with low back pain. Spine J 2001;1:198-204.

93. Cobo SorianoJ, Sendino Revuelta M, Fabregate Fuente M, et al. Predictors of outcome after decompressive lumbar surgery and instrumented posterolateral fusion. Eur Spine J 2010;19:1841-1848.

94. Allen RT, Rihn JA, Glassman SD, et al. An evidence-based approach to spine surgery. Am J Med Qual 2009;24(6 Suppl):S15-S24.

95. Patel N, Bagan B, Vadera S, et al. Obesity and spine surgery: relation to perioperative complications. J Neurosurg Spine 2007;6:291-297.

96. Knaub MA, Won DS, McGuire R, et al. Lumbar spinal stenosis: indications for arthrodesis and spinal instrumentation. Instr Course Lect 2005;54:313-319.

97. Mummaneni PV, Haid RW, Rodts GE. Lumbar interbody fusion: state-of-the-art technical advances. Invited submission from the Joint Section Meeting on Disorders of the Spine and Peripheral Nerves, March 2004. J Neurosurg Spine 2004;1:24-30.

98. Benefits and Risks—Infuse Bone Graft and LT-Cage Device. 2010. Available at: http://www.medtronic.com/your-health/lumbar-degenerative-disc-disease/surgery/benefits-and-risks/index.htm.

99. Huang RC, Lim MR, Girardi FP, et al. The prevalence of contraindications to total disc replacement in a cohort of lumbar surgical patients. Spine 2004;29:2538-2541.

100. Resnick DK, Watters WC. Lumbar disc arthroplasty: a critical review. Clin Neurosurg 2007;54:83-87.

101. Panthong A, Norkaew P, Kanjanapothi D, et al. Anti-inflammatory, analgesic and antipyretic activities of the extract of gamboge from Garcinia hanburyi Hook f. J Ethnopharmacol 2007;111:335-340.

102. Wong DA, Annesser B, Birney T, et al. Incidence of contraindications to total disc arthroplasty: a retrospective review of 100 consecutive fusion patients with a specific analysis of facet arthrosis. Spine J 2007;7:5-11.

103. Huang RC, Lim MR, Girardi FP, et al. The prevalence of contraindications to total disc replacement in a cohort of lumbar surgical patients. Spine 2004;29:2538-2541.

104. Carragee EJ, Lincoln T, Parmar VS, et al. A gold standard evaluation of the "discogenic pain" diagnosis as determined by provocative discography. Spine 2006;31:2115-2123.

105. Swan J, Hurwitz E, Malek F, et al. Surgical treatment for unstable low-grade isthmic spondylolisthesis in adults: a prospective controlled study of posterior instrumented fusion compared with combined anterior-posterior fusion. Spine J 2006;6:606-614.

106. Fairbank J, Frost H, Wilson-MacDonald J, et al. Randomised controlled trial to compare surgical stabilisation of the lumbar spine with an intensive rehabilitation programme for patients with chronic low back pain: the MRC spine stabilisation trial. BMJ 2005;330:1233.

107. Brox JI, Reikeras O, Nygaard O, et al. Lumbar instrumented fusion compared with cognitive intervention and exercises in patients with chronic back pain after previous surgery for disc herniation: a prospective randomized controlled study. Pain 2006;122:145-155.

108. Fritzell P, Hagg O, Nordwall A. Complications in lumbar fusion surgery for chronic low back pain: comparison of three surgical techniques used in a prospective randomized study. A report from the Swedish Lumbar Spine Study Group. Eur Spine J 2003;12:178-189.

109. Kalanithi PS, Patil CG, Boakye M. National complication rates and disposition after posterior lumbar fusion for acquired spondylolisthesis. Spine 2009;34:1963-1969.

110. Medtronic. Benefits and risks—Infuse bone graft and LT-cage device. 2008. Available at: http://www.medtronic.com/your-health/lumbar-degenerative-disc-disease/surgery/benefits-and-risks/index.htm.

111. Brower RS, Vickroy NM. A case of psoas ossification from the use of BMP-2 for posterolateral fusion at L4-L5. Spine 2008;33:E653-E655.

112. Stryker Biotech OP-1 Putty: package insert. Available at: http://www.stryker.com/stellent/groups/public/documents/web_prod/127024.pdf. (It is also a document: Literature Number V260223 Rev. 01 Stryker, 2009.)

113. Mardjetko SM, Connolly PJ, Shott S, et al. Degenerative lumbar spondylolisthesis. A meta-analysis of literature 1970-1993. Spine 1994;19:2256-2265.

114. Yuan HA, Garfin SR, Dickman CA, et al. A historical cohort study of pedicle screw fixation in thoracic, lumbar, and sacral spinal fusions. Spine 1994;19:2279-2296.

115. Wood GW 2nd, Boyd RJ, Carothers TA, et al. The effect of pedicle screw/plate fixation on lumbar/lumbosacral autogenous bone graft fusions in patients with degenerative disc disease. Spine 1995;20:819-830.

116. Salehi SA, Tawk R, Ganju A, et al. Transforaminal lumbar interbody fusion: surgical technique and results in 24 patients. Neurosurgery 2004;54:368-374.

117. Lowe TG, Coe JD. Resorbable polymer implants in unilateral transforaminal lumbar interbody fusion. J Neurosurg 2002;97(4 Suppl):S464-S467.

118. Humphreys SC, Hodges SD, Patwardhan AG, et al. Comparison of posterior and transforaminal approaches to lumbar interbody fusion. Spine 2001;26:567-571.

119. Harms J, Rolinger H. [A one-stager procedure in operative treatment of spondylolistheses: dorsal traction-reposition and anterior fusion (author's transl).] Z Orthop Ihre Grenzgeb 1982;120:343-347.

120. Kim DH, Rhim R, Li L, et al. Prospective study of iliac crest bone graft harvest site pain and morbidity. Spine J 2009;9:886-892.

121. Schwartz CE, Martha JF, Kowalski P, et al. Prospective evaluation of chronic pain associated with posterior autologous iliac crest bone graft harvest and its effect on postoperative outcome. Health Qual Life Outcomes 2009;7:49.

122. Gibson S, McLeod I, Wardlaw D, et al. Allograft versus autograft in instrumented posterolateral lumbar spinal fusion: a randomized control trial. Spine 2002;27:1599-1603.

123. Juratli SM, Mirza SK, Fulton-Kehoe D, et al. Mortality after lumbar fusion surgery. Spine 2009;34:740-747.

124. Jansson KA, Blomqvist P, Granath F, et al. Spinal stenosis surgery in Sweden 1987-1999. Eur Spine J 2003;12:535-541.

125. Deyo RA, Ciol MA, Cherkin DC, et al. Lumbar spinal fusion. A cohort study of complications, reoperations, and resource use in the Medicare population. Spine 1993;18:1463-1470.

126. Fenton JJ, Mirza SK, Lahad A, et al. Variation in reported safety of lumbar interbody fusion: influence of industrial sponsorship and other study characteristics. Spine 2007;32:471-480.

127. Rosen C, Kiester PD, Lee TQ. Lumbar disk replacement failures: review of 29 patients and rationale for revision. Orthopedics 2009;32:562.

128. Patel AA, Brodke DS, Pimenta L, et al. Revision strategies in lumbar total disc arthroplasty. Spine 2008;33:1276-1283.

129. Laban MM, Riutta JC. Idiopathic arm pain. J Bone Joint Surg Am 2005;87:677-678.

130. van OA, Oner FC, Verbout AJ. Complications of artificial disc replacement: a report of 27 patients with the SB Charite disc. J Spinal Disord Tech 2003;16:369-383.

131. Mayer HM, Wiechert K, Korge A, et al. Minimally invasive total disc replacement: surgical technique and preliminary clinical results. Eur Spine J 2002;11(Suppl 2):124-130.

132. Elabbadi N, Ancelin ML, Vial HJ. Use of radioactive ethanolamine incorporation into phospholipids to assess in vitro antimalarial activity by the semiautomated microdilution technique. Antimicrob Agents Chemother 1992;36:50-55.

133. McAfee PC, Cunningham B, Holsapple G, et al. A prospective, randomized, multicenter Food and Drug Administration investigational device exemption study of lumbar total disc replacement with the CHARITE artificial disc versus lumbar fusion: part II: evaluation of radiographic outcomes and correlation of surgical technique accuracy with clinical outcomes. Spine 2005;30:1576-1583.

134. Guyer RD, McAfee PC, Banco RJ, et al. Prospective, randomized, multicenter Food and Drug Administration investigational device exemption study of lumbar total disc replacement with the CHARITE artificial disc versus lumbar fusion: five-year follow-up. Spine J 2009;9:374-386.

135. Dagenais S, Roffey DM, Wai EK, et al. Can cost utility evaluations inform decision making about interventions for low back pain? Spine J 2009;9:944-957.

136. van der Roer N, Goossens MEJB, Evers SMAA, et al. What is the most cost-effective treatment for patients with low back pain? A systematic review. Best Pract Res Clin Rheumatol 2005;19:671-684.

137. Soegaard R, Bunger CE, Christiansen T, et al. Circumferential fusion is dominant over posterolateral fusion in a long-term perspective: cost-utility evaluation of a randomized controlled trial in severe, chronic low back pain. Spine 2007;32:2405-2414.

138. Freeman BJC, Steele NA, Sach TH, et al. ISSLS prize winner: cost-effectiveness of two forms of circumferential lumbar fusion: a prospective randomized controlled trial. Spine 2007;32:2891-2897.

139. North RB, Kidd D, Shipley J, et al. Spinal cord stimulation versus reoperation for failed back surgery syndrome: a cost effectiveness and cost utility analysis based on a randomized, controlled trial. Neurosurgery 2007;61:361-368.

SCOTT HALDEMAN
SIMON DAGENAIS

Conclusion

This textbook presents numerous approaches that are currently available for the management of low back pain, each of which could reasonably be considered a viable option to relieve this common and often debilitating symptom. An attempt was made to group similar interventions into sections describing somewhat related approaches, each of which may have a number of variations. Collectively, the chapters in this textbook present data from hundreds of studies related to dozens of interventions, many of which evaluated very specific treatment protocols for a highly selected group of patients with low back pain. Our natural inclination as clinicians is to formulate broad, sweeping statements that could easily be remembered and applied in clinical settings, whereas our tendency as researchers is to emphasize that findings from individual studies may not be reproducible when the setting, population, or clinical protocol is changed. The main challenge in presenting the information in this textbook was to generalize findings to facilitate their interpretation while maintaining the details necessary to ensure their accuracy; achieving such a perfect balance can often be elusive.

We have previously described the current management of low back pain as the "supermarket approach," whereby the many approaches available are grouped into aisles (categories), within which products (treatments) differentiated by brands (clinicians) attempt to gain market share through advertising. This scenario has resulted in the seemingly haphazard heterogeneity observed in the management of low back pain, which has led to increases in the utilization and costs of all interventions without a corresponding improvement in outcomes. When considering that patients confronted with the vast array of available interventions often have chronic pain and other comorbidities influencing their psychological well-being, the previous analogy can be extended to shopping in a foreign supermarket while hungry and tired. This is clearly not an ideal vantage point from which to make an important medical decision such as choosing a treatment for low back pain.

When we elected to develop the January/February 2008 special focus issue of *The Spine Journal* on this topic into a textbook, we attempted to level the playing field by ensuring that each chapter would provide clinicians, patients, third-party payers, and other stakeholders with the information each required to make a more informed decision. This necessitated that all chapters follow the prescribed format, methods, content, and writing style to facilitate comparison of different interventions. Because this textbook is based on scientific evidence, it was also necessary for each chapter to review the best available literature in a similar fashion, highlighting the same important concepts for the studies uncovered. Our goal was to provide decision makers with a trustworthy source of information to educate them about the most common treatment options for low back pain using a standardized framework blending scientific evidence and clinical experience.

Although authors who had contributed review articles to the special focus issue in 2008 had received similar instructions at that time, this standardized approach was not strictly enforced because each manuscript also had to serve as a standalone journal article independently of the others. That limitation was not necessary when developing this textbook, in which we were able to edit the chapters in a much stricter fashion to ensure uniformity. We have attempted to create a reference source where it is possible for a reader to look at any treatment listed in this textbook and compare the information under any given section with similar information for alternative treatments they may also be considering in other chapters. Each chapter therefore focused mostly on those points that we believed were most likely to provide the information necessary for decision makers to choose among these many interventions.

The rationale for this approach should be intuitive to readers who are familiar with the types of buying guides we often turn to when making important or large purchases for any product or service. When applying the comparison shopping framework to selecting an intervention for low back pain, there are five basic questions that must be answered:

1. Exactly what is the intervention and what can I expect to happen if I decide to purchase it?
2. Is there a reasonable explanation as to how the intervention is likely to achieve the desired result and is there a body of research to support that theory?
3. What are the expected benefits of this intervention and how certain is it that I will experience these benefits?
4. What are the potential or known safety issues associated with this intervention and what is the likelihood that I may experience a harmful effect?
5. What is this intervention likely to cost and how does its cost compare to other available alternatives?

To answer these questions, each chapter is divided into five sections: (1) description, (2) theory, (3) efficacy, (4) safety, and (5) costs. Each of those sections is based on scientific evidence, supplemented by the authors' professional judgment and clinical expertise when necessary to address gaps in the literature.

In this final chapter, we have elected to review all the treatment approaches explored in this textbook, propose a simplified framework to evaluate each one, and present our personal conclusions about how we would formulate a recommendation for a patient with low back pain. Our careful and repeated review of the material presented in this textbook allows us to arrive at what we now consider a reasonable approach to the management of low back pain. Although this represents merely our opinions as clinicians and researchers, we describe how the process of editing this textbook has influenced our thinking on this matter.

BASIC ASSUMPTIONS

There are a few points that became obvious to us after reading and editing the chapters in this textbook and the scientific literature related to low back pain on which they are based. Although these statements may not be universally accepted by all spine clinicians, researchers, or those with low back pain, and will no doubt be investigated for many years to come, they offer a perspective from which to evaluate the interventions presented in this textbook, as well as those yet to be discovered that will be added to this array of options in future years:

1. The most conservative interventions are generally preferred as the starting point when seeking care for low back pain.
2. It may be necessary to gradually progress from more conservative to less conservative interventions if prior approaches have failed to produce the intended results and patients are appropriate candidates for those interventions.
3. Most clinicians and patients will prefer interventions with a clearly understood mechanism of action, strong evidence supporting their efficacy, a low incidence of reported harms, and favorable cost effectiveness.
4. When two or more interventions are similar with respect to theory, efficacy, safety, and costs, issues such as convenience, availability, and personal preference may also guide decision making.
5. Not all patients will respond to interventions in a similar manner, and a certain degree of trial and error is unavoidable when selecting interventions for low back pain.
6. All interventions for low back pain generally have diminishing returns, and persistent, severe low back pain is the least likely to completely resolve.
7. Patients and clinicians should focus more on physical function and activities of daily living rather than pain severity alone when monitoring progress.
8. Many factors (whether known, suspected, or unknown), contribute to the chronicity and disability that can be associated with low back pain.
9. A multidisciplinary management approach addressing biopsychosocial and pathoanatomic factors may be necessary when single interventions are unable to improve symptoms, physical function, and overall health.

Having identified these basic assumptions, it is now possible to discuss conclusions about each of the important aspects of evaluating the interventions presented in the preceding chapters (i.e., efficacy, safety, cost effectiveness).

EVIDENCE OF EFFICACY

The first and probably the most important thing to determine before a treatment is selected is whether that treatment is likely to be of any benefit in relieving symptoms and improving function. As noted in Chapter 1, there are a number of criteria that can be used to assess the strength and quality of the scientific evidence supporting the efficacy of a specific intervention. If one understands these criteria, it is possible to list and compare the best available evidence supporting the efficacy of the different interventions. To facilitate this process, a framework such as the hierarchy of evidence may be used to interpret findings from different study designs.

Expert Opinion

There was a time when expert opinion was the only basis necessary to consider a particular treatment approach. The opinions of clinicians are often based on their education, including the textbooks, mentors, and faculty members who influenced their opinions, as well their personal clinical experience with an intervention. Unfortunately, each of these criteria has been demonstrated to be flawed as vantage points for evaluating a treatment for low back pain. Few clinicians today receive training in more than a few of the multiple treatment approaches discussed in the text, leading to personal biases in favor of familiar interventions and against those which are unknown. Educational materials and academic experts rarely agree about which treatment is best. The natural tendency of patients with low back pain to recover with time and the strong placebo effect of any treatment for these symptoms make the personal experience of a clinician very unreliable as a predictor of the likelihood that an outcome, whether positive or negative, truly occurred as a result of a treatment offered a patient or simply occurred by chance.

Case Reports/Case Series

Reporting on the results of a small group of patients who undergo innovative treatments can be useful to alert others about new interventions or new uses of existing interventions, but offers very little information beyond the opinion and experience of a clinician using that approach. The biases that have the potential to render such observations invalid have been widely documented. They include the failure to determine and measure important outcomes, often retrospective assessment of records, failure to consider the natural history of low back pain, and the strong placebo effect of many treatments. Many case reports also lack adequate follow-up of patients, and large dropout rates are common in many of these studies. Case reports and case series are important in providing questions about the possibility that a treatment may be of value, but do not provide any definitive answers about effectiveness themselves.

Cohort Studies

Considerable information can be obtained by studying a large cohort of patients undergoing a specific treatment approach using a well-designed study protocol. This study design should include a predetermined research question, a prospective enrollment, assessment and interpretation of results by a person who is not the clinician offering the treatment, a well-defined follow-up procedure that includes multiple periods of outcomes assessment, and efforts to minimize dropout rates of subjects included in the study. These studies provide information on what we can expect to occur in a group of patients undergoing a specific treatment, which gives us good insight into prognosis, frequency of harms, and potential costs. These studies, however, cannot tell us whether a treatment is in fact responsible for the outcomes observed and generally do not compare the treatment with alternative approaches or no treatment at all.

Randomized Controlled Clinical Trials

It is only through well designed, well performed, and well reported randomized controlled trials (RCTs) that we can glean useful, meaningful, and credible information about the comparative efficacy of a treatment in a well defined group of participants who meet study eligibility criteria. This approach minimizes the influence of known or unknown confounders by selecting participants from the same pool of eligible patients and reduces the possibility that results will be biased by study personnel or other factors. It is for this reason that the RCT has become the gold standard study design to assess the efficacy of treatment. In the absence of RCTs, it is not possible to state that a treatment, however convincing its theoretical construct, is in fact effective, or to make any statements comparing the effectiveness of that to an alternative treatment approach.

Systematic Reviews with Meta-Analysis

Meta-analysis is a statistical method of combining the results of multiple RCTs to estimate treatment effects. It generally requires that many RCTs have used assessment methods, and is especially useful when there are multiple RCTs where the number of patients enrolled in each study is relatively small. Combining the results of multiple RCTs increases statistical power to estimate effects in a larger population. There are, however, very few examples of successful meta-analyses of interventions for low back pain due to heterogeneity in study protocols, variation in outcomes measures, differences in populations of patients studied, and different follow-up periods reported in the available studies. Where possible, however, meta-analyses can give greater confidence on the efficacy of a treatment than is possible from smaller RCTs.

Findings

It should be stated that none of the treatments described in this textbook stand out as so superior to all others as to be the obvious approach for all patients with low back pain. In fact, it is quite challenging on the basis of scientific evidence alone to select one specific intervention in the textbook as none is overwhelmingly convincing in all of the aspects considered (i.e., theory, efficacy, safety, cost effectiveness). Some of the interventions presented are somewhat similar in nature in one or more aspects, stem from the same basic science, have been subjected to somewhat comparable clinical studies, have equivalent safety profiles, and roughly equal costs, whereas others suffer from the same lack of clear supporting scientific evidence in any of those areas.

EVIDENCE OF SAFETY

Whereas the majority of studies summarized in this textbook have examined the efficacy of interventions, comparatively little research has been conducted on their safety. Although everyone hopes for a technically flawless procedure that will lead to a positive clinical outcome, this cannot always be achieved for a variety of reasons. An intervention carried out perfectly on a poorly selected patient with contraindications or predictors of poor outcomes is not likely to achieve favorable results. Even when the patient is selected appropriately, adverse events can occur during demanding procedures that may be self-limiting and minor, or could be much more serious. Occasionally, even a carefully selected patient and correctly performed procedure may yield poor clinical outcomes for unknown reasons.

It is only in recent years that the importance of safety and harms related to treatments for low back pain has begun to be recognized and investigated. For years, and to a large extent even today, most adverse events to treatment for low back pain have been presented as case reports and small case series. Many of the reported harms from treatments discussed in this book are based on isolated case reports, surveys of the personal experience of a group of clinicians, or speculation on perceived harms, rather than being based on well-documented prospective cohort or population based studies. As one would expect, we have greater information on harms for those treatments that have been the subject of clinical trials using larger study populations than for those treatments that have not been the subject of extensive clinical research.

The two main types of harms that have been reported for interventions related to low back pain are minor adverse events (AEs) and serious adverse events (SAEs). Minor AEs are by nature temporary and self-limiting, and would encompass symptoms such as short-lived delayed onset muscle soreness following exercise, temporary increases in local symptoms following mobilization, spinal manipulation therapy (SMT), massage, or acupuncture, or temporary systemic reactions such as dizziness, headache, or anxiety that may accompany injection procedures or other treatments. SAEs are those that may be life-threatening, require hospitalization, or result in permanent disability or death. This group of harms includes lumbar puncture related headaches following injections that may be severe enough to require hospitalization, cardiovascular events related to general anesthesia, gastrointestinal bleeding with the use of nonsteroidal anti-inflammatory drugs (NSAIDs), detoxification for opioid related addiction, nerve root injuries, spinal cord injuries, and systemic or local infections following injections or surgery.

Findings

It should be clear upon reviewing the evidence presented in this textbook related to the safety of interventions that virtually all treatment approaches have been associated with some AEs. Patients who choose noninvasive treatments such as exercise, SMT, acupuncture, or physical modalities can still expect to experience minor AEs on a fairly frequent basis but SAEs are extremely rare. All medications have well-defined AEs that have to be considered, including dependence, gastrointestinal bleeding, hepatic toxicity, and renal toxicity, some of which may be fatal. Virtually all patients who undergo invasive treatments can expect some AEs whether they are related to the invasive nature of the puncture of the skin, the medication injected or administered for anesthesia, perioperative AEs such as infection, or AEs related to incorrectly performed procedures. As a general rule, the more invasive the treatment approach, the greater the likelihood and severity of AEs.

EVIDENCE OF COST EFFECTIVENESS

Upon reviewing the evidence summarized in this textbook related to cost effectiveness, it should be clear that most of the published studies have evaluated treatment protocols with multiple interventions and different control groups, making it difficult to interpret their results for specific treatment approaches. Further complicating the interpretation of cost effectiveness analyses (CEAs) and cost utility analyses (CUAs) is that studies do not consistently report the same categories of costs, do not consider costs borne by all payers, and often exclude nonmedical indirect costs such as lost productivity. The cost perspective taken in CEAs and CUAs is often narrow, which may result in excluding relevant costs that are borne by others not considered in the analysis (e.g., government, employer, patient).

There are a number of other points that must be considered when examining costs. The first is the cost per unit of treatment. This may be the cost of a single dose of care such as the cost of a consultation and prescription of medication, an office visit that includes a treatment such as manipulation or acupuncture or the cost of an injection or surgical procedure. The second is the cost of a course of treatment. This includes the entire cost of prescribing and monitoring a medication over the average period of time for the prescription, which could be 2 weeks to a month or longer. It may include a course of 5 to 10 exercise and education sessions or 5 to 10 manipulation or acupuncture treatments. In the case of invasive treatments it could include hospitalization, the use

of a surgical unit, the cost of an anesthesiologist and post-treatment follow-up visits.

The payment for treatment, however, varies greatly depending on government policy, insurance coverage, contracts with providing physicians and even between cities, counties, and states. For the purpose of this discussion we have made assumptions, where possible, based on Medicare rates in the United States and reported average number of treatments or doses for an episode of back pain. The third and probably most important aspect of cost determination is cost effectiveness. It is only in recent years that some effort is being expended in the clinical and scientific communities to examine cost effectiveness. If done properly, CEAs would not only include the actual direct costs of care but also the costs of dealing with serious harms, the likelihood of recurrence, the likelihood that the pain will become chronic after care, and the impact of the treatment on disability or loss of productivity. Although the amount of available research on cost effectiveness is limited, we have included the results of a few of the studies that have been published and discussed in this book, though no firm conclusions can be drawn at this time.

CATEGORIES OF LOW BACK PAIN

To provide a framework for this discussion, the assumptions described above can be applied to the broad categories of low back pain that appear to exist, recognizing that any attempt to simplify such a challenging clinical condition will also have limitations. For the purposes of determining an evidence-based assessment and management approach to patients who present to a health care provider with low back pain, it appears possible to divide these patients into three categories:

1. Low back pain with serious spinal pathology such as tumor, infection, unstable fracture, cauda equina syndrome, or systemic inflammatory disease
2. Low back pain with substantial neurologic involvement, including a confirmed diagnosis of radiculopathy with sensory or motor deficits in the lower extremities
3. Low back pain without serious spinal pathology or substantial neurologic involvement, which may otherwise be (misleadingly) termed uncomplicated, common, nonspecific, or mechanical low back pain

ASSESSMENT OF LOW BACK PAIN

It is increasingly clear and evident from this textbook and other literature on this subject that there is simply no consistent explanation for the etiology of low back pain in most patients. Furthermore, there is no consensus that it is even beneficial to attempt to determine the precise anatomic structure that may have produced the original nociceptive signal which, once initiated, may be felt throughout the lumbosacral region. Most diagnostic testing commonly used for low back pain, including provocative orthopedic or manual testing, diagnostic imaging such as x-rays, computed tomography (CT), and magnetic resonance imaging (MRI), challenge injections such as selective nerve root blocks, facet blocks, and discography, or electrodiagnostic testing such as electromyography (EMG) or nerve conduction velocity (NCV), has simply not been subjected to the type of research that is necessary to state definitively that its results can be used to make a conclusive decision about the most appropriate treatment to consider next. The role of routine diagnostic testing, beyond that which may be required to place a patient into one of the three aforementioned categories of low back pain, is therefore questionable and may delay recovery.

For the extremely small minority of patients with low back pain and several red flags indicative of potentially serious spinal or other pathology, a combination of x-rays and blood tests or CT and MRI may be required to rule out the underlying etiology. For the small minority of patients with low back pain with substantial neurologic involvement who fail to improve following an appropriate period of conservative management and who are interested in pursuing more invasive treatment options, CT or MRI is likely appropriate. If results from those studies are inconclusive or cannot be reconciled with other clinical findings, EMG or NCV may be appropriate. For the remaining majority of patients with low back pain who do not present with red flags for serious spinal pathology or substantial neurologic involvement, additional diagnostic testing does not appear worthwhile. More useful information may be learned through trial and error with conservative approaches that do not require advanced or invasive diagnostic testing.

MANAGEMENT OF LOW BACK PAIN BY CATEGORY

Low Back Pain with Serious Spinal Pathology

Patients who have low back pain and red flags for serious spinal pathology that is then confirmed by advanced imaging represent a very small fraction of those who present with this condition. Although their existence must always be considered by health care providers who conduct an assessment of low back pain, the management of serious spinal pathology cannot easily be summarized as each etiology may require complex and individualized management to address the underlying pathology. For example, vertebral body fracture may require fusion surgery if unstable, or simply palliative care if stable, while a spinal tumor impinging on a nerve root may require both decompression surgery and chemotherapy depending on the origin of the cancer.

Low Back Pain with Substantial Neurologic Involvement

Patients who have low back pain with substantial neurologic involvement excluding severe, progressive, or diffuse neurologic deficits that may indicate cauda equina syndrome or myelopathy constitute a serious spinal pathology (see above). Others with substantial neurological involvement should receive the same initial management approach as those without serious spinal pathology or substantial neurologic involvement (see below), although these patients may require more regular and comprehensive follow-up to ensure that there is no progression of neurologic deficits. The precise length and nature of conservative treatment options that should be attempted depends on several factors, including the nature of the underlying pathology and the availability of effective, safe, and cost-effective interventions to address that specific pathology. Providers should also consider the length and severity of symptoms, their impact on a patient's physical function, personal life, and ability to work, when making their recommendations Other factors to consider include a patient's personal preference for delaying progression to other interventions based on tolerance, patience, and concerns about safety, finances, or other considerations, even when deemed appropriate by a health care provider. There is, however, very little research on the effectiveness of the nonsurgical treatment approaches for radiculopathy on which to base one's choice of treatment.

Instances of low back pain with substantial neurologic involvement in which a more rapid progression from conservative treatments to invasive approaches such as injections or surgery may be warranted include: (1) focal disc herniation with nerve root entrapment and definite neurologic deficits consistent with severe radiculopathy, (2) spinal stenosis with well-described and debilitating neurogenic claudication, and (3) vertebral segment instability due to severe degeneration or spondylolisthesis. In such instances, it may be reasonable to first undergo an epidural steroid injection (ESI) with the goal of delaying surgery if the temporary pain relief obtained is sufficient to resume normal activities. It is not yet clear that one method of ESI is superior to all others. Should an ESI be successful at substantially reducing or eliminating symptoms for several weeks or months, it may be reasonable to try another ESI to further delay surgery. The maximum number of ESIs that may be administered periodically has not been determined but series of there does not appear to be any basis for the commonly prescribed series of three ESIs if the first is unsuccessful. An adjunctive analgesic such as an anticonvulsant medication may also be considered for chronic neuropathic pain.

Should ESIs fail to provide adequate relief of symptoms or not be indicated for a particular patient with substantial neurologic involvement, it appears appropriate to consider decompression surgery. This is particularly true if the patient is experiencing severe incapacitating pain as there is evidence of rapid short-term relief of severe radicular pain following surgery. There is, however, no clear evidence that one form of decompression surgery is preferred over the others, and the decision as to the type of decompression is commonly dictated by the experience and training of the spine surgeons who will perform the procedure. Although decompression surgery performed for disc herniation often improves both pain and disability associated with radicular pain, there is no evidence that it has a significant impact on axial low back pain. Decompression surgery appears superior to rehabilitation over the short term, with long-term outcomes being similar to those that may be obtained with multidisciplinary approaches combining education, exercise, analgesic medication, and behavioral interventions. Decompression surgery also appears to be beneficial at relieving leg symptoms due to neurogenic claudication associated with spinal stenosis.

Low Back Pain without Serious Spinal Pathology or Substantial Neurologic Involvement

The remaining category of low back pain without serious spinal pathology or substantial neurologic involvement contains the vast majority of patients who present with this complaint. This broad category can further be divided into three subgroups:

1. Those who have occasional low back pain and are interested in lifestyle modifications that may help prevent or minimize future occurrences of low back pain (subgroup A)
2. Those who have more frequent but mild low back pain that does not interfere with their normal activities and wish to receive temporary pain relief (subgroup B)
3. Those who have frequent and severe low back pain that interferes with their normal activities and are hoping to obtain long lasting pain relief or improve their ability to function (subgroup C)

Because this category represents the largest number of patients with low back pain and is the most clinically challenging group for which injections or surgery are not clearly indicated, we will explore the evidence presented in this textbook to compare the relative efficacy, safety, and costs of various interventions that may be considered for each subgroup of patients.

Subgroup A

Epidemiologic studies have shown that virtually the entire population can anticipate experiencing low back pain at some time in their lives and are therefore always at risk for an episode of low back pain. The current literature suggests that there is nothing we can do to guarantee that a person will not experience low back pain in the future. It does, however, appear that engaging in a regular exercise program, maintaining an active life, not being overweight, not smoking, and avoiding psychosocial stressors can reduce the likelihood that a person will develop low back pain, or at least make it much less likely that any low back pain that is experienced will interfere with normal work and home activities. Furthermore, it does not appear that any specific treatment approach is of any benefit in reducing the likelihood of developing low back pain in the future and claims to that effect have not been adequately proven.

Subgroup B

The majority of us can expect to experience low back pain at some point during our life. Fortunately, most of the episodes of low back pain experienced by the population are self-limiting and do not result in any interference in activities of daily living. At times, however, the pain may reach the point where the person will seek some relief from the discomfort of this type of pain. Most people with this type of pain will not seek the care of a clinician but will simply use at-home methods of obtaining relief and wait for the pain to pass. The chapter on watchful waiting and brief education provides some indication on what these patients could consider. Again, the maintenance of normal activities, regular exercise, avoidance of excessive psychological stress and understanding the natural course of low back pain offers the best chance of preventing the symptoms from getting worse. If relief from symptom is needed, a person in this subgroup might consider a home heating pad or over-the-counter analgesics such as acetaminophen or a mild NSAID such as ibuprofen. Some people with this form of low back pain will seek a few sessions of SMT, massage, or acupuncture to get relief. Other treatments do not appear to offer much benefit to this subgroup of patients.

Subgroup C

In a number of people, low back pain can reach a point where it begins to interfere with normal work or home activities. It is this subgroup of people that is most likely to seek care from one of the many clinicians who offer treatment for low back pain. The person whose low back pain begins to interfere with normal activity has a number of choices. The natural history for most episodes of nonspecific low back pain is gradual improvement over several days or weeks, with or without treatment. Many people with bothersome low back pain find they can manage symptoms with over-the-counter analgesics or NSAIDs and slightly reduced activity for a short period of time. It is, however, reasonable for people with bothersome low back pain to seek the opinion or care of a clinician to be informed of treatment options that can be considered to reduce symptoms and improve function. The options include several sessions of SMT, acupuncture, or massage, combined with a supervised exercise therapy program to increase cardiovascular fitness, muscle strength, stabilization, and flexibility, which can then be continued as a home exercise program. After consideration of the harms and costs of these interventions, it should be up to the patient to decide which of these treatments to pursue, since the effectiveness of these treatment approaches appears to be somewhat similar. It is, however, possible that a patient may respond to or tolerate one treatment approach more than another and it may be necessary to try different treatments. If the pain is severe then a brief period of opioid analgesics may be indicated, but rarely for more than 1 or 2 weeks. The patient should also be made aware of the adverse side effects or harms associated with these medications, including the possibility of dependence and addiction.

What is clear from the literature is that educating a patient so that he or she understands the nature of the problem and what can be expected from treatment is crucial to recovery. The patient should be made aware that bed rest is detrimental to low back pain and will prolong recovery, whereas maintaining normal activities and exercise within their tolerance will not harm them. Failure to educate patients about appropriate activities may lead them to worry that there is something more seriously wrong and reduce their activities, which could delay their recovery. This could also lead them to demand further investigation and more invasive treatments that are not likely to be helpful and which carry significant chances of harms or prolonged disability. To date, there is no convincing evidence that any of the injection or surgical treatment approaches in this category and subgroup of patients with nonspecific low back pain is likely to reduce symptoms meaningfully in the long term. The single exception to this rule is the rare person with incapacitating low back pain who is not responsive to the common treatments and in whom a standard x-ray reveals an unstable vertebral segment due to severe spondylolisthesis that can be developmental or due to severe degenerative changes. Under such circumstances, surgical fusion may be indicated.

CONCLUSION

We have reached a point in history where it is now possible to look at the scientific literature and determine the level of evidence to support or reject specific treatment approaches to low back pain. We have reasonable evidence to support certain treatments and reject others on the basis of efficacy, safety, and costs. We hope that readers of this textbook will come away with a better understanding of some of the most popular, as well as the less widely used, methods of treating low back pain and will be able to understand the theoretical and experimental basis for the different treatment approaches. We also hope that this textbook will allow readers to compare the different treatments in sufficient detail to determine whether a specific treatment should be considered when faced with low back pain.

Although this textbook was centered on scientific evidence, it was neither feasible nor possible to present all of the details regarding each study that was referenced. Our goal was to succinctly present the information related to the theory, efficacy, safety, and costs of various interventions for our intended core audience of spine clinicians, researchers, and third-party payers. Researchers may have wished for a more meticulous description of study methodology, clinicians may have wanted further details about various short- and long-term outcome measures, and payers may have longed for definitive conclusions from cost effectiveness analyses. Those requiring additional information about the scientific literature discussed in this textbook are hence referred to the various clinical practice guidelines, systematic reviews, randomized controlled trials, observational studies, and cost effectiveness analyses cited herein to learn more. We hope that our focus on the strengths and weaknesses of the current scientific evidence will spur dialogue between the various stakeholders to undertake research required to address important gaps in our knowledge about the optimal methods for managing low back pain.

Finally, we have presented our own interpretation of the information to develop an evidence-informed approach to low back pain. This approach is consistent with most of the evidence-based, multidisciplinary clinical practice guidelines that have been published. The readers of this textbook should be able to determine whether we have interpreted the evidence appropriately and modify their approach based on any difference in the interpretation of the evidence they feel is appropriate. More than anything, however, we believe that it is possible to offer patients an evidence-informed approach to the care of their low back pain to rectify the current supermarket approach based on excessive or misleading claims, advertising, ignorance of the underlying literature, or interventions promoted solely on the basis of the individual experience of clinicians or the biases of an insurance carrier. If we have achieved this objective, even partially, patients who seek the advice of a clinician who has studied this textbook should feel they are receiving the highest level of evidence-informed treatment for their low back pain.

Answers to Review Questions

CHAPTER 5

1. a
2. c
3. b
4. c
5. a
6. c
7. b

CHAPTER 6

1. a
2. c
3. d
4. d
5. false
6. true
7. true

CHAPTER 7

1. a
2. c
3. d
4. c
5. true
6. true

CHAPTER 8

1. a
2. a
3. c
4. d
5. c
6. b
7. d

CHAPTER 9

1. d
2. b
3. d
4. b
5. b
6. c
7. d
8. c

CHAPTER 10

1. d
2. a
3. b
4. false
5. d
6. true

CHAPTER 11

1. d
2. c
3. a
4. true
5. a
6. c
7. d

CHAPTER 12

1. b
2. a
3. b
4. a
5. c
6. false
7. false

CHAPTER 13

1. c
2. a
3. c
4. false
5. true
6. d
7. d

CHAPTER 14

1. a
2. d
3. b
4. c
5. c
6. false
7. false

CHAPTER 15

1. d
2. c
3. b
4. c
5. d
6. a

CHAPTER 16

1. c
2. a
3. e
4. e
5. e
6. false
7. c
8. false

CHAPTER 17

1. b
2. c
3. a
4. d
5. false
6. false
7. a
8. a

CHAPTER 18

1. d
2. false
3. false
4. false
5. false
6. b
7. d
8. c

CHAPTER 19

1. false
2. true
3. b
4. b
5. b
6. d
7. a

CHAPTER 20

1. d
2. a
3. c
4. b
5. c
6. true
7. false

CHAPTER 21

1. b
2. c
3. d
4. b
5. d
6. false

CHAPTER 22

1. b
2. c
3. true
4. e
5. e
6. true
7. c

CHAPTER 23

1. c
2. a

3. c
4. false
5. a
6. d
7. b
8. d

CHAPTER 24

1. a
2. d
3. c
4. c
5. d
6. d
7. a
8. b

CHAPTER 25

1. a
2. d
3. c
4. false
5. a
6. d
7. false

CHAPTER 26

1. c
2. c
3. b
4. b
5. d
6. a
7. true
8. false

CHAPTER 27

1. c
2. a
3. a
4. d
5. b
6. b
7. false
8. c

CHAPTER 28

1. d
2. false
3. true
4. b
5. c
6. a
7. b
8. false

CHAPTER 29

1. d
2. b
3. a
4. c
5. false
6. false
7. d

CHAPTER 30

1. c
2. d
3. d
4. a
5. true
6. false
7. false

Glossary

A

acetazolamide Third-generation antiepileptic medication; brand name Diamox.

active release therapy (ART) Type of manual therapy in which manual pressure is applied to a specific muscle while the patient slowly and actively moves a joint adjacent to that muscle through its full range of motion.

acupressure Type of massage therapy technique in which manual pressure is applied to acupuncture points to stimulate them using fingers rather than needles; also known as massage acupuncture.

acupuncturist Licensed health provider trained to administer needle acupuncture. May be a standalone license or additional certification for traditional Chinese medicine practitioners, physicians, chiropractors, and physical therapists.

acute low back pain Episode of low back pain where current symptoms have lasted less than 6 weeks.

adaptive coping Type of response to chronic pain in which symptoms are coherent, pain is consistent with underlying pathology, function is concordant with impairment, and mood is appropriate to levels of pain and function.

addiction Neurobiological disease characterized by behaviors such as compulsive use of a psychoactive substance despite the harms endured.

adjunctive analgesics Category of medications whose primary indication is not related to pain but that are also used for pain relief.

adverse events (AEs) Unfavorable medical occurrence in a clinical research participant, including abnormal signs, symptoms, or diseases, even if not related to the research intervention.

algometer Instrument used to measure the amount of compression required to elicit a painful response in trigger points; also called dolorimeter.

allograft fusion Type of fusion surgery in which small bone chips are obtained from a person other than the patient to aid with the fusion process.

amitriptyline Tricyclic antidepressant medication; brand name Elavil.

amoxapine Tricyclic antidepressant medication; brand name Asendin.

anesthesiologist Physician who specializes in the administration of anesthesia.

ankylosing spondylitis Arthritic condition in which systemic inflammation affects the vertebrae and sacroiliac joints, causing premature degeneration and possible instability; often accompanied by other symptoms, including changes in vision and urination.

anticonvulsants Category of medication whose primary indication is management of epileptic seizures. Subcate-gories of interest to low back pain include first-generation, second-generation, and third-generation antiepileptics, which are occasionally used as adjunctive analgesics; also known as antiepileptics.

antidepressants Category of medication whose primary indication is depression. Subcategories of interest to low back pain include tricyclic antidepressants (TCAs), selective serotonin reuptake inhibitors (SSRIs), and serotonin-norepinephrine reuptake inhibitors (SNRIs), which are occasionally used as adjunctive analgesics.

antiepileptics Category of medication whose primary indication is management of epileptic seizures. Subcategories of interest to low back pain include first-generation, second-generation, and third-generation antiepileptics, which are occasionally used as adjunctive analgesics; also known as anticonvulsants.

antispasmodic muscle relaxants Type of muscle relaxant whose primary indication is muscle spasm.

antispastic muscle relaxants Type of muscle relaxant whose primary indication is muscle spasticity.

arthrodesis Type of surgery in which adjacent bony anatomical structures are surgically joined because they are thought to have excessive mobility, or are otherwise contributing to the presenting symptoms; also known as fusion surgery. The main types of fusion surgery for low back pain are defined according to their use of surgical instrumentation (e.g., plates, screws, cages) and approaches (e.g., anterior, posterior, circumferential).

arthroplasty Surgical procedure in which an anatomical structure is surgically removed and replaced with an artificial joint, prosthesis, or medical device.

aspirin Type of nonsteroidal anti-inflammatory drug; brand names include Bayer Aspirin and Bufferin.

autogenous bone graft fusion Type of fusion surgery in which small bone chips are harvested from the patient, usually the iliac crest, to aid with the fusion process; also known as autograft fusion or autologous bone graft fusion.

autograft fusion Type of fusion surgery in which small bone chips are harvested from the patient, usually the iliac crest, to aid with the fusion process; also known as autologous or autogenous bone graft fusion.

autologous bone graft fusion Type of fusion surgery in which small bone chips are harvested from the patient, usually the iliac crest, to aid with the fusion process; also known as autograft fusion or autogenous bone graft fusion.

B

back school Type of intervention that typically includes group education about low back pain (LBP), appropriate self-management of LBP, training about how to live with LBP, how to adapt activities of daily living for those with

LBP, and recommendations for general and back-specific therapeutic exercises.

balneotherapy Type of modality used in physical therapy that involves immersing the body in hot or cold water, with or without bath salts or other substances, to promote relaxation or stimulation; also known as spa therapy.

bio-psychosocial approach to low back pain Approach to managing low back pain (LBP) that recognizes that symptoms are influenced by a host of psychosocial and economic factors, including prior experiences with LBP, beliefs about LBP, general and psychological health, job satisfaction, economic status, education, involvement in litigation, and social well-being at home. Often contrasted with the bio-medical or anatomical approach to LBP, which focuses more on identifying specific pathologies.

bipolar radiofrequency energy Type of energy used in intradiscal thermal therapies, in which an electrical current passes directly from the positive pole of the instrument to its negative pole. This energy is thought to decrease the collateral damage that may occur when electrical energy must first travel through the body to an external grounding pad.

bone morphogenic protein Substance used in fusion surgery to enhance the body's natural bone growth process, which can be used instead of, or in addition to, autograft or allograft bone chips; also known as recombinant human bone morphogenic protein.

breakthrough pain Type of pain that can occur even while a patient is taking opioid analgesics or other medications intended to control pain.

brief education Type of intervention that typically includes a consultation with a health care provider who discusses the basic etiology, expected prognosis, and treatment options for low back pain, gives tips for self-management of low back pain, and lists circumstances in which medical care should be considered.

C

carbamazepine First-generation antiepileptic medication; brand names include Carbatrol, Epitol, Equetro, and Tegretol.

case report/series Type of clinical research study in which a clinician describes the clinical characteristics of one patient (case report) or several patients (case series) in whose management the clinician was involved.

cauda equina syndrome Neurologic condition in which spinal nerves in the lower portion of the spinal cord are compressed, causing various pathognomonic signs and symptoms in the pelvis and lower extremities. Often represents a medical emergency in which surgical intervention may be required.

caudal epidural steroid injection Type of epidural injection in which the needle is placed in the caudal epidural space to deliver medication.

celecoxib Type of nonsteroidal anti-inflammatory drug; brand name Celebrex.

centralization Phenomenon observed in the McKenzie approach in which radicular pain decreases and is focused in the axial lumbar spine region.

challenge facet blocks Type of interventional diagnostic procedure in which symptoms are monitored following injection of local anesthetics or other substances near the lumbar medial branch suspected of contributing to low back pain. Often used as a screening procedure to identify patients who may benefit from lumbar medial branch neurotomy; also known as diagnostic facet injections or lumbar medial branch blocks.

chi Life energy that flows throughout the body along meridians, and whose disruption is thought to result in disease according to traditional Chinese medicine, which includes needle acupuncture; also known as life energy or qi. The two main types of chi are yin and yang.

chiropractor Type of health care practitioner focused on the diagnosis and treatment of neuromusculoskeletal disorders, primarily with spinal manipulation therapy; also known as a doctor of chiropractic.

chronic low back pain (CLBP) Episode of low back pain where current symptoms have lasted more than 12 weeks.

citalopram Selective serotonin reuptake inhibitor antidepressant medication; brand name Celexa.

claudication Intermittent pain, fatigue, or cramping in the legs that is often worse after walking or standing and is usually relieved by sitting or leaning forward. The two main types of claudication are neurogenic and vascular.

clinical practice guideline (CPG) Type of clinical research study in which a multidisciplinary panel of expert clinicians, scientists, decision makers, and patients interpret the best available scientific evidence to make recommendations about the most appropriate use of therapeutic or diagnostic interventions for a particular medical condition such as low back pain.

clomipramine Tricyclic antidepressant medication; brand name Anafranil.

coblation Type of energy used in intradiscal therapies in which a plasma of high-energy ionized particles is used to remove targeted tissues. The plasma is thought to disrupt organic bonds between molecules and minimize the damage that could occur if heat energy were used.

cognitive behavioral therapy (CBT) Type of intervention in which a therapist helps a patient to recognize, confront, and change any irrational thoughts that could be contributing to undesired behaviors and replace them with more appropriate thoughts and behaviors.

common analgesics Category of medication whose primary indication is pain. Subcategories of interest to low back pain include nonsteroidal anti-inflammatory drugs (NSAIDs) and simple analgesics.

common low back pain Term used to describe low back pain (LBP) in which no specific anatomical structure or pathology can be identified as being responsible for symptoms; also known as nonspecific LBP or simple LBP.

complementary and alternative medicine (CAM) Term used to indicate interventions, practices, products, and health care systems that are not generally considered part of conventional medicine. Categories of interest to low back pain include acupuncture and massage therapy.

computed tomography (CT) Type of advanced diagnostic imaging procedure in which a patient lies in a machine that uses ionizing radiation to produce cross-sectional images of the body.

continuous release opioids Type of opioid analgesic in which the active ingredients are absorbed slowly from the gastrointestinal tract or transdermally, which may prolong their effect; also known as extended-release opioids or sustained-release opioids.

contraindication Sign, symptom, or other patient characteristic suggesting that a particular intervention is not appropriate for a patient, often due to an increased risk of experiencing poor outcomes or harms.

cost effectiveness analysis (CEA) Type of health economic evaluation in which both the costs and the effectiveness outcomes associated with an intervention are evaluated and compared to other available alternatives.

cost of illness Type of health economic study in which the economic costs of a particular illness or medical condition are examined from various perspectives, including those of the patient, payers, or society; also known as economic burden of illness.

cost utility analysis (CUA) Type of health economic evaluation in which both the costs and the utility outcomes associated with an intervention are evaluated and compared to other available alternatives; the outcomes of interest are health-related utility.

COX-2 inhibitors Newer type of nonsteroidal anti-inflammatory drugs (NSAIDs) that selectively inhibits only the COX-2 isoenzyme and is thought to decrease the risk of gastrointestinal bleeding associated with prolonged used of traditional NSAIDs, which also inhibit the COX-1 isoenzyme important to the gastrointestinal lining. Also known as selective NSAIDs, and includes medications such as celecoxib and rofecoxib, some of which were removed from the United States market due to concerns about the risk of cardiovascular adverse events.

coxibs Subgroup of nonselective nonsteroidal anti-inflammatory drugs that includes celecoxib, rofecoxib, valdecoxib, and etoricoxib.

current procedural terminology (CPT) codes Codes used by health care practitioners to inform third-party payers about the specific type of diagnostic or therapeutic intervention performed for a particular patient; used for billing and reimbursement purposes.

craniosacral therapy Type of massage therapy technique in which light pressure is applied along the sacrum, spine, and cranial sutures while the patient performs deep breathing to promote relaxation.

D

dapoxetine Selective serotonin reuptake inhibitor antidepressant medication; brand name Priligy.

decompression surgery Type of spinal surgery in which the primary goal is to remove structures in the neural canal that are thought to cause neural impingement. The two main types of decompression surgery for low back pain are standard/traditional/open and microscopic/minimally invasive/endoscopic.

deep friction massage Type of massage therapy technique in which strong, prolonged pressure is applied to a small area of pain to temporarily decrease blood flow before releasing the pressure to stimulate reperfusion and removal of chemical mediators of inflammation.

degenerative cascade Structural changes that may occur in the discs, facet joints, and ligamentum flavum as a result of degenerative disc disease, and which may eventually lead to neural impingement if severe.

dependence Phenomenon in which the body, through physiological adaptation induced by chronic use, requires a particular psychoactive substance in order to function. This phenomenon can occur independently of addiction.

derangement syndrome Type of pain syndrome in the McKenzie approach in which centralization can be achieved with directional preference movements.

desipramine Tricyclic antidepressant medication; brand name Norpramin.

desvenlafaxine Serotonin-norepinephrine reuptake inhibitor antidepressant medication; brand name Pristiq.

diabetic peripheral neuropathy Type of damage that can occur in peripheral nerves secondary to long-term diabetes, and which may be associated with neurologic symptoms such as pain, numbness, tingling, or burning along the distribution of a peripheral nerve.

diagnostic classifications for low back pain Four main categories that can be used to describe patients with low back pain (LBP): (1) common, nonspecific, and nondisabling LBP, (2) common, nonspecific, disabling LBP, (3) LBP with substantial neurologic deficits, and (4) LBP related to serious spinal pathology.

diagnostic facet injections Type of interventional diagnostic procedure in which symptoms are monitored following injection of local anesthetics or other substances near the lumbar medial branch suspected of contributing to low back pain. Often used as a screening procedure to identify patients who may benefit from additional interventions aimed at the facet joints; preferred terminology is controlled diagnostic lumbar medial branch blocks.

diagnostic related group (DRG) Codes used by hospitals to inform third-party payers about the specific medical condition and type of diagnostic or therapeutic intervention performed for a particular patient. The codes can be derived from combinations of ICD-9 and CPT codes and are often used for billing and reimbursement purposes.

diagnostic testing Type of procedures performed to detect anatomical or physiologic abnormalities, to clarify the etiology of a condition, and to formulate a diagnosis. Categories of interest to low back pain include diagnostic imaging, electrodiagnostic testing, laboratory testing, and invasive testing.

dibenzepin Tricyclic antidepressant medication; brand names include Noveril, Anslopax, Deprex, Ecatril, Neodit, and Victoril.

diclofenac Type of nonsteroidal anti-inflammatory drug; brand names include Cambia, Cataflam, Voltaren, and Zipsor.

differential diagnosis List of potential diagnoses created by health practitioners who are uncertain about the specific etiology of a condition; the list can later be modified based on newly available information.

diflunisal Type of nonsteroidal anti-inflammatory drug; brand name Dolobid.

direct health care costs Term used in health economics to describe costs that are directly related to health care services such as office visits, medications, hospital services, and diagnostic tests; frequently estimated from charges or prices, though these may differ from true costs.

direct nonmedical costs Term used in health economics to describe costs that are directly related to an illness but which are not considered health care, including travel and incidental costs to attend appointments or modifications made to a house to facilitate access for the disabled; frequently estimated from charges or prices, though these may differ from true costs.

directional preference Phenomenon observed in the McKenzie approach in which movement or a sustained posture in a particular direction decreases pain and improves range of motion.

disc arthroplasty Type of surgery in which an intervertebral disc is removed and replaced with a device intended to function as a replacement disc; also known as disc replacement or artificial disc replacement.

discectomy Type of decompression surgery in which an intervertebral disc is partially or completely removed.

discography Type of interventional diagnostic procedure in which radiopaque material is injected into an intervertebral disc suspected of contributing to low back pain. The main goals are to assess the integrity of the disc by observing the distribution of radiopaque material and to determine the level of pressure required to reproduce or increase symptoms from that disc; also known as provocative discography.

distraction manipulation Type of traction therapy in which distraction is applied along specific planes of motion to optimize the position of specific spinal structures to receive mobilization or spinal manipulation therapy.

diversion Phenomenon that can occur when medications (usually stronger opioid analgesics) that are prescribed by physicians are used or sold to someone other than the intended patient.

doctor of chiropractic (DC) Type of health care practitioner focused on the diagnosis and treatment of neuromusculoskeletal disorders, primarily with spinal manipulation therapy; also known as a chiropractor.

doctor of naturopathy (ND) Type of health care practitioner focused on the diagnosis and treatment of conditions using primarily herbal remedies, nutritional supplements, acupuncture, homeopathy, manual therapy, and other forms of complementary and alternative medicine; also known as a naturopath.

doctor of physical therapy Type of health care practitioner focused on the management of a variety of medical conditions primarily using education, therapeutic exercises, and physical modalities to improve physical function; also known as physical therapists or physiotherapists.

dosulepin hydrochloride Tricyclic antidepressant medication; brand names include Prothiaden, Dothep, Thaden and Dopress.

doxepin Tricyclic antidepressant medication; brand names include Sinequan, Prudoxin, and Zonalon.

duloxetine Serotonin-norepinephrine reuptake inhibitor antidepressant medication; brand names include Cymbalta and Yentreve.

dysfunction syndrome Type of pain syndrome in the McKenzie approach in which intermittent pain is produced only at the end-range in a single direction of restricted movement.

dysfunctional patient Type of patients with chronic pain who are more likely to respond poorly to all biomedical interventions aimed at specific anatomical structures, and whose symptoms may appear out of proportion to the suspected pathology, possibly due to psychological comorbidities.

E

economic burden of illness Type of health economic study in which the economic costs of a particular illness or medical condition are examined from various perspectives, including those of the patient, payers, or society; also known as cost of illness.

effectiveness Ability of an intervention to achieve clinically meaningful outcomes in uncontrolled settings (e.g., general practice settings); often answers the research question "does it actually work?"

efficacy Ability of an intervention to achieve clinically meaningful outcomes in controlled settings (e.g., randomized controlled trial); often answers the research question "could it potentially work?"

effleurage Type of massage therapy technique in which light, long, slow, soothing strokes are applied along a broad area of the body using the palms and fingers; often used at the beginning of the massage.

electrical muscle stimulation (EMS) Type of electrotherapeutic modality used in physical therapy that delivers an electrical current through superficial electrodes placed on the skin to target specific motor nerve fibers and stimulate muscle contractions.

electroacupuncture Type of intervention in which acupuncture needles are stimulated with electricity using high frequency transcutaneous electrical nerve stimulation.

electrotherapeutic modalities Types of modalities used in physical therapy in which electricity is used for therapeutic purposes (e.g., transcutaneous electrical nerve stimulation, electrical muscle stimulation, interferential current therapy); often intended to reduce pain, swelling, or tissue restriction, or increase strength, muscle activity, coordination, or rate of healing.

epidemiology Scientific discipline concerned with the study of the distribution and determinants of health and disease in populations; two main branches of interest to low back pain include classical epidemiology, which focuses on etiology of disease, and clinical epidemiology, which focuses on clinical management of disease.

epidural steroid injections (ESIs) Type of intervention in which injections are used to introduce corticosteroids into the epidural space; three main subtypes of interest to low back pain include caudal, interlaminar, and transforaminal.

episodic low back pain Longstanding low back pain in which symptoms can disappear completely and then reappear.

ergonomics Scientific discipline concerned with the study of workers and their environment; examples of activities of interest to low back pain include the health effects of repetitive or monotonous movements and the physical design of work settings.

escitalopram Selective serotonin reuptake inhibitor antidepressant medication; brand names include Lexapro, Cipralex, Seroplex, and Lexamil.

ethosuximide First-generation antiepileptic medication; brand names include Emeside and Zarontin.

ethotoin First-generation antiepileptic medication; brand name Peganone.

etiology Cause or origin of a particular medical condition or illness.

etodolac Type of nonsteroidal anti-inflammatory drug; brand name Lodine.

etoricoxib Type of nonsteroidal anti-inflammatory drug; brand name Arcoxia.

evidence-based medicine (EBM) Field of study within clinical epidemiology focused on using the best available scientific evidence to optimize clinical decisions.

expert opinion Type of clinical research study in which a clinician or scientific expert offers opinions, theories, or personal philosophies to support the assessment or management of a particular medical condition without offering supporting scientific data.

extended-release opioids Type of opioid analgesic in which the active ingredients are absorbed slowly from the gastrointestinal tract or transdermally, which may prolong their effect; also known as continuous-release opioids or sustained-release opioids.

F

Faber's procedure Provocative test in which the hip is passively placed in maximal flexion, abduction, and external rotation to assess the integrity of the hip capsule; acronym for hip Flexion ABduction External Rotation (FABER) test.

facet denervation Type of intervention in which the sensory nerves supplying a zygapophysial joint are destroyed using radiofrequency (e.g., rhizotomy) or chemicals (e.g., neurolysis) to prevent transmission of nociceptive signals from that anatomical structure; preferred terminology is lumbar medial branch neurotomy.

facet rhizotomy Type of percutaneous intervention in which a radiofrequency electrode is placed on a lumbar medial branch suspected of contributing to low back pain and an electrical current is delivered to coagulate sensory nerves and prevent conduction of nociceptive impulses; preferred terminology is lumbar medial branch neurotomy.

fear avoidance behavior Type of behavior in which patients develop a fear that normal movements or activities of daily living will cause or aggravate their pain; can occur with chronic, longstanding low back pain in which patients mistakenly develop associations between various activities and their symptoms.

fear avoidance training Type of behavioral intervention in which patients with fear avoidance behavior are taught to confront their fears of normal movements or activities by engaging in the activities repeatedly in supervised settings.

felbamate Second-generation antiepileptic medication; brand name Felbatol.

flavectomy Type of surgical intervention used in decompression surgery that involves surgical removal of the ligamentum flavum, usually to expose the spinal cord, cauda equina, and spinal nerve roots.

fluoxetine Selective serotonin reuptake inhibitor antidepressant medication; brand names include Prozac and Sarafem.

fluvoxamine Selective serotonin reuptake inhibitor antidepressant medication; brand name Luvox.

foraminotomy Type of surgical procedure used in decompression surgery that involves surgical removal of a portion of the facet joint near the intervertebral foramen, often to reduce stenosis or compression that may occur secondary to disc herniations or degenerative disc disease.

fosphenytoin Second-generation antiepileptic medication; brand names include Cerebyx and Prodilantin.

French energetic acupuncture Type of needle acupuncture in which needles are placed along meridians to restore the optimal flow of chi.

friction period approach Method used in health economic evaluations to estimate the value of lost productivity due to absenteeism based on the assumption that disabled workers will eventually be replaced. Values lost productivity according to the time necessary to find and train replacements to restore productivity (known as the friction period), which varies according to the scarcity of the worker involved.

functional restoration Type of intervention based on the biopsychosocial approach to low back pain that combines education, physical rehabilitation, behavioral, and other interventions to decrease symptoms and improve function.

fusion surgery Type of surgery in which adjacent bony anatomical structures are surgically joined because they are thought to have excessive mobility, or are otherwise contributing to the presenting symptoms; also known as arthrodesis. The main types of fusion surgery for low back pain are defined according to their use of surgical instrumentation (e.g., plates, screws, cages) and approaches (e.g., anterior, posterior, circumferential).

G

gabapentin Second-generation antiepileptic medication; brand name Neurontin.

general practitioner (GP) Type of medical physician focused on the diagnosis and treatment of all medical conditions in primary care settings; often mistakenly referred to as a family doctor, which is now a recognized primary care specialty.

geographical adjustment factor Process used by Medicare to modify payments for covered services according to the cost of living in different parts of the country.

goal-oriented assessment of low back pain Assessment of low back pain (LBP) to achieve specific goals: (1) rule out serious spinal pathology, (2) rule out rare but specific causes of LBP, (3) identify substantial neurologic involvement, (4) evaluate the severity of symptoms and functional limitations, and (5) acknowledge the presence of risk factors for chronicity. Term is used to differentiate itself from diagnosis, since assessment of LBP may not result in a specific anatomical diagnosis.

H

herbal medicines Products derived from plants, herbs, flowers, or trees that are thought to contain one or more active ingredients that may be beneficial for specific symptoms or medical conditions. Can be administered in a variety of methods, including tablets, capsules, poultices, teas, and tinctures.

homeopath Type of health care practitioner who specializes in the practice of homeopathy.

homeopathic remedy Interventions used in homeopathy which consist of one or more products derived from herbal, mineral, or animal substances, which are then diluted with water or alcohol in a 1:10 ratio (e.g., 1X) several times until the final product contains the desired concentration or potency (e.g., 10X is 1:10,000,000,000).

homeopathy System of healing established by Samuel Hahnemann in the late 1700s based on the law of similars, which proposes that a substance capable of inducing specific symptoms in a healthy person can also cure those symptoms when administered in infinitesimally small doses as a homeopathic remedy.

human capital approach Method used in health economic evaluations to estimate the value of lost productivity due to absenteeism based on the assumption that permanently disabled workers would otherwise have worked until a fixed retirement age (e.g., 65 years old). Values lost productivity according to length of time spent on disability until the expected age of retirement.

hydrocodone Opioid analgesic medication; brand names include Vicodin, Hydrococet, and Symtan.

I

ibuprofen Type of nonsteroidal anti-inflammatory drug; brand names include Advil, Midol, Motrin, and Nuprin.

imipramine Tricyclic antidepressant medication; brand name Tofranil.

immediate-release opioids Type of opioid analgesic in which the active ingredients are absorbed immediately from the gastrointestinal tract, which produces a rapid onset of analgesia; these opioids are often short acting and used specifically for breakthrough pain.

incremental cost effectiveness ratio (ICER) Result of a health economic evaluation in which the costs and effectiveness of two or more interventions are evaluated and compared to each other. The ratio usually expresses the additional costs per quality-adjusted life-year that result from selecting an intervention that is both more costly and more effective than an alternative intervention.

indirect health care costs Term used in health economics to describe costs that are not directly related to health care services or other expenses incurred as a result of an illness or medical condition, but occur as a consequence of that condition (e.g., lost productivity due to missed work, lost household productivity).

indoleacetic acids Subgroup of nonsteroidal anti-inflammatory drugs that includes etodolac, indomethacin, sulindac, and tolmetin.

indomethacin Type of nonsteroidal anti-inflammatory drug; brand name Indocid.

instrumentation Term used in fusion surgery to describe surgical instruments such as plates, screws, hooks, cables and cages; also known as surgical hardware.

interferential current (IFC) therapy Type of electrotherapeutic modality used in physical therapy in which a high frequency electrical current is administered through superficial electrodes and delivered over a large area, allowing for deeper penetration of the current to the underlying muscles.

International Classification of Disease (ICD) codes Codes used by health care practitioners to inform third-party payers about the specific medical condition or illness that was diagnosed in a particular patient; often used for reimbursement purposes. The most commonly used version in the United States is ICD-9, although the latest version is ICD-10.

interlaminar epidural steroid injection Type of epidural injection in which the needle is placed between spinous processes and into the epidural space to deliver medication; also known as translaminar.

interpersonally distressed patients Type of patients with chronic pain who are more likely to respond poorly to all biomedical interventions aimed at specific anatomical structures and whose symptoms may appear out of proportion to the suspected pathology, possibly due to psychological co-morbidities or addiction.

interventional diagnostic testing Type of diagnostic testing in which a needle is placed on or near a specific anatomical structure and stimulated with medications (e.g., local anesthetic) or radiopaque substances (e.g., discography) to help determine if that structure is contributing to specific symptoms.

intradiscal biacuplasty Type of percutaneous intervention that uses two bipolar, cooled, radiofrequency energy electrodes positioned on either side of the annulus fibrosus to ablate the targeted tissues (e.g., outer annulus).

intradiscal electrothermal annuloplasty (IDEA) Type of percutaneous intervention that uses heat energy applied with a catheter to target structures within the intervertebral disc (e.g., outer annulus); also known as intradiscal thermal annuloplasty and intradiscal electrothermal therapy.

intradiscal electrothermal therapy (IDET) Type of percutaneous intervention that uses heat energy applied with a catheter to target structures within the intervertebral disc (e.g., outer annulus); also known as intradiscal thermal annuloplasty and intradiscal electrothermal annuloplasty.

intradiscal radiofrequency thermocoagulation (IRFT) Type of percutaneous intervention that uses radiofrequency energy applied with a catheter to target various structures within the intervertebral disc (e.g., outer annulus); also known as intradiscal radiofrequency treatment and percutaneous intradiscal radiofrequency thermocoagulation.

intradiscal radiofrequency treatment (IRFT) Type of percutaneous intervention that uses radiofrequency energy applied with a catheter to target various structures within the intervertebral disc (e.g., outer annulus); also known as intradiscal radiofrequency thermocoagulation and percutaneous intradiscal radiofrequency thermocoagulation.

intradiscal thermal annuloplasty (IDTA) Type of percutaneous intervention that uses heat energy applied with a catheter to target structures within the intervertebral disc (e.g., outer annulus); also known as intradiscal electrothermal annuloplasty and intradiscal electrothermal therapy.

intradiscal thermal therapies Term used to describe percutaneous interventions using heat energy applied with a catheter to target structures within the intervertebral disc (e.g., outer annulus); also known as intradiscal electrothermal therapy, intradiscal electrothermal annuloplasty, and intradiscal thermal annuloplasty.

isokinetic exercise Type of strengthening exercise in which muscles contract at a fixed speed.

isotonic exercise Type of strengthening exercise in which muscles contract against a fixed resistance that provides constant tension.

J

Japanese meridian therapy Type of needle acupuncture developed in Japan based on identifying and correcting life energy imbalance through palpation and examination of the pulse, and focused on precise needle technique.

Japanese Orthopaedic Association scale Patient-reported outcome measure intended to assess the severity of myelopathy as reflected in upper and lower extremity function and sensory deficits, as well as bladder function.

joint sclerotherapy Type of injection in which various solutions (e.g., dextrose, glycerin, phenol) are administered into ligaments to promote connective tissue growth and repair by stimulating the acute inflammatory cascade. Derived from sclerotherapy injections for varicose veins; also known as regenerative injection therapy, joint sclerotherapy, or prolotherapy.

K

ketorolac Type of nonsteroidal anti-inflammatory drug; brand name Toradol.

Korean constitutional acupuncture Type of needle acupuncture developed in Korea based on recognizing and correcting imbalances in life energy throughout 12 meridians that control bodily functions, which may be expressed differently in individuals based on their body type (e.g., constitution).

L

lacosamide Third-generation antiepileptic medication; brand name Vimpat.

laminectomy Type of decompression surgery in which a lamina is partially or completely removed.

laminoplasty Type of decompression surgery in which one side of a lamina is partially severed to allow the other side to swing posteriorly as if on a hinge, thereby relieving some neural compression.

laminotomy Type of decompression surgery in which part of the lamina is removed to reduce neural compression, while preserving the posterior aspect (e.g., spinous process) of the vertebra.

lamotrigine Second-generation antiepileptic medication; brand name Lamictal.

Leamington five elements acupuncture Type of needle acupuncture developed by J. R. Worsley in the 20th century in Leamington, United Kingdom, based on the five traditional elements (fire, earth, metal, water, and wood) as well as the five seasons in nature (fall, winter, spring, summer, and Indian summer). This type of acupuncture uses color, sound, smell, and pulse to diagnose imbalance in chi that may cause disease.

levetiracetam Second-generation antiepileptic medication; brand name Keppra.

levorphanol Opioid analgesic medication; brand name Levo-Dromoran.

life energy Life energy that flows throughout the body along meridians and whose disruption is thought to result in disease according to traditional Chinese medicine, which includes needle acupuncture; also known as chi or qi. The two main types of life energy are yin and yang.

lofepramine Tricyclic antidepressant medication; brand names include Gamanil, Tymelyt, and Lomont.

long-acting opioids Type of opioid analgesic in which the active ingredients or dosing produces a longer analgesia; these opioids are often taken on a time-contingent schedule to minimize fluctuations in pain relief.

long-lever spinal manipulation therapy Type of spinal manipulation therapy in which the thrust is applied by a hand placed on the targeted spinal segment, as well as by rotating the patient's thigh or torso.

low back pain (LBP) Pain located in the lumbar region of the spine below the ribcage and above the pelvis; also used as a generic term that encompasses all symptoms of low back pain, including numbness, tingling, burning, or weakness.

lumbar extension dynamometer Instrument used to measure strength during active lumbar extension.

lumbar medial branch block (LMBB) Type of interventional diagnostic procedure in which symptoms are monitored following injection of local anesthetics or other substances near the lumbar medial branch suspected of contributing to low back pain. Often used as a screening procedure to identify patients who may benefit from lumbar medial branch neurotomy; also incorrectly known as diagnostic facet injections or challenge facet blocks.

lumbar medial branch neurotomy (LMBN) Type of percutaneous intervention in which a radiofrequency electrode is placed on a lumbar medial branch suspected of contributing to low back pain and an electrical current is delivered to coagulate sensory nerves and prevent conduction of nociceptive impulses; also incorrectly known as facet rhizotomy.

lumbar spine Lower section of the spine below the thoracic spine and above the sacrum, which consists of five vertebrae, named lumbar 1-5 (e.g., L1-L5).

lumbar stabilization exercise Type of therapeutic exercise focused on improving the neuromuscular control, strength, and endurance of muscles responsible for maintaining dynamic and static spinal and trunk stability; examples include dead bug and cat/camel exercises.

lumbar strengthening exercise Type of therapeutic exercise focused on improving the strength and endurance of the lumbar extensor muscles (e.g., iliocostalis lumborum, longissimus thoracis, and spinalis thoracis); examples include the Roman chair exercises.

M

magnetic resonance imaging (MRI) Type of advanced diagnostic imaging procedure in which a patient lies in a machine that uses magnetic energy to produce cross-sectional images of the body.

manipulation under anesthesia (MUA) Type of manual therapy in which spinal manipulation therapy is performed while the patient is maintained under general anesthesia.

manipulation under epidural steroid injections (MUESI) Type of manual therapy in which spinal manipulation therapy is performed after the patient has received an epidural steroid injection.

manipulation under joint anesthesia (MUJA) Type of manual therapy in which spinal manipulation therapy is performed after the patient has received a local anesthetic or steroid injections in the spine.

maprotiline Tetracyclic antidepressant medication; brand names include Deprilept, Ludiomil, and Psymion.

massage acupuncture Type of massage therapy technique in which manual pressure is applied to acupuncture points to stimulate them using fingers rather than needles; also known as acupressure.

massage therapist Type of health care practitioner focused on delivering massage therapy, either for the treatment of musculoskeletal disorders or for general relaxation.

massage therapy Type of manual therapy focused on soft tissues (e.g., muscles) that uses a variety of techniques such as deep friction, effleurage, kneading, myofascial release, tapotement, and vibration to target specific structures or achieve therapeutic goals (e.g., increased blood flow, relaxation); usually given by a licensed massage therapist.

McKenzie method Type of approach to low back pain that includes a method of assessment focused on identifying directional preferences, and therapy using exercises based on directional preference.

mechanical low back pain Term used to describe nonspecific low back pain in which symptoms are usually exacerbated by physical activity and relieved by rest, and in which provocative tests are able to reproduce or exacerbate symptoms by applying a mechanical load to the lumbar spine.

medial facetectomy Type of decompression surgery that involves removal of the medial portion of a facet, often secondary to bony hypertrophy that may contribute to neural compression.

medicine-assisted manipulation (MAM) Term used to describe manual therapy in which spinal manipulation therapy is performed while, or shortly after, the patient has received medication for anesthesia (e.g., manipulation under anesthesia) or analgesia (e.g., epidural steroid injection).

meloxicam Type of nonsteroidal anti-inflammatory drug; brand name Mobic.

meperidine Opioid analgesic medication; brand name Demerol.

meridians Concept used in traditional Chinese medicine to describe the flow of life energy along specific paths throughout the body, consisting of 12 primary meridians and 8 secondary meridians, along which points stimulated in acupressure or acupuncture are located.

methadone Opioid analgesic medication; brand names include Symoron, Dolphine, Amidone, and Methadose.

methsuximide First-generation antiepileptic medication; brand name Celontin.

minerals Substances derived from elements that are naturally occurring on earth (e.g., sodium, calcium) and are essential to promote or regulate biochemical reactions related to cellular metabolism, growth, development, structure, function, and balance.

morphine Opioid analgesic medication; brand names include MS Contin, MSIR, Avinza, and Kadian.

moxibustion Type of intervention used in traditional Chinese medicine that involves burning the herb *Artemisia vulgaris* (e.g., moxa, mugwort) to regulate the flow of life energy.

multidisciplinary approach to low back pain Approach to managing low back pain that incorporates multiple health care practitioners from a variety of disciplines, most commonly combining physical rehabilitation, behavioral, and pain management interventions.

muscle spasm Involuntary, short, and occasionally painful muscle contraction often secondary to musculoskeletal injuries.

muscle spasticity Involuntary, persistent muscle contraction often secondary to central nervous system disorders.

myofascial release Type of massage therapy technique in which the therapist applies slow, deep pressure with the fingers to target specific muscles, tendons, or connective tissues.

N

naproxen Type of nonsteroidal anti-inflammatory drug; brand names include Aleve, Anaprox, and Naprosyn.

naturopath Type of health care practitioner focused on the diagnosis and treatment of conditions using primarily herbal remedies, nutritional supplements, acupuncture, homeopathy, manual therapy, and other forms of complementary and alternative medicine; also known as a doctor of naturopathy.

needle acupuncture Type of intervention in which very thin metallic needles are placed at specific points in the body to restore the flow of life energy or achieve other therapeutic purposes; needles can be stimulated manually or with electrical current; term is also used to differentiate this intervention from acupressure.

neural impingement Clinical phenomenon in which neurologic sensory (e.g., pain, numbness, tingling, burning) or motor (e.g., reduced strength, atrophy) changes occur as result of compressing structures within the neural canal (e.g., spinal nerve root), often secondary to intervertebral foramen stenosis, spinal stenosis, or large disc herniations.

neurologic involvement Term used to describe neurologic signs (e.g., deep tendon reflexes, muscle strength, atrophy) or symptoms (e.g., radicular pain, burning, numbness, tingling) that may occur in the lower extremities with low back pain secondary to neural compression from intervertebral foramen stenosis or spinal stenosis.

neuropathic pain Type of pain that occurs from actual damage or injury to a nerve; term used to differentiate this type of pain from nociceptive pain.

nociceptive pain Type of pain that occurs from stimulation of nociceptive receptors that are sensitive to thermal, mechanical, or chemical changes in surrounding tissues; term used to differentiate this type of pain from neuropathic pain.

nonrandomized controlled trials (non-RCTs) Type of clinical research study in which willing participants with a particular medical condition who meet stated eligibility criteria are assigned by researchers or by choice to an intervention and whose outcomes are compared with those of participants assigned to another intervention designated as a control group.

nonselective nonsteroidal anti-inflammatory drugs (NSAIDs) Type of medication that inhibits the cyclooxygenase isoenzymes 1 (e.g., COX-1) and 2 (e.g., COX-2); main categories include nonselective and selective NSAIDs; also known as traditional NSAIDs.

nonspecific low back pain Term used to describe low back pain (LBP) in which no specific anatomical structure or pathology can be identified as being responsible for symptoms; also known as simple LBP or common LBP.

nortriptyline Tricyclic antidepressant medication; brand name Pamelor.

nutritional supplement Products derived from ingredients that may naturally occur in food sources that are often used to supplement dietary intake, correct deficiencies, or achieve other therapeutic goals; main types include herbal remedies, vitamins, minerals, and homeopathic remedies.

O

opioid analgesics Type of medication used primarily for pain relief that act on opioid receptors; main types include weaker opioid analgesics and stronger opioid analgesics, though other classification systems also exist.

opioid-induced hyperalgesia Phenomenon that can occur with prolonged use of opioid analgesics in which patients experience an increased sensitivity to nociceptive signals resulting in greater pain symptoms than originally present, often secondary to rapid dose escalation or excessive use of opioid analgesics.

Oswestry disability index (ODI) Patient-reported outcome measure intended to assess physical function related to various activities of daily living that can be impacted by low back pain.

oxaprozin Type of nonsteroidal anti-inflammatory drug; brand name Daypro.

oxcarbazepine Second-generation antiepileptic medication; brand name Trileptal.

oxicams Subgroup of nonselective nonsteroidal anti-inflammatory drugs that includes piroxicam and meloxicam.

oxycodone Opioid analgesic medication; brand name OxyContin.

oxymorphone Opioid analgesic medication; brand name Opana.

P

pain management physician Physician with additional training in the management of pain; this board certification is often obtained by anesthesiologists or physiatrists who wish to specialize in this clinical area.

pain-contingent medication use Method of taking medication as needed for symptomatic relief; term used to differentiate this use from time-contingent use. Also known as *pro re nata* (PRN), the Latin term for "as needed".

paroxetine Selective serotonin reuptake inhibitor antidepressant medication; brand names include Paxil and Pexeva.

percutaneous intradiscal radiofrequency thermocoagulation (PIRFT) Type of percutaneous intervention that uses radiofrequency energy applied with a catheter to target various structures within the intervertebral disc (e.g., outer annulus); also known as intradiscal radiofrequency thermocoagulation and intradiscal radiofrequency treatment.

peripheralization Phenomenon observed in the McKenzie approach in which radicular pain increases when performing repeated or sustained movement in a particular direction.

petrissage Type of massage technique that involves forceful kneading with stiff fingers or knuckles to press and release muscle tissue in circular motions, often with multiple passes over a small area.

pharmacy benefits manager (PBM) Commercial organization hired by health plans to administer prescription medication benefits; often responsible for approving and processing payment of claims for prescription medications according to an approved formulary listing the generic and brand name medications approved in various drug classes.

phenobarbital First-generation antiepileptic medication; brand name Luminal.

phenylacetics Subgroup of nonsteroidal anti-inflammatory drugs that includes diclofenac.

phenytoin First-generation antiepileptic medication; name brands include Dilantin and Phenytek.

phonophoresis Type of modality used in physical therapy in which therapeutic ultrasound is used to facilitate the absorption of topical products such as analgesic or anti-inflammatory creams.

physical agents Types of modalities used in physical therapy that involve thermal, acoustic, or radiant energy (e.g., therapeutic ultrasound, and superficial heat and ice); intended to reduce pain, swelling, or tissue restriction, and increase strength, muscle activity, coordination, or rate of healing.

physical modalities Types of intervention used in physical therapy for a variety of therapeutic purposes; the main types include electrotherapeutic modalities (e.g., transcutaneous electrical nerve stimulation) and physical agents (e.g., ice, heat).

physical therapist Type of health care practitioner focused on the management of a variety of medical conditions primarily using education, therapeutic exercises, and physical modalities to improve physical function; also known as physiotherapists or doctors of physical therapy.

physical therapy (PT) Health profession focused on the management of a variety of medical conditions primarily using education, therapeutic exercises, and physical modalities to improve physical function; also known as physiotherapy.

physiotherapist Type of health care practitioner focused on the management of a variety of medical conditions primarily using education, therapeutic exercises, and physical modalities to improve physical function; also known as physical therapists or doctors of physical therapy.

physiotherapy (PT) Health profession focused on the management of a variety of medical conditions primarily using education, therapeutic exercises, and physical modalities to improve physical function; also known as physical therapy.

piroxicam Type of nonsteroidal anti-inflammatory drug; brand name Feldene.

placebo Type of intervention used in clinical research studies which is thought to be completely inert (e.g., has no therapeutic effect) and can be used to as a control group to assess the efficacy of an active intervention in a randomized controlled trial; also known as a sham or simulated intervention.

point prevalence Prevalence of a medical condition at any given point in time; often reported as prevalence within a very narrow time frame (e.g., past 7 days) from the survey or study in which it is measured.

postherpetic neuropathy Clinical condition in which persistent neuropathic pain occurs in one or more spinal nerve roots after an acute episode of shingles due to an infection with the herpes zoster virus.

postural syndrome Type of pain syndrome in the McKenzie approach in which pain is intermittent, often in the midline, and is exacerbated by sustained postures such as slouching and relieved by correcting posture (e.g., restoring the lumbar lordosis).

pregabalin Second-generation antiepileptic medication; brand name Lyrica.

pressure pain threshold (PPT) Minimum amount of physical pressure required to produce pain on a trigger point; often measured with an algometer and reported as pounds per square inch.

prevalence Rate of individuals affected by a particular medical condition of interest compared to the broader population that is at risk; must also specify the time frame of interest (e.g., 80% lifetime prevalence of low back pain in the general adult population).

primary care management of low back pain Phase of care for low back pain (LBP) in which patients first present with symptoms to a primary care provider (e.g., general practitioner). The main goals of this phase of management are to conduct a goal-oriented assessment of LBP, educate patients about LBP, and recommend appropriate interventions to manage symptoms.

primidone First-generation antiepileptic medication; brand name Mysoline.

pro re nata **(PRN)** Method of taking medication as needed (its Latin meaning) for symptomatic relief; term used to differentiate this use from time-contingent use. Also known as pain-contingent use.

progressive resistance exercise Type of exercise that involves muscle contraction against resistance that is slowly increased over time to develop muscular strength and endurance; based on the principles of muscle overload, specificity, reversibility, frequency, intensity, repetitions, volume, duration, and mode.

prolotherapy Type of injection in which various solutions (e.g., dextrose, glycerin, phenol) are administered into ligaments to promote connective tissue growth and repair by stimulating the acute inflammatory cascade. Derived from sclerotherapy injections for varicose veins; also known as regenerative injection therapy or joint sclerotherapy.

proprioception Ability to recognize precise joint position, orientation, and movement, and use that information to modify muscle function accordingly; based on nerve impulses received from mechanical and other receptors in surrounding tissues.

proprionic acids Subgroup of nonsteroidal anti-inflammatory drugs that includes ibuprofen, naproxen, ketorolac, and oxaprozin.

prospective observational study Type of clinical research study in which willing participants with a particular medical condition who meet stated eligibility criteria receive a particular intervention, and their results are measured over time by researchers.

protriptyline Tricyclic antidepressant medication; brand name Vivactil.

provocative discography Type of interventional diagnostic procedure in which radiopaque material is injected into an intervertebral disc suspected of contributing to low back pain. The main goals are to assess the integrity of the disc by observing the distribution of radiopaque material and to determine the level of pressure required to reproduce or increase symptoms from that disc; also known as discography.

psychotherapy Term used to describe various behavioral interventions in which a behavioral health practitioner attempts to manage mental illness, mood disorders, or undesired behaviors using a variety of communication techniques.

pyramid of evidence Graphical method of categorizing scientific evidence used in evidence-based medicine in which study designs that are less prone to confounding and bias (e.g., randomized controlled trials) are placed at the top of the pyramid, while those of less robust study designs (e.g., case series) are placed at the bottom. This concept is used to emphasize that although all evidence may be considered when making medical decisions, results from different study designs should not necessarily be given equal weight; does not take methodological quality of studies within a particular study design into account.

Q

qi Life energy that flows throughout the body along meridians, and whose disruption is thought to result in disease according to Traditional Chinese Medicine, which includes needle acupuncture; also known as chi or life energy. The two main types are yin and yang.

quality-adjusted life-year (QALY) Unit of measurement used in health economic evaluations focused on health related quality of life (e.g., cost utility analysis); incorporates both length of life (e.g., year) and quality of life (e.g., utility) to project outcomes into the future.

R

radiculopathy General term used to describe neurologic symptoms involving a spinal nerve root.

randomized controlled trial (RCT) Type of clinical research study in which willing participants with a particular medical condition who meet stated eligibility criteria are assigned by chance to an intervention and their outcomes are compared with those of participants assigned to another intervention designated as a control group; often considered the gold standard study design to assess the efficacy of interventions.

recombinant human bone morphogenic protein Substance used in fusion surgery to enhance the body's natural bone growth process, which can be used instead of, or in addition to, autograft or allograft bone chips; also known as bone morphogenic protein.

recurrent low back pain Type of longstanding low back pain in which symptoms can disappear completely for long periods of time and then reappear.

red flags Signs, symptoms, or patient characteristics that may indicate the need for additional screening to eliminate the possibility of serious underlying medical conditions (e.g., serious spinal pathology).

reflexology Type of massage therapy technique focused on applying slow, deep pressure with the fingers to specific points along the hands and feet that are thought to influence the flow of life energy in specific organs.

regenerative injection therapy Type of injection in which various solutions (e.g., dextrose, glycerin, phenol) are administered into ligaments to promote connective tissue growth and repair by stimulating the acute inflammatory cascade. Derived from sclerotherapy injections for varicose veins; also known as prolotherapy or joint sclerotherapy.

relative value unit (RVU) Unit of measurement used by third-party payers such as Medicare to determine the relative value of covered services based on required physician time, skill, training and intensity, practice overhead, and costs of malpractice. Relative value units are then multiplied by a geographic adjustment factor and a conversion factor to calculate reimbursement levels.

resource based relative value scale (RBRVS) Method used by third-party payers such as Medicare to establish the value of covered services based on the actual resources consumed when delivering that service as determined by its relative value unit.

retrospective observational study (OBS) Type of clinical research study in which the outcomes of participants with a particular medical condition who meet stated eligibility criteria and have already received a particular intervention are measured over time based on information available in their medical records or from subsequent questionnaires or interviews.

rofecoxib Type of nonsteroidal anti-inflammatory drug; brand name Vioxx.

Roland-Morris disability questionnaire (RMDQ) Patient-reported outcome measure intended to assess physical function related to various activities of daily living that can be impacted by low back pain.

Rolfing Type of manual therapy in which slow, deep friction massage is applied to connective tissue throughout the body to release fibrous adhesions and restore mobility to surrounding muscles and joints.

rufinamide Third-generation antiepileptic medication; brand name Banzel.

S

salicylates Subgroup of nonsteroidal anti-inflammatory drugs that includes aspirin (e.g., salicylic acid), diflunisal, and salsalate.

salsalate Type of nonsteroidal anti-inflammatory drug; brand names include Disalcid, Salsitab, and Salflex.

sciatica Term given to radiculopathy involving the sciatic nerve; symptoms may include radicular pain, burning, numbness, or tingling along the distribution of the sciatic nerve, which extends from the buttocks to the posterior thigh, leg, and foot.

secondary care management of low back pain One of the three phases of care for low back pain focused on a small portion of patients whose symptoms can be attributed to specific anatomical structures or pathologies that may be addressed through focused interventions such as injections, percutaneous procedures, or surgery; often involves consultations with nonsurgical and surgical spine specialists.

selective nonsteroidal anti-inflammatory drugs Newer type of nonsteroidal anti-inflammatory drugs (NSAIDs) that selectively inhibits only the COX-2 isoenzyme and is thought to decrease the risk of gastrointestinal bleeding associated with prolonged used of traditional NSAIDs, which also inhibit the COX-1 isoenzyme important to the gastrointestinal lining. Also known as COX-2 inhibitors, and includes medications such as celecoxib and rofecoxib, some of which were removed from the United States market due to concerns about the risk of cardiovascular adverse events.

selective serotonin reuptake inhibitors (SSRI) Newer type of antidepressant medications thought to act on serotonergic pathways which are occasionally used off-label as adjunctive analgesics for low back pain; includes medications such as fluoxetine and citalopram.

serious spinal pathology Very rare medical conditions that can occasionally present with symptoms of low back pain (LBP), including spinal tumors, spinal fracture, spinal infection, cauda equina syndrome, and systemic inflammatory disease; these conditions may require surgical management of the underlying pathology to improve the LBP.

serotonin-norepinepherine reuptake inhibitors (SNRI) Newer type of antidepressant medications thought to act on both serotonergic and norepinephrine pathways and which are occasionally used off-label as adjunctive analgesics for low back pain; includes medications such as venlafaxine and duloxetine.

sertraline Selective serotonin reuptake inhibitor antidepressant medication; brand name Zoloft.

sham intervention Type of intervention used in clinical research studies which is thought to be completely inert (e.g., has no therapeutic effect) and can be used to as a control group to assess the efficacy of an active intervention in a randomized controlled trial; also known as a placebo or simulated intervention.

short-form 12 (SF-12) Patient-reported outcome measure consisting of 12 questions intended to reflect health related quality of life, including levels of physical and mental functioning. Has been validated as an outcome measure for a variety of conditions and represents a shorter version of the more comprehensive short-form 36.

short-form 36 (SF-36) Patient-reported outcome measure consisting of 36 questions intended to reflect health related quality of life, including the following 8 aspects: vitality, physical functioning, bodily pain, general health perceptions, physical role functioning, emotional role functioning, social role functioning, and mental health. Has been validated as an outcome measure for a variety of conditions.

short-lever spinal manipulation therapy Type of spinal manipulation therapy in which the thrust is applied by the hand placed directly on the targeted spinal segment.

sibutramine Serotonin-norepinephrine reuptake inhibitor antidepressant medication; brand name Meridia.

simple analgesics Type of medication used primarily for pain relief, including acetaminophen; term is often used to differentiate these medications from opioid or adjunctive analgesics.

simple low back pain Term used to describe low back pain (LBP) in which no specific anatomical structure or pathology can be identified as being responsible for the symptoms; also known as nonspecific LBP or common LBP.

simulated intervention Type of intervention used in clinical research studies which is thought to be completely inert (e.g., has no therapeutic effect) and can be used to as a control group to assess the efficacy of an active intervention in a randomized controlled trial; also known as a placebo or sham intervention.

spa therapy Type of modality used in physical therapy that involves immersing the body in hot or cold water, with or without bath salts or other substances, to promote relaxation or stimulation; also known as balneotherapy.

spinal manipulation therapy (SMT) Type of manual therapy in which a high-velocity, low-amplitude manual thrust is applied to a specific spinal joint or segment to temporarily move it beyond its passive range of motion.

spinal mobilization (MOB) Type of manual therapy in which manual force is applied to a specific spinal joint or segment to move it within its passive range of motion; term is often used to differentiate this approach from spinal manipulation therapy, which involves a thrust.

spinal stenosis Medical condition in which the neural canal is narrowed, often as a result of advanced degenerative changes in the surrounding structures. If substantial, stenosis can result in compression of the spinal cord, cauda equina, or spinal nerve roots, which can produce neurologic symptoms in the lower extremities, particularly neurogenic claudication.

stiripentol Third-generation antiepileptic medication; brand name Diacomit.

stronger opioid analgesics Subcategory of opioid analgesics used to differentiate from weaker opioids; consists of more potent medications such as morphine or fentanyl.

subacute low back pain Episode of low back pain where current symptoms have lasted from 6 to 12 weeks.

substantial neurologic involvement Moderate, severe, or progressive neurologic signs (e.g., deep tendon reflexes, muscle strength, atrophy) or symptoms (e.g., radicular pain, burning, numbness, tingling) that may occur in the lower extremities with low back pain secondary to neural compression from intervertebral foramen stenosis or spinal stenosis.

sulindac Type of nonsteroidal anti-inflammatory drug; brand name Clinoril.

surgical hardware Term used in fusion surgery to describe surgical instruments such as plates, screws, hooks, cables and cages; also known as instrumentation.

sustained-release opioids Type of opioid analgesic in which the active ingredients are absorbed slowly from the gastrointestinal tract or transdermally, which may prolong their effect; also known as continuous-release opioids or extended-release opioids.

systematic review (SR) Type of clinical research study in which the scientific literature pertaining to a specific research question is searched, evaluated, summarized, and synthesized to help guide decision making.

T

tapotement Type of massage therapy technique in which a broad area is rhythmically or rapidly tapped or hacked using cupped hands.

tertiary care management of low back pain One of the three phases of care for low back pain focused on a very small portion of patients who do not improve following primary care or secondary care. The goal of this phase of care is to integrate education, exercise, medications, and behavioral interventions to manage longstanding symptoms that are unlikely to be completely cured with interventions focuses on specific pathologies alone.

therapeutic exercise Type of exercise intended to treat or manage a specific medical condition; mainly differentiated from recreational exercise by its intent.

third-party payers Commercial (e.g., health plan, employer) or government (e.g., Medicare, worker's compensation) organization that is financially responsible for the costs of health care received by a patient (first party) from their health care provider (second party).

tiagabine Second-generation antiepileptic medication; brand name Gabitril.

time-contingent medication use Method of taking medication on a regular schedule (e.g., every 4 hours) based on the expected duration of symptomatic relief, rather than taking medication as needed; often recommended with analgesics taken for low back pain.

tolmetin Type of nonsteroidal anti-inflammatory drug; brand name Tolectin.

topiramate Second-generation antiepileptic medication; brand name Topamax.

traction therapy Type of intervention in which the goal is to temporarily separate the vertebrae along the longitudinal axis of the spine (e.g., caudad and cephalad) by using mechanical forces created by counterweights, manual pressure, or by lying on a table with top and bottom sections that can move apart from each other. The main types of traction therapy for low back pain are intermittent, sustained, and continuous.

traditional Chinese medicine (TCM) System of healing that originated in China thousands of years ago that is based on recognizing and correcting imbalance in chi with therapies such as herbs, needle acupuncture, and massage.

traditional nonsteroidal anti-inflammatory drugs (NSAIDs) Type of medication that inhibits the cyclo-oxygenase isoenzymes 1 (e.g., COX-1) and 2 (e.g., COX-2); main categories include nonselective and selective NSAIDs; also known as nonselective NSAIDs.

traditional Thai massage (TTM) Type of massage therapy technique that involves applying deep and prolonged pressure (e.g., 5-10 seconds) with fingers or knuckles on specific areas of the body.

Tramadol Opioid analgesic medication; brand names include Rybix ODT, Ryzolt, and Ultram.

transcutaneous electrical nerve stimulations (TENS) Type of electrotherapeutic modality used in physical therapy that delivers an electrical current through superficial electrodes placed on the skin around the area of symptoms. Depending on the settings, it can cause a tingling sensation by stimulating sensory nerve fibers, or muscle contractions.

transdermal fentanyl Opioid analgesic which is applied topically via a skin patch; brand name Duragesic.

transforaminal epidural steroid injection Type of epidural injection in which the needle is placed in the intervertebral foramen near the spinal nerve root to deliver medication; usually performed under radiographic guidance.

transversalis muscle Skeletal muscle in the trunk area with its origins on the sternum, lower ribcage, and inguinal ligament and its insertions on the pubic and iliac bones that is responsible for flexion of the trunk; also known as transverse abdominis or transversus abdominis.

transverse abdominis Skeletal muscle in the trunk area with its origins on the sternum, lower ribcage, and inguinal ligament and its insertions on the pubic and iliac bones that is responsible for flexion of the trunk; also known as transversus abdominis or transversalis muscle.

transversus abdominis Skeletal muscle in the trunk area with its origins on the sternum, lower ribcage, and inguinal ligament and its insertions on the pubic and iliac bones that is responsible for flexion of the trunk; also known as transverse abdominis or transversalis muscle.

triage Process used in health care to prioritize or categorize patients according to the severity of their condition; can be used with low back pain (LBP) to classify patients with serious spinal pathology, substantial neurologic involvement, disabling nonspecific LBP, or non-disabling LBP.

tricyclic antidepressants (TCAs) Older type of antidepressant medications thought to act on serotonergic and nor-epinephrine pathways that are occasionally used off-label as adjunctive analgesics for low back pain; includes medications such as amitriptyline and amoxapine.

trigger point injection (TPI) Type of injection that involves introducing medications such as corticosteroids, local anesthetics, or other substances directly into trigger points.

trigger points Painful areas within skeletal muscle in which external pressure on a palpable "taut band" can produce an involuntary twitch response termed a "jump sign" that provokes referred pain in distant structures; the two main types of trigger points are active, which can cause pain with movement, and latent, which can cause pain in response to direct compression.

trimipramine Tricyclic antidepressant medication; brand name Surmontil.

U

ultrasound Type of physical modality in which sound waves are produced and applied to a specific body region using a hand-held probe and conductive gel; can be delivered in pulsed or continuous waves with different amplitudes expressed in watts per square centimeter.

unipolar radiofrequency energy Type of energy used in intradiscal thermal therapies in which an electrical current passes through a probe and then to a grounding pad, similar to electrocautery.

utility Short form for health related utility, which is a concept used in health economics to describe the value or preference that someone expresses for a particular state of health that can then be converted to a number on a scale from 0 (e.g., death) to 1 (e.g., perfect health).

V

valdecoxib Type of nonsteroidal anti-inflammatory drug; brand name Bextra.

valproic acid First-generation antiepileptic medication; brand names include Depacon, Depakene, Depakote, and Stavzor.

variable resistance exercise Type of exercise that involves a muscular contraction performed against a changing level of resistance that attempts to mimic the strength curve of the targeted muscle.

variable-angle roman chair (VARC) Type of exercise equipment used to perform lumbar extensor strengthening exercises, composed of a platform to stand on, cushions for the feet and waist, and handles. The inclination of the platform can be adjusted vertically to change the degree of difficulty.

vascular claudication Type of claudication caused by insufficient blood flow, often related to peripheral artery disease.

venlafaxine Serotonin-norepinephrine reuptake inhibitor antidepressant medication; brand name Effexor.

vibration Type of massage therapy technique in which a body region is grasped gently with the hands and fingers and shaken or vibrated lightly and quickly.

vigabatrin Second-generation antiepileptic medication; brand name Sabril.

visual analog scale (VAS) Type of patient-reported outcome measure in which the severity of symptoms (usually pain) is indicated by placing a mark on 100mm line, which is then measured to find the corresponding number (e.g., mark placed halfway through 100mm line indicates 50/100).

vitamins Category of chemical substances found to be essential for normal functioning of the body, including cell metabolism, growth, development, and regulation. Often work together with enzymes and cofactors to produce required biochemical reactions.

W

watchful waiting Type of passive intervention involving minimal care that often includes activity modification, education, monitoring changes in severity or nature of symptoms, and waiting for low back pain to resolve itself over time.

weaker opioid analgesics Subcategory of opioid analgesics used mainly to differentiate from stronger opioids; often consists of simple analgesics such as acetaminophen combined with low doses of codeine or tramadol.

X

x-rays Type of diagnostic imaging procedure that uses ionizing radiation to produce images of the internal structures of the body, most particularly bone.

Y

yang Concept used in traditional Chinese medicine to describe the fast, hot, or excited energy found in the body; imbalance of yang is thought to result in specific signs or symptoms.

yellow flags Factors that may increase the risk of prolonged or disabling low back pain, including those related to socioeconomics (e.g., age, gender, marital status, income), work (e.g., job satisfaction, work autonomy, supervisor empathy), litigation (e.g., worker's compensation, personal injury), behavior (e.g., anxiety, depression, fear avoidance), or general health (e.g., obesity).

yin Concept used in traditional Chinese medicine to describe the slow, cold, or passive energy found in the body; imbalance of yin is thought to result in specific signs or symptoms.

Z

zonisamide Second-generation antiepileptic medication; brand name Zonegran.

Index

Page numbers followed by "f" denote figures; "t," tables; "b," boxes

McARDLE LIBRARY
0151 604 7223